## TEXTBOOK EDITION

# PHARMACEUTICAL BIOTECHNOLOGY
## FUNDAMENTALS AND APPLICATIONS
### Third Edition

Edited by

**Daan J. A. Crommelin**
*Dutch Top Institute Pharma*
*Leiden, The Netherlands*

*Utrecht University*
*Utrecht, The Netherlands*

**Robert D. Sindelar**
*University of British Columbia*
*Vancouver, British Columbia, Canada*

**Bernd Meibohm**
*University of Tennessee Health Science Center*
*Memphis, Tennessee, USA*

**informa**
healthcare

New York   London

Informa Healthcare USA, Inc.
52 Vanderbilt Avenue
New York, NY 10017

International Standard Book Number-10: 1-4200-4437-0 (Softcover)
International Standard Book Number-13: 978-1-4200-4437-9 (Softcover)

---

### Library of Congress Cataloging-in-Publication Data

---

Pharmaceutical biotechnology: fundamentals and applications / edited by
Daan J.A. Crommelin, Robert D. Sindelar, Bernd Meibohm.—3rd ed.
    p. ; cm.
  Includes bibliographical references and index.
  ISBN-13: 978-1-4200-4437-9 (pb : alk. paper)
  ISBN-10: 1-4200-4437-0 (pb : alk. paper)  1.  Pharmaceutical biotechnology.  I. Crommelin,
D. J. A. (Daan J. A.) II. Sindelar, Robert D. III. Meibohm, Bernd.
  RS380.P484 2007a
  615'.19—dc22                                  2007025744

---

**Visit the Informa web site at**
**www.informa.com**

**and the Informa Healthcare Web site at**
**www.informahealthcare.com**

AL

GY

# Preface

In recent years, biotechnology drug products have gained a major share of prescribed pharmaceuticals. These drug products include peptides and proteins, including monoclonal antibodies and antibody fragments, as well as antisense oligonucleotides and DNA preparations for gene therapy. From 2000 to 2006, biologics accounted for 33% of all New Active Substances that were launched, and are reflected to a similar degree in the current development pipelines of the pharmaceutical industry. Drug products such as epoetin-α (Epogen®, Eprex®, Procrit®), abciximab (ReoPro®), interferons-α (Intron®A, Roferon®A), interferons -β (Avonex®, Rebif®, Betaseron®), anti-TNF-α agents (Enbrel®, Remicade®, Humira®), and trastuzumab (Herceptin®) are all examples of highly successful biotech drugs that have revolutionized the pharmacotherapy of previously unmet medical needs.

The techniques of biotechnology are a driving force of modern drug discovery as well. Due to this rapid growth in the importance of biopharmaceuticals and the techniques of biotechnologies to modern medicine and the life sciences, the field of pharmaceutical biotechnology has become an increasingly important component in the education of today's and tomorrow's pharmacists and pharmaceutical scientists. We believe that there is a critical need for an introductory textbook on pharmaceutical biotechnology that provides well-integrated, detailed coverage of both the basic science and clinical application of biotechnology-product pharmaceuticals.

Previous editions of *Pharmaceutical Biotechnology* have provided a well-balanced framework for education in various aspects of pharmaceutical biotechnology, including production, dosage forms, administration, and therapeutic application. Rapid growth and advances in the field of pharmaceutical biotechnology, however, made it necessary to revise this textbook in order to provide up-to-date information and introduce students to the cutting edge knowledge and technology of this field.

This third edition of the textbook builds on the successful concept used in the preceding editions. It is structured into three major sections. An initial basic science section introduces the reader to key concepts at the foundation of the technology relevant for protein therapeutics including molecular biology, production and analysis procedures, formulation development, pharmacokinetics and pharmacodynamics, and evolving new technologies and applications. The subsequent section discusses the various therapeutic classes of biologics. A final section concludes with chapters including regulatory, economic and pharmacy practice considerations.

All chapters of the previous edition were revised and regrouped according to therapeutic application. Specifically, the section on monoclonal antibodies was completely revised and structured according to therapeutic application in order to allow for a comprehensive discussion of the substantial number of recently approved antibody drugs. In addition, new chapters on immunogenicity of therapeutic proteins, oligonucleotides, and regulatory issues and drug product approval for biopharmaceuticals have been added.

In order to achieve an easier integration of the textbook into the curricula of pharmacy education programs, all chapters on therapeutically used proteins or protein classes are cross-referenced with the current editions of the three major pharmacotherapy textbooks that form the cornerstone of applied therapeutics learning in most pharmacy schools in North America. *Pharmaceutical Biotechnology, third edition* is intended to complement these textbooks in pharmacy education with its specific emphasis on biopharmaceuticals. Thus, pharmaceutical aspects of biotech drugs presented in this textbook are linked to their pharmacotherapeutic application and enable an easy integration of this textbook into existing pharmacy programs.

In accordance with previous editions, this new edition has as a primary target students in undergraduate and professional pharmacy programs as well as graduate students in pharmaceutical sciences. A secondary audience is pharmaceutical scientists in industry and academia, particularly those that have not received formal training in pharmaceutical biotechnology and are inexperienced in this field.

We are convinced that *Pharmaceutical Biotechnology* makes an important contribution to the education of pharmaceutical scientists, pharmacists, and other healthcare professionals as well as serving as a ready resource on biotechnology. By increasing the knowledge and expertise in the development, application and therapeutic use of biotech drugs, we hope to help facilitate a widespread, rational, and safe application of protein therapeutics.

*Daan J. A. Crommelin*
*Robert D. Sindelar*
*Bernd Meibohm*

# Contents

# Contributors

**Rita R. Alloway**  Department of Internal Medicine/Division of Nephrology, University of Cincinnati, Cincinnati, Ohio, U.S.A.

**Banmeet Anand**  Genentech, Inc., South San Francisco, California, U.S.A.

**Tsutomu Arakawa**  Alliance Protein Laboratories, Thousand Oaks, California, U.S.A.

**John M. Beals**  Eli Lilly & Company, Lilly Research Laboratories, Indianapolis, Indiana, U.S.A.

**Ronald W. Bordens**  Schering-Plough Corporation, Kenilworth, New Jersey, U.S.A.

**Rene Braeckman**  Reliance Clinical Research Services, Newtown, Pennsylvania, U.S.A.

**Daan J. A. Crommelin**  Utrecht University, Utrecht and Dutch Top Institute Pharma, Leiden, The Netherlands

**Maria A. Croyle**  College of Pharmacy, The University of Texas at Austin, Austin, Texas, U.S.A.

**Michael R. DeFelippis**  Eli Lilly & Company, Lilly Research Laboratories, Indianapolis, Indiana, U.S.A.

**Rong Deng**  Genentech, Inc., South San Francisco, California, U.S.A.

**Paul Fielder**  Genentech, Inc., South San Francisco, California, U.S.A.

**MaryAnn Foote**  MaryAnn Foote Associates, Westlake Village, California, U.S.A.

**Thomas Gelzleichter**  Genentech, Inc., South San Francisco, California, U.S.A.

**Mic Hamers**  SynCo Bio Partners BV, Amsterdam, The Netherlands

**Jennifer Hanje**  The Ohio State University Medical Center and James Cancer Hospital, Columbus, Ohio, U.S.A.

**Jeffrey M. Harris**  Genentech, Inc., South San Francisco, California, U.S.A.

**Wiel P. M. Hoekstra**  Department of Biology, Utrecht University, Utrecht, The Netherlands

**Paul Ives**  SynCo Bio Partners BV, Amsterdam, The Netherlands

**Wim Jiskoot**  Division of Drug Delivery Technology, Leiden/Amsterdam Center for Drug Research, Leiden University, Leiden, The Netherlands

**Terreia S. Jones**  Department of Clinical Pharmacy, University of Tennessee College of Pharmacy, Memphis, Tennessee, U.S.A.

**Amita Joshi**  Genentech, Inc., South San Francisco, California, U.S.A.

**Shasha Jumbe**  Genentech, Inc., South San Francisco, California, U.S.A.

**Farida Kadir**  Postacademic Education Pharmacists (POA), Bunnik, The Netherlands

**Saraswati Kenkare-Mitra**  Genentech, Inc., South San Francisco, California, U.S.A.

**Gideon F. A. Kersten**  Netherlands Vaccine Institute (NVI), Bilthoven, The Netherlands

**Eugene M. Kolassa**    Medical Marketing Economics, LLC, and Department of Pharmacy, University of Mississippi, Oxford, Mississippi, and University of the Sciences, Philadelphia, Pennsylvania, U.S.A.

**Paul M. Kovach**    Eli Lilly & Company, Lilly Research Laboratories, Indianapolis, Indiana, U.S.A.

**Peter Kuebler**    Genentech, Inc., South San Francisco, California, U.S.A.

**John C. Kuth**    Medical College of Georgia Health, Inc., Augusta, Georgia, U.S.A.

**Robert A. Lazarus**    Genentech, Inc., South San Francisco, California, U.S.A.

**Jing Li**    Genentech, Inc., South San Francisco, California, U.S.A.

**Melinda Marian**    Schering-Plough Biopharma, Palo Alto, California, U.S.A.

**Enrico Mastrobattista**    Department of Pharmaceutical Sciences, Utrecht University, Utrecht, The Netherlands

**Bernd Meibohm**    University of Tennessee Health Science Center, College of Pharmacy, Department of Pharmaceutical Sciences, Memphis, Tennessee, U.S.A.

**Nishit B. Modi**    ALZA Corporation, Mountain View, California, U.S.A.

**Susannah E. Motl Moroney**    Roche Laboratories Inc., Nutley, New Jersey, U.S.A.

**James Q. Oeswein**    Genentech, Inc. (Retired), South San Francisco, California, U.S.A.

**Michael A. Panzara**    Biogen-Idec, Inc., Cambridge, Massachusetts, U.S.A.

**Sidney Pestka**    Department of Molecular Genetics, Microbiology and Immunology, University of Medicine and Dentistry of New Jersey–Robert Wood Johnson Medical School, Piscataway, New Jersey, U.S.A.

**John S. Philo**    Alliance Protein Laboratories, Thousand Oaks, California, U.S.A.

**Peggy Piascik**    University of Kentucky College of Pharmacy, Lexington, Kentucky, U.S.A.

**Jean-Charles Ryff**    Biotech Research and Innovation Network, Basel, Switzerland

**Tom Sam**    Global Regulatory Affairs, N.V. Organon, Oss, The Netherlands

**Huub Schellekens**    Departments of Pharmaceutical Sciences and Innovation Studies, Utrecht University, Utrecht, The Netherlands

**Raymond M. Schiffelers**    Department of Pharmaceutical Sciences, Utrecht University, Utrecht, The Netherlands

**Vinod P. Shah**    Pharmaceutical Consultant, North Potomac, Maryland, U.S.A.

**Robert D. Sindelar**    The University of British Columbia, Vancouver, British Columbia, Canada

**Sjef C. M. Smeekens**    Department of Biology, Utrecht University, Utrecht, The Netherlands

**Frank-Peter Theil**    Genentech, Inc., South San Francisco, California, U.S.A.

**Jeffrey S. Wagener**    Department of Pediatrics, University of Colorado Medical School, Denver, Colorado, U.S.A.

**Nicole A. Weimert**    Department of Pharmacy Services, Medical University of South Carolina, Charleston, South Carolina, U.S.A.

# Abbreviations

| | | | |
|---|---|---|---|
| $^{125}$I-hGH | iodine labeled human growth hormone | BCGFII | B-cell growth factor |
| $5HT_{2a}$ | serotonergic receptor subtype | BDNF | brain-derived neurotrophic factor |
| A | adenine | BHK | baby hamster kidney |
| Å | angstroms | BMD | bone mineral density |
| AA | amino acid(s) | BMT | bone marrow transplantation |
| AAV | adeno-associated virus | bp | base pairs of DNA |
| Ab | antibody | BRCA1 | breast cancer gene 1 |
| ABO | blood group antigens | BRMs | biological response modifiers |
| ACT | activated clotting time | | |
| ADA | adenosine deaminase | BSA | bovine serum albumin |
| ADCC | antibody-dependent cellular cytotoxicity | C | cytosine |
| | | CAM | cell adhesion molecules |
| ADME | absorption, distribution, metabolism, excretion | CAR | Coxsackie adenovirus receptor |
| ADP | adenosine diphosphate | CCK | cholecystokinin |
| Ag | antigen | CD | circular dichroism |
| AG-LCR | asymmetric gap ligation chain reaction | CDC | complement-dependent cytotoxicity |
| AHF | antihemophiliac factor/ factor VIII | CDL | lytic complement pathway |
| ALS | amyotrophic lateral sclerosis | cDNA | copy DNA/ complementary deoxyribonucleic acid (sometimes also "cloned DNA") |
| AMI | acute myocardial infarction | | |
| AML | acute myelogenous leukemia | CDR | complementarity determining region |
| ANC | absolute neutrophil count | CEA | cost-effectiveness analysis |
| AP | alkaline phosphatase | | |
| APC | antigen presenting cell | CETP | cholesterol (cholesteryl) ester transfer protein |
| aPCC | activated prothrombin complex concentrate | CF | cystic fibrosis |
| apoE | apolipoprotein E | CFTR | cystic fibrosis transmembrane conductance regulator |
| APSAC | acylated plasminogen-streptokinase activator | | |
| ARDS | adult respiratory distress syndrome | CFU | colony-forming unit |
| | | CFU-GM | granulocyte-macrophage progenitor cells |
| Asn | asparagine | | |
| Asp | aspartic acid | | |
| ATP | adenosine 5′-triphosphate | CG | chorionic gonadotropin |
| | | CGD | chronic granulomatous disease |
| ATPase | adenosine triphosphatase | | |
| AUC | area under the curve | $C_H(1,2,3)$ | constant region(s) of heavy chain of lgG |
| B | biotin | | |
| BCG | bacille Calmette-Guérin | CHO | Chinese hamster ovary |

| | | |
|---|---|---|
| **CL** | elimination clearance from central compartment | maximum inhibition or stimulation |
| **CMI** | cell-mediated immunity | **ECD** extracellular domain |
| **CML** | chronic myelogenous leukemia | **EDF** eosinophil differentiation factor |
| **CMV** | cytomegalovirus | **EDTA** ethylenediaminetetra-acetic acid |
| **CNS** | central nervous system | **EGF** epidermal growth factor |
| **Con A** | concanavalin A | **EGFR** epidermal growth factor receptor |
| **COPD** | chronic obstructive pulmonary disease | **Ei** electrospray ionization |
| **CRI** | chronic renal insufficiency | **ELISA** enzyme-linked immunosorbent assay |
| **CRS** | cytokine release syndrome | $E_{max}$ maximum inhibition or stimulation |
| **CSF(s)** | colony stimulating factor(s) | **EMBL** European Molecular Biology Laboratory |
| **cSNPs** | SNPs occurring in gene coding regions | **EMEA** European Medicine Evaluation Agency |
| **CT** | cholera toxin | **EPO** erythropoietin |
| **CTCL** | cutaneous T-cell lymphoma | **ERK/MAP** extracellular signal-regulated kinase/ mitogen activated protein kinase |
| **CTL** | cytotoxic T-lymphocyte | |
| **CTP** | cytidine 5'-triphosphate | |
| **CUA** | cost utility analysis | **ES** embryonic stem cells |
| **D2** | dopaminergic D2 receptors | **EU** endotoxin unit |
| | | **FACS** fluorescence activated cell sorter |
| $D_5W$ | dextrose 5% in water | |
| **dATP** | deoxyadenosine 5'-triphosphate | **Fc** constant fragment (of immunoglobulins) |
| **dCTP** | deoxycytidine 5'-triphosphate | **FcRN** Brambell receptor/$F_c$ salvage receptor |
| **DDA** | dioctadecyldimethyl-ammoniumbromide | **FDA** Food and Drug Administration |
| **DDBJ** | DNA Data Bank of Japan | $FEV_1$ mean forced expiratory volume in one second |
| **ddNTP** | dideoxyribonucleotide triphosphate | |
| **DF** | diafiltration | **FGF** fibroblast growth factor |
| **dGTP** | deoxyguanosine 5'-triphosphate | **FH** familial hypercholesterolemia |
| $\Delta G_U$ | free energy | **fMLP** formyl-methionyl-leucyl-phenylalanine |
| **DLS** | dynamic light scattering | |
| **DNA** | deoxyribonucleic acid | **FPLC** fast protein liquid chromarography |
| **DNase** | deoxyribonuclease (I) | |
| **dNTP** | deoxyribonucleotide triphosphate | **FSH** follicle-stimulating hormone |
| **DSC** | differential scanning calorimetry | **FTIR** Fourier transform infrared spectroscopy |
| **DTP** | diphtheria-tetanus-pertussis | $F_v$ variable domains of light and heavy chains |
| **dTTP** | Deoxythymidine-5'-triphosphate | **FVC** forced vital capacity |
| | | **G** guanine |
| **E** | enzyme | **G-CSF** granulocyte colony-stimulating factor |
| $E_o$ | baseline effect | |
| **EBV** | Epstein-Barr virus | **G-LCR** gap ligation chain reaction |
| $EC_{50}$ | concentration that produces 50% of | **Ga-DF** gallium-desferal |

| | | | |
|---|---|---|---|
| GCV | gancyclovir | | antigen |
| GDNF | glial-derived neurotrophic growth factor | HMWP | high molecular weight protein |
| GEMM | granulocyte, erythrocyte, monocyte and megakaryocyte | HPLC | high-performance liquid chromatography |
| GERD | gastroesophageal reflux disease | HPRT | hypoxanthine phosphoribosyl transferase |
| GF | growth factor | HRP | horseradish peroxidase |
| GFR | glomerular filtration rate | HSA | human serum albumin |
| GH | growth hormone | HSCs | hematopoietic stem cells |
| GHBP | growth hormone binding protein | HSV | herpes simplex virus |
| | | HTS | high-throughput screening |
| GHD | growth hormone deficiency | IA | intra-arterial |
| GHRH | growth hormone releasing hormone | IC | intracoronary |
| | | ICAM-1 | intracellular adhesion molecule-1 |
| GIFT | gamete infra-fallopian transfer | ICSI | intracytoplasmic sperm injection |
| GIcNAc | N-acetyl-glucosamine | IEF | iso-electric focusing |
| GLP | good laboratory practice | iep | iso-electric point |
| GM-CSF | granulocyte-macrophage colony-stimulating factor | IFN | interferon(s) |
| | | Ig | immunoglobulin(s) |
| | | IGF | insulin-like growth factor |
| GMP | good manufacturing practice | IGFBP | IGF binding protein |
| GnRH | gonadotropin releasing hormone | IL | interleukin(s) |
| | | IM | intramuscular |
| GO | glucose-oxidase | IO | intra-orbital |
| GP | glycoprotein | IP | intraperitoneal |
| GRF | growth hormone releasing factor | IPTG | iso-propyl-$\beta$-thiogalactoside |
| GTP | guanosine 5'-triphosphate | IPV | inactivated polio vaccine |
| | | ISS | idiopathic short stature |
| GvHD | graft versus host disease | ITP | idiopathic thrombocytopenic purpura |
| h | human | | |
| HACA | human anti-chimeric antibody | ITR | inverted terminal repeat |
| HAMA | humane anti-mouse antibodies | IUGR | intrauterine growth retardation |
| HB(sAg) | hepatitis B (surface antigen) | IV | intravenous |
| | | IVF | in vitro fertilization |
| Hct | hematocrit | Kb | thousand base pairs of DNA |
| HEPA | high efficiency particulate air filters | Kd | dissociation rate constant |
| HER2 | human epidermal growth factor receptor gene | kDa | kilodalton |
| | | KGF | keratinocyte growth factor |
| HGF | hematopoietic growth factor | $K_m$ | Michaelis Menten constant |
| HIC | hydrophobic interaction chromatography | LAF | lymphocyte activating factor |
| His | histidine | LAK | leucocyte activated killer (cells) |
| HIV | human immunodeficiency virus | | |
| HLA | humane leukocyte | LAtTP | long acting tissue plasminogen activator |

| | | | |
|---|---|---|---|
| LCR | ligation chain reaction | | phosphatidyl- |
| LDL | low-density lipoprotein | | ethanolamine |
| LDLR | low-density lipoprotein | MuLV | murine leukemia virus |
| | receptor | mUPA | murine urokinase-type |
| LH | luteinizing hormone | | plasminogen activator |
| LHRH | luteinizing hormone | $M_w$ | relative molecular mass |
| | releasing hormone | NBP | non-ionic block |
| LIF | leukemia inhibitory | | copolymers |
| | factor | NCBI | National Center for |
| LPD | lymphoproliferative | | Biotechnology |
| | disorders | | Information |
| LPS | lipopolysaccharide | NCS | neocarzinostatin |
| LRP | (low-density) | NESP | novel erythropoiesis |
| | lipoprotein receptor- | | stimulating protein |
| | related protein | NF | natural form |
| LTR | long terminal repeat | NF-kB | transcription factor in |
| LYZ | lysozyme | | B- and T-cells |
| M1 | nauscarinic receptor | NFs | neurotrophic factors |
| | subtype | NGF | nerve growth factor |
| M3 | muscarinic receptor | NIH | National Institutes of |
| | subtype | | Health |
| M cells | microfold cells | NK | natural killer cell(s) |
| MAb(s) | monoclonal antibody(s) | NMR | nuclear magnetic |
| MAC | membrane attack | | resonance spectroscopy |
| | complex | NOESY | 2-D nuclear Overhauser |
| MALDI | matrix-assisted laser | | effect NMR technique |
| | desorption ionization | NPH | neutral protamine |
| MAP | multiple antigen peptide | | Hagedorn |
| Mb | million base pairs of | NPL | neutral protamine lispro |
| | DNA | NSAIDs | non-steroidal anti- |
| MCB | master cell bank | | inflammatory drugs |
| M-CSF | macrophage colony- | NZS | neocarzinostatin |
| | stimulating factor | ODNs | oligodeoxynucleotides |
| MDR-1 | multiple drug resistance | OLA | oligonucleotide ligation |
| Meg | megakaryocyte | | assay |
| Met-GH | methionine human | OMP | outer membrane protein |
| | growth hormone | ON | oligonucleotide |
| met-rhGH | methionyl recombinant | ori | origin of replication |
| | human growth | PAGE | polyacrylamide gel |
| | hormone, contains | | electrophoresis |
| | N-terminal methionine | PAI | plasminogen activator |
| MGDF | megakaryocyte growth | | inhibitors |
| | and development | PBPCs | peripheral blood |
| | factor | | progenitor cells |
| MHC | major histocompatibility | PCI | percutaneous coronary |
| | complex | | intervention |
| MI | myocardial infarction | PCR | polymerase chain |
| MMAD | mean mass aerodynamic | | reaction |
| | diameter | PCTA | percutaneous |
| MMR | measles-mumps-rubella | | transluminal coronary |
| MPS | mononuclear phagocyte | | angioplasry |
| | system | PD | pharmacodynamics |
| $M_r$ | relative molecular mass | PDGF | platelet-derived growth |
| mRNA | messenger ribonucleic | | factor |
| | acid/messenger RNA | PEG | polyoxyethylene = |
| MTP-PE | muramyltripeptide- | | polyethyleneglycol |

| | | | |
|---|---|---|---|
| PEG IL-2 | PEGylated interleukin-2 (polyethylene glycol modified interleukin-2) | rhG-CSF | recombinant human granulocyte colony-stimulating factor |
| PEG-rhMGDF | pegylated-recombinant human megakaryocyte growth and development factor | rhGH | recombinant human growth hormone, natural sequence |
| PEI | polyethylene imines | RIA | radioimmunoassay |
| PG | peptidoglycans | rBPI | recombinant bactericidal/ permeability increasing protein |
| P$^1$ | iso-electric point, negative logarithm | | |
| pit-hGH | pituitary-derived human growth hormone | RME | receptor mediated endocytosis |
| PK | pharmacokinetics | RMS | root mean square |
| PLGA | polylactic-coglycolic acid | RNA | ribonucleic acid |
| | | RNase P | ribonuclease P |
| PNA | peptide nucleic acid | RNase H | ribonuclease H |
| PP | polypropylene | RP-HPLC | reversed-phase high performance liquid chromatography |
| PT | prothrombin time | | |
| PTCA | percutaneous transluminal coronary angioplasty | | |
| | | rRNA | ribosomal RNA |
| | | RSV | respiratory syncytial virus |
| PTH | parathyroid hormone | | |
| PTT | partial thromboplastin time | RT | reverse transcriptase |
| | | rt-PA | recombinant tissue-type plasminogen activator |
| PVC | polyvinyl chloride | | |
| PVDF | polyvinylidine difluoride | | |
| QALY | quality-adjusted life year | RT-PCR | reverse transcription polymerase chain reaction |
| r | recombinant | | |
| rAAT | recombinant α1-antitrypsin | RTU | ready to use solution |
| RAC | U.S. Recombinant DNA Advisory Committee | SA | streptavidin |
| | | SBS | short bowel syndrome |
| rAHF | recombinant anti-hemophilia factor | SC | suspension culture or subcutaneous |
| RBC | red blood cells | SCF | stem cell factor (also known as c-kit ligand and steel factor) |
| rBPI | recombinant bactericial/ permeability-increasing protein | | |
| | | ScF$_v$ | single chain variable fragments |
| rDNA | recombinant deoxyribonucleic acid/ recombinant-DNA | SCI | subcutaneous infusion |
| | | SCN | severe chronic neutropenia |
| rG-CSF | recombinant granulocyte colony-stimulating factor (filgrastim) | scu PA | single chain urokinase plasminogen activator |
| RGD | amino acid sequence Arg-Gly-Asp (arginine-glycine-aspartic acid) | SDS-PAGE | sodium dodecyl sulfate polyacrylamide-gel electrophoresis |
| rhGM-CSF | recombinant granulocyte-macrophage colony-stimulating factor | SEC | size-exclusion chromatography |
| | | Ser | serine |
| | | SLE | systemic lupus erythematosus |
| rhDNase | recombinant human deoxyribonuclease I | SNP(s) | single nucleotide polymorphism(s) |
| rh-EPO | recombinant human erythropoietin | SOD | superoxide dismutase |

| | | | |
|---|---|---|---|
| SSC | large scale suspension culture process | TPO | thrombopoietin |
| STI | soy bean trypsin inhibitor | TR | terminal repeats |
| | | TRAP | thrombin receptor activating peptide |
| T/dTTP | deoxythymidine 5'-triphosphate | TRF | T cell replacement factor |
| T | thymine | tRNA | transfer RNA |
| t-PA | tissue plasminogen activator | TSE | transmissible spongiphormous encephalitis |
| T3,T4 | thyroid hormones | | |
| TAC | T-cell activating antigen | TSH | thyroid-stimulating hormone |
| TAS | transcription-based amplification system | TSP | thrombospondin |
| TCGF | T-cell growth factor | U | uracil |
| TDTH | delayed type hypersensitivity T-cells | UF | ultrafiltration |
| | | uPA | urokinase-type plasminogen activator |
| $T_e$ | eutectic temperature | | |
| TFF | tangential flow filtration | UTP | uridine 5'-triphosphate |
| TFPI | tissue factor pathway inhibitor | UV | ultraviolet |
| | | VEGF | vascular endothelial growth factor |
| $T_g$ | glass transition temperature | | |
| | | VLP | virus like particles |
| TGF | tissue growth factor | VSV | vesicular stomatitis virus |
| $T_h$-cell | T-helper cell | | |
| $TH_{1,2}$ | Type 1 or 2 T-helper cell | W | weight |
| TIL | tumor infiltrating lymphocytes | WCB | working cell bank |
| | | WHO | World Health Organization |
| TIMI | thrombolysis in myocardial infraction | WHO-IUIS | World Health Organization-International Union of Immunologic Societies |
| TNF-α | tumor necrosis factor α | | |
| tPA | tissue-type plasminogen activator | | |
| TPMT | thiopurine methyltransferase | X-FEL | x-ray free electron laser |

# 1

# Molecular Biotechnology

*Wiel P. M. Hoekstra and Sjef C. M. Smeekens*
*Department of Biology, Utrecht University, Utrecht, The Netherlands*

## INTRODUCTION

Biotechnology has been defined in many different ways. Specific definitions for pharmaceutical biotechnology can be deduced directly from these definitions. In general biotechnology implies the use of microorganisms, plants, and animals or parts thereof for the production of useful compounds. Consequently, pharmaceutical biotechnology should be considered as biotechnological manufacturing of pharmaceutical products.

Various forms of biotechnology existed already in ancient times. The Bible documents this ancient origin of biotechnology, informing us about Noah who apparently knew how to make wine from grapes. Based merely on experience but without understanding of the underlying principles, bioproducts were for many ages homemade in a traditional fashion.

Insight into the nature of the traditional processes was achieved about 1870 when Pasteur made clear that chemical conversions in these processes are performed by living cells and should thus be considered as biochemical conversions. Biotechnology became science! In the decades after Pasteur knowledge increased when the role of enzymes as catalysts for most of the biochemical conversions became apparent. Based on that knowledge, tools became available to control and optimize the traditional processes to a certain extent.

A further and very important breakthrough took place after the development of molecular biology. The notion, brought forward by the pioneers in molecular biology around 1950, that DNA encodes proteins and in this way controls all cellular processes was the impetus for a new period in biotechnology. The fast evolving DNA technologies, after the development of the recombinant DNA technology in the seventies, allowed biotechnologists to control gene expression in the organisms used for biotechnological manufacturing. Moreover, the developed technologies opened ways to introduce foreign DNA into all kinds of organisms. As will be shown later, genetically modified organisms constructed in that way opened up complete new possibilities for biotechnology. The new form of biotechnology, based on profound knowledge of the DNA molecule and the availability of manipulation technologies of DNA, is frequently described as "molecular biotechnology." The possibilities of the molecular approaches for further development of biotechnology were immediately apparent, albeit that the expectations sometimes were overestimated. At the same time biotechnology became the subject of public debate. An important question in the debate deals with potential risks: Do genetically modified organisms as used in production facilities pose unknown risks for an ecosystem and for the human race itself? Moreover, a profound ethical question was brought forward: Is it right to modify the genetic structure of living organisms?

In this chapter we will focus mainly on the new biotechnology by describing its means and goals. As to the question concerning potential risks of the technology, we will confine ourselves to stating that all sorts of measurements are taken to avoid risks while using genetically modified organisms. The ethical aspects, interesting as they are, are beyond the scope of this chapter.

## THE CELL

Although biotechnology does not exclusively make use of cells but also of complete organisms or of cell constituents, knowledge of basic cell biology is required to understand biotechnology to its full extent.

Cells from all sorts of organisms are used in biotechnology. Not only prokaryotic cells like simple unicellular bacteria are used, but also eukaryotic cells, like cells of higher microorganisms, plants, and animals, are exploited. Those cell types are not dealt with in detail. The unifying concepts in cell biology and the diversification as far as relevant for pharmaceutical biotechnology will be the main topic of discussion in this chapter.

### ■ The Prokaryotic Cell

The prokaryotes, to which the bacteria belong, represent the simplest cells in nature. A schematic illustration (Fig. 1) depicts a prokaryotic cell. Such a cell is in fact no more than cytoplasm surrounded by some surface layers, generally described as the cell envelope. In the bacterial world one distinguishes two main types of organisms. They are called Gram-positive or Gram-negative based on different behavior in a classical cell staining technique. The fundamental differences between these two prokaryotic types are mainly apparent in the structure of the cell envelope.

The bacterial cell envelope consists of a cytoplasmic membrane and of a very characteristic wall structure called the peptidoglycan layer. The cells of Gram-positive organisms are multilayered with peptidoglycan while only one or two such layers are found in cells of Gram-negative organisms. However, the clearest distinction between the two types of bacterial cells is that in Gram-negative organisms the cell is surrounded by a very specific extra membrane layer, called outer membrane (OM) (Fig. 2). Next to the cytoplasmic membrane, also called the inner membrane (IM), the OM is a permeation barrier for substances that are transported into or out of the cell.

A prominent and very particular chemical constituent of the OM is the compound named lipopolysaccharide (LPS). Biopharmaceutical products gained from Gram-negative organisms must be extensively purified especially when they are used as a pharmaceutical for man or animal (Chapters 3 and 4), since LPS set free during the isolation of the product has, even in a very low concentration, severe toxic effects to man and animals.

In the bacterial cell DNA is generally organized in one large circular molecule. The bacterial DNA is not surrounded by a nuclear membrane and is not as complex in organization as DNA in eukaryotic cells. One generally refers to bacterial DNA as chromosomal DNA, analogous to the nomenclature in eukaryotic cells. Bacteria may, apart from the chromosomal DNA, harbor autonomously replicating small DNA molecules, called plasmids. Functions that are essential for a bacterial cell are usually encoded by the chromosome, whereas functions encoded by plasmids are generally in no way essential. Nevertheless, plasmids endow the bacterial cell with properties that may be very important for the survival of the bacteria. Antibiotic resistances and production of toxic proteins, for example, are well-known plasmid encoded traits. As we will see later, plasmids are used in biotechnology as important and basic tools for the recombinant DNA technology.

When we refer to plasmids as small DNA molecules, this is of course in comparison to the size of the chromosomal DNA. Besides, one has to realize that plasmids vary in size. Small plasmids, generally the relevant ones for biotechnology, harbor about 6000 DNA building units, called nucleotides. Chromosomal DNA of a bacterium contains at least 1000 times more nucleotides. The DNA content of an animal or plant cell on the other hand exceeds several hundred times that of a bacterial cell. Moreover, the DNA of the former cells is no longer organized in one molecule, but in several linear chromosomes. A popular way to illustrate this fast growing

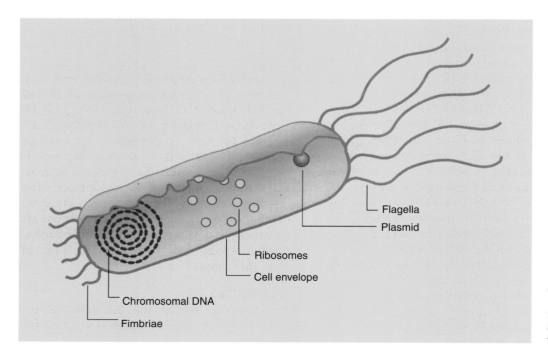

Flagella
Plasmid
Ribosomes
Cell envelope
Chromosomal DNA
Fimbriae

**Figure 1** ■ Cross section (*artificial*) through a bacterial cell. The surface structures (*fimbriae and flagella*) are not essential structures but allow the cells to adhere and to move.

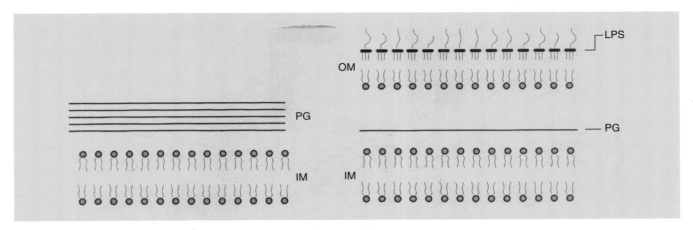

**Figure 2** ■ Cell envelope G$^+$ cell (*left*) and G$^-$ cell (*right*). *Abbreviations*: G$^+$, Gram positive; G$^-$, Gram negative; PG, peptido-glycans; LPS, lipopolysaccharide; OM, outer membrane; IM, inner membrane.

complexity of DNA molecules in nature is based on pages and books. One can easily write on one page the composition of the DNA of a small plasmid by its nucleotide composition, using the symbols A, C, G, and T for the various nucleotides in the DNA. To do the same for the bacterial chromosome, a book with about 1000 pages is needed. For an animal cell or a plant cell it requires a few hundred books, each containing about 1000 pages to describe the DNA.

Bacterial cells, like all cells, harbor in their cytoplasm the ribosomes as essential structures for protein synthesis, as well as a great variety of enzymes and other (macro)molecules required for the proper physiology of the cell. Most important, however, is that, apart from chromosome, ribosomes and sometimes plasmids, generally no other distinct structures are visible in the cytoplasm of the bacterial cell, even when studied with an electron microscope. Furthermore, there are no compartments present in the cytoplasm of the prokaryotic cell.

### ■ The Eukaryotic Cell

Figure 3 presents a schematic picture of a plant cell as an example of an eukaryotic cell. The eukaryotic cell has a very complex structure, not only by the presence of cell organelles like the nucleus, mitochondria, and chloroplast (exclusively found in plant cells), but also by the presence of specific internal membranes and of vacuoles. This complex and compartmentalized structure implies a complicated functional behavior and is one of the reasons that in the initial phase of modern biotechnology simple bacterial cells, easier to handle and more simple to modify, were prominently used. Nowadays, molecular biotechnologists use all sorts of eukaryotic cells, exploiting the fast growing insights in cell biology.

### GENE EXPRESSION

Genetic information, chemically determined by the DNA structure, is transferred during cell division to daughter cells by DNA replication and is expressed by transcription (conversion of DNA into RNA) followed by translation (conversion of RNA into protein). This set of processes is found in all cells and proceeds generally in similar ways. It is one of the main unifying concepts in cell biology. The pioneers of molecular biology called that series of events the "central dogma" of biology. It was found later that retroviruses, a special class of animal RNA viruses, encode an enzyme that catalyzes the conversion of RNA into complementary DNA. This enzyme, called the reverse transcriptase since it directs, so to say, the reverse of the transcription, therefore enables an information flow from RNA into DNA. Reverse transcriptase became, as will be shown later, a very important tool for DNA technology.

The various DNA linked processes are schematically depicted below:

$$DNA \leftrightarrow RNA \rightarrow protein$$

The "central dogma" was based on investigations done with bacteria and viruses. Later it was found that in eukaryotic organisms many genes are expressed differently from what was predicted by the dogma in the strict sense. In some cases the RNA derived by transcription of an eukaryotic DNA segment is subject to a process called splicing before it leaves the nucleus. During this process certain parts, the so-called introns, of the nascent RNA molecules are removed, after which the other parts (the exons) are linked together and form the effective RNA for the protein synthesis (Fig. 4).

Furthermore, it is important to realize that a nascent protein, the direct result of the translation, is

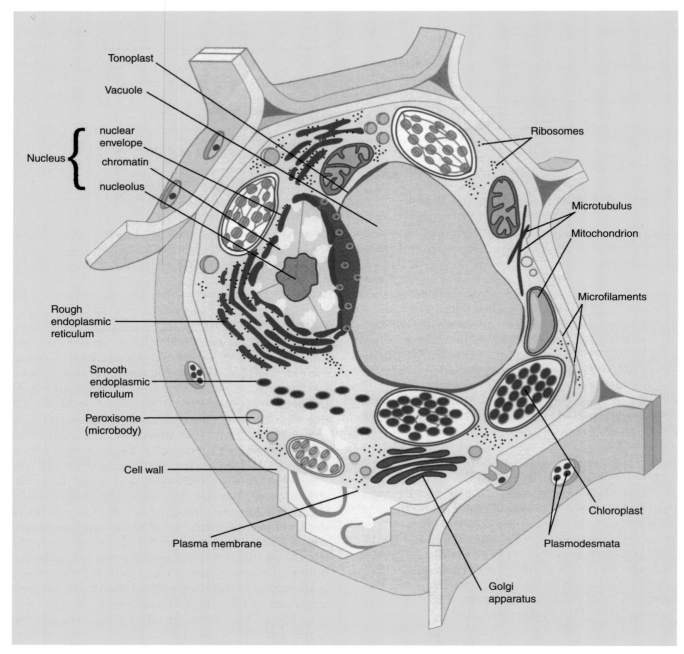

**Figure 3** ■ Plant cell, schematic view.

not necessarily identical to the protein functional in the cell as enzyme or structural protein. Most proteins as we find them in the cell are modified by post-translational events. Nascent polypeptides are, for example, trimmed by peptidases; in some cases lipidic groups are linked to the protein, while in eukaryotic cells modification through linking of sugar groups (glycosylation) is a common event. Such post-translational modifications are important features with regard to the specific function of the protein.

Precise knowledge of the information flow in the cell is very important for biotechnology, since it offers possibilities to control cellular processes at the level of gene expression. Therefore, the essentials of elements and processes involved in the flow of genetic information will be described below.

■ **DNA Replication**
Although DNA may be differently organized in various organisms one or more double-stranded

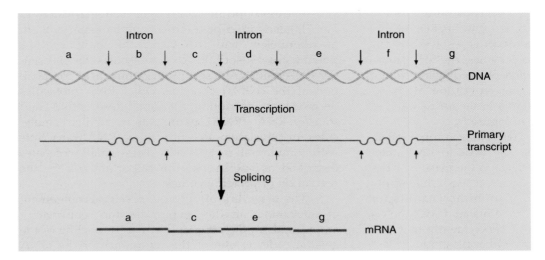

**Figure 4** ■ RNA splicing.

DNA molecules in a helix conformation are the predominant structures. Strands of DNA are composed of four specific building elements (shortly written as A, C, G, and T), the deoxyribonucleotides deoxyadenosine 5'-triphosphate, (dATP) deoxycytidine 5'-triphosphate (dCTP), deoxyguanosine 5'-triphosphate (dGTP), and deoxythymidine 5'-triphosphate (dTTP) linked by phosphodiester bonds. The two strands in the DNA helix are held together through hydrogen bonds between the nucleotides in the various strands. The DNA strands in the helix are complementary in their nucleotide composition: an A in one strand is always facing a T in the other one, while a C is always facing a G (Fig. 5). Moreover, the strands in double-stranded DNA run antiparallel: the 5'-P end of the one strand faces the 3'-OH end of the complementary strand and the other way round.

During cell division the genetic information in a parental cell is transferred to the daughter cells by DNA replication. Essential in the very complex DNA replication process is the action of DNA polymerases. During replication each DNA strand is copied into a complementary strand that runs antiparallel. The topological constraint for replication due to the double helix structure of the DNA is solved by unwinding of the helix, catalyzed by the enzyme helicase. In a set of biochemical events deoxyribonucleotide monomers are added one by one to the end of a growing DNA strand in a 5' to 3' direction.

DNA replication starts from specific sites, called origins of replication (*ori*). The bacterial chromosome and many plasmids have only one such site. In the much larger eukaryotic genomes there can be hundreds of *ori*s present. For circular DNA molecules like bacterial chromosomes and plasmids there are two possible ways for the replication. Semi conservative replication (Fig. 6A) proceeding in the closed circle as

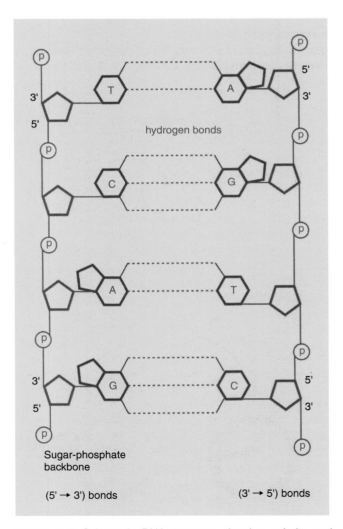

**Figure 5** ■ Schematic DNA structure showing polarity and complementarity.

such (Fig. 6B) is one way. The constraint brought forward by the rotation as a consequence of the unwinding (there is no free end!) is resolved by the activity of a special class of enzymes, the topoisomerases. Alternatively, replication proceeds via a rolling circle model. In that case the replication starts by cutting one of the DNA strands in the *ori* region and then proceeds as indicated in Figure 6C.

Bacterial plasmids are defined as autonomously replicating DNA molecules. The basis for that statement is the presence of an *ori* site in the plasmids. The qualification autonomous, however, does not imply that a plasmid is independent from host factors for replication and expression. Some plasmids depend on very specific host factors and consequently they can only replicate in specific hosts. Other plasmids are less specific as to their host factor requirements and are able to replicate in a broad set of hosts. As will be demonstrated later, this difference in host range is meaningful when plasmids are exploited in biotechnology.

### ■ Transcription

Genetic information is located in the genes formed by discrete segments of the cellular DNA. In a process called transcription (presented schematically in Fig. 7), genes are copied into a complementary length of ribonucleic acid (RNA) by the enzyme RNA polymerase. Most of the RNA molecules, the messenger RNAs (mRNAs), specify the amino acid composition of the cellular proteins. Other RNA molecules derived by transcription, ribosomal RNA (rRNA) and transfer RNA (tRNA), participate as auxiliary molecules for translation. Recently, micro-RNA transcripts were found in all sorts of cells. These small molecules described as siRNA play an important role in the regulation of protein synthesis.

The discovery of how the specific arrangement of nucleotides in the gene codes the sequence of amino acids in the polypeptide, the unraveling of the genetic code, is one of the milestones of the DNA époque. It was found that triplets of nucleotides in the DNA, and consequently in the mRNA, code for the amino acid composition of a protein. Most important was finding that the genetic code was (almost) universal in nature. A given triplet of nucleotides, a so-called codon, in mRNA codes for the same amino acid in nearly all organisms.

In the mRNA molecules there is more information than merely the triplets required for the encoded protein. The protein encoding information is preceded by a piece of RNA that allows binding to the ribosome, while after the triplet encoding the C-terminal amino acid there is some RNA that functioned in the termination of the transcription process. Thus, signals are required to guarantee within this mRNA molecule a proper start and finish for the polypeptide synthesis. Near the 5'-end of the mRNA a specific triplet, coding for the amino acid methionine, dictates the proper start of the polypeptide synthesis and near the 3'-end a specific triplet (a stop codon) dictates a proper finish of the polypeptide synthesis. The genetic code, on the basis of the triplets in the mRNA, is presented in Table 1. One may see that there are three different stop codons. Moreover, it is clear from this Table 1 that the code is highly redundant: for certain amino acids there are several codons. Whenever there is a choice between various codons for one amino acid, different organisms tend to show different preferences. Later it will become clear that this organism dependent codon preference has consequences for certain biotechnological processes.

Transcription starts with the binding of the enzyme RNA polymerase at a specific site, called promoter, immediately upstream from a gene or from a set of genes transcribed as an operational unit (an operon). Promoters vary in their efficiency to bind RNA polymerase. Some promoters, the strong promoters, are highly efficient while others are weak and often require additional factors for effective binding of RNA polymerase. Promoter structures, in prokaryotes as

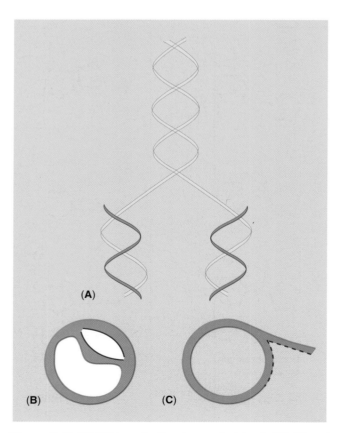

**Figure 6** ■ **(A)** DNA replication (general picture). **(B)** Closed circle replication. **(C)** Rolling circle model.

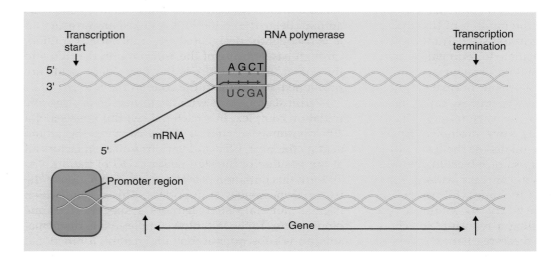

**Figure 7** ▪ Transcription. Upper part shows ongoing transcription. Lower part depicts the start, involving specific binding of RNA polymerase to the promoter region.

well as in eukaryotes, have been studied in great detail. Based on such studies it is now feasible in biotechnology, as shown later, to fuse very effective promoter structures to any gene that one wishes to be expressed.

After binding of the RNA polymerase, the DNA helix is partially unwound and subsequently the transcription process starts. RNA synthesis then proceeds with the ribonucleotides ATP, GTP, CTP and UTP (uridine 5′-triphosphate) as building units. One DNA strand in the gene, the so-called template strand, serves as the matrix for this RNA synthesis.

Like in the DNA synthesis, the RNA synthesis runs antiparallel in the direction 5′ to 3′ and proceeds in a complementary way. The latter implies that a G in the matrix DNA leads to C in the RNA, a C leads to a G, a T to an A while an A in the DNA shows up as a U in the RNA. The transcription may stop either on the basis of intrinsic structural features of the RNA at the end of the gene or the operon or by the intervention of a specific terminating protein factor at this site.

Transcription can be regulated at various stages in the process. The intrinsic properties of the

| First position (5′-end) | Second position | | | | Third position (3′-end) |
|---|---|---|---|---|---|
| | **U** | **C** | **A** | **G** | |
| **U** | Phe | Ser | Tyr | Cys | **U** |
| | Phe | Ser | Tyr | Cys | **C** |
| | Leu | Ser | Stop | Stop | **A** |
| | Leu | Ser | Stop | Trp | **G** |
| **C** | Leu | Pro | His | Arg | **U** |
| | Leu | Pro | His | Arg | **C** |
| | Leu | Pro | Gln | Arg | **A** |
| | Leu | Pro | Gln | Arg | **G** |
| **A** | Lle | Thr | Asn | Ser | **U** |
| | Lle | Thr | Asn | Ser | **C** |
| | Lle | Thr | Lys | Arg | **A** |
| | **Met** | Thr | Lys | Arg | **G** |
| **G** | Val | Ala | Asp | Gly | **U** |
| | Val | Ala | Asp | Gly | **C** |
| | Val | Ala | Glu | Gly | **A** |
| | **Val** | Ala | Glu | Gly | **G** |

*Note*: The bold codons are used for initiation.

**Table 1** ▪ The "universal" genetic code.

promoter, next to various kinds of proteins that can either repress or stimulate the binding of RNA polymerase, regulate the transcription start. Transcription termination can also be regulated. Termination may, under the influence of physiological factors, occur at a premature stage. Alternatively, the normal termination signal could be ignored (a process called read-through). This may lead to various lengths of transcripts starting from the same promoter. Finally gene activity can also be regulated at the level of the formed mRNA. All transcripts are subject to degradation, but rates of degradation can vary widely: Some transcripts have a short half-life time while others are very stable. Biotechnologists try to influence the expression of a gene encoding a relevant biotechnological protein at each of these regulation levels in order to achieve optimal production.

## ■ Translation

Translation, presented schematically in Figure 8, is a complex cellular process where mRNA molecules, ribosomes, tRNA molecules, amino acids, aminoacyl synthetases and a number of translation factors act together in a highly coordinated way. The ribosome, an organelle built from rRNA molecules and proteins, is the cellular structure where the various compounds for the protein synthesis assemble.

The building elements of the proteins, the amino acids, are used in the protein synthesis in a form adapted for a convenient interaction with the mRNA. The adaptation of the amino acid is achieved by coupling it to a specific tRNA molecule through the catalytic action of specific aminoacyl synthetases. The adapted amino acid is linked to the 3'-OH terminus of a specific tRNA molecule. Each tRNA molecule contains in a characteristic loop of the molecule a

specific triplet. This triplet is complementary and runs antiparallel to the codon for the linked amino acid and is consequently designated the anticodon. Coupling through base pairing of the anticodon in the tRNA to the codon in the mRNA is the way amino acids are positioned according to the code in the mRNA.

Translation starts with the formation of a specific initiation complex. In a bacterial cell this consists of a 30S ribosomal subunit, a tRNA carrying the amino acid methionine, GTP and various initiation factors all at the position of the start codon AUG of the mRNA. To form this initiation complex the 5'-end region of the bacterial messenger is important. This region, which itself is not translated, harbors a specific ribosome binding site. To the initiation complex a 50S ribosomal subunit is subsequently bound, creating a functional 70S ribosome. Translation then proceeds, with the help of specific elongation factors, in such a way that the 70S ribosomes are transported along the mRNA molecule stepwise over a distance of one triplet. This stepwise transport guarantees that protein synthesis proceeds in a coordinated way dictated by the (triplet) codons. The amino acids, delivered by the specific tRNA molecules, are linked together, one after the other, by peptide bond formation. Meanwhile the tRNA carriers are set free again.

At the end of a mRNA molecule there are one or more stop codons. These triplets do not accept any tRNA-aminoacyl molecule and are therefore terminating signals for protein synthesis. After termination the protein is released from the 70S ribosome. The ribosomes then fall apart in their 30S and 50S subunits which may be used in a further translation cycle.

Although there is a common general picture for translation in prokaryotes and eukaryotes there are nevertheless various distinct differences, especially in the nature of initiation and elongation factors. A very clear distinction is a direct consequence of the difference in DNA organization between pro- and eukaryotes. In the prokaryotic cell, mRNA is already available for the ribosomes while it is still in the process of transcription. In the eukaryotic cell, on the other hand, the mRNA is only available for translation after it is completely synthesized and after it is transported through the nuclear membrane. Consequently, transcription and translation are coupled processes in the prokaryotic cell, while these processes occur separately in the eukaryotic cell.

## RECOMBINANT DNA TECHNOLOGY

After it was established that DNA is the chemical constituent for the hereditary properties of the cell and after the discovery that (bacterial) cells can spontaneously take up DNA, investigators immediately tried to manipulate the genetic properties of all

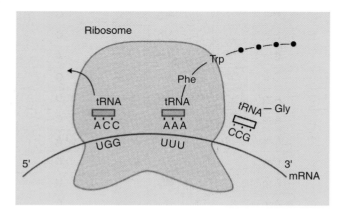

**Figure 8** ■ Schematic picture of ongoing translation. The amino acid Phe is linked to the growing peptide chain. The tRNA that delivered the previous amino acid Trp is leaving the ribosome complex. The next amino acid to be linked will be Gly, according to the mRNA code.

kinds of cells. To achieve this, they simply added foreign DNA to microbial cells, plant cells or animal cells. All these attempts failed. There are two reasons for this lack of success. First of all, only a limited number of bacterial species is able to take up DNA spontaneously; most bacteria and certainly animal and plant species are unable to do this. Secondly, foreign DNA, if at all taken up, is in general not maintained in the receptor cell. DNA brought into a cell from outside will only be maintained if it is able to replicate autonomously, or if it is integrated in the recipient genome. In all other cases foreign DNA will not be propagated in the cell culture and will eventually disappear by degradation through the activity of cellular nucleases.

Genetic modification of organisms became feasible later on when recombinant DNA technologies were developed. This enabled the fusion of any DNA fragment to DNA molecules able to maintain themselves by autonomous replication (such molecules are called replicons). The various specific techniques developed to introduce recombinant DNA molecules into all sorts of biological cells led to successful genetic modification strategies.

Replicons used as carriers for foreign DNA fragments are termed vectors. The vectors exploited in the DNA technology include mainly plasmids from bacteria or yeast, or DNA from bacterioviruses, animal viruses or plant viruses. Especially small microbial plasmids are very popular as vectors in biotechnology, since they can easily be isolated as intact circular double-stranded molecules. Plasmids with a broad host range, mentioned before, are very attractive since they can be used in various hosts and consequently enable a flexible application of the DNA technology.

For the application of plasmids in biotechnology, one has to fuse foreign DNA to the isolated plasmid in order to create a recombinant DNA molecule. The technology for this, the so-called recombinant DNA technology or DNA cloning technology, became feasible after the discovery of a specific class of nucleases, the so-called restriction endonucleases. Next to nucleases able to cleave any phosphodiester bond in DNA, nucleases which only cleave DNA at very specific sites are present in nature. These enzymes, the restriction enzymes, were discovered around 1970 in microorganisms. Their function is to discriminate between foreign DNA and self DNA. Microbial cells may in real life be confronted with DNA from an unrelated cell via various genetic transfer systems. Although all DNA is built likewise, DNA can be marked specifically at particular sites by a characteristic pattern of methylated or glucosylated nucleotides. This DNA marking, which does not interfere with the coding and replicating functions, is host specific. Restriction enzymes have the remarkable property to recognize DNA on the basis of the specific host marking. When DNA is transferred and the marking does not fit with the recipient cell, such DNA will be recognized and cut at specific sites by the restriction enzyme. Once the DNA is cut it will be further degraded in the cell. As is the case in many biological systems, things are never absolute: some DNA molecules may escape from the action of the restriction enzymes and by getting a proper marking they can be rescued.

The very selective action of the restriction enzymes is the basis for their application in the recombinant DNA technology. Addition of a restriction enzyme to a plasmid without proper marking will convert the closed circular molecule to linear fragments, provided that the plasmid harbors recognition sites for the chosen restriction enzyme. In Figure 9 this is depicted for a special, but representative case. A plasmid with only one recognition site for

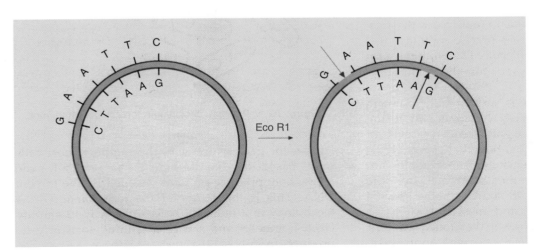

**Figure 9** ■ Treatment of a plasmid with an unique EcoR1 site. This restriction enzyme will open the plasmid and make it amenable for manipulation.

the restriction enzyme *Eco*R1 is treated with this enzyme. The double-stranded DNA is then asymmetrically cut at the recognition site, encompassing six bases namely GAATTC, which leads to linear DNA with typical short single-stranded ends. If foreign DNA—isolated either from microbial, plant or animal cells—with recognition sites for the enzyme *Eco*R1 is likewise cut with this enzyme, fragments with single-stranded ends characteristic for *Eco*R1 in the vector are formed. When the open vector and the foreign DNA fragments are brought together under appropriate physicochemical conditions, the various single-stranded ends may recombine due to the presence of complementary bases. A possible reaction product could be a plasmid to which a specific foreign DNA fragment, as a passenger, is linked. Although the DNA pieces in such construct are interlinked by base pairing, they do not form a closed circular molecule. The enzyme DNA ligase, present in all sorts of cells and able to catalyze the formation of phosphodiester bonds, is used to create a closed circular recombinant DNA molecule. Although DNA fragments with complementary single-stranded ends (so-called cohesive ends) are the most favorable ones for linking, DNA ligase is also able to link fragments with blunt ends.

According to the technology presented schematically in Figure 10, recombinant DNA molecules consisting of vector and passenger DNA can be created. A great number of restriction enzymes with very specific recognition sites is available to cut DNA at a specific site. Some enzymes, like *Eco*R1, recognize a sequence of six base pairs, other enzymes recognize just four bases. Some, again like *Eco*R1, cut the DNA asymmetrically while others create blunt ends when cutting DNA. In Table 2 some representative restriction enzymes are listed.

Recombinant DNA molecules are biologically of no interest as long as they reside in the reaction tube. Transfer of the construct to a living cell, however, may change the situation drastically. If the vector that served for the construct is able to replicate in the host, all daughter cells will inherit a precise copy (a clone) of the recombinant DNA molecule. Therefore the term "cloning" is frequently used for the technology described above.

The cloning technique is very suitable to obtain large amounts of a specific DNA fragment, by fusing such a fragment to an appropriate vector and transferring the construct to a host that can easily be cultivated to high cell densities. The recombinant DNA molecules, which can then be isolated from the cell mass, form an abundant source for the specific DNA fragment. Moreover and most important for pharmaceutical biotechnology, if the cloned piece of foreign DNA harbors an intact gene with appropriate

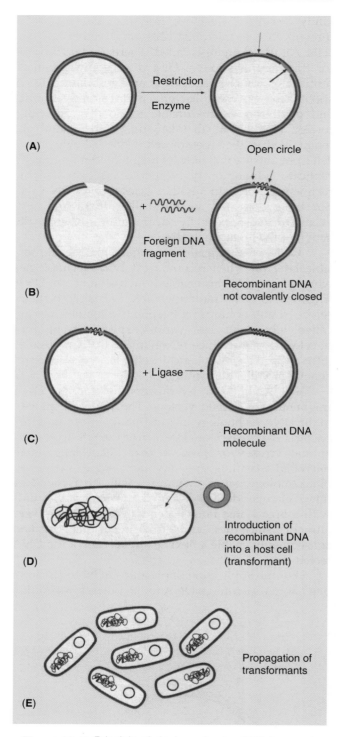

**Figure 10** ▪ Principle of cloning a foreign DNA fragment.

signals for gene expression, the modified host cells may, based on the universal character of gene expression, produce proteins encoded by the foreign DNA. This is the power of the recombinant DNA technology in a nutshell: an efficient way to amplify DNA fragments and a way to gain all sorts of gene products from hosts that one can choose.

| Enzyme | Source | Cutting sequence[a] |
|--------|--------|---------------------|
| EcoR1 | *Escherichia coli* | G↓AATT C |
| | | C TTAA↑G |
| Pst1 | *Providencia stuartii* | C TGCA↓G |
| | | G↑ACGT C |
| Taq1 | *Thermus aquaticus* | T↓CG A |
| | | A GC↑T |
| Hinf1 | *Hemophilus influenzae* | G↓ANT C |
| | | C TNA↑G |
| Msp1 | *Moraxella species* | C↓CG G |
| | | G GC↑C |
| HaeIII | *Hemophilus aegyptus* | GG↓CC |
| | | CC↑GG |

[a] N, no base preference.
*Note*: Open space in the recognition site indicates the endonucleolytic cut by the enzyme.

**Table 2** ■ Some restriction enzymes, their origin, and their recognition site.

## ■ DNA Transfer

As stated above, transfer of a recombinant DNA molecule to a cell is an essential step in DNA technology. Some bacterial cells, like those of the species *Bacillus subtilis* which are frequently used in industrial biotechnology, are able to take up DNA under physiological conditions. This process is described as natural transformation. In most cases, however, microbial cells have to be forced by an unusual regimen to take up DNA. For example, in the case of microorganisms such non-physiological conditions are created by applying a heat shock to the host cells in the presence of high amounts of $Ca^{2+}$ ions. An alternative technique used to force DNA uptake is electroporation. For that purpose DNA and cells are brought together in a cuvette which is then subjected to a vigorous electrical discharge. Under those artificial conditions the cell envelope is forced to open itself, after which DNA may enter through the "holes" that are created. The brute force in these techniques kills a large fraction of the cells, but sufficient cells survive, among which are several that took up DNA. The technique of electroporation is widely applicable and frequently used.

Next to direct transfer of recombinant DNA molecules as such, there is at least for transfer to bacterial cells the possibility to package DNA in a bacteriophage capsid and then to mimic the normal bacteriophage infection procedure (Fig. 11). Transfer to bacterial cells can also be achieved by making use of conjugation. Conjugation is a process where DNA transfer takes place by cell–cell mating. For conjugation a special class of plasmids is required, so-called conjugative plasmids. If a cell with such a plasmid—the donor—meets a cell without such plasmid—the recipient—they may form together cell aggregates. In the so-called mating aggregate the

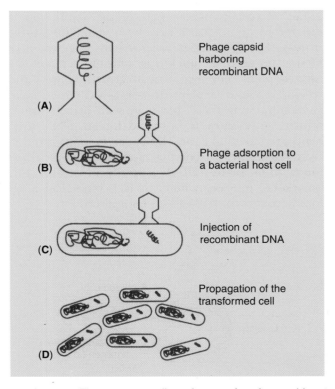

Phage capsid harboring recombinant DNA

(A)

Phage adsorption to a bacterial host cell

(B)

Injection of recombinant DNA

(C)

Propagation of the transformed cell

(D)

**Figure 11** ■ Phage as a mediator for transfer of recombinant DNA.

plasmid from the donor has the ability to transfer itself, as a consequence of a conjugative replication process according to the rolling circle model, to the recipient cell. By manipulating the conjugative plasmids one may create donors harboring recombinant DNA molecules which can then rather efficiently be transferred by cell–cell contact.

If an animal virus or a plant virus is used as vector for the recombinant DNA technology, one may exploit natural virus infection processes to transfer DNA to an animal or a plant cell (see Chapter 8). Like the case in microorganisms, DNA transfer to animal cells can be forced by a treatment with high amounts of $Ca^{2+}$ ions or by another chemical treatment. Next to that, it is possible to inject DNA with a syringe into the nucleus of the cell. The latter technique (one could speak of a kind of micro-surgery) is feasible due to the relative large dimensions of the animal cells compared to bacteria and is also applied to plant cells. The technique is illustrated in Figure 12. The cell is brought on the tip of a thin glass tube and is fixed to the tube by suction at the other end of the tube. By means of a micromanipulator a small syringe filled with DNA is directed to the nucleus of the fixed cell and then the DNA is injected into the nucleus.

A very successful way to transfer DNA into plant systems is based on a special type of conjugation. The soil bacterium, *Agrobacterium tumefaciens*, harbors a conjugative plasmid called Ti (acronym for tumor inducing). If such a bacterium infects wounded tissues of certain plants, part of the Ti-plasmid is transferred to a plant cell in a conjugation-like process. This transfer is followed by integration of the transferred DNA into the genome of the plant. The infected plant cells lose normal growth control and develop a tumor (a plant disease called crown gall). By manipulating the Ti-plasmid, such that its tumor inducing properties are lost and foreign DNA fragments are linked to it, any DNA can be transferred in a convenient way from the modified *Agrobacterium* donor to a plant cell. Figure 13 illustrates this remarkable process, where, in fact, biological kingdom barriers are crossed in a natural fashion.

Since the wall of the plant cell is the main barrier for uptake of DNA, one has exploited protoplasts of plant cells (i.e., plant cells lacking walls) to introduce DNA. Protoplasts can take up DNA quite easily. It is feasible to regenerate from genetically modified protoplasts intact plant cells. Finally, a very artificial method to introduce DNA in plant tissue has been developed. Microprojectiles covered with DNA are shot with a gun into plant cells. In fact, many plant species that can not readily be genetically modified with any of the methods mentioned above can be modified using this rather bizarre gun method.

The various techniques that are used to transfer DNA are generally not very efficient and may cause, as stated before, extensive killing of cells. Moreover, the fate of the transferred DNA is not always predictable. For example, in some cases the introduced DNA is subject to nuclease-mediated breakdown, while in animal or plant cells the introduced DNA does not always reach the nucleus, nor is it always integrated in a proper way. All methods to transfer DNA yield, in general, only a few cells that are vital and stable. Therefore, selection techniques are highly desirable to find these rare cells. Most selection techniques use a marker on the vector that codes for a selective property. Markers which code for a resistance towards a specific antibiotic substance are frequently used. If the cell that has to be modified is sensitive towards that antibiotic, the few modified cells from the transfer trial can easily be selected by bringing samples of the treated cells (either microbial cells, plant cells or animal cells) in a medium containing the relevant antibiotic. Only the cells that took up DNA and do maintain that DNA in their progeny will proliferate, all other cells are killed or, at least, do not grow. An alternative selection method uses recipient cells with specific growth deficiencies

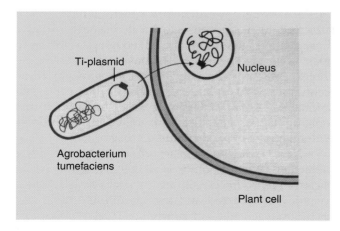

**Figure 13** ■ Plant cell modification by Ti-plasmid. Part of the Ti-plasmid (*marked*) is transferred to the plant cell and may be stably integrated in the plant DNA.

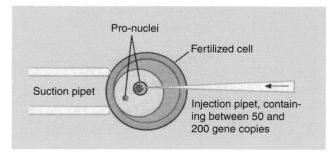

**Figure 12** ■ Injection of foreign DNA into a fertilized cell.

and vectors carrying genes which overcome such deficiencies.

## ■ DNA Sources

As stated before, any DNA can be used to construct recombinant DNA molecules. In protein production based on recombinant DNA technology very distinct pieces of DNA are required. Referring to the metaphor described before in this chapter, only a few lines on a specific page in one of the many books are required. Isolation of specific pieces of DNA directly from the DNA of a bacterial cell and, certainly, of a plant or an animal cell implies a very tedious search. Can one find a DNA fragment of interest in a more convenient way? There are several strategies.

### Synthetic DNA

It is feasible to use synthetic DNA as a source for the desired recombinant DNA sequence. If one seeks DNA that codes for a specific protein, the amino acid sequence of that protein is sometimes known. With the genetic code as guide one may synthesize the coding DNA by organic synthesis and use that DNA (called oligonucleotide) to construct an appropriate recombinant DNA molecule. Although the technique to unravel the amino acid composition of proteins and the possibilities of the organic DNA synthesis have improved over the past years, the organic DNA synthesis approach is only feasible to clone genes coding small proteins. For example, the synthetic approach has been used successfully for large scale production of human insulin, as will be described later.

The synthetic DNA approach allows the choice, whenever there are more triplets available for a certain amino acid, of the triplet that is used most frequently in the host that is selected for the production. In other words this technique allows one to master the codon usage problem, mentioned earlier in this chapter.

### cDNA

An alternative for direct isolation of cellular DNA coding for a specific protein is the copy DNA (cDNA) approach. This important development in DNA technology became apparent when the enzyme reverse transcriptase was exploited as a tool.

Genes are not always expressed in the cell, nor are they expressed everywhere in the organism. Some genes are only expressed in a certain stage of cell growth, or under very specific environmental conditions, or expressed only in very specific tissues of an organism. The mRNA molecules in a cell thus represent a minority of all the available genes, namely those that are actually expressed. Knowledge of the

cell physiology or knowledge of the specific biological tasks of animal and plant tissues, enables the isolation of a particular and characteristic set of mRNA molecules. Conversion of these mRNA molecules by the enzyme reverse transcriptase into DNA leads to synthesis of the genes that were expressed. These DNA molecules, called cDNA molecules, to distinguish them from the natural DNA molecules, can be used for gene cloning. Provided that the search starts with the right kind of cell culture conditions or with the appropriate tissues the cDNA strategy can be very efficient. It is illustrated in Figure 14.

cDNA cloning has some obvious consequences. In contrast to a gene that is directly isolated from the chromosome, cDNA lacks a promoter region. Furthermore, in the case of genes harboring exons and introns, cDNA is built only from exons. The lack of the authentic promoter requires that in the cloning strategy a promoter should be fused to the cDNA in order to achieve gene expression. Mostly a strong promoter that can be switched on and off, depending on environmental or tissue conditions, is fused to cDNA.

Control over foreign gene expression by using a suitable promoter is very essential as foreign proteins may disturb the physiology of the host cell and cause a premature stop of cell development. Therefore, a promoter like the *lac* promoter well-known from molecular pioneer work with *Escherichia coli* is frequently used in bacterial cells to direct the synthesis of a foreign protein. This promoter is only switched on when an appropriate inducer like iso-propyl-β-thiogalactoside (IPTG) is added to the

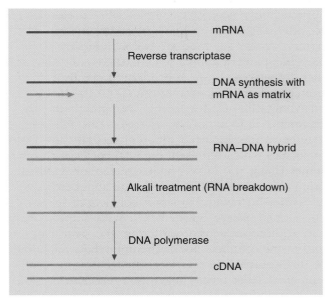

**Figure 14** ■ Synthesis of cDNA.

medium. Cultivation of the cells in the absence of the inducer allows optimal cell growth since the possible deleterious foreign gene product is not produced. When high cell numbers are present in the culture, the inducer is added and consequently the foreign gene product is produced. Possible negative effects of the foreign protein on the cell are minimal in their consequences since high cell numbers, often near to the maximum yield, are present when the harmful production is started.

In an animal or a plant a foreign gene should preferably be expressed only in certain tissues to keep the animal or the plant vital or to be able to isolate the protein efficiently. In those biotechnological applications where mammals like sheep, goat or cow are used as host for pharmaceutical products (an approach called "pharmaceutical farming"), the mammary gland is frequently used as an expression tissue. The cDNA for a product protein is therefore fused to a promoter that is only expressed in that tissue. Transferring such a DNA construct into embryos of the host animal may lead to genetically modified animals that exclusively deliver the pharmaceutical product as part of their milk. This production route enables an efficient isolation and allows relatively simple purification strategies (see Chapter 7).

The lack of introns in the cDNA has the advantage that cDNA may lead to a functional gene product even in organisms where splicing does not occur (like in prokaryotic cells) or where splicing is ambiguous or unreliable.

### DNA Libraries

The mRNA approach is not feasible if precise knowledge of gene expression is lacking and does not allow cloning of DNA that is not expressed. A general approach to master very complex DNA molecules for recombinant DNA technology is to create a DNA library. To do so, random DNA fragments from a bacterial, plant or animal cell are fused to a vector and then transferred to an appropriate host. By isolating from a bacterial cell, for example, DNA fragments that on average amount 1% of total DNA and linking these fragments individually to a vector, one may create together a few hundred different recombinant DNA molecules which represent the total bacterial chromosome. Using the "DNA-book" metaphor again: the original bacterial "DNA-book" with about 1000 pages is divided in about 150 small booklets of let say 10 pages each. These booklets tell, with some overlap and without an a priori ordering, the same story as told in the complete book. The immediate advantage of this approach is that large molecules are split in suitable smaller pieces linked to a replicon.

An individual host with a specific recombinant DNA molecule thus harbors a fragment of the total DNA on a replicating vector. By preselecting from the library the cells carrying gene(s) or DNA of interest, one may obtain a smaller molecule harboring little more than the DNA of interest by trimming the fragment isolated from these cells. By subsequent cloning of such smaller fragments one may achieve the final goal: a recombinant DNA molecule with a very distinct piece of foreign DNA. It is noteworthy to mention in this respect that DNA libraries are available from many organisms. Likewise cDNA libraries exist from many tissues such as the human brain. By analysis of the various fragments, insight into the genetic structure of all sorts of organisms is rapidly growing. In this respect the unraveling of the human genome revealed to the world in the year 2000 is worth mentioning.

### ■ Production by Recombinant DNA Technology

Only two of the many examples available of the production of biopharmaceuticals by the recombinant DNA technology will be treated here: the production of human insulin and the production of the human growth hormone (hGH). The pharmaceutical aspects of both proteins are discussed in more detail in Chapters 12 and 13, respectively.

The large scale production of human insulin nicely illustrates the synthetic DNA approach. Moreover, this example shows clearly that, besides knowledge of the coding gene, detailed knowledge of the protein to be produced is required.

The structural gene for human insulin is 1430 nucleotides long, while the gene is intervened by intron sequences of 179 and 786 nucleotides. The protein encoded by the gene is 110 amino acids in length. However, the mature protein encompasses a total of 51 amino acids. It consists of two separate chains: an A chain of 21 amino acids and a B chain of 30 amino acids. Chains A and B are held together by S bonds between the amino acids cysteine on the adjacent chains. The human insulin protein is apparently extensively processed after translation. Processing proceeds in two steps. The primary product, called preproinsulin, is 110 amino acids long in accordance with the prediction from the DNA sequence. During the membrane translocation of the protein the "pre" part of the protein, a stretch of 24 amino acids serving as the leader sequence for membrane translocation, is cleaved off. The remaining protein, 86 amino acids long, is called proinsulin. This protein is further processed in pancreatic cells, while an internal fragment (called the C or connecting chain) of 33 amino acids together with a few assorted amino acids is enzymatically removed. The A and B chains that are left are associated through S bonds and form the mature and biologically active insulin.

The strategy for the gene cloning according to the detailed knowledge of the mature protein, was to clone and produce the chains A and B separately. The information for the fragment A was assembled by linking a set of appropriate oligonucleotides. This DNA was then by ligation fused to the end of the gene *lacZ*, controlled by the *lac*-promoter, in the plasmid pBR322, a very well-known *E. coli* cloning vector. At the fusion point between *lacZ* and the information for chain A a codon for the amino acid methionine was built in, for reasons that will be explained later on. The information for fragment B was (for strategic reasons) synthesized in two steps. Firstly, the N-terminal coding part was synthesized by linking oligonucleotides. This fragment was fused to the plasmid pBR322 and propagated in *E. coli* as such. Secondly, the C-terminal coding part was synthesized and also propagated after ligating it to pBR322. The two DNA fragments were then isolated from the respective recombinant DNA molecules. Both parts were linked together and fused at the end of the *lacZ* gene in the plasmid pBR322. Again the codon for the amino acid methionine was built in at the fusion point.

The linking of the information for A and B to the *lacZ* gene, part of the well-known lactose-operon, has two advantages. First of all, both fragments depend for their expression on the regimen of the *lac*-promoter and the *lacZ* gene, which allows an effective and controlled expression. Secondly, the peptides A and B are synthesized as products fused to β-galactosidase. Since especially small foreign peptides in a bacterial cell are very vulnerable to proteolytic breakdown, the fusion strategy is an effective mean to prevent breakdown. Treatment of the isolated fusion proteins with the agent cyanogen bromide allows the isolation of the fragments A and B. This agent has the ability to cleave peptides whenever the amino acid methionine is present and cleaves immediately after this amino acid. Since neither fragment A nor B of insulin contain methionine and the cloning strategy guaranteed the presence of methionine at the fusion point, the isolation of peptides A and B as such is relatively simple. The final step consists of mixing A and B and allowing the S bonds to form spontaneously. Figure 15 presents the procedure of insulin production with the help of synthetic DNA.

The strategy to clone and produce hGH shows some other interesting features. First of all, the production was initiated by making cDNA out of an mRNA pool derived from the human pituitary, the tissue where this peptide hormone is synthesized. The cDNA molecule coding for the hGH was isolated and, since it contained information of 24 amino acids that should guarantee transport in the human cell, it was reduced with an appropriate restriction enzyme. However, in this procedure the coding information for some of the amino acids essential for the activity of

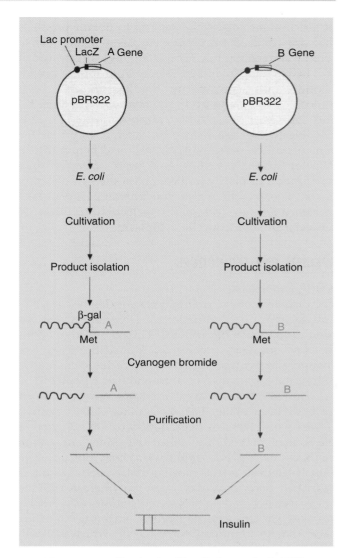

**Figure 15** ▪ Synthesis of insulin by synthetic DNA.

the mature hormone was lost. This missing part of information lost from the original cDNA molecule was chemically synthesized and fused to the fragmented cDNA molecule in order to get the full information for the mature hGH. Next, the construct was linked to a bacterial vector in such a way that it was fused to a strong promoter. In some constructs information coding for a bacterial leader sequence was linked to the hGH gene. Then, sequences coding for a bacterial leader peptide (a N-terminal sequence of about 20 amino acids) were added to induce translocation of the protein over the cytoplasmic membrane. This additional translocation sequence has rather specific physicochemical properties. The leader peptide signal enables a protein to cross the cytoplasmic membrane barrier during which the leader peptide is cleaved off. The reason for attaching an additional signal in this case is that in certain production strategies one wishes to obtain products that are released from the cytoplasm to be able to select a convenient purification strategy afterwards. If the hGH gene is linked to an appropriate leader peptide and expressed in the host *E. coli*, hGH molecules will show up in the space between the IM and the OM, the so-called periplasmic space. It is possible to damage the OM in such a way that the contents of the periplasm are set free. Then, purification of hGH is rather easy and cheaper than purification of hGH as a product in the cytoplasm of *E. coli*. Cloning strategies that guarantee membrane translocation are frequently selected in order to release a protein from the cytoplasm.

## SPECIFIC DNA TECHNIQUES

### ■ DNA Sequencing

The development of technologies for detailed nucleotide sequence determination of DNA molecules has been of immense importance. This knowledge opens the way for very precise DNA modifications, like changing individual nucleotides in order to change an individual amino acid in a protein (see Chapter 7).

In 1977 two different methods were published for DNA sequencing. The Maxam and Gilbert method is based on chemical degradation of DNA, whereas the Sanger method, also called the chain termination method, uses DNA replication enzymology. The Sanger method is the most popular method and is described here. It uses a DNA polymerase enzyme normally involved in DNA replication. DNA polymerases are template dependent, meaning that they need a single-stranded DNA molecule which they will copy according to the A-T and G-C base pairing rules, and are primer dependent, meaning that they need a free 3'-hydroxyl group of an oligonucleotide as a starting point for the incorporation of deoxyribonucleotide triphosphates (dATP, dCTP, dTTP, and dGTP). The primer is a short, chemically synthesized molecule, about 20 nucleotides in length which is complementary and antiparallel to a segment in the single-stranded DNA molecule to be sequenced. Under the right conditions it will hybridize and thus provide a specific starting point for the elongation reaction by the polymerase.

The method depends in essence on the inclusion in the reaction mixture of a so-called dideoxyribonucleotide triphosphate (ddNTP). These molecules not only lack the 2' hydroxyl group on the ribose as is normal in DNA, but also the 3' hydroxyl group; hence the name *di*-deoxy. These ddNTP's can be incorporated into DNA strands by DNA polymerase. However, since the lacking 3'-hydroxyl group is required for DNA elongation, the DNA molecules which have incorporated such a ddNTP are no longer substrate for

further chain elongation: the chain terminates with a ddNTP and this principle is used for the sequencing reaction. Per reaction four tubes are set up which contain template, primer and the four dNTPs. To the four tubes ddNTP is added. To the first tube ddATP is added, to the second tube ddTTP, to the third tube ddCTP and to the fourth tube ddCTP. The ratio of dNTP versus ddNTP in each tube is chosen in such a way that a small number of templates in each tube will incorporate the specific ddNTP and will no longer be substrates for elongation (chain termination). Therefore in each tube a fraction of the strands will terminate with the specific ddNTP present in that particular tube. The length of the terminated strands is determined by the oligonucleotide primer, which sets a fixed starting point, and the ddNTP incorporated. In the first reaction tube, for example, fragment lengths are determined by the position of the various A nucleotides in the template. After the synthesis reaction the contents of the four individual sequencing tubes are applied to a high resolution polyacrylamide gel electrophoresis system which separates individual elongation products based on their length. Tube 1 reveals the positions of A, tube 2 of C, tube 3 of T and tube 4 of G. The reaction products can be visualized either by autoradiography in case a small aliquot of radioactively labeled dNTP has been incorporated in all reactions (usually alpha-$^{32}$P-dCTP) or by fluorography in case a fluorescent group has been chemically added to the sequencing primer during its synthesis. The latter method is especially very well suited for automation. Currently sequencing machines are commercially available which, in one run, can sequence over 800 nucleotides. In such machines 20 to 40 runs can be loaded and analyzed simultaneously which tremendously enhances productivity. Needless to say, sequences are handled, analyzed and stored electronically. Three interlinked computer sequence databases are operational in the world, which are freely accessible via Internet.

### ■ Genome Sequencing

In recent years whole genomes of various organisms have been sequenced and sequencing of all sorts of organisms is going on all over the world. Such projects started with sequencing the genome of microorganisms, various prokaryotes as well as eukaryotes, but was extended to higher organisms like the nematode *Caenorhabditis elegans*, the insect *Drosophila melanogaster*, the plant *Arabidopsis thaliana* and finally, considered as the most prominent achievement in this respect, the genome of man, *Homo sapiens*.

The detailed knowledge of genome structures ("genomics") has a great impact on biotechnology, not in the least on pharmaceutical biotechnology. However, knowing the genome sequence is only a start. But, it enables researchers to approach in a direct way functional aspects of the genome: when and how genes are expressed, in what way genes cooperate during their expression which enables us to understand gene networks, etc. Such an integrative genetic approach is generally called "functional genomics." Functional genomics together with the detailed studies on the proteins that the cell produces (called "proteomics") will give pharmaceutical biotechnology a new outlook.

As an example, the new future for pharmaceutical biotechnology can be illustrated by the development of new antibiotics. Classical antibiotics are isolated from nature as secondary metabolites produced by various microorganisms. Their antibiotic properties are based on the interference with vital processes in pathogenic microorganisms. The number of target molecules in the bacterial cells which are affected by the classical antibiotics are rather limited (Note the different meaning of "target" in this context as compared to "drug targeting" discussed in Chapter 4.) For example, *Mycobacterium tuberculosis* causes tuberculosis, a disease with a great impact in the world. Detailed knowledge of the genome structure of pathogenic bacteria might reveal all kinds of specific vital target molecules in this pathogen. Detailed knowledge of new target molecules will enable the pharmaceutical scientist to synthesize chemical compounds which interfere with (the products of) vital target genes. The problem of the prevalence of pathogenic microorganisms resistant to classical antibiotics is now in principle open for a solution by synthesizing new target-directed chemical compounds.

Moreover, the human genome knowledge is the basis for recognition of all kinds of genetic polymorphisms that distinguish individual people. In the near future, insight in the individual genes of a patient opens ways for more effective therapies based on a patient's individual characteristics and needs. This emerging field in the pharmaceutical sciences with direct implications for the practitioner is called "pharmacogenetics."

The pharmaceutical industry is highly interested in the possibilities arising from more detailed genome knowledge and is investing in functional genomics, proteomics and pharmacogenetics. In Chapter 7 the technological background and implications of functional genomics, proteomics and pharmacogenetics will be discussed in more detail.

## ■ DNA Hybridization

To gain insight in the DNA composition, sequencing is the final approach. There is, however, a possibility to acquire information about DNA structure by hybridization with the help of so-called DNA probes.

In essence the probe is a specific single-stranded DNA fragment. Such a probe will form double-stranded DNA (in other words will hybridize) whenever it encounters a single-stranded complementary piece of DNA under appropriate conditions. There are many applications for DNA probes.

If, for example, one wishes to see which recombinant DNA molecule in an extensive DNA library harbors a gene of interest, one might use a DNA probe. DNAs from the library are converted into single-stranded DNA and then confronted with a probe that reflects a very characteristic segment of the desired gene. Hybridization will, provided that the probe has the required specificity, only occur with target DNA molecules that harbor the gene of interest.

The use of DNA hybridization probes in diagnostic testing in humans can be illustrated by using cystic fibrosis (CF) as an example. The frequency of this heritable and deadly disease is approximately once in 2000 live births making it the most frequent genetic disorder among Caucasians. The cloning of the gene in 1989 based on its position on the human genetic map was a *tour de force* involving several laboratories. It enabled the molecular analysis of the genetic defect, revealing that approximately 70% of the diseased genes contain an identical mutation: a three base pair deletion in the protein coding gene resulting in the loss of a phenylalanine amino acid at position 508 of the 1480 amino acid-long protein. This mutation was named CFdel 508 and the knowledge gained was used to design oligonucleotide probes for rapid screening purposes.

These single-strand DNA probes are complementary to the normal and CFdel 508 regions of the CF gene shown below. The symbols L, E, etc. represent various amino acids (see Chapter 2); F, e.g., stands for phenylalanine.

*Normal:*
```
      L   E   N   I   I   F   G   V
5'-AAA GAA AAT ATC ATC TTT GGT GTT-3'
```

*Mutant (CFdel508):*
```
      L   E   N   I       G   V
5'-AAA GAA AAT ATC AT---T GGT GTT-3'
```

DNA, isolated, e.g., from white blood cells of suspected carriers or amnion fluid in which embryos are suspended, is boiled to make it single stranded and then immobilized on filter paper. Next, hybridization with normal and CFdel 508 specific probes clarifies whether one has the disease, in which case both the maternal and the paternal genes are affected, or whether one is a carrier of the disease in which one of the two genes is affected (heterozygosy) and the other is normal at this genomic position.

Variation on this technology allows for the automated and simultaneous screening for many genetic diseases for which the molecular lesions are known. Kits which contain all the reagents necessary for a particular test are commercially available.

## ■ PCR Technology

For the detection of DNA or for testing the presence of mutations in DNA the probe method described above is very powerful. Within the current probe techniques, however, a substantial amount of DNA is required to allow the detection of target DNA. The PCR (polymerase chain reaction) technology became very popular in recent years to acquire large amounts of DNA.

In the PCR technology target DNA is amplified by in vitro DNA synthesis, occurring in a number of fast repeating steps. The reaction starts with the conversion of the double-stranded target DNA to single-stranded DNA and uses specific oligonucleotides as primers to allow DNA polymerase to do its job. The choice of the oligonucleotide primers, hybridizing with each of both target strands, will determine the left and right limits of the DNA to be amplified.

Each PCR cycle (illustrated in Fig. 16) consists of three steps each requiring only 1 to 3 minutes. In the first step the target DNA must be made single stranded and this is done by heating the sample to 92°C. The second step involves the specific hybridization of the two primers to the complementary single-stranded DNA. The optimal temperature for this process is about 55°C. In the third step DNA polymerase will extend the primer sequence using the single stranded DNA as a template. The optimal extension temperature is about 72°C since the DNA polymerase chosen is derived from a thermophilic bacterium, *Thermus aquaticus*, which normally grows in hot springs at temperatures above 80°C. This DNA polymerase is extremely resistant against heat denaturing and survives the 92°C DNA denaturing step. All reagents (target DNA, primers, dNTPs and polymerase) are put in a tube which is sealed and usually 20 to 30 PCR cycles are performed. The procedure can be automated and PCR machines are available which control the temperature for each of the three separate steps of a PCR cycle. Such machines can process hundreds of tubes simultaneously and produce results within 2 to 4 hours.

Ideally each cycle of DNA replication doubles the amount of DNA which is located in-between the chosen primers. Thirty PCR cycles will give an amplification of $2^{30}$ times. This means that minute quantities of DNA can be amplified with specific primers to easily detectable levels. It should be realized that the specificity of the reaction is fully determined by the PCR primers and these primers

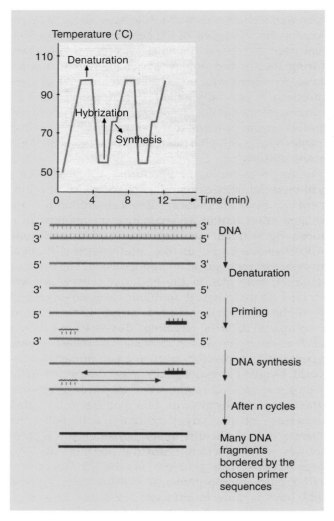

**Figure 16** ■ PCR method. *Upper panel*: Sequence of heating, hydridizing, synthesis. *Lower panel*: Synthesis events.

will also determine the length of the amplified fragment. The tremendous sensitivity of the technique has sparked the development of a great number of applications where such sensitivity is of paramount importance. Also, compared to many other detection methods, the PCR procedure is very fast.

For example, the presence of microbial pathogens in raw and processed food products can be unequivocally determined using this technology. DNA is extracted from this material and the PCR reaction is performed using primers which are specific for the suspected pathogen(s). Detailed knowledge of DNA sequences of all sorts of genes in all sorts of organisms allows the development of such specific primers, the main prerequisite for diagnostic PCR technology. If specific amplified DNA products can be detected, this is proof that the pathogen is present in the material. Also in clinical material (blood, urine, etc.) the technique is used extensively as a rapid and sensitive test for the presence of bacterial and viral pathogens. A third area where PCR has become standard technology is in forensic science. At a crime scene often minute quantities of potentially important evidence is found (single hairs, blood drops, semen stains, etc.) and PCR technology can be used to get enough DNA to show the origin of this material. These are only a few examples of the use of PCR technology. PCR is often an essential step in elaborate diagnostic and detection procedures and novel applications are continuously being developed.

As for the application of the PCR technology for diagnosis of pathogens, one has to realize that for most purposes the intent is to detect viable pathogens. The PCR technology obviously cannot distinguish DNA from vital or dead material and in that respect it is not always an adequate technique. The PCR technique is a very sensitive one since minute amounts of DNA are highly amplified. This high sensitivity may limit the discriminative power of the technique when applied for diagnostic purposes. For example, it may detect minor contaminants in the samples. Moreover, DNA contaminants may be introduced during the performance of the tests. It is therefore a major concern in the application of PCR to avoid DNA contaminations that could cause false positive reactions.

Modified PCR techniques and related methodologies are discussed in Chapter 7.

## CELL CULTURES

Biotechnology depends heavily on techniques to cultivate pro- and eukaryotic cells, since these cells are sources of bioproducts or of mediators of various bioconversions. The scale of culturing is an important issue in biotechnology. Experience from small scale cultures is not directly transferable to large scale culturing in manufacturing industries. What can be cultivated in small flasks in a research laboratory cannot always be cultivated efficiently on an industrial scale. Simply enlarging the culture devices from small flasks to tanks containing many thousand liters is not enough. Cultivation on an industrial level requires very sophisticated and delicate process technologies (see Chapter 3).

### ■ Cultivation of Microbes

Some microbial species are very popular in biotechnology since they can be cultivated in an easy and safe way. To microbial species with a long lasting tradition in biotechnology belong bacterial species like *Clostridium acetobutyricum*, *Corynebacterium* sp., *Xanthomonas* sp., *Bacillus* sp., *Lactobacillus* sp. as well as the fungi *Saccharomyces cerevisiae* (baker's yeast), *Penicillium* sp. and *Aspergillus* sp.

In general, microbes can be cultivated either in vessels or tanks filled with an appropriate liquid growth medium or on plates containing a growth medium solidified with agar (see Chapter 3). Culturing in this way implies that the conditions for the growing cells gradually diminish, since nutrients are depleted by the growing cells and growth inhibiting metabolites gradually accumulate. Consequently, microbial growth under these conditions will stop after a while. However, there are culture devices, the continuous culture apparatus, which allow indefinite growth of the microorganisms. This is achieved by continuously adding fresh medium to the culture, meanwhile removing growing cells and metabolites by an overflow device. Under a proper regimen of addition and removal, a "steady state" situation where cells continuously grow is created. The suggestive name for such cultures is "continuous culture." Most industrial biotechnology, however, is based on culturing in tanks without a supply and overflow device. Such culture devices are called "batch cultures."

Figure 17 presents a typical picture of bacterial growth in a batch culture. There are several characteristic phases in the so-called bacterial growth curve. Bacteria generally do not immediately start multiplying when they are inoculated in a fresh medium. A phase, called the lag phase, where cells do not divide but gradually adapt to the specific growth conditions in the medium precedes the phase where all cells start to divide. This phase, the actual growth phase, is called the logarithmic or exponential phase. The exponential growth phase is for many biotechnological applications very relevant since most of the genes are then optimally expressed. The exponential phase is followed by the stationary phase, where active growth comes to an end due to depletion and spoilage of the medium.

The stage where the exponential growth is about to end is of interest for some biotechnological purposes. At that stage, for reasons that are not completely understood, some microorganisms start the synthesis of so-called secondary metabolites. These metabolic products are, according to their name, not essential for the basic cellular metabolism, but may be very relevant as bioproducts. Secondary metabolites relevant for pharmaceutical biotechnology are for example antibiotics as produced by some microorganisms.

After some time the stationary phase is followed by a phase where the bacteria die off. This stage is clearly not of great interest for biotechnology.

The bacterial growth curve is not directly applicable for microbes that do not reproduce by binary fission. However, a lag phase preceding a phase of active growth and followed by a stationary phase is generally found.

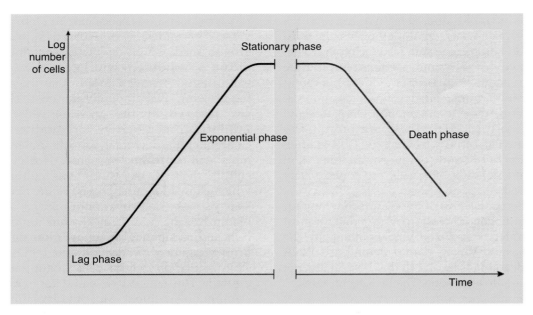

**Figure 17** ■ Bacterial growth curve.

Also in biotechnology time is money and maximum cell yields are therefore required. Thus one tries to keep the lag phase as short as possible and to postpone the onset of the stationary phase. The first goal is achieved by inoculating the tank with cells that, by proper preculturing, are optimally adapted to the medium in the tank. The second goal is achieved in various ways. A successful approach, especially when cells are limited in outgrowth by medium depletion, consists of adding fresh medium near the end of the exponential phase. This technique is called "fed batch culture."

To achieve optimal growth of microorganisms it is not only essential to provide a medium with the proper nutrients, but also conditions like pH, oxygen tension and temperature have to be chosen appropriately and should be controlled while cultivating. Last but not least, infection with other microorganisms should be prevented. This requires strict sterility measures and work protocols.

To give an idea about the impressive performance of fast growing microbial cells, such cells may grow with doubling times of about 30 minutes and cultures can easily reach densities of $10^9$ cells per mL. If one cultivates bacterial cells on plates, a colony on such plate, appearing after one day or so, might easily harbor millions of cells.

■ **Animal Cell Cultures**

Animal cells can be isolated out of a particular tissue after a protease (trypsin) treatment. When such cells are transferred to glass or plastic they will adhere and start growing, if supplied with a suitable liquid growth medium. A cell culture of this type is called a "primary" culture. Such cultures will die after a while and are thus not very useful for biotechnology.

Some animal cell types, however, become exceptional in their growth characteristics when they are cultivated. The main characteristic is that the cell becomes immortal. Such cells are used to prepare "continuous" cell lines. They may survive for months or even years, as long as they are diluted and recultured at frequent intervals. Some cells of malignant origin or originating from normal cells transformed by a virus like the Epstein Barr virus are immortal and grow to high cell densities. For pharmaceutical biotechnology the latter cell lines may be of limited value since they are of malignant nature and may release transforming viruses as a contaminant for the pharmaceutical product. Most useful are non-malignant immortalized cell lines, e.g., 3T3 fibroblasts.

Some cell lines depend on a solid support for their growth; others can be cultivated in suspension which may be advantageous for biotechnology. Successful cultivation of animal cells in vitro requires a suitable, in general very complex, growth medium providing not only all nutritional requirements for the cells but also a number of specific growth factors and hormones. The pH must be buffered around 7.0 and proper osmotic conditions isotonic with the cell cytoplasm are required (see Chapter 3).

Animal cell cultivation is certainly much more complicated than cultivation of common microorganisms. For pharmaceutical biotechnology there are various safe cell lines available, each with their specific characteristics.

## ▪ Plant Cell Cultures

Plants have always been an important source of pharmacologically active compounds. The complex structure of many of these compounds precludes their chemical synthesis, certainly on a commercial scale. Many active compounds are extracted from intact plants or plant parts. Such compounds usually are present in very low quantities and this has triggered research into the use of alternative production methods.

Cell biologists have tried to produce high levels of active compounds in plant cell cultures but this has not been an easy task. Next to the problems associated with large scale cell cultures, a major problem with plant cells is that they can not be kept in the differentiated state. When fully differentiated plant tissues are excised to initiate a cell culture this differentiated state is usually lost. Often the compound of interest is made only in specialized tissues in the intact plants. Use of these tissues for cell culture initiation results in a significant decrease in the production of the compound of interest. The addition of plant hormones (e.g., auxins and cytokinins) may alleviate this problem, but up until now efficient production of pharmaceutically interesting compounds in plant cell culture systems is rare. Systems that are available are usually based on procedures involving repeated selection of cell lines with the highest production potential.

Production capacity of cell lines can be further improved by feeding to the culture strategically chosen cheaply available precursors for the compound of interest. The cells then perform the final and chemically most demanding biosynthetic steps. A better understanding of cellular differentiation processes combined with genetic modification technology of plant cells may help in overcoming these problems and allow for a more efficient use of plant cell cultures in pharmaceutical biotechnology. To circumvent the plant culturing problems one might exploit the recombinant DNA technology, described before. Several of the plant genes which encode enzymes involved in biosynthesis of pharmaceutically active compounds have been cloned. Expression of such genes in heterologous host systems opens an *ex planta* way for enzymatic synthesis of active compounds.

## CONCLUSION

Growing knowledge in the physiology of microbial, animal and plant cells together with detailed insight in gene structure and function has opened new ways for pharmaceutical biotechnology. This chapter is merely an introductory illustration of new approaches based on DNA technology. In order to appreciate and exploit the achievements of cell biology and recombinant DNA technology, further reading is required. The books listed below are just a few out of a large number of excellent books available.

## FURTHER READING

Alberts B, Johnson HA, Lewis J, Raff M,. Roberts K, Walter P (2002). Molecular Biology of the Cell. 4th edn. New York: Garland Publ. Inc.

Alcamo IE (1999). DNA Technology: The Awesome Skill. 2nd edn. Harcourt-Academic Press.

Bourgaize D, Jewell TR, Buiser RG (2000). Biotechnology: Demystifying the Concepts. Addison Wesley-Longman Inc.

Brown TA (2002). Genomes. 2nd ed. Oxford, UK: Wisley-Liss.

Watson J, Gilman M, Wikowski J, Zolle M (1992). Recombinant DNA. 2nd ed. New York: Freeman and Company.

# 2

# Biophysical and Biochemical Analysis of Recombinant Proteins

*Tsutomu Arakawa and John S. Philo*
Alliance Protein Laboratories, Thousand Oaks, California, U.S.A.

## INTRODUCTION

For a recombinant protein to become a human therapeutic, its biophysical and biochemical characteristics must be well understood. These properties serve as a basis for comparison of lot-to-lot reproducibility, for establishing the range of conditions to stabilize the protein during production, storage and shipping, and for identifying characteristics useful for monitoring stability during long-term storage.

A number of techniques can be used to determine the biophysical properties of proteins and to examine their biochemical and biological integrity. Where possible, the results of these experiments are compared with those obtained using naturally occurring proteins in order to be confident that the recombinant protein has the desired characteristics of the naturally occurring one.

## PROTEIN STRUCTURE

### ■ Primary Structure

Most proteins which are developed for therapy perform specific functions by interacting with other small and large molecules, e.g., cell surface receptors, binding proteins, nucleic acids, carbohydrates and lipids. The functional properties of proteins are derived from their folding into distinct three-dimensional structures. Each protein fold is based on its specific polypeptide sequence in which different amino acids are connected through peptide bonds in a specific way. This alignment of the 20 amino acids, called a primary sequence, has in general all the information necessary for folding into a distinct tertiary structure comprising different secondary structures such as α-helices and β-sheets (see below). Because the 20 amino acids possess different side chains, polypeptides with widely diverse properties are obtained.

All of the 20 amino acids consist of a $C_\alpha$ carbon to which an amino group, a carboxyl group, a hydrogen, and a side chain bind in L configuration (Fig. 1). These amino acids are joined by condensation to yield a peptide bond consisting of a carboxyl group of an amino acid joined with the amino group of the next amino acid (Fig. 2).

The condensation gives an amide group, NH, at the N-terminal side of $C_\alpha$, and a carbonyl group, C=O, at the C-terminal side. These groups, as well as the amino acyl side chains, play important roles in protein folding. Due to their ability to form hydrogen bonds, they make major energetic contributions to the formation of two important secondary structures, α-helix and β-sheet. The peptide bonds between various amino acids are very much equivalent, however, so that they do not determine which part of a sequence should form an α-helix or β-sheet. Sequence-dependent secondary structure formation is determined by the side chains.

The twenty amino acids commonly found in proteins are shown in Figure 3. They are described by their full names and three- and one-letter codes. Their side chains are structurally different in such a way that at neutral pH, aspartic and glutamic acid are negatively charged and lysine and arginine are positively charged. Histidine is positively charged to an extent that depends on the pH. At pH 7.0, on average about half of the histidine side chains are positively charged. Tyrosine and cysteine are protonated and uncharged at neutral pH, but become negatively charged above pH 10 and 8, respectively.

Polar amino acids consist of serine, threonine, asparagine, and glutamine, as well as cysteine, while nonpolar amino acids consist of alanine, valine, phenylalanine, proline, methionine, leucine, and isoleucine. Glycine behaves neutrally while cystine, the oxidized form of cysteine, is characterized as hydrophobic. Although tyrosine and tryptophan often enter into polar interactions, they are better characterized as nonpolar, or hydrophobic, as described later.

These twenty amino acids are incorporated into a unique sequence based on the genetic code, as the

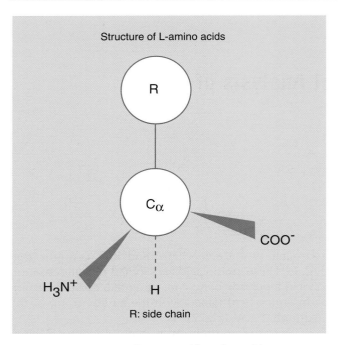

**Figure 1** Structure of L-amino acids.

acid composition, as shown in Table 1; i.e., a list of the total number of each type of amino acid contained in this protein molecule.

Using the $pK_a$ values of these side chains and one amino and carboxyl terminus, one can calculate total charges (positive plus negative charges) and net charges (positive minus negative charges) of a protein as a function of pH, i.e., a titration curve. Since cysteine can be oxidized to form a disulfide bond or can be in a free form, accurate calculation above pH 8 requires knowledge of the status of cysteinyl residues in the protein. The titration curve thus obtained is only an approximation, since some charged residues may be buried and the effective pKa values depend on the local environment of each residue. Nevertheless, the calculated titration curve gives a first approximation of the overall charged state of a protein at a given pH and hence its solution property. Other molecular parameters, such as isoelectric point (pI; where the net charge of a protein becomes zero), molecular weight, extinction coefficient, partial specific volume and hydrophobicity, can also be estimated from the amino acid composition, as shown in Table 1.

The primary structure of a protein, i.e., the sequence of the twenty amino acids, can lead to the three-dimensional structure because the amino acids have diverse physical properties. First, each type of amino acid has the tendency to be more preferentially incorporated into certain secondary structures. The frequencies with which each amino acid is found in α-helix, β-sheet and β-turn, secondary structures

example in Figure 4 shows. This is an amino acid sequence of granulocyte-colony stimulating factor (G-CSF), which selectively regulates proliferation and maturation of neutrophils. Although the exact properties of this protein depend on the location of each amino acid and hence the location of each side chain in the three-dimensional structure, the average properties can be estimated simply from the amino

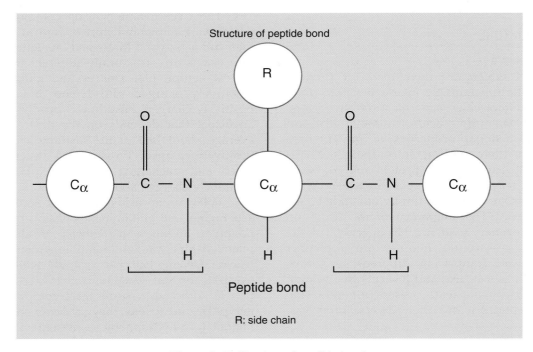

**Figure 2** Structure of peptide bond.

## Structure of 20 amino acids

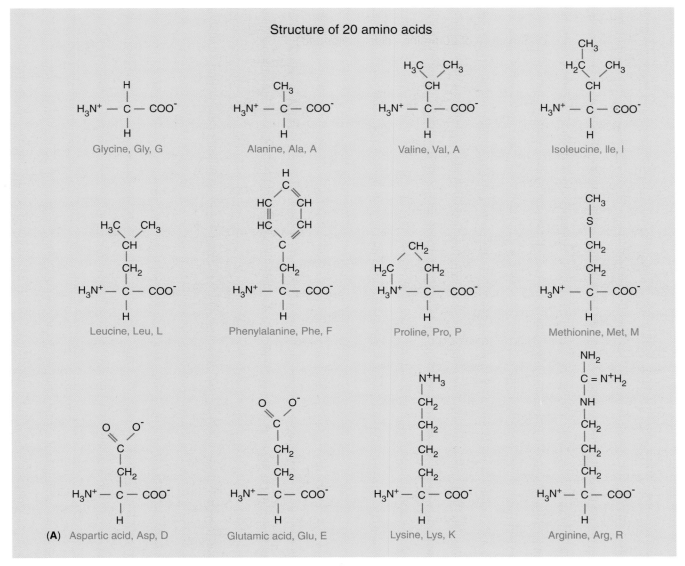

**Figure 3A** ■ Structure of 20 amino acids.

that are discussed later in this chapter, can be calculated as an average over a number of proteins whose three-dimensional structures have been solved. These frequencies are listed in Table 2. The β-turn has a distinct configuration consisting of four sequential amino acids and there is a strong preference for specific amino acids in these four positions. For example, asparagine has an overall high frequency of occurrence in a β-turn and is most frequently observed in the first and third position of a β-turn. This characteristic of asparagine is consistent with its side chain being a potential site of N-linked glycosylation. Effects of glycosylation on the biological and physicochemical properties of proteins are extremely important; however, their contribution to structure is not readily predictable based on the amino acid composition.

Based on these frequencies, one can predict for particular polypeptide segments which type of

secondary structure they are likely to form. As shown in Figure 5A, there are a number of methods developed to predict the secondary structure from the primary sequence of the proteins. Using G-CSF (Fig. 5B) as an example, regions of α-helix, β-sheets, turns, hydrophilicity, and antigen sites can be suggested.

Another property of amino acids, which impacts on protein folding, is the hydrophobicity of their side chains. Although nonpolar amino acids are basically hydrophobic, it is important to know how hydrophobic they are. This property has been determined by measuring the partition coefficient or solubility of amino acids in water and organic solvents and normalizing such parameters relative to glycine. Relative to the side chain of glycine, a single hydrogen, such normalization shows how strongly the side chains of nonpolar amino acids

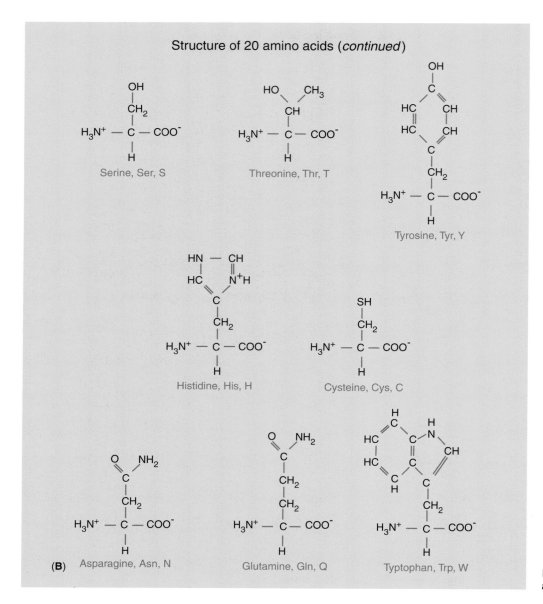

## Structure of 20 amino acids (continued)

Serine, Ser, S

Threonine, Thr, T

Tyrosine, Tyr, Y

Histidine, His, H

Cysteine, Cys, C

**(B)**   Asparagine, Asn, N

Glutamine, Gln, Q

Typtophan, Trp, W

**Figure 3B** ▪ Structure of 20 amino acids.

prefer the organic phase to the aqueous phase. A representation of such measurements is shown in Table 3. The values indicate that the free energy increases as the side chain of tryptophan and tyrosine are transferred from an organic solvent to water and that such transfer is thermodynamically unfavorable. Although it is unclear how comparable the hydrophobic property is between an organic solvent and the interior of protein molecules, the hydrophobic side chains favor clustering together, resulting in a core structure with properties similar to an organic solvent. These hydrophobic characteristics of nonpolar amino acids and hydrophilic characteristics of polar amino acids generate a partition of amino acyl residues into a hydrophobic core and hydrophilic surface, resulting in overall folding.

## ▪ Secondary Structure

### α-Helix

Immediately evident in the primary structure of a protein is that each amino acid is linked by a peptide bond. The amide, NH, is a hydrogen donor and the carbonyl, C=O, is a hydrogen acceptor, and they can form a stable hydrogen bond when they are

```
TPLGPASSLPQSFLLKCLEQVRKIQGDGAALQEKLCATYK      40
LCHPEELVLLGHSLGIPWAPLSSCPSQALQLAGCLSQLHS      80
GLFLYQGLLQALEGISPELGPTLDTLQLDVADFATTIWQQ     120
MEELGMAPALQPTQGAMPAFASAFQRRAGGVLVASHLQSF     160
LEVSYRVLRHLAQP
```

**Figure 4** ▪ Amino acid sequence of G-CSF.

| Parameter | Value |
|---|---|
| Molecular weight | 18673 |
| Total number of amino acids | 174 |
| 1 microgram | 53.5 picomoles |
| Molar extinction coefficient | 15820 |
| 1 A (280) | 1.18 mg/ml |
| Isoelectric point | 5.86 |
| Charge at pH 7 | −3.39 |

**Table 1A** ▪ Amino acid composition and structural parameters

positioned in an appropriate configuration of the polypeptide chain. Such structures of the polypeptide chain are called secondary structure. Two main structures, α-helix and β-sheet, accommodate such

| Amino acid | Number | % by weight | % by frequency |
|---|---|---|---|
| A Ala | 19 | 7.23 | 10.92 |
| C Cys | 5 | 2.76 | 2.87 |
| D Asp | 4 | 2.47 | 2.30 |
| E Glu | 9 | 6.22 | 5.17 |
| F Phe | 6 | 4.73 | 3.45 |
| G Gly | 14 | 4.28 | 8.05 |
| H His | 5 | 3.67 | 2.87 |
| 1 Me | 4 | 2.42 | 2.30 |
| K Lys | 4 | 2.75 | 2.30 |
| L Leu | 33 | 20.00 | 18.97 |
| M Met | 3 | 2.11 | 1.72 |
| N Asn | 0 | 0.00 | 0.00 |
| P Pro | 13 | 6.76 | 7.47 |
| Q Gin | 17 | 11.66 | 9.77 |
| R Arg | 5 | 4.18 | 2.87 |
| S Ser | 14 | 6.53 | 8.05 |
| T Thr | 7 | 3.79 | 4.02 |
| V Val | 7 | 3.71 | 4.02 |
| W Trp | 2 | 1.99 | 1.15 |
| Y Tyr | 3 | 2.62 | 1.72 |

**Table 1B** ▪ Amino acid composition and structural parameters

stable hydrogen bonds. The main chain forms a right-handed helix, because only the L-form of amino acids are in proteins, and makes one turn per 3.6 residues. The overall length of α-helices can vary widely. Figure 6 shows an example of a short α-helix. In this case, the C=O group of residue 1 forms a hydrogen bond to the NH group of residue 5 and C=O group of residue 2 forms a hydrogen bond with the NH group of residue 6. Thus, at the start of an α-helix, four amide groups are always free and at the end of an α-helix four carboxyl groups are also free. As a result, both ends of an α-helix are highly polar.

Moreover, all the hydrogen bonds are aligned along the helical axis. Since both peptide NH and C=O groups have electric dipole moments pointing in the same direction, they will add to a substantial dipole moment throughout the entire α-helix, with the negative partial charge at the C-terminal side and the positive partial charge at the N-terminal side.

The side chains project outward from the α-helix. This projection means that all the side chains surround the outer surface of an α-helix and interact both with each other and with side chains of other regions which come in contact with these side chains. These interactions, so-called long-range interactions, can stabilize the α-helical structure and help it to act as a folding unit. Often an α-helix serves as a building block for the three-dimensional structure of globular proteins by bringing hydrophobic side chains to one side of a helix and hydrophilic side chains to the opposite side of the same helix. Distribution of side chains along the α-helical axis can be viewed using the helical wheel. Since one turn in an α-helix is 3.6 residues long, each residue can be plotted every $360°/3.6 = 100°$ around a circle (viewed from the top of α-helix), as shown in Figure 7. Such a plot shows the projection of the position of the residues onto a plane perpendicular to the helical axis. One of the predicted helices in erythropoietin is shown in Figure 7, using an open circle for hydrophobic side chains and an open rectangle for hydrophilic side chains. It becomes immediately obvious that one side of the α-helix is highly hydrophobic, suggesting that this side forms an internal core, while the other side is relatively hydrophilic and is hence most likely exposed to the surface. Since many biologically important proteins function by interacting with other macromolecules, the information obtained from the helical wheel is extremely useful. For example, mutations of amino acids in the solvent-exposed side may lead to identification of regions responsible for biological activity, while mutations in the internal core may lead to altered protein stability.

### β-Sheet

The second major secondary structural element found in proteins is the β-sheet. In contrast to the α-helix,

| α-helix | | β-sheet | | β-turn | | β-turn position 1 | | β-turn position 2 | | β-turn position 3 | | β-turn position 4 | |
|---|---|---|---|---|---|---|---|---|---|---|---|---|---|
| Glu | 1.51 | Val | 1.70 | Asn | 1.56 | Asn | 0.161 | Pro | 0.301 | Asn | 0.191 | Trp | 0.167 |
| Met | 1.45 | Lie | 1.60 | Gly | 1.56 | Cys | 0.149 | Ser | 0.139 | Gly | 0.190 | Gly | 0.152 |
| Ala | 1.42 | Tyr | 1.47 | Pro | 1.52 | Asp | 0.147 | Lys | 0.115 | Asp | 0.179 | Cys | 0.128 |
| Leu | 1.21 | Phe | 1.38 | Asp | 1.46 | His | 0.140 | Asp | 0.110 | Ser | 0.125 | Tyr | 0.125 |
| Lys | 1.16 | Trp | 1.37 | Ser | 1.43 | Ser | 0.120 | Thr | 0.108 | Cys | 0.117 | Ser | 0.106 |
| Phe | 1.13 | Leu | 1.30 | Cys | 1.19 | Pro | 0.102 | Arg | 0.106 | Tyr | 0.114 | Gin | 0.098 |
| Gin | 1.11 | Cys | 1.19 | Tyr | 1.14 | Gly | 0.102 | Gin | 0.098 | Arg | 0.099 | Lys | 0.095 |
| Trp | 1.08 | Thr | 1.19 | Lys | 1.01 | Thr | 0.086 | Gly | 0.085 | His | 0.093 | Asn | 0.091 |
| Ile | 1.08 | Gin | 1.10 | Gin | 0.98 | Tyr | 0.082 | Asn | 0.083 | Glu | 0.077 | Arg | 0.085 |
| Val | 1.06 | Met | 1.05 | Thr | 0.96 | Trp | 0.077 | Met | 0.082 | Lys | 0.072 | Asp | 0.081 |
| Asp | 1.01 | Arg | 0.93 | Trp | 0.96 | Gin | 0.074 | Ala | 0.076 | Tyr | 0.065 | Thr | 0.079 |
| His | 1.00 | Asn | 0.89 | Arg | 0.95 | Arg | 0.070 | Tyr | 0.065 | Phe | 0.065 | Leu | 0.070 |
| Arg | 0.98 | His | 0.87 | His | 0.95 | Met | 0.068 | Glu | 0.060 | Trp | 0.064 | Pro | 0.068 |
| Thr | 0.83 | Ala | 0.83 | Glu | 0.74 | Val | 0.062 | Cys | 0.053 | Gin | 0.037 | Phe | 0.065 |
| Ser | 0.77 | Ser | 0.75 | Ala | 0.66 | Leu | 0.061 | Val | 0.048 | Leu | 0.036 | Glu | 0.064 |
| Cys | 0.70 | Gly | 0.75 | Met | 0.60 | Ala | 0.060 | His | 0.047 | Ala | 0.035 | Ala | 0.058 |
| Tyr | 0.69 | Lys | 0.74 | Phe | 0.60 | Phe | 0.059 | Phe | 0.041 | Pro | 0.034 | Ile | 0.056 |
| Asn | 0.67 | Pro | 0.55 | Leu | 0.59 | Glu | 0.056 | Ile | 0.034 | Val | 0.028 | Met | 0.055 |
| Pro | 0.57 | Asp | 0.54 | Val | 0.50 | Lys | 0.055 | Leu | 0.025 | Met | 0.014 | His | 0.054 |
| Gly | 0.57 | Glu | 0.37 | Ile | 0.47 | Ile | 0.043 | Trp | 0.013 | Ile | 0.013 | Val | 0.053 |

*Source*: Taken and edited from Chou PY and Fasman GD, (1978), Ann. Rev. Biochem. 47, 251–276 with permission from Annual Reviews, Inc.

**Table 2** ■ Frequency of occurrence of 20 amino acids in α-helix, β-sheet, and β-turn.

which is built up from a continuous region with a peptide hydrogen bond linking every fourth amino acid, the β-sheet is comprised of peptide hydrogen bonds between different regions of the polypeptide that may be far apart in sequence. β-strands can interact with each other in one of the two ways shown in Figure 8, i.e., either parallel or antiparallel. In a parallel β-sheet, each strand is oriented in the same direction with peptide hydrogen bonds formed between the strands, while in antiparallel β-sheets, the polypeptide sequences are oriented in the opposite direction. In both structures, the C=O and NH groups project into opposite sides of the polypeptide chain, and hence a β-strand can interact from either side of that particular chain to form peptide hydrogen bonds with adjacent strands. Thus, more than two β-strands can contact each other either in a parallel or in an antiparallel manner, or even in combination. Such clustering can result in all the β-strands lying in a plane as a sheet. The β-strands which are at the edges of the sheet have unpaired alternating C=O and NH groups.

Side chains project perpendicularly to this plane in opposite directions and can interact with other side chains within the same β-sheet or with other regions of the molecule, or may be exposed to the solvent.

In almost all known protein structures, β-strands are right-handed twisted. This way, the β-strands adapt into widely different conformations. Depending on how they are twisted, all the side chains in the same strand or in different strands do not necessarily project in the same direction.

## Loops and Turns

Loops and turns form more or less linear structures, and interact with each other to form a folded three-dimensional structure. They are comprised of an amino acid sequence which is usually hydrophilic and exposed to the solvent. These regions consist of β-turns (reverse turns), short hairpin loops, and long loops. Many hairpin loops are formed to connect two antiparallel β-strands.

As shown in Figure 5A, the amino acid sequences which form β-turns are relatively easy to predict, since turns must be present periodically to fold a linear sequence into a globular structure. Amino acids found most frequently in the β-turn are

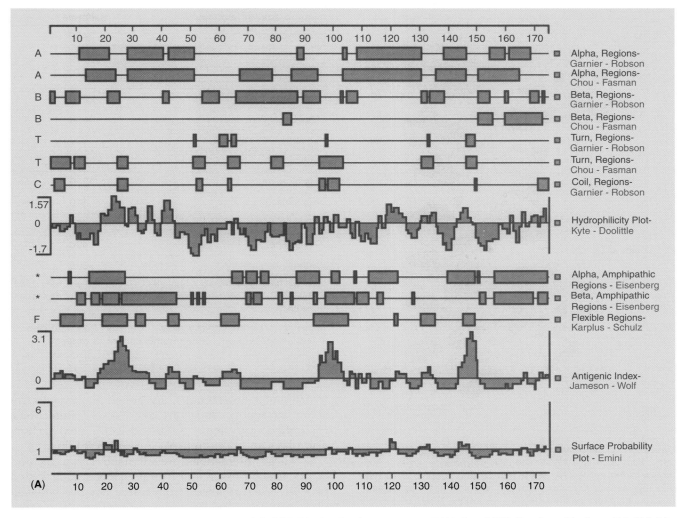

**Figure 5A** ■ Predicted secondary structure of G-CSF. Obtained using a program DNA Star (DNA Star Inc., Madison, WI, U.S.A.).

usually not found in α-helical or β-sheet structures. Thus, proline and glycine represent the least observed amino acids in these typical secondary structures. However, proline has an extremely high frequency of occurrence at the second position in the β-turn while glycine has a high preference at the third and fourth position of a β-turn.

Although loops are not as predictable as β-turns, amino acids with high frequency for β-turns also can form a long loop. Even though difficult to predict, loops are an important secondary structure, since they form a highly solvent exposed region of the protein molecules and allow the protein to fold onto itself.

■ **Tertiary Structure**

Combination of the various secondary structures in a protein results in its three-dimensional structure. Many proteins fold into a fairly compact, globular structure.

The folding of a protein molecule into a distinct three-dimensional structure determines its function. Enzyme activity requires the exact coordination of catalytically important residues in the three-dimensional space. Binding of antibody to antigen and binding of growth factors and cytokines to their receptors all require a distinct, specific surface for high affinity binding. These interactions do not occur if the tertiary structures of antibodies, growth factors and cytokines are altered.

A unique tertiary structure of a protein can often result in the assembly of the protein into a distinct quaternary structure consisting of a fixed stoichiometry of protein chains within the complex. Assembly can occur between the same proteins or between different polypeptide chains. Each molecule in the complex is called a subunit. Actin and tubulin self-associate into F-actin and microtubule, while hemoglobin is a tetramer consisting of two α and two β subunits. Among the cytokines and growth factors, interferon-γ is a homodimer, while platelet-derived growth factor is a homodimer of either A or B chains or a heterodimer of the

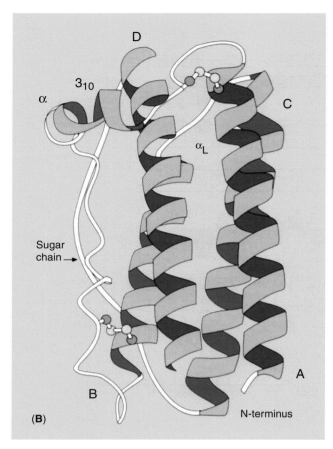

| Amino acid side chain | cal/mole |
|---|---|
| Tryptophan | 3400 |
| Norleucine | 2600 |
| Phenylalanine | 2500 |
| Tyrosine | 2300 |
| Dihydroxyphenylalanine | 1800 |
| Leucine | 1800 |
| Valine | 1500 |
| Methionine | 1300 |
| Histidine | 500 |
| Alanine | 500 |
| Threonine | 400 |
| Serine | −300 |

*Source*: Taken from Nozaki Y, Tanford C. (1971). J. Biol. Chem. 246, 2211–2217 with permission from American Society of Biological Chemists.

**Table 3** ▪ Hydrophobicity scale: transfer free energies of amino acid side chains from organic solvent to water.

**Figure 5B** ▪ Secondary structure of filgrastim (*recombinant* G-CSF). Filgrastim is a 175-amino acid polypeptide. Its four anti-parallel alpha helices (**A**, **B**, **C**, and **D**) and short 3 to 10 type helix ($3_{10}$) form a helical bundle. The two biologically active sites ($\alpha$ and $\alpha_L$) are remote from modifications at the N terminus of the A helix and the sugar chain attached to loop C–D. *Note*: Filgrastim is not glycosylated; the sugar chain is included to illustrate its location in endogenous G-CSF.

A and B chain. The formation of a quaternary structure occurs via non-covalent interactions or through disulfide bonds between the subunits.

## ▪ Forces

Interactions occurring between chemical groups in proteins are responsible for formation of their specific secondary, tertiary and quaternary structures. Either repulsive or attractive interactions can occur between different groups. Repulsive interactions consist of steric hindrance and electrostatic effects. Like-charges repel each other and bulky side chains, although they do not repel each other, cannot occupy the same space. Folding is also against the natural tendency to move toward randomness, i.e., increasing entropy. Folding leads to a fixed position of each atom and hence a decrease in entropy. For folding to occur this decrease in entropy, as well as the repulsive interactions, must be overcome by attractive interactions, i.e.,

hydrophobic interactions, hydrogen bonds, electrostatic attraction, and van der Waals interactions. Hydration of proteins, discussed in the next section, also plays an important role in protein folding.

These interactions are all relatively weak and can be easily broken and formed. Hence, each folded protein structure arises from a fine balance between these repulsive and attractive interactions. The stability of the folded structure is a fundamental concern in developing protein therapeutics.

### Hydrophobic Interactions

The hydrophobic interaction reflects a summation of the van der Waals attractive forces among nonpolar groups in the protein interior, which change the surrounding water structure necessary to accommodate these groups if they become exposed. The transfer of nonpolar groups from the interior to the surface requires a large decrease in entropy so that hydrophobic interactions are essentially entropically driven. The resulting large positive free energy change prevents the transfer of nonpolar groups from the largely sheltered interior to the more solvent exposed exterior of the protein molecule. Thus, nonpolar groups preferentially reside in the protein interior while the more polar groups are exposed to the surface and surrounding environment. The partitioning of different amino acyl residues between the inside and outside of a protein correlates well with the hydration energy of their side chains, i.e., their relative affinity for water.

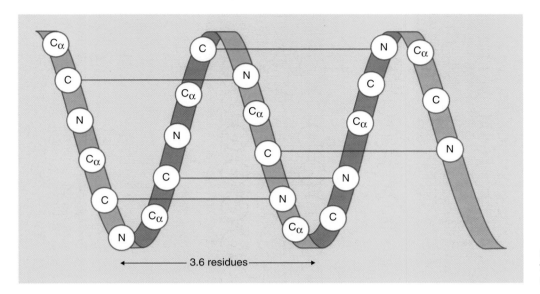

**Figure 6** ■ Schematic illustration of the structure of α-helix.

## Hydrogen Bonds

The hydrogen bond is ionic in character since it depends strongly on the sharing of a proton between two electronegative atoms (generally oxygen and nitrogen atoms). Hydrogen bonds may form either between a protein atom and a water molecule or exclusively as protein intramolecular hydrogen bonds. Intramolecular interactions can have

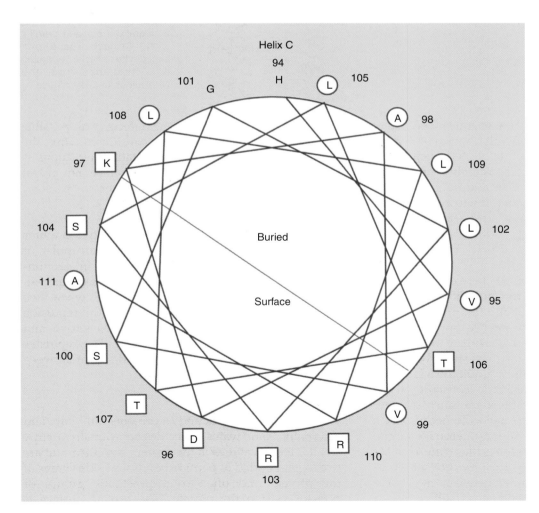

**Figure 7** ■ Helical wheel analysis of erythropoietin sequence, from His94 to Ala111. *Source*: Elliott S, personal communication.

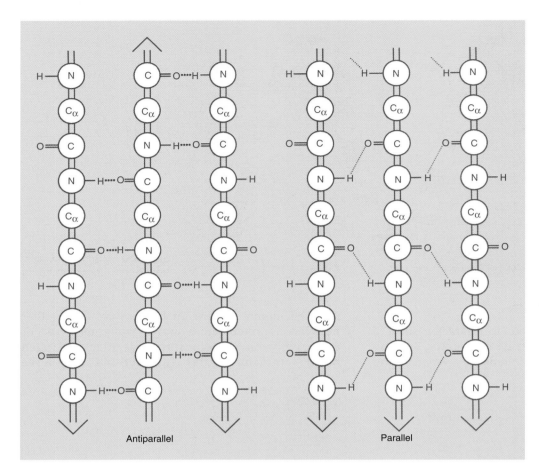

Antiparallel                                    Parallel

**Figure 8** ■ Schematic illustration of the structure of antiparallel (*left*) and parallel (*right*) β-sheet. The arrows indicate the direction of amino acid sequence from the N-terminus to C-terminus.

significantly more favorable free energies (because of entropic considerations) than intermolecular hydrogen bonds, so the contribution of all hydrogen bonds in the protein molecule to the stability of protein structures can be substantial. In addition, when the hydrogen bonds occur in the interior of protein molecules, the bonds become stronger due to the hydrophobic environment.

*Electrostatic Interactions*
Electrostatic interactions occur between any two charged groups. According to Coulomb's law, if the charges are of the same sign, the interaction is repulsive with an increase in energy, but if they are opposite in sign it is attractive, with a lowering of energy. Electrostatic interactions are strongly dependent upon distance, according to Coulomb's law, and inversely related to the dielectric constant of the medium. Electrostatic interactions are much stronger in the interior of the protein molecule because of a lower dielectric constant. The numerous charged groups present on protein molecules can provide overall stability by the electrostatic attraction of opposite charges, for example, between negatively charged carboxyl groups and positively charged

amino groups. However, the net effects of all possible pairs of charged groups must be considered. Thus, the free energy derived from electrostatic interactions is actually a property of the whole structure, not just of any single amino acid residue or cluster.

*van der Waals Interactions*
Weak van der Waals interactions exist between atoms (except the bare proton), whether they are polar or nonpolar. They arise from net attractive interactions between permanent dipoles and/or induced (temporary and fluctuating) dipoles. However, when two atoms approach each other too closely, the repulsion between their electron clouds becomes strong and counterbalances the attractive forces. The repulsive force is even more sensitive to the distance between two atoms.

■ **Hydration**
Water molecules are bound to proteins internally and externally. Some water molecules occasionally occupy small internal cavities in the protein structure, and are hydrogen-bonded to peptide bonds and side chains of the protein and often to a prosthetic group, or cofactor, within the protein. The protein surface is

large and consists of a mosaic of polar and nonpolar amino acids, and it binds a large number of water molecules, i.e., it is hydrated, from the surrounding environment. As described in the previous section, water molecules trapped in the interior of protein molecules are bound more tightly to hydrogen-bonding donors and acceptors because of a lower dielectric constant.

Solvent around the protein surface clearly has a general role in hydrating peptide and side chains but might be expected to be rather mobile and non-specific in its interactions. Well-ordered water molecules can make significant contributions to protein stability. One water molecule can hydrogen-bond to two groups distant in the primary structure on a protein molecule, acting as a bridge between these groups. Such a water molecule may be highly restricted in motion, and can contribute to the stability, at least locally, of the protein, since such tight binding may exist only when these groups assume the proper configuration to accommodate a water molecule that is present only in the native state of the protein. Such hydration can also decrease the flexibility of the groups involved.

There is also evidence for solvation over hydrophobic groups on the protein surface. So-called hydrophobic hydration occurs because of the unfavorable nature of the interaction between water molecules and hydrophobic surfaces, resulting in the clustering of water molecules. Since this clustering is energetically unfavorable, such hydrophobic hydration does not contribute to the protein stability. However, this hydrophobic hydration facilitates hydrophobic interaction. This unfavorable hydration is diminished as the various hydrophobic groups come in contact either intramolecularly or intermolecularly, leading to the folding of intrachain structures or to protein–protein interactions.

Both the loosely and strongly bound water molecules can have an important impact, not only on protein stability but also on protein function. For example, certain enzymes function in non-aqueous solvent provided that a small amount of water, just enough to cover the protein surface, is present. Bound water can modulate the dynamics of surface groups, and such dynamics may be critical for enzyme function. Dried enzymes are, in general, inactive and become active after they absorb 0.2 g water per g protein. This amount of water is only sufficient to cover surface polar groups, yet may give sufficient flexibility for function.

Evidence that water bound to protein molecules has a different property from bulk water can be demonstrated by the presence of non-freezable water. Thus, when a protein solution is cooled below –40°C, a fraction of water, ~0.3 g water/g protein, does not freeze and can be detected by high resolution NMR. Several other techniques also detect a similar amount of bound water. This unfreezable water reflects the unique property of bound water that prevents it from adopting an ice structure.

## PROTEIN FOLDING

Proteins become functional only when they assume a distinct tertiary structure. Many physiologically and therapeutically important proteins present their surface for recognition by interacting with molecules such as substrates, receptors, signaling proteins and cell–surface adhesion macromolecules. When recombinant proteins are produced in *Escherichia coli*, they often form inclusion bodies into which they are deposited as insoluble proteins. Formation of such insoluble states does not naturally occur in cells where they are normally synthesized and transported. Therefore, an in vitro process is required to refold insoluble recombinant proteins into their native, physiologically active state. This is usually accomplished by solubilizing the insoluble proteins with detergents or denaturants, followed by the purification and removal of these reagents concurrent with refolding the proteins (see Chapter 3).

Unfolded states of proteins are usually highly stable and soluble in the presence of denaturing agents. Once the proteins are folded correctly, they are also relatively stable. During the transition from the unfolded form to the native state, the protein must go through a multitude of other transition states in which it is not fully folded and denaturants or solubilizing agents are at low concentrations or even absent.

The refolding of proteins can be achieved in various ways. The dilution of proteins at high denaturant concentration into aqueous buffer will decrease both denaturant and protein concentration simultaneously. The addition of an aqueous buffer to a protein–denaturant solution also causes a decrease in concentrations of both denaturant and protein. The difference in these procedures is that, in the first case, both denaturant and protein concentrations are the lowest at the beginning of dilution and gradually increase as the process continues. In the second case, both denaturant and protein concentrations are highest at the beginning of dilution and gradually decrease as the dilution proceeds. Dialysis or the diafiltration of protein in the denaturant against an aqueous buffer resembles the second case, since the denaturant concentration decreases as the procedure continues. In this case, however, the protein concentration remains unchanged. Refolding can also be achieved by first binding the protein in denaturants to a solid phase, i.e., to a column matrix, and then equilibrating it with an aqueous buffer. In this case, protein concentrations are not well defined. Each procedure has advantages and disadvantages and may be applicable for one protein, but not to another.

If proteins in the native state have disulfide bonds, cysteines must be correctly oxidized. Such oxidation may be done in various ways, e.g., air oxidation, glutathione catalyzed disulfide exchange, or adduct formation followed by reduction and oxidation or by disulfide reshuffling.

Protein folding has been a topic of intensive research since Anfinsen's demonstration that ribonuclease can be refolded from the fully reduced and denatured state in in vitro experiments. This folding can be achieved only if the amino acid sequence itself contains all information necessary for folding into the native structure. This is the case, at least partially, for many proteins. However, a lot of other proteins do not refold in a simple one-step process. Rather, they refold via various intermediates which are relatively compact and possess varying degrees of secondary structures, but which lack a rigid tertiary structure. Intrachain interactions of these preformed secondary structures eventually lead to the native state. However, the absence of a rigid structure in these preformed secondary structures can also expose a cluster of hydrophobic groups to those of other polypeptide chains, rather than to their own polypeptide segments, resulting in intermolecular aggregation. High efficiency in the recovery of native protein depends to a large extent on how this aggregation of intermediate forms is minimized. The use of chaperones or polyethylene glycol has been found quite effective for this purpose. The former are proteins, which aid in the proper folding of other proteins by stabilizing intermediates in the folding process and the latter serves to solvate the protein during folding and diminishes interchain aggregation events.

Protein folding is often facilitated by co-solvents, such as polyethylene glycol. As described above, proteins are functional and highly hydrated in aqueous solutions. True physiological solutions, however, contain not only water but also various ions and low and high molecular weight solutes, often at very high concentrations. These ions and other solutes play a critical role in maintaining the functional structure of the proteins. When isolated from their natural environment, the protein molecules may lose these stabilizing factors and hence must be stabilized by certain compounds, often at high concentrations. These solutes are also used in vitro to assist in protein folding, and to help stabilize proteins during large-scale purification and production as well as for long-term storage. Such solutes are often called co-solvents when used at high concentrations, since at such high concentrations they also serve as a solvent along with

water molecules. These solutes encompass sugars, amino acids, inorganic and organic salts, and polyols. They may not strongly bind to proteins, but instead typically interact weakly with the protein surface to provide significant stabilizing energy without interfering with their functional structure.

When recombinant proteins are expressed in eukaryotic cells and secreted into media, the proteins are generally folded into the native conformation. If the proteins have sites for N-linked or O-linked glycosylation, they undergo varying degrees of glycosylation depending on the host cells used and level of expression. For many glycoproteins, glycosylation is not essential for folding, since they can be refolded into the native conformation without carbohydrates, nor is glycosylation often necessary for receptor binding and hence biological activity. However, glycosylation can alter important biological and physicochemical properties of proteins, such as pharmacokinetics, solubility, and stability.

## ■ Techniques Specifically Suitable for Characterizing Protein Folding

Conventional spectroscopic techniques used to obtain information on the folded structure of proteins are circular dichroism (CD), fluorescence, and Fourier transform infrared spectroscopies (FTIR). CD and FTIR are widely used to estimate the secondary structure of proteins. The α-helical content of a protein can be readily estimated by CD in the far UV region (180–260 nm) and by FTIR. FTIR signals from loop structures, however, occasionally overlap with those arising from an α-helix. The β-sheet gives weak CD signals, which are variable in peak positions and intensities due to twists of interacting β-strands, making far-UV CD unreliable for evaluation of these structures. On the other hand, FTIR can reliably estimate the β-structure content as well as distinguish between parallel and antiparallel forms.

CD in the near-UV region (250–340 nm) reflects the environment of aromatic amino acids, i.e., tryptophan, tyrosine and phenylalanine, as well as that of disulfide structures. Fluorescence spectroscopy yields information on the environment of tyrosine and tryptophan residues. CD and fluorescence signals in many cases are drastically altered upon refolding and hence can be used to follow the formation of the tertiary structure of a protein.

None of these techniques can give the folded structure at the atomic level, i.e., they give no information on the exact location of each amino acyl residue in the three-dimensional structure of the protein. This information can only be determined by X-ray crystallography or NMR. However, CD, FTIR, and fluorescence spectroscopic methods are fast and require lower protein concentrations than either NMR or X-ray crystallography, and are amenable for the examination of the protein under widely different conditions. When a naturally occurring form of the protein is available, these techniques, in particular near-UV CD and fluorescence spectroscopies, can quickly address whether the refolded protein assumes the native folded structure.

Temperature dependence of these spectroscopic properties also provides information about protein folding. Since the folded structures of proteins are built upon cooperative interactions of many side chains and peptide bonds in a protein molecule, elimination of one interaction by heat can cause cooperative elimination of other interactions, leading to the unfolding of protein molecules. Thus, many proteins undergo a cooperative thermal transition over a narrow temperature range. Conversely, if the proteins are not fully folded, they may undergo non-cooperative thermal transitions as observed by a gradual signal change over a wider range of temperature.

Such a cooperative structure transition can also be examined by differential scanning calorimetry. When the structure unfolds, it requires heat. Such heat absorption can be determined using this highly sensitive calorimetry technique.

Hydrodynamic properties of proteins change greatly upon folding, going from elongated and expanded structures to compact globular ones. Sedimentation velocity and size exclusion chromatography (see the section entitled Analytical Techniques) are two frequently used techniques for the evaluation of hydrodynamic properties, although the latter is much more accessible. The sedimentation coefficient (how fast a molecule migrates in a centrifugal field) is a function of both the molecular weight and hydrodynamic size of the proteins, while elution position in size exclusion chromatography (how fast it migrates through pores) depends only on the hydrodynamic size (see Chapter 3). In both methods, comparison of the sedimentation coefficient or elution position with that of a globular protein with an identical molecular weight (or upon appropriate molecular weight normalization) gives information on how compactly the protein is folded.

For oligomeric proteins, the determination of molecular weight of the associated states and acquisition of the quaternary structure can be used to assess the folded structure. For strong interactions, specific protein association requires that intersubunit contact surfaces perfectly match each other. Such an associated structure, if obtained by covalent bonding, may be determined simply by sodium dodecylsulfate polyacrylamide gel electrophoresis (PAGE). If protein association involves non-covalent interactions,

sedimentation equilibrium or light scattering experiments can assess this phenomenon. Although these techniques have been used for many decades with some difficulty, emerging technologies in analytical ultracentrifugation and laser light scattering, and appropriate software for analyzing the results, have greatly facilitated their general use, as described in detail below.

Two fundamentally different light scattering techniques can be used in characterizing recombinant proteins. "Static" light scattering measures the intensity of the scattered light. "Dynamic" light scattering measures the fluctuations in the scattered light intensity as molecules diffuse in and out of a very small scattering region (Brownian motion).

Static light scattering is often used on-line in conjunction with size-exclusion chromatography (SEC). The scattering signal is proportional to the product of molecular mass times weight concentration. Dividing this signal by one proportional to the concentration, such as obtained from an UV absorbance or refractive index detector, then gives a direct and absolute measure of the mass of each peak eluting from the column, independent of molecular conformation and elution position. This SEC-static scattering combination allows rapid identification of whether the native state of a protein is a monomer or an oligomer and the stoichiometry of multi-protein complexes. It is also very useful in identifying the mass of aggregates which may be present, and thus is useful for evaluating protein stability.

Dynamic light scattering (DLS) measures the diffusion rate of the molecules, which can be translated into the Stokes radius, a measure of hydrodynamic size. Although the Stokes radius is strongly correlated with molecular mass, it is also strongly influenced by molecular shape (conformation) and thus DLS is far less accurate than static scattering for measuring molecular mass. The great strength of DLS is its ability to cover a very wide size range in one measurement, and to detect very small amounts of large aggregates (<0.01% by weight). Other important advantages over static scattering with SEC are a wide choice of buffer conditions and no potential loss of species through sticking to a column.

An analytical ultracentrifuge incorporates an optical system and special rotors and cells in a high speed centrifuge to permit measurement of the concentration of a sample versus position within a spinning centrifuge cell. There are two primary strategies: analyzing either the sedimentation velocity or the sedimentation equilibrium. When analyzing the sedimentation velocity the rotor is spun at very high speed, so the protein sample will completely sediment and form a pellet. The rate at which the protein pellets is measured by the optical system to derive the sedimentation coefficient, which depends on both mass and molecular conformation. When more than one species is present (e.g., a monomer plus a covalent dimer degradation product), a separation is achieved based on the relative sedimentation coefficient of each species.

Because the sedimentation coefficient is sensitive to molecular conformation, and can be measured with high precision (~0.5%), sedimentation velocity can detect even fairly subtle differences in conformation. This ability can be used, for example, to confirm that a recombinant protein has the same conformation as the natural wild-type protein, or to detect small changes in structure with changes in the pH or salt concentration that may be too subtle to detect by other techniques, such as CD or differential scanning calorimetry.

In sedimentation equilibrium a much lower rotor speed and milder centrifugal force is used than for sedimentation velocity. The protein still accumulates toward the outside of the rotor, but no pellet is formed. This concentration gradient across the cell is continuously opposed by diffusion, which tries to restore a uniform concentration. After spinning for a long times (usually 12–36 hours) an equilibrium is reached where sedimentation and diffusion are balanced and the distribution of protein no longer changes with time. At sedimentation equilibrium the concentration distribution depends only on the molecular mass and is independent of molecular shape. Thus, self-association for the formation of dimers or higher oligomers (whether reversible or irreversible) is readily detected, as are binding interactions between different proteins. For reversible association, it is possible to determine the strength of the binding interaction by measuring samples over a wide range of protein concentrations.

In biotechnology applications, sedimentation equilibrium is often used as the "gold standard" for confirming that a recombinant protein has the expected molecular mass and biologically active state of oligomerization in solution. It can also be used to determine the average amount of glycosylation or conjugation of moieties such as polyethylene glycol. The measurement of binding affinities for receptor–cytokine, antigen–antibody, or other interaction can also sometimes serve as a functional characterization of recombinant proteins (although some of these interactions are too strong to be measured by this method).

Site specific chemical modification and proteolytic digestion are also powerful techniques for studying the folding of proteins. The extent of chemical modification or proteolytic digestion depends on whether the specific sites are exposed to the solvent or are buried in the interior of the protein molecules and are thus inaccessible to these modifications. For example, trypsin cleaves peptide bonds on the C-terminal side of basic residues. Although most proteins contain several basic residues, brief exposure of the native protein to trypsin usually generates only a few peptides, as cleavage occurs only at the accessible basic residues, whereas the same treatment can generate many more peptides when done on the denatured (unfolded) protein, since all the basic residues are now accessible (see also peptide mapping in section Mass Spectrometry).

## PROTEIN STABILITY

Although freshly isolated proteins may be folded into a distinct three-dimensional structure, this folded structure is not necessarily retained indefinitely in aqueous solution. The reason is that proteins are neither chemically nor physically stable. The protein surface is chemically highly heterogeneous and contains reactive groups. Long-term exposure of these groups to environmental stresses causes various chemical alterations. Many proteins, including growth factors and cytokines, have cysteine residues. If some of them are in a free or sulfhydryl form, they may undergo oxidation and disulfide exchange. Oxidation can also occur on methionyl residues. Hydrolysis can occur on peptide bonds and on amides of asparagine and glutamine residues. Other chemical modifications can occur on peptide bonds, tryptophan, tyrosine, and amino and carboxyl groups. Table 4 lists both a number of reactions that can occur during purification and storage of proteins and methods that can be used to detect such changes.

Physical stability of a protein is expressed as the difference in free energy, $\Delta G_U$, between the native and denatured states. Thus, protein molecules are in equilibrium between the above two states. As long as this unfolding is reversible and $\Delta G_U$ is positive, it does not matter how small the $\Delta G_U$ is. In many cases, this reversibility does not hold. This is often seen when $\Delta G_U$ is decreased by heating. Most proteins denature upon heating and subsequent aggregation of the denatured molecules results in irreversible denaturation. Thus, unfolding is made irreversible by aggregation:

$$\text{Native state} \xleftrightarrow{\Delta G_U} \text{Denatured state} \xrightarrow{k} \text{Aggregated state}$$

Therefore, any stress that decreases $\Delta G_U$ and increases k will cause the accumulation of irreversibly inactivated forms of the protein. Such stresses may include chemical modifications as described above and physical parameters, such as pH, ionic strength, protein concentration, and temperature. Development of a suitable formulation that prolongs the shelf-life of

| | Physical property affected | Method of analysis |
|---|---|---|
| Oxidation<br>Cys<br>Disulfide<br>Intrachain<br>Interchain<br>Met, Trp, Tyr | Hydrophobicity<br>Size<br>Hydrophobicity | RP-HPLC, SDS-PAGE<br>Size exclusion chromatography<br>Mass spectrometry |
| Peptide bond<br>hydrolysis | Size | Size exclusion chromatography<br>SDS-PAGE |
| N to O migration<br>Ser, Thr | Hydrophobicity<br>Chemistry | RP-HPLC inactive in Edman reaction (used to determine amino acid sequence in peptide fragments of enzymatically degraded proteins) (Fig. 15) |
| α-Carboxy to<br>β-carboxy<br>migration<br>Asp, Asn | Hydrophobicity<br>Chemistry | RP-HPLC inactive in Edman reaction (used to determine amino acid sequence in peptide fragments of enzymatically degraded proteins) (Fig. 15) |
| Deamidation<br>Asn, Gln | Charge | Ion exchange chromatography |
| Acylation<br>α-amino group,<br>ε-amino group | Charge | Ion exchange chromatography<br>Mass spectrometry |
| Esterification/<br>carboxylation<br>Glu, Asp, C-terminal | Charge | Ion exchange chromatography<br>Mass spectrometry |
| Secondary structure<br>changes | Hydrophobicity<br>Size<br>Sec/tert structure<br>Sec/tert structure<br>Aggregation<br>Sec/tert structure,<br>aggregation | RP-HPLC<br>Size exclusion chromatography<br>CD<br>FTIR<br>Light scattering<br>Analytical ultracentrifugation |

**Table 4** Common reactions affecting stability of proteins.

a recombinant protein is essential when it is to be used as a human therapeutic.

The use of protein stabilizing agents to enhance storage stability of proteins has become customary. These compounds affect protein stability by increasing $\Delta G_U$. These compounds, however, may also increase k and hence their net effect on long-term storage of proteins may vary among proteins, as well as on the storage conditions.

When unfolding is irreversible due to aggregation, minimizing the irreversible step should increase the stability, and often this may be attained by the addition of mild detergents. Prior to selecting the proper detergent concentration and type, however, their effects on $\Delta G_U$ must be carefully evaluated.

Another approach for enhancing storage stability of proteins is to lyophilize, or freeze-dry, the proteins (see Chapter 4). Lyophilization can minimize the aggregation step during storage, since both chemical modification and aggregation is reduced in the absence of water. The effects of a lyophilization process itself on $\Delta G_U$ and k are not fully understood

and hence such a process must be optimized for each protein therapeutic.

## ANALYTICAL TECHNIQUES

In one of the previous sections on "Techniques Specifically Suitable for Characterizing Folding" a number of (spectroscopic) techniques were mentioned that can be specifically used to monitor protein folding. These were: CD, FTIR, fluorescence spectroscopy, and DSC. Moreover, analytical ultracentrifugation and light scattering techniques were discussed in more detail. In this section other techniques will be discussed.

### ■ Blotting Techniques
Blotting methods form an important niche in biotechnology. They are used to detect very low levels of unique molecules in a milieu of proteins, nucleic acids, and other cellular components. They can detect aggregates or breakdown products occurring during long-term storage and they can be used to detect components from the host cells used in producing recombinant proteins.

Biomolecules are transferred to a membrane ("blotting"), and this membrane is then probed with specific reagents to identify the molecule of interest. Membranes used in protein blots are made of a variety of material including nitrocellulose, nylon, and polyvinylidine difluoride (PVDF), all of which avidly bind protein.

Liquid samples can be analyzed by methods called dot blots or slot blots. A solution containing the biomolecule of interest is filtered through a membrane which captures the biomolecule. The difference between a dot blot and a slot blot is that the former uses a circular or disk format, while the latter is a rectangular configuration. The latter method allows for a more precise quantification of the desired biomolecule by scanning methods and relating the integrated results to that obtained with known amounts of material.

Often the sample is subjected to some type of fractionation, such as PAGE, prior to the blotting step. An early technique, Southern blotting, named after the discoverer, E.M. Southern, is used to detect DNA fragments. When this procedure was adapted to RNA fragments and to proteins, other compass coordinates were chosen as labels for these procedures, i.e., northern blots for RNA and western blots for proteins. Western blots involve the use of labeled antibodies to detect specific proteins.

*Transfer of Proteins*
Following PAGE, the transfer of proteins from the gel to the membrane can be accomplished in a number of ways. Originally, blotting was achieved by capillary action. In this commonly used method, the membrane is placed between the gel and absorbent paper. Fluid from the gel is drawn toward the absorbent paper and the protein is captured by the intervening membrane. A blot, or impression, of the protein within the gel is thus made.

The transfer of proteins to the membrane can occur under the influence of an electric field, as well. The electric field is applied perpendicularly to the original field used in separation so that the maximum distance the protein needs to migrate is only the thickness of the gel, and hence the transfer of proteins can occur very rapidly. This latter method is called electroblotting.

*Detection Systems*
Once the transfer has occurred, the next step is to identify the presence of the desired protein. In addition to various colorimetric staining methods, the blots can be probed with reagents specific for certain proteins, as for example, antibodies to a protein of interest. This technique is called immunoblotting. In the biotechnology field, immunoblotting is used as an identity test for the product of interest. An antibody that recognizes the desired protein is used in

1. ■ Transfer protein to membrane, e.g., by electroblotting.
2. ■ Block residual protein binding sites on membrane with extraneous proteins such as milk proteins.
3. ■ Treat membrane with antibody which recognizes the protein of interest. If this antibody is labeled with a detecting group then go to step 5.
4. ■ Incubate membrane with secondary antibody which recognizes primary antibody used in step 3. This antibody is labeled with a detecting group.
5. ■ Treat the membrane with suitable reagents to locate the site of membrane attachment of the labeled antibody in step 4 or step 5.

**Table 5**  ■  Major steps in blotting proteins to membranes.

this instance. Secondly, immunoblotting is sometimes used to show the absence of host proteins. In this instance, the antibodies are raised against proteins of the organism in which the recombinant protein has been expressed. This latter method can attest to the purity of the desired protein.

Table 5 lists major steps needed for the blotting procedure to be successful. Once the transfer of proteins is completed, residual protein binding sites on the membrane need to be blocked so that antibodies used for detection react only at the location of the target molecule, or antigen, and not at some non-specific location. After blocking, the specific antibody is incubated with the membrane.

The antibody reacts with a specific protein on the membrane only at the location of that protein because of its specific interaction with its antigen. When immunoblotting techniques are used, methods are still needed to recognize the location of the interaction of the antibody with its specific protein. A number of procedures can be used to detect this complex (Table 6).

The antibody itself can be labeled with a radioactive marker such as $^{125}$I and placed in direct contact with X-ray film. After exposure of the membrane to the film for a suitable period, the film is developed and a photographic negative is made of the location of radioactivity on the membrane. Alternatively, the antibody can be linked to an enzyme which, upon the addition of appropriate reagents, catalyzes a color or light reaction at the site of the antibody. These procedures entail purification of the antibody and specifically label it. More often, "secondary" antibodies are used. The primary antibody is the one which recognizes the protein of interest. The secondary antibody is then an antibody that specifically recognizes the primary antibody. Quite commonly, the primary antibody is raised in rabbits. The secondary antibody may then be an antibody raised in another animal, such as goat, which recognizes rabbit antibodies. Since this secondary antibody recognizes rabbit antibodies in general, it can be used as a generic reagent to detect rabbit antibodies in a number of different

- Antibodies are labeled with radioactive markers such as [125]I.
- Antibodies are linked to an enzyme such as HRP or AP. On incubation with substrate an insoluble colored product is formed at the location of the antibody. Alternatively, the location of the antibody can be detected using a substrate which yields a chemiluminescent product, an image of which is made on photographic film.
- Antibody is labeled with biotin. Streptavidin or avidin is added to strongly bind to the biotin. Each streptavidin molecule has four binding sites. The remaining binding sites can combine with other biotin molecules which are covalently linked to HRP or to AP.

**Table 6**  Detection methods used in blotting techniques.

proteins of interest that have been raised in rabbits. Thus, the primary antibody specifically recognizes and complexes a unique protein, and the secondary antibody, suitably labeled, is used for detection (see the section entitled ELISA and Fig. 10).

The secondary antibody can be labeled with a radioactive or enzymatic marker group and used to detect several different primary antibodies. Thus, rather than purifying a number of different primary antibodies, only one secondary antibody needs to be purified and labeled for recognition of all the primary antibodies. Because of their wide use, many common secondary antibodies are commercially available in kits containing the detection system and follow routine, straightforward procedures.

In addition to antibodies raised against the amino acyl constituents of proteins, specific antibodies can be used which recognize unique post-translational components in proteins, such as phosphotyrosyl residues, which are important during signal transduction, and carbohydrate moieties of glycoproteins.

Figure 9 illustrates a number of detection methods that can be used on immunoblots. The primary antibody, or if convenient, the secondary antibody, can have an appropriate label for detection. They may be labeled with a radioactive tag as mentioned previously. Secondly, these antibodies can be coupled with an enzyme such as horseradish peroxidase (HRP) or alkaline phosphatase (AP). Substrate is added and is converted to an insoluble, colored product at the site of the protein–primary antibody–secondary antibody–HRP product. An alternative substrate can be used which yields a chemiluminescent product. A chemical reaction leads to the production of light which can expose photographic or X-ray film. The chromogenic and chemiluminescent detection systems have comparable sensitivities to radioactive methods. The former detection methods are displacing the latter method, since problems associated with handling radioactive material and radioactive waste solutions are eliminated.

As illustrated in Figure 9, streptavidin, or alternatively avidin, and biotin can play an important role in detecting proteins on immunoblots. This is because biotin forms very tight complexes with streptavidin and avidin. Secondly, these proteins are multimeric and contain four binding sites for biotin. When biotin is covalently linked to proteins such as antibodies and enzymes, streptavidin binds to the covalently bound biotin, thus recognizing the site on the membrane where the protein of interest is located.

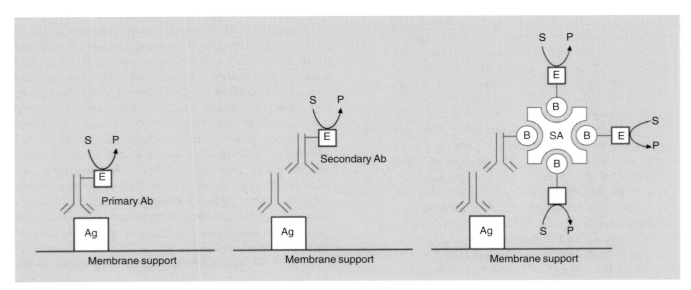

**Figure 9**  Common immunoblotting detection systems used to detect antigens (Ag) on membranes. *Abbreviations*: Ab, antibody; E, enzyme (*such as HRP or AP*); S, substrate; P, product (*either colored and insoluble or chemiluminescent*); B, biotin; Sa, streptavidin.

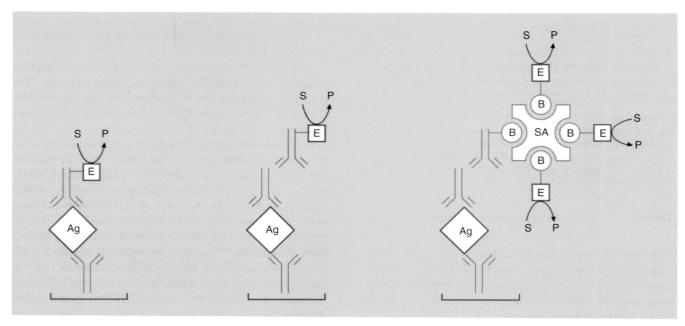

**Figure 10** ▪ Examples of several formats for ELISA in which the specific antibody is adsorbed to the surface of a microtitration plate. (See Fig. 9 for *abbreviations.*) The antibody is represented by the Y type structure. The product P is colored and the amount generated is measured with a spectrometer or plate reader.

## ▪ Immunoassays

### *ELISA*

Enzyme-linked immunosorbent assay (ELISA) provides a means to quantitatively measure extremely small amounts of proteins in biological fluids and serves as a tool for analyzing specific proteins during purification. This procedure takes advantage of the observation that plastic surfaces are able to adsorb low but detectable amounts of proteins. This is a solid phase assay. Therefore, antibodies against a certain desired protein are allowed to adsorb to the surface of microtitration plates. Each plate may contain up to 96 wells so that multiple samples can be assayed. After incubating the antibodies in the wells of the plate for a specific period of time, excess antibody is removed and residual protein binding sites on the plastic are blocked by incubation with an inert protein. Several microtitration plates can be prepared at one time since the antibodies coating the plates retain their binding capacity for an extended period. During the ELISA, sample solution containing the protein of interest is incubated in the wells and the protein (Ag) is captured by the antibodies coating the well surface. Excess sample is removed and other antibodies which now have an enzyme (E) linked to them are added to react with the bound antigen.

The format described above is called a sandwich assay since the antigen of interest is located between the antibody on the titer well surface and the antibody containing the linked enzyme. Figure 10 illustrates a number of formats that can be used in an ELISA. A suitable substrate is added and the enzyme linked to the antibody–antigen–antibody well complex converts this compound to a colored product. The amount of product obtained is proportional to the enzyme adsorbed in the well of the plate. A standard curve can be prepared if known concentrations of antigen are tested in this system, and the amount of antigen in unknown samples can be estimated from this standard curve. A number of enzymes can be used in ELISAs. However, the most common ones are HRP and AP. A variety of substrates for each enzyme are available which yield colored products when catalyzed by the linked enzyme. Absorbance of the colored product solutions is measured on plate readers, instruments which rapidly measure the absorbance in all 96 wells of the microtitration plate, and data processing can be automated for rapid throughput of information. Note that detection approaches partly parallel those discussed in the section on Blotting. The above ELISA format is only one of many different methods. For example, the microtitration wells may be coated directly with the antigen rather than having a specific antibody attached to the surface. Quantitation is made by comparison with known quantities of antigen used to coat individual wells.

Another approach, this time subsequent to the binding of antigen either directly to the surface or to an antibody on the surface, is to use an antibody specific to the antibody binding the protein antigen, that is, a secondary antibody. This latter, secondary, antibody contains the linked enzyme used for detection. As already discussed in the section on blotting, the advantage to this approach is that such antibodies can be obtained in high purity and with the desired enzyme linked to them from commercial sources. Thus, a single source of enzyme-linked antibody can be used in assays for different protein antigens. Should a sandwich assay be used, then antibodies from different species need to be used for each side of the sandwich. A possible scenario is that rabbit antibodies are used to coat the microtitration wells; mouse antibodies, possibly a monoclonal antibody, are used to complex with the antigen and then a goat anti-mouse immunoglobulin containing linked HRP or AP is used for detection purposes.

As with immunoblots discussed above, streptavidin or avidin can be used in these assays if biotin is covalently linked to the antibodies and enzymes (Fig. 10).

If a radioactive label is used in place of the enzyme in the above procedure, then the assay is a solid phase radioimmunoassay (RIA). Assays are moving away from the use of radioisotopes, because of problems with safety and disposal of radioactive waste and since non-radioactive assays have comparable sensitivities.

## ■ Electrophoresis

Analytical methodologies for measuring protein properties stem from those used in their purification. The major difference is that systems used for analysis have a higher resolving power and detection limit than those used in purification. The two major methods for analysis have their bases in chromatographic or electrophoretic techniques.

### PAGE

One of the earliest methods for analysis of proteins is PAGE. In this assay, proteins, being amphoteric molecules with both positive and negative charge groups in their primary structure, are separated according to their net electrical charge. A second factor which is responsible for the separation is the mass of the protein. Thus, one can consider more precisely that the charge to mass ratio of proteins determines how they are separated in an electrical field. The charge of the protein can be controlled by the pH of the solution in which the protein is separated. The farther away the protein is from its pI value, that is, the pH at which it has a net charge of zero, the greater is the net charge and hence the greater is its charge to mass ratio. Therefore, the direction and speed of migration of the protein depend on the pH of the gel. If the pH of the gel is above its pI value, then the protein is negatively charged and hence migrates toward the anode. The higher the pH of

the gel the faster the migration. This type of electrophoresis is called native gel electrophoresis.

The major component of polyacrylamide gels is water. However, they provide a flexible support so that after a protein has been subjected to an electrical field for an appropriate period of time, it provides a matrix to hold the proteins in place until they can be detected with suitable reagents. By adjusting the amount of acrylamide that is used in these gels, one can control the migration of material within the gel. The more acrylamide, the more hindrance for the protein to migrate in an electrical field.

The addition of a detergent, sodium dodecyl sulfate (SDS), to the electrophoretic separation system allows for the separation to take place primarily as a function of the size of the protein. Dodecyl sulfate ions form complexes with proteins, resulting in an unfolding of the proteins, and the amount of detergent that is complexed is proportional to the mass of the protein. The larger the protein, the more detergent that is complexed. Dodecyl sulfate is a negatively charged ion. When proteins are in a solution of SDS, the net effect is that the own charge of the protein is overwhelmed by that of the dodecyl sulfate complexed with it, so that the proteins take on a net negative charge proportional to their mass.

PAGE in the presence of SDS is commonly known as SDS-PAGE. All the proteins take on a net negative charge, with larger proteins binding more SDS but with the charge to mass ratio being fairly constant among the proteins. An example of SDS-PAGE is shown in Figure 11. Here, SDS-PAGE is used to monitor expression of G-CSF receptor and of G-CSF (panel B) in different culture media.

Since all proteins have essentially the same charge to mass ratio, how can separation occur? This is done by controlling the concentration of acrylamide in the path of proteins migrating in an electrical field. The greater the acrylamide concentration, the more difficult it is for large protein molecules to migrate relative to smaller protein molecules. This is sometimes thought of as a sieving effect, since the greater the acrylamide concentration, the smaller the pore size within the polyacrylamide gel. Indeed, if the acrylamide concentration is sufficiently high, some high molecular weight proteins may not migrate at all within the gel. Since in SDS-PAGE the proteins are denatured, their hydrodynamic size, and hence the degree of retardation by the sieving effects, is directly related to their mass. Proteins containing disulfide bonds will have a much more compact structure and higher mobility for their mass unless the disulfides are reduced prior to electrophoresis.

As described above, native gel electrophoresis and SDS-PAGE are quite different in terms of the mechanism of protein separation. In native gel

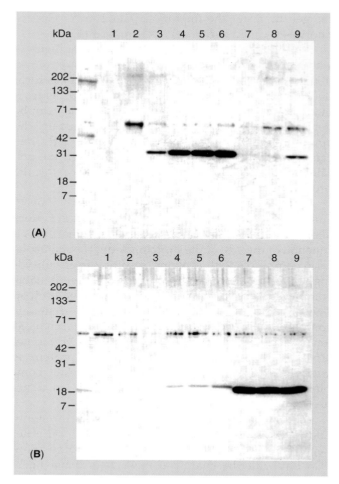

**Figure 11** ▇ SDS-PAGE of G-CSF receptor, about 35 kDa (**A**) and G-CSF, about 20 kDa (**B**). These proteins are expressed in different culture media (lane 1–9). Positions of molecular weight standards are given on the left side. The bands are developed with antibody against G-CSF receptor (**A**) or G-CSF (**A**) after blotting.

electrophoresis, the proteins are in the native state and migrate on their own charges. Thus, this electrophoresis can be used to characterize proteins in the native state. In SDS-PAGE, proteins are unfolded and migrate based on their molecular mass. As an intermediate case, Blue native electrophoresis is developed, in which proteins are bound by a dye, Coomassie blue, used to stain protein bands. This dye is believed to bind to the hydrophobic surface of the proteins and to add negative charges to the proteins. The dye-bound proteins are still in the native state and migrate based on the net charges, which depend on the intrinsic charges of the proteins and the amounts of the negatively charged dye. This is particularly useful for analyzing membrane proteins, which tend to aggregate in the absence of detergents. The dye prevents the proteins from aggregation by binding to their hydrophobic surface.

### Isoelectric Focusing (IEF)

Another method to separate proteins based on their electrophoretic properties is to take advantage of their isoelectric point. In a first run a pH gradient is established within the gel using a mixture of small molecular weight ampholytes with varying pI values. The high pH conditions are established at the site of the cathode. Then, the protein is brought on the gel, e.g., at the site where the pH is 7. In the electrical field the protein will migrate until it reaches the pH on the gel where its net charge is zero. If the protein were to migrate away from this pH value it could gain a charge and migrate toward its pI value again, leading to a focusing effect.

### Two-Dimensional Gel Electrophoresis

The above methods can be combined into a procedure called 2-D gel electrophoresis. Proteins are first fractionated by IEF based upon their pI values. They are then subjected to SDS-PAGE perpendicular to the first dimension and fractionated based on the molecular weights of proteins. SDS-PAGE cannot be performed before IEF, since once SDS binds to and denatures the proteins they no longer migrate based on their pI values.

### Detection of Proteins within Polyacrylamide Gels

Although the polyacrylamide gels provide a flexible support for the proteins, with time the proteins will diffuse and spread within the gel. Consequently, the usual practice is to fix the proteins or trap them at the location where they migrated to. This is accomplished by placing the gels in a fixing solution in which the proteins become insoluble.

There are many methods for staining proteins in gels, but the two most common and well-studied methods are either staining with Coomassie blue or by a method using silver. The latter method is used if increased sensitivity is required. The principle of developing the Coomassie blue stain is the hydrophobic interaction of a dye with the protein. Thus, the gel takes on a color wherever a protein is located. Using standard amounts of proteins, the amount of protein or contaminant may be estimated. Quantification using the silver staining method is less precise. However, due to the increased sensitivity of this method, very low levels of contaminants can be detected. These fixing and staining procedures denature the proteins. Hence, proteins separated under native conditions, as in native or Blue native gel electrophoresis, will be denatured. To maintain the native state, the gels can be stained with copper or other metal ions.

### Capillary Electrophoresis

With recent advances in instrumentation and technology, capillary electrophoresis has gained an increased presence in the analysis of recombinant proteins. Rather than having a matrix, as in PAGE through which the proteins migrate, they are free in solution in an electric field within the confines of a capillary tube with a diameter of 25 to 50 micrometers. The capillary tube passes through an ultraviolet light or fluorescence detector that measures the presence of proteins migrating in the electric field. The movement of one protein relative to another is a function of the molecular mass and the net charge on the protein. The latter can be influenced by pH and analytes in the solution. This technique has only partially gained acceptance for routine analysis, because of difficulties in reproducibility of the capillaries and in validating this system. Nevertheless, it is a powerful analytical tool for the characterization of recombinant proteins during process development and in stability studies.

## ■ Chromatography

Chromatography techniques are used extensively in biotechnology not only in protein purification procedures (see Chapter 3), but also in assessing the integrity of the product. Routine procedures are highly automated so that comparisons of similar samples can be made. An analytical system consists of an autosampler which will take a known amount (usually a known volume) of material for analysis and automatically places it in the solution stream headed toward a separation column used to fractionate the sample. Another part of this system is a pump module which provides a reproducible flow rate. In addition, the pumping system can provide a gradient which changes properties of the solution such as pH, ionic strength, and hydrophobicity. A detection system (or possibly multiple detectors in series) is located at the outlet of the column. This measures the relative amount of protein exiting the column. Coupled to the detector is a data acquisition system which takes the signal from the detector and integrates it into a

value related to the amount of material (Fig. 12). When the protein appears, the signal begins to increase, and as the protein passes through the detector, the signal subsequently decreases. The area under the peak of the signal is proportional to the amount of material which has passed through the detector. By analyzing known amounts of protein, an area versus amount of protein plot can be generated and this may be used to estimate the amount of this protein in the sample under other circumstances. Another benefit of this integrated chromatography system is that low levels of components which appear over time can be estimated relative to the major desired protein being analyzed. This is a particularly useful function when the long-term stability of the product is under evaluation.

Chromatographic systems offer a multitude of different strategies for successfully separating protein mixtures and for quantifying individual protein components (see Chapter 3). The following describes some of these strategies.

### Size Exclusion Chromatography

As the name implies, this procedure separates proteins based on their size or molecular weight or shape. The matrix consists of very fine beads containing cavities and pores accessible to molecules of a certain size or smaller, but inaccessible to larger molecules. The principle of this technique is the distribution of molecules between the volume of solution within the beads versus the volume of solution surrounding the beads. Small molecules have access to a larger volume than do large molecules. As solution flows through the column, molecules can diffuse back and forth, depending upon their size, in and out of the pores of the beads. Smaller molecules can reside within the pores for a finite period of time whereas larger molecules, unable to enter these spaces, continue along in the fluid stream. Intermediate-sized molecules spend an intermediate

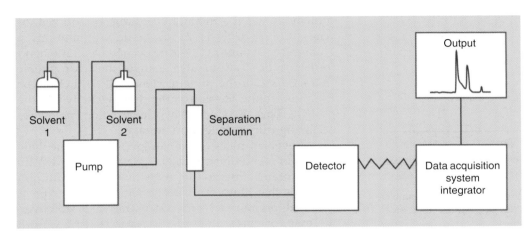

**Figure 12** ■ Components of a typical chromatography station. The pump combines solvents 1 and 2 in appropriate ratios to generate a pH, salt concentration, or hydrophobic gradient. Proteins that are fractioned on the column pass through a detector which measures their occurrence. Information from the detector is used to generate chromatograms and the relative amount of each component.

amount of time within the pores. They can be fractionated from large molecules that cannot access the matrix space at all and from small molecules that have free access to this volume and spend most of the time within the beads. Protein molecules can distribute between the volume within these beads and the excluded volume based on the mass and shape of the molecule. This distribution is based on the relative concentration of the protein in the beads versus the excluded volume.

Size exclusion chromatography can be used to estimate the mass of proteins by calibrating the column with a series of globular proteins of known mass. However, the separation depends on molecular shape (conformation) as well as mass, and highly elongated proteins—proteins containing flexible, disordered regions—and glycoproteins will often appear to have masses as much as two to three times the true value. Other proteins may interact weakly with the column matrix and be retarded, thereby appearing to have a smaller mass. Thus, sedimentation or light scattering methods are preferred for accurate mass measurement. Over time, proteins can undergo a number of changes that affect their mass. A peptide bond within the protein can hydrolyze, yielding two smaller polypeptide chains. More commonly, size exclusion chromatography is used to assess aggregated forms of the protein. Figure 13 shows an example of this. The peak at 22 minutes represents the native protein. The peak at 15 minutes is aggregated protein and that at 28 minutes depicts degraded protein yielding smaller polypeptide chains. Aggregation can occur when a protein

molecule unfolds to a slight extent and exposes surfaces that are attracted to complementary surfaces on adjacent molecules. This interaction can lead to dimerization or doubling of molecular weight or to higher molecular weight oligomers. From the chromatographic profile, the mechanism of aggregation can often be implicated. If dimers, trimers, tetramers, etc. are observed, then aggregation occurs by stepwise interaction of a monomer with a dimer, trimer, etc. If dimers, tetramers, octamers, etc. are observed, then aggregates can interact with each other. Sometimes, only monomers and high molecular weight aggregates are observed, suggesting that intermediate species are kinetically of short duration and protein molecules susceptible to aggregation combine into very large molecular weight complexes.

### Reversed-Phase High Performance Liquid Chromatography

Reversed-phase high performance liquid chromatography (RP-HPLC) takes advantage of the hydrophobic properties of proteins. The functional groups on the column matrix contain from one to up to eighteen carbon atoms in a hydrocarbon chain. The longer this chain, the more hydro-phobic is the matrix. The hydrophobic patches of proteins interact with the hydrophobic chromatographic matrix. Proteins are then eluted from the matrix by increasing the hydrophobic nature of the solvent passing through the column. Acetonitrile is a common solvent used, although other organic solvents such as ethanol also may be employed. The solvent is made acidic by the addition of trifluoroacetic acid, since proteins have increased solubility at pH values further removed from their pI. A gradient with increasing concentration of hydrophobic solvent is passed through the column. Different proteins have different hydrophobicities and are eluted from the column depending on the "hydrophobic potential" of the solvent.

This technique can be very powerful. It may detect the addition of a single oxygen atom to the protein, as when a methionyl residue is oxidized, or when the hydrolysis of an amide moiety on a glutamyl or asparginyl residue occurs. Disulfide bond formation or shuffling also changes the hydrophobic characteristic of the protein. Hence, RP-HPLC can be used not only to assess the homogeneity of the protein, but also to follow degradation pathways occurring during long term storage.

Reversed-phase chromatography of proteolytic digests of recombinant proteins may serve to identify this protein. Enzymatic digestion yields unique peptides that elute at different retention times or at different organic solvent concentrations. Moreover, the map, or chromatogram, of peptides arising from

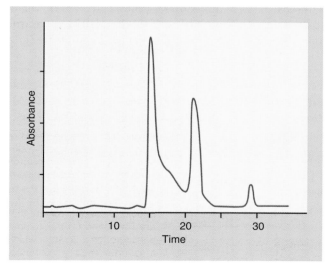

**Figure 13** ▪ Size exclusion chromatography of a recombinant protein which, on storage, yields aggregates and smaller peptides.

enzymatic digestion of one protein is quite different from the map obtained from another protein. Several different proteases, such as trypsin, chymotrypsin and other endoproteinases, are used for these identity tests (see below under Mass Spectrometry).

## Hydrophobic Interaction Chromatography

A companion to RP-HPLC is hydrophobic interaction chromatography (HIC), although in principle this latter method is normal-phase chromatography, i.e., here an aqueous solvent system rather than an organic one is used to fractionate proteins. The hydrophobic characteristics of the solution are modulated by inorganic salt concentrations. Ammonium sulfate and sodium chloride are often used since these compounds are highly soluble in water. In the presence of high salt concentrations (up to several molar), proteins are attracted to hydrophobic surfaces on the matrix of resins used in this technique. As the salt concentration decreases, proteins have less affinity for the matrix and eventually elute from the column. This method lacks the resolving power of RP-HPLC, but is a more gentle method, since low pH values or organic solvents as used in RP-HPLC can be detrimental to some proteins.

## Ion Exchange Chromatography

This technique takes advantage of the electronic charge properties of proteins. Some of the amino acyl residues are negatively charged and others are positively charged. The net charge of the protein can be modulated by the pH of its environment relative to the pI value of the protein. At a pH value lower than the pI, the protein has a net positive charge, whereas at a pH value greater than the pI, the protein has a net negative charge. Opposites attract in ion-exchange chromatography. The resins in this procedure can contain functional groups with positive or negative charges. Thus, positively charged proteins bind to negatively charged matrices and negatively charged proteins bind to positively charged matrices. Proteins are displaced from the resin by increasing salt, e.g., sodium chloride, concentrations. Proteins with different net charges can be separated from one another during elution with an increasing salt gradient. The choice of charged resin and elution conditions are dependent upon the protein of interest.

In lieu of changing the ionic strength of the solution, proteins can be eluted by changing the pH of the medium, i.e., with the use of a pH gradient. This method is called chromatofocusing and proteins are separated based on their pI values. When the solvent pH reaches the pI value of a specific protein, the protein has a zero net charge and is no longer attracted to the charged matrix and hence is eluted.

## Other Chromatographic Techniques

Other functional groups may be attached to chromatographic matrices to take advantage of unique properties of certain proteins. These affinity methodologies, however, are more often used in the manufacturing process than in analytical techniques (see Chapter 3). For example, conventional affinity purification schemes of antibodies use Protein-A or -G columns. Protein-A or -G specifically binds antibodies. Antibodies consist of variable regions and constant regions (see Chapter 4). The variable regions are antigen-specific and hence vary in sequence from one antibody to another, while the constant regions are common to each subgroup of antibodies. The constant region binds to Protein-A or -G.

## ■ Bioassays

Paramount to the development of a protein therapeutic is to have an assay that identifies its biological function. Chromatographic and electrophoretic methodologies can address the homogeneity of a biotherapeutic and be useful in investigating stability parameters. However, it is also necessary to ascertain whether the protein has acceptable bioactivity. Bioactivity can be determined either in vivo, i.e., by administering the protein to an animal and ascertaining some change within its body (function), or in vitro. Bioassays in vitro monitor the response of a specific receptor or microbiological or tissue cell line when the therapeutic protein is added to the system. An example of an in vitro bioassay is the increase in DNA synthesis in the presence of the therapeutic protein as measured by the incorporation of radioactively labeled thymidine. The protein factor binds to receptors on the cell surface that triggers secondary messengers to send signals to the cell nucleus to synthesize DNA. The binding of the protein factor to the cell surface is dependent upon the amount of factor present. Figure 14 presents a dose response curve of thymidine incorporation as a function of concentration of the factor. At low concentrations, the factor is too low to trigger a response. As the concentration increases, the incorporation of thymidine occurs, and at higher concentrations the amount of thymidine incorporation ceases to increase as DNA synthesis is occurring at the maximum rate. A standard curve can be obtained using known quantities of the protein factor. Comparison of other solutions containing unknown amounts of the factor with this standard curve will then yield quantitative estimates of the factor concentration. Through experience during the development of the protein therapeutic, a value is obtained for a fully functional protein. Subsequent comparisons to this value can be used to ascertain any loss in activity during stability

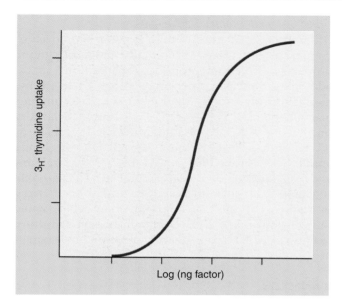

**Figure 14** ■ An in vitro bioassay showing a mitogenic response in which radioactive thymidine is incorporated into DNA in the presence of an increasing amount of a protein factor.

studies, or changes in activity when amino acyl residues of the protein are modified.

Other in vitro bioassays can measure changes in cell number or production of another protein factor in response to the stimulation of cells by the protein therapeutic. The amount of the secondary protein produced can be estimated by using an ELISA.

### ■ Mass Spectrometry

Recent advances in the measurement of the molecular masses of proteins have made this technique an important analytical tool. While this method was used in the past to analyze small volatile molecules, the molecular weights of highly charged proteins with masses of over 100 kilodaltons (kDa) can now be accurately determined.

Because of the precision of this method, post-translational modifications such as acetylation or glycosylation can be predicted. The masses of new protein forms that arise during stability studies provide information on the nature of this form. For example, an increase in mass of 16 Dalton suggests that an oxygen atom has been added to the protein as happens when a methionyl residue is oxidized to a methionyl sulfoxide residue. The molecular mass of peptides obtained after proteolytic digestion and separation by HPLC indicate from which region of the primary structure they are derived. Such HPLC chromatogram is called a "peptide map." An example is shown in Figure 15. This is obtained by digesting a protein with pepsin and by subsequently separating the digested peptides by reverse HPLC. This highly characteristic pattern for a protein is

called a "protein fingerprint." Peaks are identified by elution times on HPLC. If peptides have molecular masses differing from those expected from the primary sequence, the nature of the modification to that peptide can be implicated. Moreover, molecular mass estimates can be made for peptides obtained from unfractionated proteolytic digests. Molecular masses that differ from expected values indicate that a part of the protein molecule has been altered, that glycosylation or another modification has been altered, or that the protein under investigation still contains contaminants.

Another way that mass spectrometry can be used as an analytical tool is in the sequencing of peptides. A recurring structure, the peptide bond, in peptides tends to yield fragments of the mature peptide which differ stepwise by an amino acyl residue. The difference in mass between two fragments indicates the amino acid removed from one fragment to generate the other. Except for leucine and isoleucine, each amino acid has a different mass and hence a sequence can be read from the mass spectrograph. Stepwise removal can occur from either the amino terminus or carboxy terminus.

By changing three basic components of the mass spectrometer, the ion source, the analyzer and the detector, different types of measurement may be undertaken. Typical ion sources which volatilize the proteins are electrospray ionization (EI), fast atom bombardment and liquid secondary ion. Common analyzers include quadrupole, magnetic sector, and time of flight instruments. The function of the analyzer is to separate the ionized biomolecules based on their mass to charge ratio. The detector measures a current whenever impinged upon by charged particles. EI and matrix-assisted laser desorption (MALDI) are two sources that can generate high molecular weight volatile proteins. In the former method, droplets are generated by spraying or nebulizing the protein solution into the source of the mass spectrometer. As the solvent evaporates, the protein remains behind in the gas phase and passes through the analyzer to the detector. In MALDI, proteins are mixed with a matrix which vaporizes when exposed to laser light, thus carrying the protein into the gas phase. An example of MALDI-mass analysis is shown in Fig. 16, indicating the singly charged ion (116118 Dalton) and the doubly charged ion (58036.2) for a purified protein. Since proteins are multi-charge compounds, a number of components are observed representing mass to charge forms, each differing from the next by one charge. By imputing various charges to the mass to charge values, a molecular

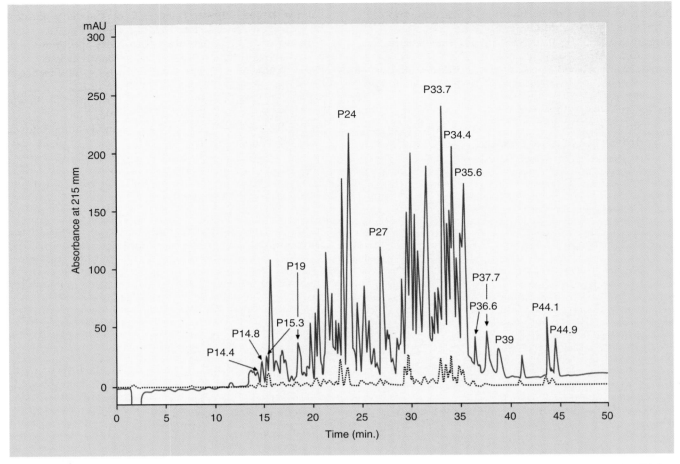

**Figure 15** ▪ Peptide map of pepsin digest of recombinant human β-secretase. Each peptide is labeled by elution time in HPLC.

mass of the protein can be estimated. The latter step is empirical since only the mass to charge ratio is detected and not the net charge for that particular particle.

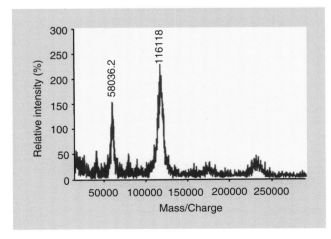

**Figure 16** ▪ MALDI mass analysis of a purified recombinant human β-secretase. Numbers correspond to the singly charged and doubly charged ions.

## CONCLUDING REMARKS

With the advent of recombinant proteins as human therapeutics, the need for methods to evaluate their structure, function, and homogeneity has become paramount. Various analytical techniques are used to characterize the primary, secondary, and tertiary structure of the protein and to determine the quality, purity and stability of the recombinant product. Bioassays establish its activity.

## FURTHER READING

Butler JE, ed. (1991). Immunochemistry of Solid-Phase Immunoassay. Boca Raton, FL: CRC Press.

Crabb JW, ed. (1995). Techniques in Protein Chemistry VI. San Diego, CA: Academic Press.

Coligan J, Dunn B, Ploegh H, Speicher D, Wingfield P, eds. (1995). Current Protocols in Protein Science. New York: J. Wiley & Sons.

Creighton TE, ed. (1989). Protein Structure: A Practical Approach. Oxford, UK: IRL Press.

Crowther JR (1995). ELISA, Theory and Practice. Totowa, NJ: Humana Press.

Dunbar BS (1994). Protein Blotting: A Practical Approach. New York: Oxford University Press.

Gregory RB, ed. (1994). Protein-Solvent Interactions. New York: Marcel Dekker.

Hames BD, Rickwood D, eds. (1990). Gel Electrophoresis of Proteins: A Practical Approach, 2nd ed. New York: IRL Press.

Jiskoot W, Crommelin DJA, eds. (2005). Methods for Structural Analysis of Protein Pharmaceuticals. Arlington, VA: AAPS Press.

Landus JP, ed. (1994). Handbook of Capillary Electrophoresis. Boca Raton, FL: CRC Press.

McEwen CN, Larsen BS, eds. (1990). Mass Spectrometry of Biological Materials. New York: Marcel Dekker.

Price CP, Newman DJ, eds. (1991). Principles and Practice of Immunoassay. New York: Stockton Press.

Schulz GE, Schirmer RH, eds. (1979). Principles of Protein Structure. New York: Springer-Verlag.

Shirley BA, ed. (1995). Protein Stability and Folding. Totowa, NJ: Humana Press.

# 3

# Production and Downstream Processing of Biotech Compounds

*Farida Kadir*
*Postacademic Education Pharmacists (POA), Bunnik, The Netherlands*

*Mic Hamers and Paul Ives*
*SynCo Bio Partners BV, Amsterdam, The Netherlands*

## INTRODUCTION

The growing therapeutic use of proteins has created an increasing need for practical and economical processing techniques. As a result, biotechnological production methods have advanced tremendously in recent years, particularly in areas where disposable, single use production technology can be applied to mitigate many of the economic and quality issues arising from manufacturing these products (Hodge, 2004).

When producing proteins for therapeutic use, a number of issues must be considered related to the manufacturing, purification and characterization of the products. Biotechnological products for therapeutic use have to meet strict specifications, especially when used via the parenteral route (Walter and Werner, 1993).

In this chapter several aspects of production and purification will be dealt with briefly. For further details the reader is referred to the literature mentioned.

## PRODUCTION

### ■ Expression Systems

#### General Considerations

Expression systems for proteins of therapeutic interest include both pro- and eukaryotic cells (bacteria, yeast, fungi, plants, insect cells, mammalian cells, and transgenic animals). The choice of a particular system will be determined to a large extent by the nature and origin of the desired protein, the intended use of the product, the amount needed, and the cost.

In principle, any protein can be produced using genetically engineered organisms, but not every type of protein can be produced by every type of cell. In the majority of cases the protein is foreign to the host cells that have to produce it and although the translation of the genetic code can be performed by the cells, the post-translation modifications of the protein might be different as compared to the original product.

At present, over 60 different post-translation modifications of proteins are known and these modifications are species and/or cell-type specific. The metabolic pathways that lead to these modifications are genetically determined by the host cell. Thus, even if the cells are capable of producing the desired post-translation modification, like glycosylation, still the resulting glycosylation pattern might be different from that of the native protein. For example, prokaryotic cells, like bacteria, are not capable of producing glycoproteins, because they lack this post-translation modification capacity. One possible solution to these problems is to use cell types that are as closely related to the original protein-producing cell type as possible, particularly when one considers that more than 50% of human proteins are glycoproteins. Therefore, for human derived proteins, mammalian cells or transgenic animals are often a better choice than bacteria or yeast. However, developments in the field of glycosylation engineering may allow bacteria to reproduce some of the post-translation modification steps common to eukaryotic cells (Borman, 2006). Although still in its infancy, this technology could have a significant impact on future production systems.

Generalized features of proteins expressed in different biological systems are listed in Table 1 (Walter et al., 1992). However, it should be kept in mind that there are exceptions to this table for specific product/expression systems.

#### Transgenic Animals

Foreign genes can be introduced into animals like mice, rabbits, pigs, sheep, goats, and cows through nuclear transfer and cloning techniques. The desired protein is expressed in the milk of the female offspring. During lactation the milk is collected, the milk fats are removed and the skimmed milk is used as the starting material for the purification of the protein.

| Protein feature | Prokaryotic bacteria | Eukaryotic yeast | Eukaryotic mammalian cells |
|---|---|---|---|
| Concentration | High | High | Low |
| Molecular weight | Low | High | High |
| S-S bridges | Limitation | No limitation | No limitation |
| Secretion | No | Yes/no | Yes |
| Aggregation state | Inclusion body | Singular, native | Singular, native |
| Folding | Misfolding | Correct folding | Correct folding |
| Glycosylation | No | Possible | Possible |
| Retrovirus | No | No | Possible |
| Pyrogen | Possible | No | No |

**Table 1** ■ Generalized features of proteins of different biological origin.

The advantage of this technology is the relatively cheap method to produce the desired proteins in vast quantities. A disadvantage is the concern about the animal health. Some proteins expressed in the mammary gland leak back into the circulation and cause serious negative health effects. An example is the expression of erythropoetin in cows. Although the protein was well expressed in the milk, it caused severe health effects and these experiments were stopped.

The purification strategies and purity requirements for proteins from milk are not different from those derived from bacterial or mammalian cell systems, with the possible exception of proteins for oral use when expressed in milk that is otherwise consumed by humans. In the latter case, the "contaminants" are known to be safe for consumption.

The transgenic animal technology for the production of pharmaceutical proteins is still under development. No products have reached the market yet. More details about this technology are presented in Chapter 7.

*Plants*
Therapeutic proteins can also be expressed in plants and plant cell cultures (see Chapter 1). For instance, human albumin has been expressed in potatoes and tobacco. Whether these production vehicles are economically feasible has yet to be established. The lack of genetic stability of plants is sometimes a drawback. Furthermore, most plants contain phenolic oxidases that can damage the expressed protein upon extraction from the plant material. A better route is the expression of the protein in edible seeds. For instance, rice and barley can be harvested and easily kept for a prolonged period of time as raw material sources. Especially for oral therapeutics or vaccines this might be the ideal solution to produce large amounts of cheap therapeutics, because the "contaminants" are known to be safe for consumption (see Chapter 21).

The use of plant systems for the production of pharmaceutical proteins is still in an experimental phase. More details about this technology are presented in Chapter 7.

■ **Cultivation Systems**
In general, cells can be cultivated in vessels containing an appropriate liquid growth medium in which the cells are either attached to microspheres, or free in suspension or in an immobilized state as monolayers, or entrapped in matrices (usually solidified with agar). The culture method will determine the scale of the separation and purification methods. Production-scale cultivation is commonly performed in fermentors or bioreactors. Bioreactor systems can be classified into four different types: stirred-tank, airlift, microcarrier (e.g., fixed-bed bioreactors) and membrane bioreactors (e.g., hollow fiber perfusion bioreactors) (Fig. 1). Because of its reliability and experience with the design and scaling up potential, the stirred tank is still the most commonly used bioreactor. The increased use of disposables in the manufacturing process has also resulted in the appearance of disposable bioreactors which take the form of large plastic bags which can be stirred or rocked to generate mixing for mass transfer. So far the application of this kind of technology for the manufacturing of commercial product has yet to be reported.

The kinetics of cell growth and product formation will not only dictate the type of bioreactor used, but also how the growth process is run. Three types of fermentation protocols are commonly employed: (1) batch, (2) fed-batch, and (3) continuous production protocols. In all cases the cells go through four distinctive phases: lag, exponential growth, stationary, and death phase (see Chapter 1). The cell culture has to be free from undesired microorganisms that may destroy the cells or present hazards to the patient. This requires strict measures for both the procedures and materials used (Berthold and Walter, 1994; WHO 1998).

Examples of animal cells that are most commonly used to produce proteins of clinical interest are Chinese hamster ovary cells (CHO), baby hamster kidney cells (BHK), lymphoblastoid tumor cells (interferon production), melanoma cells (plasminogen activator), and hybridized tumor cells (monoclonal antibodies).

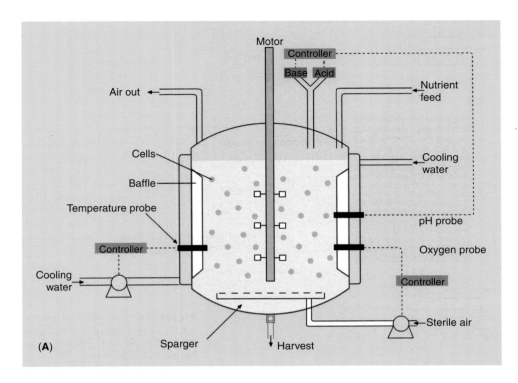

**Figure 1A** ▪ Schematic representation of stirred-tank bioreactor. *Source*: Adapted from Klegerman and Groves, 1992.

## ▪ Cultivation Medium

In order to achieve optimal growth of cells it is of great importance that not only conditions such as pH, oxygen tension and temperature are chosen and controlled appropriately, but also that a medium with the proper nutrients is provided.

The media used for mammalian cell culture are complex and consist of a mixture of diverse components, such as sugars, amino acids, electrolytes, vitamins, fetal calf serum and a mixture of peptones, growth factors, hormones, and other proteins (Table 2). Many of these ingredients are pre-blended either diluted or as homogeneous mixtures of powders. To prepare the final medium, components are dissolved in purified water before sterile filtration. Some supplements, especially fetal calf serum, contribute considerably to the presence of contaminating proteins and may seriously complicate purification procedures. Additionally, the composition of serum is variable; it depends on the individual animal, season of the year, suppliers' treatment, etc. The use of serum may introduce adventitious material such as viruses, mycoplasmas, bacteria and fungi into the culture system (Berthold and Walter, 1994). Furthermore, the possible presence of prions that can cause transmissible spongiform encephalitis (TSE) almost precludes the use bovine, sheep or goat material. However, if use of this material is inevitable, one must follow the relevant guidelines in which selective sourcing of the material is still the key measure to safety (EMEA, 1999a). Many of these potential problems when using serum in cell culture media have resulted in the creation of serum-free formulations, particularly by the medium suppliers, and a trend toward the

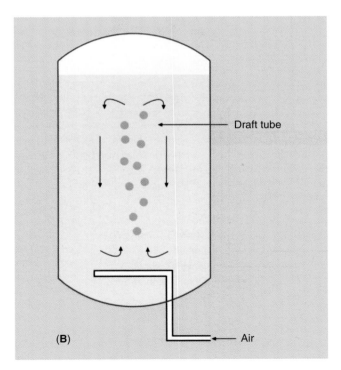

**Figure 1B** ▪ Schematic representation of airlift bioreactor. *Source*: Adapted from Klegerman and Groves, 1992.

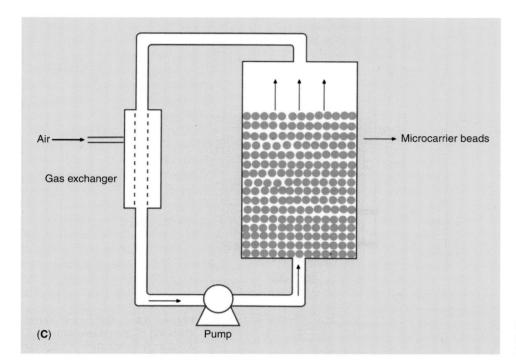

**Figure 1C** ▪ Schematic representation of fixed-bed stirred-tank bioreactor. *Source*: Adapted from Klegerman and Groves, 1992.

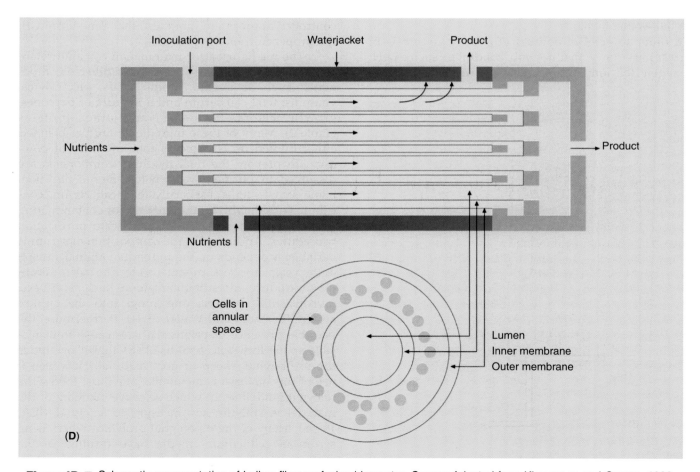

**Figure 1D** ▪ Schematic representation of hollow fiber perfusion bioreactor. *Source*: Adapted from Klegerman and Groves, 1992.

| Type of nutrient | Example(s) |
|---|---|
| Sugars | Glucose, lactose, sucrose, maltose, dextrins |
| Fat | Fatty acids, triglycerides |
| Water (high quality, sterilized) | Water for injection |
| Amino acids | Glutamine |
| Electrolytes | Calcium, sodium, potassium, phosphate |
| Vitamins | Ascorbic acid, $\alpha$-tocopherol, thiamine, riboflavine, folic acid, pyridoxin |
| Serum (fetal calf serum, synthetic serum) | Albumin, transferrin |
| Trace minerals | Iron, manganese, copper, cobalt, zinc |
| Hormones | Growth factors |

**Table 2** ▪ Major components of growth media for mammalian cell structures.

| Origin | Contaminant |
|---|---|
| Host-related | Viruses |
| | Host-derived proteins acid DNA |
| | Glycosylation variants |
| | N- and C-terminal variants |
| | Endotoxins (from Gram-negative bacterial hosts) |
| Product-related | Amino acids substitution and deletion |
| | Denatured protein |
| | Conformational isomers |
| | Dimers and aggregates |
| | Disulfide pairing variants |
| | Deamidated species |
| | Protein fragments |
| Process-related | Growth medium components |
| | Purification reagents |
| | Metals |
| | Column materials |

**Table 3** ▪ Potential contaminants in recombinant protein products derived from bacterial and non-bacterial hosts.

removal of other complex undefined medium components. Completely serum-free and chemically defined media have been shown to give satisfactory results in industrial scale production settings in certain cases, for example, in monoclonal antibody production.

### ▪ Contaminants

Quality is usually measured in terms of product purity and product consistency (reproducibility). An important consideration in the development process of the purification scheme is the ultimate purity required. For pharmaceutical applications, product purity mostly is $\geq 99\%$ when used as a parenteral (Berthold and Walter, 1994; EMEA 1999b).

Purification processes should yield potent proteins with well-defined characteristics for human use from which "all" contaminants have been removed. The purity of the drug protein in the final product will therefore largely depend upon the purification technology applied.

Table 3 lists potential contaminants that may be present in recombinant protein products from bacterial and non-bacterial sources. These contaminants can be either host-related, process-related or product-related. In the following sections special attention is paid to the detection and elimination of contamination by viruses, bacteria, cellular DNA, and undesired proteins.

### Viruses

Viruses, which require the presence of living cells to propagate, are potential contaminants of animal cell cultures and, therefore, of the final product produced by the cells (Arathoon and Birch, 1986). If present, their concentration in the purified product will be very low and it will be difficult to detect them. Although viruses such as retrovirus (type B) can be visualized under an electron microscope, a highly sensitive in vitro assay for their presence is lacking (Liptrot and Gull, 1991). The risks of some viruses (e.g., hepatitis virus) are known (Marcus-Sekura, 1991; Walter et al., 1991), but there are other viruses whose risks can not be properly judged because of lack of solid experimental data. Some virus infections, such as parvovirus, can have long latent periods before their clinical effects show up. Long-term effects of introducing viruses into a patient treated with a recombinant protein should not be overlooked. Therefore, it is required that parenterals are free from viruses. The specific virus testing regime required will depend on the cell type used for production (Löwer, 1990; Minor, 1994).

Viruses can be introduced by nutrients or they are generated by an infected production cell line. The most frequent source of virus introduction is animal serum. In addition, animal serum can introduce other unwanted agents such as bacteria, mycoplasmas, prions, fungi and endotoxins. It should be clear that appropriate screening of cell banks and growth medium constituents for viruses and other adventitious agents should be strictly regulated and supervised (Walter et al., 1991; FDA 1993; EMEA, 1997; WHO Technical Report Series 823). A validated method to remove possible viral contaminants is mandatory for licensing of all therapeutics derived from mammalian cells or transgenic animals (White et al., 1991; Minor 1994). Viruses can be inactivated by physical and chemical treatment of the product. Heat, irradiation, sonication, extreme pH, detergents, solvents, and certain disinfectants can inactivate viruses. These procedures can be harmful to the product as well and should therefore be carefully evaluated and validated (White et al., 1991; Walter et al., 1992; Minor, 1994; EMEA, 1997). Removal of viruses by nanofiltration is an elegant and effective technique and the validation aspects of this technology are extremely well described in the PDA technical report 41, 2005. Filtration through 15 nm membranes can remove even smallest non-enveloped viruses like bovine parvoviruses (Burnouf-Radosevich et al., 1994; Maerz et al., 1996). A number of methods for reducing or inactivating viral contaminants are mentioned in Table 4 (Burnouf et al., 1989; Horowitz et al., 1991; Perret et al., 1991; Horowitz et al., 1994).

### Bacteria

Unwanted bacterial contamination may be a problem for cells in culture. Usually the size of bacteria allows simple sterile filtration for adequate removal. In order to further prevent bacterial contamination during production, the raw materials used have to be sterilized and the products are manufactured under strict aseptic conditions. Production most often takes place in so-called "clean rooms" in which the chances of environmental derived contamination is reduced through careful control of the environment, for example filtration of air. Additionally, antibiotic agents can be added to the culture media in some cases, but have to be removed further downstream in the purification process. The use of beta-lactam antibiotics such as penicillin is however strictly prohibited due to over-sensitivity of some individuals to these compounds. Because of the persistence of antibiotic residues, which are difficult to eliminate from the product, appropriately designed production plants and extensive quality control systems for added reagents (medium, serum, enzymes, etc.) permitting antibiotic-free operation are preferable.

Pyrogens (usually endotoxins of gram-negative bacteria) are potentially hazardous substances (cf. Chapter 4). Humans are sensitive to pyrogen contamination at very low concentrations (picograms per mL). Pyrogens may elicit a strong fever response and can even be fatal. Simple sterile filtration does not remove pyrogens. Removal is complicated further because pyrogens vary in size and chemical composition. However, sensitive tests to detect and quantify pyrogens are commercially available. Purification schemes usually contain at least one step of ion-exchange chromatography (anionic exchange material) to remove the negatively charged endotoxins (Nolan, 1975; Berthold and Walter, 1994). Furthermore, materials used in process such as glassware are typically subjected to a depyrogenation step prior to use often by the use of elevated temperatures (180°C) in a dry heat oven.

### Cellular DNA

The application of continuous mammalian cell lines for the production of recombinant proteins might result in the presence of oncogene-bearing DNA-fragments in the final protein product (Löwer, 1990; Walter and Werner, 1993). A stringent purification protocol that is capable of reducing the DNA content to a safe level is therefore necessary (Berthold and Walter, 1994). There are a number of approaches available to validate that the purification method removes cellular DNA and RNA. One such approach involves incubating the cell line with radiolabeled nucleotides and determining radioactivity in the purified product obtained through the purification protocol. Another method is dye-binding fluorescence-enhancement assay for nucleotides. If the presence of nucleic acids persists in a final

| Category | Types | Example |
|---|---|---|
| Inactivation | Heat treatment | Pasteurization |
| | Radiation | UV-light |
| | Dehydration | Lyophilization |
| | Cross linking agents, denaturing or disrupting agents | β-propiolactone, formaldehyde, NaOH, organic solvents (e.g., chloroform), detergents (e.g., Na-cholate) |
| | Neutralization | Specific, neutralizing antibodies |
| Removal | Chromatography | Ion-exchange, immuno-affinity, chromatography |
| | Filtration | Nanofiltration |
| | Precipitation | Cyroprecipitation |

**Table 4** ▪ Methods for reducing or inactivating viral contaminants.

preparation, then additional steps must be introduced in the purification process. The question about a safe level of nucleic acids in biotech products is difficult to answer because of the lack of relevant know-how. Transfection with so-called naked DNA is very difficult and a high concentration of DNA is needed. Nevertheless, it is agreed for safety reasons that final product contamination by nucleic acids should not exceed 100 pg to 10 ng per daily dose depending on the kind of culture system (Eur Pharm III, 1997; WHO, 1998; Kung et al., 1990).

*Protein Contaminants*

As mentioned before, trace amounts of "foreign" proteins may appear in biotech products. These types of contaminants are a potential health hazard because, if present, they may be recognized as antigens by the patient receiving the recombinant protein product. On repeated use the patient may show an immune reaction caused by the contaminant while the protein of interest is performing its beneficial function. In such cases the immunogenicity may be misinterpreted as being due to the recombinant protein itself. Therefore, one must be very cautious in interpreting safety data of a given recombinant therapeutic protein.

Generally, the sources of protein contaminants are the growth medium used or the host proteins of the cells. Among the host derived contaminants, the host species' version of the recombinant protein could be present (WHO, 1998). As these proteins are similar in structure, it is possible that undesired proteins are co-purified with the desired product. For example, urokinase is known to be present in many continuous cell lines. The synthesis of highly active biological molecules such as cytokines by hybridoma cells, might be another concern (FDA, 1990; Schindler and Dinarello, 1990). Depending upon their nature and concentration these cytokines might enhance the antigenicity of the product.

"Known" or expected contaminants should be monitored at the successive stages in a purification process by suitable in-process controls, e.g., sensitive immunoassay(s). Tracing of the many "unknown" cell-derived proteins is more difficult. When developing a purification process other, less specific analyses such as SDS-PAGE are usually used in combination with various staining techniques.

## DOWNSTREAM PROCESSING

Recovering a biological reagent from a cell culture supernatant is one of the critical parts of the manufacturing procedure for biotech products and purification costs typically outweigh those of the upstream part of the production process. For the production of monoclonal antibodies, Protein A resin accounts for some 10% of the cost while virus filtration can account for some 40% of the cost (Gottschalk, 2006).

Usually, the product is available in a very dilute form, e.g., 10 to 200 mg/L, but concentrations up to 500 to 800 mg/L can be reached (Berthold and Walter, 1994; Garnick et al., 1988). The prediction is that future development in cell culture technology through application of genetics and proteomics will result in product titers in the 5 to 10 g/L range which will challenge the capacity of the downstream processing unit operations (Werner, 2005).

A concentration step is often required to reduce handling volumes for further purification. Usually, the product subsequently undergoes a series of purification steps. The first step traditionally captures and initially purifies the product, the subsequent steps remove the bulk of the contaminants, and a final step removes all trace contaminants and variant forms of the molecule. Alternatively, the reverse strategy, where the main contaminants are captured and the product is purified in subsequent steps, might result in a more economic process, especially if the product is not excreted from the cells. In the former case the product will not represent more than 1% to 5% of total cellular protein and aspecific binding of the bulk of the protein in a product specific capture step will ruin its efficiency. If the bulk contaminants can be removed first, the specific capture step will be more efficient and smaller in size, thus cheaper, and chromatographic columns could be used. After purification, additional steps like formulation and sterilization are performed on the bulk product in order to obtain the required stable final product. Formulation aspects will be dealt with in Chapter 4.

When designing a purification protocol, the possibility for scaling up should be considered carefully. A process that has been designed for small quantities is most often not suitable for large quantities for both technical and economic reasons. Developing a downstream process (i.e., the isolation and purification of the desired product) to recover a biological protein in large quantities occurs in two stages: *design* and *scale-up*.

Separating the impurities from the product protein requires a series of purification steps (*process design*), each removing some of the impurities and bringing the product closer to its final specification. In general, the starting feedstock contains cell debris and/or whole-cell particulate material that must be removed. Defining the major contaminants in the starting material is helpful in the downstream process design. This includes detailed information on the source of the material (e.g., bacterial or mammalian cell culture) and major contaminants (e.g., albumin or product analogs). Moreover, the physical characteristics of the product versus the known contaminants (thermal stability, isoelectric point, molecular weight, hydrophobicity, density, specific binding properties) largely determine the process design. Processes used for production of therapeutics should be reproducible and reliable. Methods used for recovery may expose the protein molecules to high physical stress (e.g., high temperatures and extreme pH) which alter the protein properties leading to appreciable loss in protein activity. Any substance that is used by injection must be sterile and free from pyrogens below a certain level depending on the product (limits are stated in the individual monographs which are to be consulted, such as European Pharmacopoeia: less than 0.2 mg/kg/body mass for intrathecal application). This necessitates aseptic techniques and procedures throughout with clean air and microbial control of all materials and equipment. During validation of the purification process it must also be demonstrated that potential viral contaminants can be removed (Walter et al., 1992). The purification matrices should be at least sanitizable or, if possible steam-sterilizable. For depyrogenation, the purification material must withstand either extended dry heat at 180°C or treatment with 1 to 2 M sodium hydroxide (for further information see Chapter 4). If any material in contact with the product inadvertently releases compounds, these leachables must be analyzed and their removal by subsequent purification steps must be demonstrated during process validation. The increased use of plastic film based disposable production technology (e.g., sterile bags to store liquids and filter housings) has made these aspects more significant in the last 5 years and suppliers have reacted by providing a significant body of information regarding leachables and biocompatability for typical solutions used during processing. This problem of leachables is especially hampering the use of affinity chromatography (see below) in the production of pharmaceuticals for human use. On laboratory scale affinity chromatography is an important tool for purification and the resulting product might be used for toxicity studies, but for human use the removal of any leached ligands has to be demonstrated. Because free affinity ligands will bind to the product, the removal might be very cumbersome.

*Scale-up* is the term used to describe a number of processes employed in converting a laboratory procedure into an economical, industrial process. During the scale-up phase, the process moves from the laboratory scale to the pilot plant and finally to the production plant. The objective of scale-up is to produce a product of high quality at a competitive price. Since costs of downstream processing can be as high as 50% to 80% of the total cost of a product,

practical and economical ways of purifying the product should be used. Superior protein purification methods hold the key to a strong market position (Wheelwright, 1993).

Basic operations required for a downstream purification process used for macromolecules from biological sources are shown in Figure 2.

As mentioned before, the design of downstream processing is highly product dependent. Therefore, each product requires a specific multistage purification procedure (Sadana, 1989). The basic scheme as represented in Figure 2 becomes complex. A typical example of a process flow for the downstream processing is shown in Figure 3. This scheme represents the processing of a glycosylated recombinant interferon (about 28 kDa) produced in mammalian cells. The aims of the individual unit operations are described.

Once the volume and concentration of the product can be managed, the main purification phase can start. A number of purification methods are available to separate proteins on the basis of a wide variety of different physicochemical criteria such as size, charge, hydrophobicity and solubility. Detailed information about some separation and purification methods commonly used in purification schemes is provided below.

## ■ Filtration/Centrifugation

Products from biotechnological industry must be separated from biological systems that contain suspended particulate material, including whole cells, lysed cell material, and fragments of broken cells generated when cell breakage has been necessary to release intracellular products. Most downstream

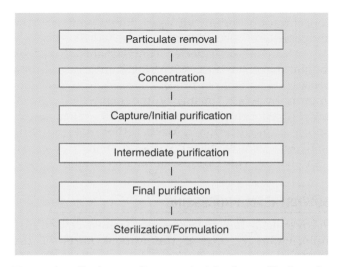

**Figure 2** ■ Basic operations required for the purification of a biopharmaceutical macromolecule.

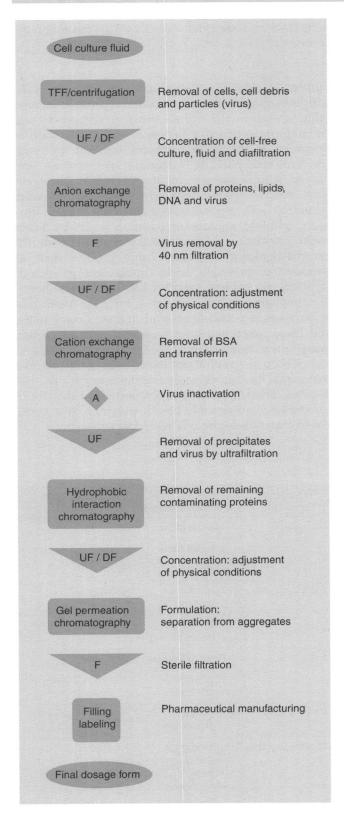

**Figure 3** ■ Downstream processing of a glycosylated recombinant interferon, describing the purpose of the inclusion of the individual unit operations. *Abbreviations*: A, adsorption; DF, diafiltration; F, filtration; TFF, tangential flow filtration; UF, ultrafiltration. *Source*: Adapted from Berthold and Walter, 1994.

processing flow sheets will, therefore, include at least one unit-operation for the removal ("clarification") or concentration, just the opposite, of particulates. Most frequently used methods are centrifugation and filtration techniques (e.g., ultrafiltration, diafiltration and microfiltration). However, the expense and effectiveness of such methods is highly dependent on the physical nature of the particulate material and of the product.

*Filtration*

Filtration can concentrate the biomass prior to further purification. Several filtration systems have been developed for separation of cells from media, the most successful being tangential flow systems (also referred to as "cross flow") where high shear across the membrane surface limits fouling, gel layer formation and concentration polarization. In ultrafiltration, mixtures of molecules of different molecular dimensions are separated by passage of a dispersion under pressure across a membrane with a defined pore size (Minton, 1990). In general, ultrafiltration achieves little purification, because of the relatively large pore size distribution of the membranes. However, this technique is widely used to concentrate macromolecules, and also to change the aqueous phase in which the particles are dispersed or in which molecules are dissolved (diafiltration) to one required for the subsequent purification steps.

*Centrifugation*

Subcellular particles and organelles, suspended in a viscous liquid (for example the particles produced when cells are disrupted by mechanical procedures) are difficult to separate either by using one fixed centrifugation step or by filtration. But, they can be isolated efficiently by centrifugation at different speeds. For instance, nuclei can be obtained by centrifugation at 400xg for 20 minutes, while plasma membrane vesicles are pelleted at higher centrifugation rates and longer centrifugation times (fractional centrifugation). In many cases, however, total biomass can easily be separated from the medium by centrifugation (e.g., continuous disc-stack centrifuge). Buoyant density centrifugation can be useful for separation of particles as well. This technique uses a viscous fluid with a continuous gradient of density in a centrifuge tube. Particles and molecules of various densities within the density range in the tube will cease to move when the isopycnic region has been reached. Both techniques of continuous (fluid densities within a range) and discontinuous (blocks of fluid with different density) density gradient centrifugation are used in buoyant density centrifugation on a laboratory scale. For application on the industrial scale, however, continuous centrifuges (e.g., tubular bowl centrifuges) are only used for discontinuous buoyant density centrifugation. This type of industrial centrifuge is mainly applied to recover precipitated proteins or contaminants.

## ■ Precipitation

The solubility of a particular protein depends on the physico-chemical environment, for example pH, ionic species and ionic strength of the solution (see Chapter 4). A slow continuous increase of the ionic strength (of a protein mixture) will selectively drive proteins out of solution. This phenomenon is known as "salting-out". A wide variety of agents, with different "salting out" potencies are available. Chaotropic series with increasing "salting out" effects of negatively (I) and positively (II) charged molecules are given below (von Hippel et al., 1964):

I $SCN^-$, $I^-$, $CLO_4^-$, $NO_3^-$, $Br^-$, $Cl^-$, $CH_3COO^-$, $PO_4^{3-}$, $SO_4^{2-}$

II $Ba^{2+}$, $Ca^{2+}$, $Mg^{2+}$, $Li^+$, $Cs^+$, $Na^+$, $K^+$, $Rb^+$, $NH_4^+$

Ammonium sulfate is highly soluble in cold aqueous solutions and is frequently used in "salting-out" purification.

Another method to precipitate proteins is to use water-miscible organic solvents (change in the dielectric constant). Examples of precipitating agents are polyethylene glycol and trichloracetic acid. Under certain conditions, chitosan and non-ionic polyoxyethylene detergents also induce precipitation (Cartwright, 1987; Homma et al., 1993; Terstappen et al., 1993). Precipitation is a scalable, simple and relatively economical procedure for the recovery of a product from a dilute feedstock. It has been widely used for the isolation of proteins from culture supernatants. Unfortunately, with most bulk precipitation methods, the gain in purity is generally limited. Moreover, extraneous components are introduced which must be eliminated later. Finally, large quantities of precipitates may be difficult to handle. Despite these limitations, recovery by precipitation has been used with considerable success for some products.

## ■ Chromatography

In preparative chromatography systems molecular species are primarily separated based on differences in distribution between two phases, one which is the stationary phase (mostly a solid phase) and the other which moves. This mobile phase may be liquid or gaseous (see Chapter 2). Nowadays, almost all stationary phases (fine particles providing a large surface area) are packed into a column. The mobile phase is passed through by pumps. Downstream purification protocols usually have at least two to three chromatography steps. Chromatographic methods used in purification procedures of biotech products are listed in Table 5 and are briefly discussed in the following sections.

### Chromatographic Stationary Phases

Chromatographic procedures often represent the rate-limiting step in the overall downstream processing. An important primary factor governing the rate of operation is the mass transport into the pores of conventional packing materials. Adsorbents employed include inorganic materials such as silica gels, glass beads, hydroxyapatite, various metal oxides (alumina) and organic polymers (cross-linked dextrans, cellulose, agarose). Separation occurs by differential interaction of sample components with the chromatographic medium. Ionic groups such as amines and carboxylic acids, dipolar groups such as carbonyl functional groups, and hydrogen bond-donating and accepting groups control the interaction of the sample components with the stationary phase and these functional groups slow down the elution rate if interaction occurs.

Chromatographic stationary phases for use on a large scale have improved considerably over the last decades. Hjerten et al. (1993) reported on the use of compressed acrylamide-based polymer structures. These materials allow relatively fast separations with

| Separation technique | Mode/principle | Separation based on |
|---|---|---|
| Membrane separation | Micofiltration | Size |
| | Ultrafiltration | Size |
| | Dialysis | Size |
| Centrifugation | Isopycnic banding | Density |
| | Non-equilibrium setting | Density |
| Extraction | Fluid extraction | Solubility |
| | Liquid/liquid extraction | Partition, change in solubility |
| Precipitation | Fractional precipitation | Change in solubility |
| Chromatography | Ion-excange Gel filtralion Affinity Hydrophobic interaction Adsorption | Charge Size Specific ligand-substrate interaction Hydrophobicity Covalent/noncovalent binding |

**Table 5** ▪ Frequently used separation processes and their physical bases.

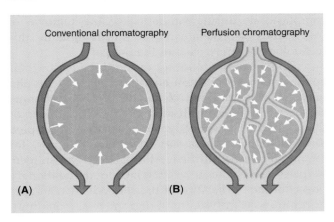

**Figure 4** ▪ The structure of conventional chromatographic particles **(A)** and perfusion or flow-though chromatographic particles **(B)**. *Source*: Adapted from Fulton, 1994.

good chromatographic performance. Another approach to the problems associated with mass transport in conventional systems is to use chromatographic particles that contain some large "through pores" in addition to conventional pores (Fig. 4). These flow-through or "perfusion chromatography" media enable faster convective mass transport into particles and allow operation at much higher speeds without loss in resolution or binding capacity (Afeyan et al., 1989; Fulton, 1994). Another development is the design of spirally wrapped columns containing the adsorption medium. This configuration permits high throughput, high capacity and good capture efficiency (Cartwright, 1987).

The ideal stationary phase for protein separation should possess a number of characteristics, among which are high mechanical strength, high porosity, no non-specific interaction between protein and the support phase, high capacity, biocompatibility and high stability of the matrix in a variety of solvents. The latter is especially true for columns used for the production of clinical materials that need to be cleaned, depyrogenized, disinfected and sterilized at regular intervals. High-performance liquid chromatography (HPLC) systems fulfill many of these criteria. Liquid phases should be carefully chosen to minimize loss of biological activity resulting from the use of some organic solvents. In HPLC small pore size stationary phases that are incompressible are used. These particles are small, rigid and regularly sized (to provide a high surface area). The mobile liquid phase is forced under high pressure through the column material. Reversed-phase HPLC systems, using less polar stationary phases than the mobile phases can be effectively integrated into large-scale purification schemes of proteins and can serve both as a means of concentration and purification (Benedek and Swadesh, 1991).

In production environments columns which operate at relatively low back pressure are often used. They have the advantage that they can be used in equipment constructed from plastics which, unlike conventional stainless steel equipment, resists all buffers likely to be employed in the separation of biomolecules (consider the effect of leachables mentioned earlier). These columns are commercially available and permit the efficient separation of proteins in a single run, making this an attractive unit operation in a manufacturing process. Results can be obtained rapidly and with high resolution. A new development is the use of stainless steel equipment that resists almost all chemicals used in protein purification including disinfection and sterilization media.

Unfortunately, HPLC equipment costs are high and this technology finds only limited application in large-scale purification schemes (Strickler and Gemski, 1987; Jungbauer and Wenisch, 1989).

### Adsorption Chromatography

In adsorption chromatography (also called "normal phase" chromatography) the stationary phase is more polar than the mobile phase. The protein of interest selectively binds to a static matrix under one condition and is released under a different condition (Chase, 1988). Adsorption chromatography methods enable high ratios of product load to stationary phase volume. Therefore, this principle is economically scalable.

### Ion-Exchange Chromatography

Ion-exchange chromatography can be a powerful step at the beginning of a purification scheme. It can be easily scaled up. Ion-exchange chromatography can be used in a negative mode, i.e., the product flows through the column under conditions that favor the adsorption of contaminants to the matrix, while the protein of interest does not bind (Tennikova and Svec, 1993). The type of the column needed is determined by the properties of the proteins to be purified (e.g., isoelectric point and charge density). Anion exchangers bind negatively charged molecules and cation exchangers bind positively charged molecules. In salt-gradient ion-exchange chromatography, the salt concentration in the perfusing elution buffer is increased continuously or in steps. The stronger the binding of an individual protein to the ion exchanger, the later it will appear in the elution buffer. Likewise, in pH-gradient chromatography, the pH is changed continuously or in steps. Here, the protein binds at one pH and is released at a different pH. As a result of the heterogeneity in glycosylation, glycosylated proteins may elute in a relatively broad pH range (up to 2 pH units).

In order to simplify purification, a specific amino acid tail can be added to the protein at the gene level to create a "purification handle". For example, a short tail consisting of arginine residues allows a protein to bind to a cation exchanger under conditions where almost no other cell proteins bind. However, this technique is only useful for laboratory scale isolation of the product and cannot be used for production scale due to regulatory problems related to the removal of the arginine or other specific tag from the protein.

*(Immuno)Affinity Chromatography*
Affinity chromatography is based on highly specific interactions between an immobilized ligand and the protein of interest. Affinity chromatography is a very powerful method for the purification of proteins. Under physiological conditions the protein binds to the ligand. Extensive washing of this matrix will remove contaminants and the purified protein can be recovered by the addition of ligands competing for the stationary phase binding sites or by changes in physical conditions (such as low or high pH of the eluent) which greatly reduce the affinity. Examples of affinity chromatography include the purification of glycoproteins, which bind to immobilized lectins and the purification of serine proteases with lysine binding sites, which bind to immobilized lysine. In these cases a soluble ligand (sugar or lysine, respectively) can be used to elute the required product under relatively mild conditions. Another example is the use of the affinity of protein A and protein G for antibodies. Protein A and protein G have a high affinity for the Fc portions of many immunoglobulins from various animals. Protein A and G matrices are commercially obtained with a high degree of purity. For the purification of e.g., hormones or growth factors, the receptors or short peptide sequence that mimic the binding site of the receptor molecule can be used as affinity ligands. Some proteins show highly selective affinity for certain dyes commercially available as immobilized ligands on purification matrices. When considering the selection of these ligands for pharmaceutical production, one must realize that some of these dyes are carcinogenic and that a fraction may leach out during the process.

An interesting approach to optimize purification is the use of a gene that codes not only for the desired protein, but also for an additional sequence that facilitates recovery by affinity chromatography. At a later stage the additional sequence is removed by a specific cleavage reaction. As mentioned before, this is a complex process that needs additional purification steps.

In general, use of affinity chromatography in the production process for therapeutics leads to complications during validation of the removal of free ligands or protein extensions. Consequently, this technology is rarely used in the industry.

The specific binding of antibodies to their epitopes is used in immunoaffinity chromatography (Chase, 1993; Kamihira et al., 1993). This technique can be applied for purification of either the antigen or the antibody. The antibody can be covalently coupled to the stationary phase and act as the "receptor" for the antigen to be purified. Alternatively, the antigen, or parts thereof, can be attached to the stationary phase for the purification of the antibody. Advantages of immunoaffinity chromatography are its high specificity and the combination of concentration and purification in one step.

A disadvantage associated with immunoaffinity methods is the sometimes very strong antibody–antigen binding. This requires harsh conditions during elution of the ligand. Under such conditions, sensitive ligands could be harmed (for example, by denaturation of the protein to be purified). This can be alleviated by (1) the selection of antibodies and environmental conditions with high specificity and sufficient affinity to induce an antibody ligand interaction, while the antigen can be released under mild conditions (Jones, 1990); (2) the use of tandem columns to change the physical conditions (e.g., pH and ionic strength) to more physiological conditions; (3) the use of a recipient solution into which the product is eluted. Another concern is disruption of the covalent bond linking the "receptor" to the matrix. This would result in elution of the entire complex. Therefore, in practice, a further purification step after affinity chromatography as well as an appropriate detection assay (e.g., ELISA) is almost always necessary. On the other hand, improved coupling chemistry that is less susceptible to hydrolysis has been developed to prevent leaching (Knight, 1990).

Scale-up of immunoaffinity chromatography is often hampered by the relatively large quantity of the specific "receptor" (either the antigen or the antibody) that is required and the lack of commercially available, ready-to-use matrices.

Examples of proteins of potential therapeutic value that have been purified using immunoaffinity chromatography are interferons, urokinase, factor VIII:C, erythropoietin, interleukin-2, human factor X, and recombinant tissue plasminogen activator.

*Hydrophobic Interaction Chromatography*
Under physiological conditions most hydrophobic amino acid residues are located inside the protein core and only a small fraction of hydrophobic amino acids is exposed on the "surface" of a protein. Their exposure is suppressed because of the presence of hydrophilic amino acids that attract large clusters of

water molecules and form a "shield". High salt concentrations reduce the hydration of a protein and the surface-exposed hydrophobic amino acid residues become more accessible. Hydrophobic interaction chromatography (HIC) is based on non-covalent and non-electrostatic interactions between proteins and the stationary phase. HIC is a mild technique, usually yielding high recoveries of proteins that are not damaged, are folded correctly and are separated from contaminants that are structurally related. HIC is ideally placed in the purification scheme after ion-exchange chromatography, where the protein usually is released in high ionic strength elution media (Heng and Glatz, 1993).

### Gel Permeation Chromatography

Gel-permeation or size-exclusion chromatography, also known as gel filtration, separates proteins according to their shape and size (Fig. 5). Inert gels with narrow pore-size distributions in the size range of proteins are available. These gels are packed into a column and the protein mixture is then loaded on top of the column and the proteins diffuse into the gel. The smaller the protein, the more volume it will have available in which to disperse. Molecules that are larger than the largest pores are not able to penetrate the gel beads and will therefore stay in the void volume of the column. When a continuous flow of buffer passes through the column, the larger proteins will elute first and the smallest molecules last. Gel permeation chromatography is a good alternative to

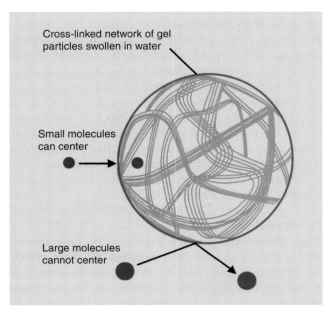

**Figure 5** ▪ Schematic representation of the principles of gel filtration. *Source*: Adapted from James, 1992.

diafiltration for buffer exchange at almost any purification stage, and it is often used in laboratory design. At production scale, the use of this technique is usually limited, because it requires relatively small sample volumes on a large column (up to one-third of the column volume in the case of "buffer exchange"). It is therefore best avoided or used late in the purification process when the protein is available in a highly concentrated form. Gel filtration is very commonly used as the final step in the purification to bring proteins in the appropriate buffer used in the final formulation. In this application, its use has little if no effect on the product purity characteristics.

### Expanded Beds

As mentioned before, purification schemes are based on multistep protocols. This not only adds greatly to the overall production costs, but also can result in significant loss of product. Therefore, there still is an interest in the development of new methods for simplifying the purification process. Adsorption techniques are popular methods for the recovery of proteins, and the conventional operating format for preparative separations is a packed column (or fixed bed) of adsorbent. Particulate material, however, can be trapped near the bed, which results in an increase in the pressure drop across the bed and eventually in clogging of the column. This can be avoided by the use of pre-column filters (0.2 μm) to save the column integrity. Another solution to this problem may be the use of expanded beds (Chase and Draeger, 1993; Fulton, 1994), also called fluidized beds (Fig. 6). In principle, the use of expanded beds enables clarification, concentration and purification to be achieved in a single step. The concept is to employ a particulate solid-phase adsorbent in an open bed with upward liquid flow. The hydrodynamic drag around the particles tends to lift them upwards, which is counteracted by gravity because of a density difference between the particles and the liquid phase. The particles remain suspended if particle diameter, particle density, liquid viscosity and liquid density are properly balanced by choosing the correct flow rate. The expanded bed allows particles (cells) to pass through, whereas molecules in solution are selectively retained (for example, by the use of ion-exchange or affinity adsorbents) on the adsorbent particles. Feedstocks can be applied to the bed without prior removal of particulate material by centrifugation or filtration, thus reducing process time and costs. Fluidized beds have been used previously for the industrial scale recovery of antibiotics such as streptomycin and novobiocin (Chase, 1994; Fulton, 1994). Stable, expanded beds can be obtained using simple equipment adapted from that used for conventional, packed bed adsorption and

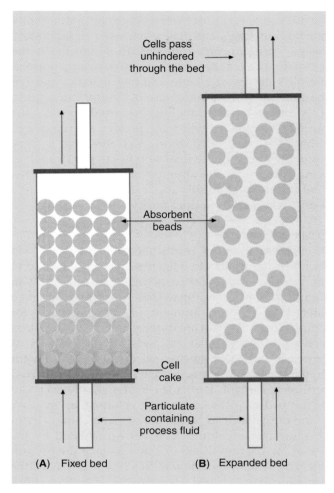

**Figure 6** ■ Comparison between **(A)** a packed bed and **(B)** an expanded bed. *Source*: Adapted from Chase and Draeger, 1993.

chromatography processes. Ion-exchange adsorbents are likely to be chosen for such separations.

## ISSUES TO CONSIDER IN PRODUCTION AND PURIFICATION OF PROTEINS

### ■ N- and C-Terminal Heterogeneity

A major problem connected with the production of biotech products is the problem associated with the amino (NH2)-terminus of the protein e.g., in *E. coli* systems, where protein synthesis always starts with f-methyl-methionine. Obviously, it has been of great interest to develop methods (Christensen et al., 1990) that generate proteins with an NH2-terminus as found in the authentic protein. When the proteins are not produced in the correct way, the final product may contain several methionyl variants of the protein in question or even contain proteins lacking one or more residues from the amino terminus. This is called the amino terminal heterogeneity. This heterogeneity can also occur with recombinant proteins (e.g.,

α-interferon) susceptible to proteases that are either secreted by the host or introduced by serum-containing media. These proteases can clip off amino acids from the C-terminal and/or N-terminal of the desired product (amino- and/or carboxy-terminal heterogeneity) (Garnick et al., 1988).

Amino- and/or carboxy-terminal heterogeneity is not desirable since it may cause difficulties in purification and characterization of the proteins. In case of the presence of an additional methionine at the N-terminal end of the protein, its secondary and tertiary structure can be altered. This could affect the biological activity and stability and may make it immunogenic. Moreover, N-terminal methionine and/or internal methionine are sensitive to oxidation (Sharma, 1990).

### ■ Chemical Modification/Conformational Changes

Although mammalian cells are able to produce proteins structurally equal to endogenous proteins, some caution is advisable. Transcripts containing the full-length coding sequence could result in conformational isomers of the protein because of unexpected secondary structures that affect translational fidelity (Sharma, 1990). Another factor to be taken into account is the possible existence of equilibria between the desired form and other forms such as dimers. The correct folding of proteins after biosynthesis is important, because it determines the specific activity of the protein (Berthold and Walter, 1994). Therefore, it is important to determine if all molecules of a given recombinant protein secreted by a mammalian expression system are folded in their native conformation. In some cases it may be relatively easy to detect misfolded structures, but in other cases it may be extremely difficult. Sometimes selection and purification of the native protein may require the development of novel preparative and analytical technologies for process development and quality assurance.

Apart from conformational changes, proteins can undergo chemical alterations, such as proteolysis, deamidation, hydroxyl and sulfhydryl oxidations during the purification process. These alterations can result in (partial) denaturation of the protein. Vice versa, denaturation of the protein may cause chemical modifications as well (e.g., as a result of exposure of sensitive groups) (Ptitsyn, 1987).

### ■ Glycosylation

Many therapeutic proteins produced by recombinant DNA technology are glycoproteins (Sharma, 1990). The presence and nature of oligosaccharide side chains in proteins affect a number of important characteristics, like the proteins' serum half-life, solubility, stability and sometimes even the pharmacological function (Cumming, 1991). Darbepoietin, a second generation, genetically modified erythropoietin, has a carbohydrate content of 80% compared to 40% for the native molecule, which increases the in vivo half-life after intravenous administration from 8 hours for erythropoietin to 25 hours for darbepoietin (Sinclair and Elliott, 2005).

As a result, the therapeutic profile may be "glycosylation" dependent. As mentioned previously, protein glycosylation is not determined by the DNA sequence. It is an enzymatic modification of the protein after translation, and can depend on the environment in the cell. Although mammalian cells are very well able to glycosylate proteins, it is hard to fully control glycosylation. Carbohydrate heterogeneity is detected by variations in the size of the chain, type of oligosaccharide, and sequence of the carbohydrates. This has been demonstrated for a number of recombinant products including interleukin-4, chorionic gonadotropin, erythropoietin and tissue plasminogen activator. Carbohydrate structure and composition in recombinant proteins may differ from their native counterparts, because the enzymes required for synthesis and processing vary among different expression systems (e.g., glycoproteins in insect cells are frequently smaller than the same glycoproteins expressed in mammalian cells) or even from one mammalian system to another.

## ■ Proteolytic Processing

Proteases play an important role in processing, maturation, modification, or isolation of recombinant proteins (Sharma and Hopkins, 1981). Proteases from mammalian cells are involved in secreting proteins into the cultivation medium. If secretion of the recombinant protein occurs co-translationally, then the intracellular proteolytic system of the mammalian cell should not be harmful to the recombinant protein. Proteases are released if cells die or break (e.g., during cell break at cell harvest) and undergo lysis. It is therefore important to control growth and harvest conditions in order to minimize this effect. Another source of proteolytic attack is found in the components of the medium in which the cells are grown. For example, serum contains a number of proteases and protease zymogens that may affect the secreted recombinant protein. If present in small amounts, and if the nature of the proteolytic attack on the desired protein is identified, appropriate protease inhibitors to control proteolysis could be used. It is best to document the integrity of the recombinant protein after each purification step.

Proteins become much more susceptible to proteases at elevated temperatures. Purification strategies should be designed to carry out all the steps at 4°C (Sharma, 1990) if proteolytic degradation occurs.

Alternatively, $Ca^{2+}$ complexing agents (e.g., citrate) can be added as many proteases depend on $Ca^{2+}$ for their activity. From a manufacturing perspective, however, providing cooling to large scale chromatographic processes, although not impossible, is a complicating factor in the manufacturing process.

## ■ Protein Inclusion Body Formation

In bacteria soluble proteins can form dense, finely granular inclusions within the cytoplasm. These "inclusion bodies" often occur in bacterial cells that overproduce proteins by plasmid expression. The protein inclusions appear in electron micrographs as large, dense bodies often spanning the entire diameter of the cell. Protein inclusions are probably formed by a build-up of amorphous protein aggregates held together by covalent and non-covalent bonds. The inability to measure inclusion body proteins directly may lead to the inaccurate assessment of recovery and yield and may cause problems if protein solubility is essential for efficient, large-scale purification (Berthold and Walter, 1994). Several schemes for recovery of proteins from inclusion bodies have been described (Krueger et al., 1989). The recovery of proteins from inclusion bodies requires cell breakage and inclusion body recovery. Dissolution of inclusion proteins is the next step in the purification scheme and typically takes place in extremely dilute solutions which tend to have the effect of increasing the volumes of the unit operations during the manufacturing phases. This can make process control more difficult if for example low temperatures are required during these steps. Generally, inclusion proteins dissolve in denaturing agents such as sodium dodecylsulfate (SDS), urea, or guanidine hydrochloride. Because bacterial systems generally are incapable of forming disulfide bonds, a protein containing these bonds has to be re-folded under oxidizing conditions to restore these bonds and to generate the biologically active protein. This so-called renaturation step is increasingly difficult if more S–S bridges are present in the molecule and the yield of renatured product could be as low as only a few percent. Once the protein is solubilized, conventional chromatographic separations can be used for further purification of the protein.

Aggregate formation at first sight may seem undesirable, but there may also be advantages as long as the protein of interest will unfold and refold properly. Inclusion body proteins can easily be recovered to yield proteins with >50% purity, a substantial improvement over the purity of soluble proteins (sometimes below 1% of the total cell protein). Furthermore, the aggregated forms of the proteins are more resistant to proteolysis (Krueger et al., 1989), because most molecules of an aggregated form are not accessible to proteolytic enzymes. Thus the high yield and relatively cheap production using a bacterial system can offset a low yield renaturation process. For a non-glycosylated, simple molecule this is still the production system of choice.

## REFERENCES

Afeyan N, Gordon N, Mazsaroff I, et al. (1989). Flow-through particles of the high-performance liquid chromatographic separation of biomolecules, perfusion chromatography. J Chromatogr 519:1–29.

Arathoon WR, Birch JR (1986). Large-scale cell culture in biotechnology. Science 232:1390–95.

Benedek K, Swadesh JK (1991). HPLC of proteins and peptides in the pharmaceutical industry. In: Fong GW, Lam SK, eds. HPLC in the Pharmaceutical Industry. New York: Dekker, 241–302.

Berthold W, Walter J (1994). Protein purification: Aspects of processes for pharmaceutical products. Biologicals 22:135–50.

Borman S (2006). Glycosylation engineering. Chem Eng News 84:13–22.

Burnouf T, Dernis D, Michalski C, Goudemand M, Huart JJ (1989). Therapeutic advantages of a high purity plasma factor IX concentrate produced by conventional chromatography. Colloque Inserm 175:25–334.

Burnouf-Radosevich M, Appourchaux P, Huart JJ, Burnouf T (1994). Nanofiltration, a new specific virus elimination method applied to high-purity Factor IX and Factor XI concentrates. Vox Sang 67:132–8.

Cartwright T (1987). Isolation and purification of products from animal cells. Trend Biotechnol 5:25–30.

Chase HA (1988). Adsorption preparation processes for protein purification. In: Mizrahi A, ed. Downstream processes: Equipment and techniques, Vol. 8. New York: A.R. Liss, 163–312.

Chase HA (1994). Purification of proteins by adsorption chromatography in expanded beds. Tibtech 12:296–303.

Chase H, Draeger N (1993). Affinity purification of proteins using expanded beds. J. Chromatogr 597:129–45.

Christensen T, Dalboge H, Snel L (1990). Postbiosynthesis modification: Human growth hormone and insulin precursors. In: Drug Manufacture, Part IV.

Cumming DA (1991). Glycosylation of recombinant protein therapeutics: Control and functional implications. Glycobiology 1(2):115–30.

European Agency for the Evaluation of Medicinal Products (EMEA, 1997), Human Medicines Evaluation Unit. ICH Topic Q5D. Quality of biotechnological products: Derivation and characterisation of cell substrates used for production of biotechnological/biological products.

European Agency for the Evaluation of Medicinal Products (EMEA, 1999a). Note for guidance on minimising the risk of transmission of animal/spongiform encephalopathy agents.

European Agency for the Evaluation of Medicinal Products (EMEA, 1999b). Human Medicines Evaluation Unit.

ICH Topic Q6B. Specifications test procedures and acceptance criteria for biotechnology/biological products.

European Pharmacopoeia (1997).3rd ed. Strasbourg: Council of Europe.

FDA, Center for Biologics Evaluation and Research (1990) Cytokine and growth factor pre-Ppivotal Ttrial information Ppackage with special emphasis on products identified for consideration under 21 CFR 312 Subpart E, Bethesda, MD, USA.

FDA, Office of Biologicals Research and Review (1993) Points to consider in the characterization of cell lines used to produce biologicals, Rockville Rike, Bethesda, MD, USA.

Fulton SP (1994). Large scale processing of macromolecules. Curr Opin Biotechnol 5:201–5.

Garnick RL, Solli NJ, Papa PA (1988). The role of quality control in biotechnology: An analytical perspective. Anal Chem 60:2546–57.

Gottschalk U (2006). The renaissance of protein purification. BioPharm Int, June.

Heng M, Glatz C (1993). Charged fusions for selective recovery of β-galactosidase from cell extract using hollow fiber ion-exchange membrane adsorption. Biotechnol Bioeng 42:333–8.

Hippel von PH, Wong K-Y (1964). Neutral salts: The generality of their effects on the stability of macromolecular conformations. Science 145:577–80.

Hjerten S, Mohammed J, Nakazato K (1993). Improvement in flow properties and pH stability of compressed, continuous polymer beds for high-performance liquid chromatography. J Chromatogr 646:121–8.

Hodge G (2004). Disposable components enable a new approach to biopharmaceutical manufacturing. BioPharm Int 15:38–49.

Homma T, Fuji M, Mori J, Kawakami T, Kuroda K, Taniguchi M (1993). Production of cellobiose by enzymatic hydrolysis: removal of β-glucosidae from cellulase by affinity precipitation using chitosan. Biotechnol Bioeng 41:405–10.

Horowitz MS, Bolmer SD, Horowitz B (1991). Elimination of disease-transmitting enveloped viruses from human blood plasma and mammalian cell culture products. Bioseperation 1:409–417.

Horowitz B, Prince AM, Hamman J, Watklevicz C (1994). Viral safety of solvent/detergent-treated blood products. Blood Coagulation and Fibrinolysis 5:S21–8.

James AM (1992). Introduction fundamental techniques. In: James AM, ed. Analysis of Amino Acids and Nucleic Acids. Oxford: Butterworth-Heinemann, 1–28.

Jones K (1990). Affinity chromatography, A technology update. Am Biotechnol Lab 8:26–30.

Jungbauer A, Wenisch E (1989). High performance liquid chromatography and related methods in purification of monoclonal antibodies. In: Advances in Biotechnological Processes. New York, Liss, pp. 161–92.

Kamihira M, Kaul R, Mattiasson B (1993). Purification of recombinant protein A by aqueous two-phase extraction integrated with affinity precipitation. Biotechnol Bioeng 40:1381–87.

Klegerman ME, Groves MJ (1992). Pharmaceutical Biotechnology. USA: Interpharm Press, Inc.

Knight P (1990). Bioseparations: Media and Modes. Biotechnology 8:200.

Krueger JK, Kulke MH, Schutt C, Stock J (1989). Protein inclusion body formation and purification. Pharmaceut Technol Int, 48–51.

Kung VT, Panfili PR, Sheldon EL, et al. (1990). Picogram quantification of total DNA using DNA-binding proteins in a silicon sensor based system. Anal Biochem 187:220–7.

Liptrot C, Gull K (1991). Detection of viruses in recombinant cells by electron microscopy. In: Spier RE, Griffiths JB, MacDonald C, eds. Animal Cell Technology, Developments, Processes and Products. Oxford: Butterworth-Heinemann Ltd, 653–6.

Löwer J (1990). Risk of tumor induction in vivo by residual cellular DNA: Quantitative Considerations. J Med Virol 31:50–3.

Maerz H, Hahn SO, Maassen A, et al. (1996). Improved removal of viruslike particles from purified monoclonal antibody IgM preparation via virus filtration. Nat Biotechnol 14:651–2.

Marcus-Sekura CJ (1991). Validation and Removal of Human Retroviruses. Center for Biologics Evaluation and Research. Bethesda, MD: FDA.

Minton AP (1990). Quantitative characterization of reversible molecular associations via analytical centrifugation. Anal Biochem 190:1–6.

Minor PD (1994). Ensuring safety and consistency in cell culture production processes: Viral screening and inactivation. TIB TECH 12:257–61.

Nolan JG, McDevitt JJ, Goldmann GS (1975). Endotoxin binding by charged and uncharged resin. Proc Soc Exp Biol Med 149:766–70.

Note for Guidance (1991). Validation of Virus Removal and Inactivation Procedure, Ad Hoc Working Party on Biotechnology/Pharmacy, European Community, DG III/8115/89-EN.

Pearson FC (1987). Pyrogens and depyrogenation, theory and practice. In: Olson WP, Groves MJ, eds. Aseptic Pharmaceutical Manufacturing. Prairie View: Interpharm Press Inc.

Perret BA, Poorbeik M, Morell A (1991). Klinische prüfung von Premogfil M SRK, einem mit monoklonalen antikörpern hochgereinigten gerinningsfaktor VIII-Konzentrat aus humanplasma. Schweiz Med Wochenschr, 121:1624–7.

PDA Journal of Pharmaceutical Science and Technology (2005), Technical report No. 41, Virus Filtration, March/April, Vol. 59, No. S-2.

Ptitsyn OB (1987). Protein folding: Hypothesis and experiments. J Protein Chem 6:273–93.

Sadana A (1989). Protein inactivation during downstream separation, Part I: The processes. Biopharm 2:14–25.

Schindler R, Dinarello CA (1990). Ultrafiltration to remove endotoxins and other cytokine-inducing materials from tissue culture media and parenteral fluids. Bio Techniques 8:408–13.

Sharma SK (1990). Key issues in the purification and characterization of recombinant proteins for therapeutic use. Adv Drug Deliv Rev 4:87–111.

Sharma SK, Hopkins TR (1981). Recent developments in the activation process of bovine chymotrypsinogen. Bioorganic Chem 10:357–74.

Sinclair AM, Elliott S (2005). Glycoengineering: The effect of glycosylation on the properties of therapeutic proteins. J. Pharm.Sci 94:1626–35.

Strickler MP, Gemski MJ (1987). Commercial production of monoclonal antibodies. New York: Marcel Dekker, 217–45.

Tennikova T, Svec F (1993). High performance membrane chromatography: Highly efficient separation method for proteins in ion-exchange, hydrophobic interaction and reversed phase modes. J Chromatogr 646:279–88.

Terstappen G, Ramelmeier R, Kula M (1993). Protein partitioning in detergent-based aqueous two-phase systems. J Biotechnol 28:263–75.

Walter J, Werner RG (1993). Regulatory requirements and economic aspects in downstream processing of biotechnically engineered proteins for parenteral application as pharmaceuticals. In: Kroner KH, Papamichael N, Schütte H, eds. Downstream Processing, Recovery and Purification of Proteins, A Handbook of Principles and Practice. New York: John Wiley Publishers Inc.

Walter J, Werz W, McGoff P, Werner RG, Berthold W (1991). Virus removal/inactivation in downstream processing. In: Spier RE, Griffiths JB, MacDonald C, eds. Animal Cell Technology: Development, Processes and Products. Linacre House, Oxford: Butterworth-Heinemann Ltd. 624–34.

Walter K, Werz W, Berthold W (1992). Virus removal and inactivation, concept and data for process validation of downstream processing. Biotech. Forum Europe 9:560–4.

Werner R (2005). The development and production of biopharmaceuticals: Technological and economic success factors. Bioprocess Int 3(9 Suppl):6–15.

Wheelwright SM (1993). Designing downstream processing for large scale protein purification. Biotechnology 5:789–93.

White EM, Grun JB, Sun C-S, Sito F (1991). Process validation for virus removal and inactivation. BioPharm 34–9.

World Health Organization (1998). Requirements for the use of animal cells as in vitro substrates for the production of biologicals (Requirements for Biological Substances No. 50). Technical Report Series 878: Biologicals 26:175–93.

World Health Organization. Guidelines for assuring the quality of pharmaceutical and biological products prepared by recombinant DNA technology. Technical Report Series 823:105–15.

# 4

# Formulation of Biotech Products, Including Biopharmaceutical Considerations

*Daan J. A. Crommelin*
Utrecht University, Utrecht and Dutch Top Institute Pharma, Leiden, The Netherlands

## INTRODUCTION

This chapter deals with formulation aspects of pharmaceutical proteins. Both technological questions and biopharmaceutical issues such as the choice of the delivery systems, the route of administration and possibilities for target site-specific delivery of proteins are considered.

## MICROBIOLOGICAL CONSIDERATIONS

### ■ Sterility

Most proteins are administered parenterally and have to be sterile. In general, proteins are sensitive to heat and other regularly used sterilization treatments; they cannot withstand autoclaving, gas sterilization, or sterilization by ionizing radiation. Consequently, sterilization of the end product is not possible. Therefore, protein pharmaceuticals have to be assembled under aseptic conditions, following the established and evolving rules in the pharmaceutical industry for aseptic manufacture. The reader is referred to standard textbooks for details (Halls, 1994; Groves, 1988; Klegerman and Groves, 1992).

Equipment and excipients are treated separately and autoclaved, or sterilized by dry heat ($>160°C$), chemical treatment or gamma radiation to minimize the bioburden. Filtration techniques are used for removal of microbacterial contaminants. Prefilters remove the bulk of the bioburden and other particulate materials. The final "sterilizing" step before filling the vials is filtration through 0.2 or 0.22 µm membrane filters. Assembly of the product is done in class 100 (maximum 100 particles $>0.5$ µm per cubic foot) rooms with laminar airflow that is filtered through high efficiency particulate air (HEPA) filters. Last but not least, the "human factor" is a major source of contamination. Well-trained operators wearing protective cloths (face masks, hats, gowns, gloves, or head-to-toe overall garments) should operate the facility. Regular exchange of filters, regular validation of HEPA equipment and thorough cleaning of the room plus equipment are critical factors for success.

### ■ Viral Decontamination

As recombinant DNA products are grown in microorganisms, these organisms should be tested for viral contaminants and appropriate measures should be taken if viral contamination occurs. In the rest of the manufacturing process, no (unwanted) viral material should be introduced. Excipients with a certain risk factor such as blood-derived human serum albumin should be carefully tested before use and their presence in the formulation process should be minimized (see Chapter 3).

### ■ Pyrogen Removal

Pyrogens are compounds that induce fever. Exogenous pyrogens (pyrogens introduced into the body, not generated by the body itself) can be derived from bacterial, viral or fungal sources. Bacterial pyrogens are mainly endotoxins shed from gram-negative bacteria. They are lipopolysaccharides. A general structure is shown in Figure 1. The basic, conserved structure in the full array of thousands of different endotoxins is the lipid A-moiety. Another general property shared by endotoxins is their high, negative electrical charge. Their tendency to aggregate and to form large units with MW of over $10^6$ in water and their tendency to adsorb to surfaces indicate that these compounds are amphipathic in nature. They are stable under standard autoclaving conditions, but break down when heated in the dry state. For this reason equipment and container are treated at temperatures above 160°C for prolonged periods (e.g., 30 minutes dry heat at 250°C).

Pyrogen removal of recombinant products derived from bacterial sources should be an integral part of the preparation process. Ion exchange chromatographic procedures (utilizing its negative charge) can effectively reduce endotoxin levels in solution (see Chapter 3).

Excipients used in the protein formulation should be essentially endotoxin free. For solutions "Water for Injection" (compendial standards) is (freshly) distilled or produced by reverse osmosis.

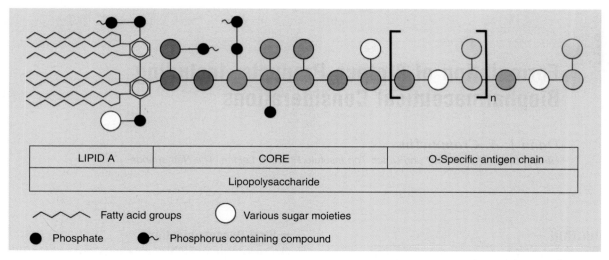

LIPID A | CORE | O-Specific antigen chain

Lipopolysaccharide

~~ Fatty acid groups ○ Various sugar moieties

● Phosphate ●~ Phosphorus containing compound

**Figure 1** ■ Generalized structure of endotoxins. Most properties of endotoxins are accounted for by the active, insoluble "lipid A" fraction being solubilized by the various sugar moieties (*different colored circles*). Although the general structure is similar, individual endotoxins vary according to their source and are characterized by the O-specific antigenic chain. *Source*: Adapted from Groves, 1988.

The aggregated endotoxins cannot pass through the reverse osmosis membrane. Removal of endotoxins immediately before filling the final container can be accomplished by using activated charcoal or other materials with large surfaces offering hydrophobic interactions. Endotoxins can also be inactivated on utensil surfaces by oxidation (e.g., peroxide) or dry heating (e.g., 30 minutes dry heat at 250°C).

## EXCIPIENTS USED IN PARENTERAL FORMULATIONS OF BIOTECH PRODUCTS

In a protein formulation one finds, apart from the active substance, a number of excipients selected to serve different purposes. This process of formulation design should be carried out with great care to ensure therapeutically effective and safe products. The nature of the protein (e.g., lability) and its therapeutic use (e. g., multiple injection systems) can make these formulations quite complex in terms of excipient profile and technology (freeze-drying, aseptic preparation). Table 1 lists components that can be found in the presently marketed formulations. In the following sections this list is discussed in more detail.

### ■ Solubility Enhancers

Proteins, in particular those that are non-glycosylated, may have a tendency to aggregate and precipitate. Approaches that can be used to enhance solubility include selection of the proper pH and ionic strength conditions. Addition of amino acids such as lysine or arginine (used to solubilize tissue plasminogen activator, t-PA), or surfactants such as sodium dodecylsulfate to solubilize non-glucosylated IL-2 can also help to increase the solubility. The

mechanism of action of these solubility enhancers depends on the type of enhancer and the protein involved and is not always fully understood.

Figure 2 shows the effect of arginine concentration on the solubility of t-PA (alteplase) at pH 7.2 and 25°C. This figure clearly indicates the dramatic effect of this basic amino acid on the apparent solubility of t-PA.

In the above examples, aggregation is physical in nature, i.e. based on hydrophobic and/or electrostatic interactions between molecules. However, aggregation based on the formation of covalent bridges between molecules through disulfide bonds, and ester or amide linkages has been described as well (see Table 4). In those cases, proper conditions should be found to avoid these chemical reactions.

### ■ Anti-Adsorption and Anti-Aggregation Agents

Anti-adsorption agents are added to reduce adsorption of the active protein to interfaces. Some proteins tend to expose hydrophobic sites, normally present in

---

■ Active ingredient
■ Solubility enhancers
■ Anti-adsorption and anti-aggregation agents
■ Buffer components
■ Preservatives and antioxidants
■ Lyoprotectants/cake formers
■ Osmotic agents
■ Carrier system (see later in this chapter)

**Table 1** ■ Components found in parenteral formulations of biotech products. All of the above are not necessarily present in one particular protein formulation.

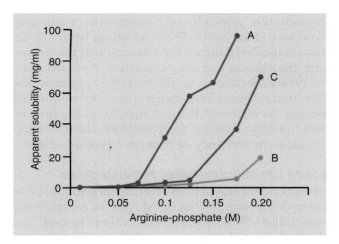

**Figure 2** ■ Effect of arginine on type I and type II alteplase at pH 7.2 and 25°C. A, type I alteplase; B, type II alteplase; C, 50:50 mixture of type I and type II alteplase. *Source*: From Nguyen and Ward, 1993.

the core of the native protein structure when an interface is present. These interfaces can be water/air, water/container wall or interfaces formed between the aqueous phase and utensils used to administer the drug (e.g., catheter, needle). These adsorbed, partially unfolded protein molecules form aggregates, leave the surface, return to the aqueous phase, form larger aggregates and precipitate. As an example, the proposed mechanism for aggregation of insulin in aqueous media through contact with a hydrophobic surface (or water–air interface) is presented in Figure 3 (Thurow and Geisen, 1984).

Native insulin in solution is in an equilibrium state between monomeric, dimeric tetrameric, and hexameric forms (see Chapter 12). The relative abundance of the different aggregation states depends on the pH, insulin concentration, ionic strength, and specific excipients (e.g., $Zn^{2+}$ and phenol). It has been suggested that the dimeric form of insulin adsorbs to hydrophobic interfaces and subsequently forms larger

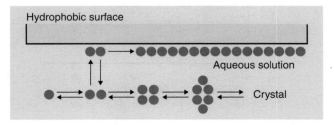

**Figure 3** ■ Reversible self-association of insulin, its adsorption to the hydrophobic interface and irreversible aggregation in the adsorbed protein films. Each circle represents a monomeric insulin molecule. *Source*: Adapted from Thurow and Geisen, 1984.

aggregates at the interface. This explains why anti-adhesion agents can also act as anti-aggregation agents. Albumin has a strong tendency to adsorb to surfaces and is therefore added in relatively high concentrations (e.g., 1%) to protein formulations as an anti-adhesion agent. Albumin competes with the therapeutic protein for binding sites and supposedly prevents adhesion of the therapeutically active agent by a combination of its binding tendency and abundant presence.

Insulin is one of the many proteins that can form fibrillar precipitates (long rod-shaped structures with diameters in the 0.1 μm range). Low concentrations of phospholipids and surfactants have been shown to exert a fibrillation-inhibitory effect. The selection of the proper pH can also help to prevent this unwanted phenomenon (Brange and Langkjaer, 1993).

Apart from albumin, surfactants can also prevent adhesion to interfaces and precipitation. These molecules readily adsorb to hydrophobic interfaces with their own hydrophobic groups and render this interface hydrophilic by exposing their hydrophilic groups to the aqueous phase.

### ■ Buffer Components

Buffer selection is an important part of the formulation process, because of the pH dependence of protein solubility and physical and chemical stability. Buffer systems regularly encountered in biotech formulations are phosphate, citrate, and acetate. A good example of the importance of the isoelectric point (its negative logarithm is equal to pI) is the solubility profile of human growth hormone (hGH, pI around 5) as presented in Figure 4.

Even short, temporary pH changes can cause aggregation. These conditions can occur, for example during the freezing step in a freeze-drying process, when one of the buffer components is crystallizing and the other is not. In a phosphate buffer, $Na_2HPO_4$ crystallizes faster than $NaH_2PO_4$. This causes a pronounced drop in pH during the freezing step. Other buffer components do not crystallize, but form amorphous systems and then pH changes are minimized.

### ■ Preservatives and Antioxidants

Methionine, cysteine, tryptophan, tyrosine, and histidine are amino acids that are readily oxidized (Table 4 in Chapter 2). Proteins rich in these amino acids are liable to oxidative degradation. Replacement of oxygen by inert gases in the vials helps to reduce oxidative stress. Moreover, the addition of antioxidants such as ascorbic acid or acetylcysteine can be considered. Interestingly, destabilizing effects on proteins have been described for antioxidants as well (Vemuri et al., 1993b). Ascorbic acid, for example, can

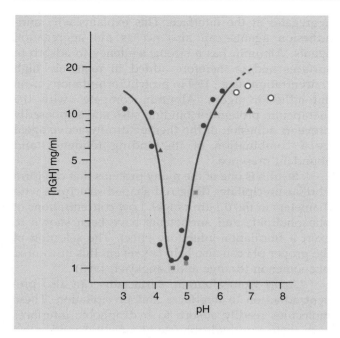

**Figure 4** ▢ A plot of the solubility of various forms of hGH as a function of pH. Samples of hGH were either recombinant hGH (*circles*), Met-hGH (*triangles*) or pituitary hGH (*squares*). Solubility was determined by dialyzing an approximately 11 mg/ml solution of each protein into an appropriate buffer for each pH. Buffers were citrate, pH 3–7, and borate, pH 8–9, all were at 10 mM buffer concentrations. Concentrations of hGH were measured by UV absorbance as well as by RP-HPLC, relative to an external standard. Closed symbols indicate that precipitate was present in the dialysis tube after equilibration; open symbols mean that no solid material was present, and thus the solubility is at least this amount. *Source*: From Pearlman and Bewley, 1993.

act as an oxidant in the presence of a number of heavy metals.

Certain proteins are formulated in containers designed for multiple injection schemes. After administering the first dose, contamination with microorganisms may occur and preservatives are needed to minimize growth. Usually, these preservatives are present in concentrations that are bacteriostatic rather than bactericidal in nature. Antimicrobial agents mentioned in the USP 29 are the mercury-containing phenylmercuric nitrate and thimerosal and p-hydroxybenzoic acids, phenol, benzyl alcohol and chlorobutanol (USP 29; Groves, 1988; Pearlman and Bewley, 1993). The use of mercury containing preservatives is presently under discussion (FDA, 2006).

## ■ Osmotic Agents

For proteins the regular rules apply for adjusting the tonicity of parenteral products. Saline and mono- or disaccharide solutions are commonly used. These excipients may not be inert; they may influence protein structural stability. For example, sugars and polyhydric alcohols can stabilize the protein structure

through the principle of "preferential exclusion" (Arakawa et al., 1991). These additives (water structure promoters) enhance the interaction of the solvent with the protein and are themselves excluded from the protein surface layer; the protein is preferentially hydrated. This phenomenon can be monitored through an increased thermal stability of the protein. Unfortunately, a strong "preferential exclusion" effect enhances the tendency of proteins to self-associate.

## ■ Shelf Life of Protein-Based Pharmaceuticals

Proteins can be stored (*i*) as an aqueous solution, (*ii*) in freeze-dried form, (*iii*) in dried form in a compacted state (tablet). Some mechanisms behind chemical and physical degradation processes have been briefly discussed in Chapter 2.

Stability of protein solutions strongly depends on factors such as pH, ionic strength, temperature, and the presence of stabilizers. For example, Figure 5 shows the pH dependence of $\alpha_1$-antitrypsin and clearly demonstrates the critical importance of pH for the shelf life of proteins.

## ■ Freeze Drying of Proteins

Proteins in solution often do not meet the preferred stability requirements for industrially produced pharmaceutical products (>2 years), even when kept permanently under refrigerator conditions (cold chain). The abundant presence of water promotes chemical and physical degradation processes.

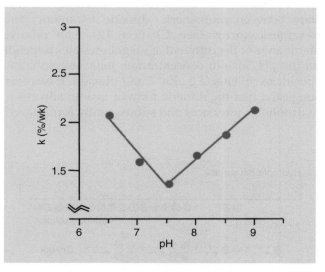

**Figure 5** ▢ pH stability profile (at 25°C) of monomeric recombinant $\alpha_1$-antitrypsin (rAAT) by size exclusion-HPLC assay (*k* = *degradation rate constant*). Monomeric rAAT decreased rapidly in concentration both under acidic and basic conditions. Optimal stability occurred at pH 7.5. *Source*: Adapted from Vemuri et al., 1993.

Freeze drying may provide the requested stability. During freeze-drying water is removed through sublimation and not by evaporation. Three stages can be discerned in the freeze-drying process: (*i*) a freezing step, (*ii*) the primary drying step, and (*iii*) the secondary drying step (Fig. 6). Table 2 explains what happens during these stages.

Freeze drying of a protein solution without the proper excipients causes, as a rule, irreversible damage to the protein. Table 3 lists excipients typically encountered in successfully freeze-dried protein products.

### ■ Freezing

In the freezing step (Fig. 6) the temperature of the aqueous system in the vials is lowered. Ice crystal formation does not start right at the thermodynamic or equilibrium freezing point, but supercooling occurs. That means that crystallization often only occurs when temperatures of –15°C or lower have been reached. During the crystallization step the temperature may temporarily rise in the vial, because of the generation of crystallization heat. During the cooling stage, concentration of the protein and excipients occurs because of the growing ice crystal mass at the expense of the aqueous water phase. This can cause precipitation of one or more of the excipients, which may consequently result in pH shifts (see above and Fig. 7) or ionic strength changes. It may also induce protein denaturation. Cooling of the vials is done through lowering the temperature of the shelf. Selecting the proper cooling scheme for the shelf, and consequently vial, is important as it dictates the degree of supercooling and ice crystal size. Small crystals are formed during fast cooling; large crystals form at lower cooling rates. Small ice crystals are required for porous solids and fast sublimation rates (Pikal, 1990a).

■ **Freezing**
The temperature of the product is reduced from ambient temperature to a temperature below the eutectic temperature ($T_e$), or below the glass transition temperature ($T_g$) of the system. A $T_g$ is encountered if amorphous phases are present.

■ **Primary drying**
Crystallized and water not bound to protein/excipient is removed by sublimation. The temperature is below the $T_e$ or $T_g$ (e.g., –40°C) and reduced pressures are used.

■ **Secondary drying**
Removal of water interacting with the protein and excipients. The temperature in the chamber is kept below $T_g$ and rises gradually, e.g., from –40°C to 20°C.

**Table 2** ■ Three stages in the freeze-drying process of protein formulations.

If the system does not (fully) crystallize but forms an amorphous mass upon cooling, the temperature in the "freezing stage" should drop below $T_g$, the glass transition temperature. In amorphous systems the viscosity changes dramatically in the temperature range around the $T_g$: a "rubbery" state exists above and a glass state below the $T_g$.

At the start of the primary drying stage no "free and fluid" water should be present in the vials. Minus forty degrees Celsius is a typical freezing temperature before sublimation is initiated through pressure reduction.

### ■ Primary Drying

In the primary drying stage (Fig. 6) sublimation of the water mass in the vial is initiated by lowering the pressure. The water vapor is collected on a condenser, with a (substantially) lower temperature than the shelf with the vials. Sublimation costs energy (about 2500 kJ/gram ice). Temperature drops are avoided by

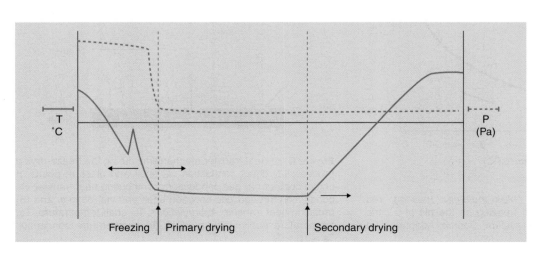

**Figure 6** ■ Example of freeze-drying protocol for systems with crystallizing water. *Abbreviations*: T, temperature; P, pressure.

| ■ *Bulking agents*: <br> Mannitol/glycine | *Reason*: <br> Elegance/blowout prevention[a] |
|---|---|
| ■ *Collapse temperature modifier*: <br> Dextran, albumin/gelatine | *Reason*: <br> Increase collapse temperature |
| ■ *Lyoprotectant*: <br> Sugars, albumin | *Reason*: <br> Protection of the physical structure of the protein[b] |

[a] Blowout is the loss of material taken away by the water vapor that leaves the vial. It occurs when little solid material is present in the vial.

[b] Mechanism of action of lyoprotectants is not fully understood. Factors that might play a role are: (1) lyoprotectants replace water as stabilizing agent (water replacement theory); (2) lyoprotectants increase the $T_g$ of the cake/frozen system; (3) lyoprotectants will absorb moisture from the stoppers; (4) lyoprotectants slow down the secondary drying process and minimize the chances for overdrying of the protein. Overdrying might occur when residual water levels after secondary drying become too low. Pikal (1990b) considers the chance for overdrying "in real life" small.

**Table 3** ■ Typical excipients in a freeze-dried protein formulation.

the supply of heat from the shelf to the vial, so the shelf is heated during this stage.

Heat is transferred to the vial through (*i*) direct shelf-vial contact (conductance), (*ii*) radiation, and (*iii*) gas conduction (Fig. 8). Gas conduction depends on the pressure: if one selects relatively high gas pressures, heat transport is promoted because of a high conductivity. But, it reduces mass transfer, because of a low driving force: the pressure between equilibrium vapor pressure at the interface between the frozen mass/dried cake and the chamber pressure (Pikal, 1990a).

During the primary drying stage one transfers heat from the shelf through the vial bottom and the frozen mass to the interface frozen mass/dry powder, to keep the sublimation process going. During this drying stage the vial content should never reach or exceed the eutectic temperature or glass transition temperature range. Typically a safety margin of $2°C$ to $5°C$ is used, otherwise

the cake will collapse. Collapse causes a strong reduction in sublimation rate and poor cake formation. Heat transfer resistance decreases during the drying process as the transport distance is reduced by the retreating interface. With the mass transfer resistance (transport of water vapor), however, the opposite occurs. Mass transfer resistance increases during the drying process as the dry cake becomes thicker.

This situation makes it clear that parameters such as chamber pressure and shelf heating are not necessarily constant during the primary drying

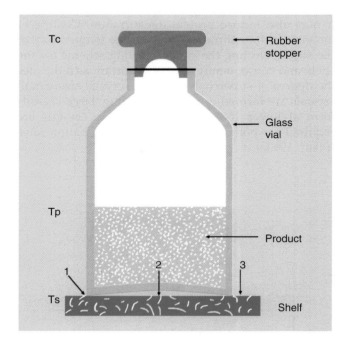

**Figure 8** ■ Heat transfer mechanisms during the freeze-drying process: (1) direct conduction via shelf and glass at points of actual contact, (2) gas conduction: contribution heat transfer via conduction through gas between shelf and vial bottom, and (3) radiation heat transfer. *Abbreviations*: Ts, shelf temperature; Tp, temperature sublimating product; Tc, temperature condensor. Ts > Tp > Tc.

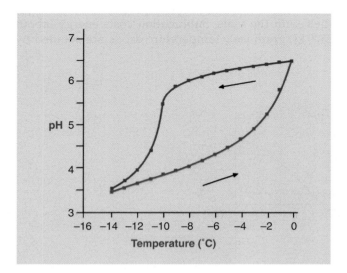

**Figure 7** ■ Thawing/cooling (*blue indicates thawing; red indicates cooling*). The effect of freezing on the pH of a citric acid-disodium phosphate buffer system. *Source*: Adapted from Pikal, 1990a.

process. They should be carefully chosen and adjusted as the drying process proceeds.

The eutectic temperature or glass transition temperature are parameters of great importance to develop a rationally designed freeze-drying protocol. Information about these parameters can be obtained by microscopic observation of the freeze-drying process, differential scanning calorimetry (DSC), or electrical resistance measurements.

An example of a DSC scan providing information on the $T_g$ is presented in Figure 9 (Franks et al., 1991). The $T_g$ heavily depends on the composition of the system: excipients and water content. Lowering the water content of an amorphous system causes the $T_g$ to shift to higher temperatures.

### ■ Secondary Drying
When all frozen or amorphous water that is non-protein and non-excipient bound is removed, the secondary drying step starts (Fig. 6). The end of the primary drying stage is reached when product temperature and shelf temperature become equal, or when the partial water pressure drops (Pikal, 1990a). As long as the "non-bound" water is being removed, the partial water pressure almost equals the total pressure. In the secondary drying stage the temperature is slowly increased to remove "bound" water; the chamber pressure is still reduced. The temperature should stay all the time below the collapse/eutectic temperature, which continues to rise when residual water contents drop. Typically, the secondary drying step ends when the product has been kept at 20°C for some time. The residual water content is a critical, endpoint indicating parameter. Values as low as 1% residual water in the cake have been recommended.

Figure 10 (Pristoupil, 1985; Pikal, 1990a) exemplifies the decreasing stability of freeze-dried hemoglobin with increasing residual water content.

When stored in the presence of reducing lyoprotectants such as glucose and lactose the Maillard reaction may occur: amino groups of the proteins react with the lyoprotectant in the dry state and the cake color turns yellow-brown. The use of non-reducing sugars such as sucrose or trehalose may avoid this problem.

### ■ Other Approaches to Stabilize Proteins
Compacted forms of proteins are being used for certain veterinary applications, such as sustained release formulations of growth hormones. The pellets should contain as few additives as possible. They can be applied subdermally or intramuscularly when the compact pellets are introduced by compressed air-powered rifles into the animals (Klegerman and Groves, 1992).

## DELIVERY OF PROTEINS: ROUTES OF ADMINISTRATION AND ABSORPTION ENHANCEMENT

### ■ The Parenteral Route of Administration
Parenteral administration is here defined as administration via those routes where a needle is used, including intravenous (IV), intramuscular (IM), subcutaneous (SC) and intraperitoneal (IP) injections. More information on the pharmacokinetic behavior of recombinant proteins is provided in Chapter 5. It suffices here to state that the blood half-life of biotech products can vary over a wide range. For example, the circulation half-life of t-PA is a few minutes, while

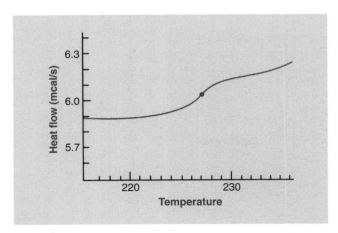

**Figure 9** ■ 9 DSC heating trace for a frozen solution of sucrose and sodium chloride, showing the glass transition temperature of the freeze concentrate at 227 K. For pure freeze-concentrated sucrose, $T_g = 241$ K (1 Cal = 4.2 J). *Source*: Adapted from Franks et al., 1991.

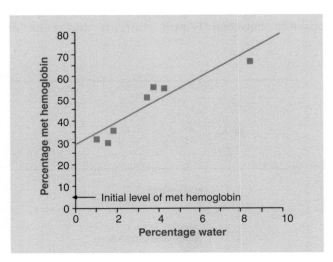

**Figure 10** ■ The effect of residual moisture on the stability of freeze-dried hemoglobin (~6%) formulated with 0.2 M sucrose; decomposition to met hemoglobin during storage at 23°C for 4 years. *Source*: From Pikal, 1990a; data reported by Pritoupil et al., 1985.

monoclonal antibodies (MAb) reportedly have half-lives of a few days. Obviously, one reason to develop modified proteins through site directed mutagenesis is to enhance circulation half-life. A simple way to expand the mean residence time for short half-life proteins is to switch from IV to IM or SC administration. One should realize that by doing that, changes in disposition may occur, with a significant impact on the therapeutic performance of the drug. These changes are related to: (i) the prolonged residence time at the IM or SC site of injection compared to IV administration and the enhanced exposure to degradation reactions (peptidases) and (ii) differences in disposition.

*Regarding point 1*: Prolonged residence time at the IM or SC site of injection and the enhanced exposure to degradation reactions. For instance, diabetics can become "insulin resistant" through high tissue peptidase activity (Maberly et al., 1982). Other factors that can contribute to absorption variation are related to differences in exercise level of the muscle at the injection site and also massage and heat at the injection site. The state of the tissue, for instance the occurrence of pathological conditions, may be important as well.

*Regarding point 2*: Differences in disposition. Upon administration, the protein may be transported to the blood through the lymphatics or may enter the blood circulation through the capillary wall at the site of injection (Figs. 11 and 12). The fraction of the administered dose taking this lymphatic route is molecular weight dependent (Supersaxo et al., 1990). Lymphatic transport takes time (hours) and uptake in the blood circulation is highly dependent on the injection site. On its way to the blood, the lymph passes through draining lymph nodes and contact is possible between lymph contents and cells of

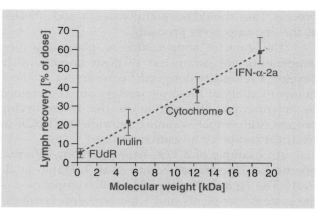

**Figure 12** ■ Correlation between the molecular weight and the cumulative recovery of rIFN alpha-2a ($M_w$ 19 kDa), cytochrome C ($M_w$ 12.3 kDa), inulin ($M_w$ 5.2 kDa), and FUDR ($M_w$ 256.2 Da) in the efferent lymph from the right popliteal lymph node following SC administration into the lower part of the right hind leg of sheep. Each point and bar show the mean and standard deviation of three experiments performed in separate sheep. The line drawn is the best fit by linear regression analysis calculated with the four mean values. The points have a correlation coefficient $r$ of 0.998 ($p < 0.01$). *Source*: Adapted from Supersaxo et al., 1990.

the immune system such as macrophages, B- and T-lymphocytes residing in the lymph nodes.

### ■ The Oral Route of Administration

Oral delivery of protein drugs would be preferable, because it is patient friendly and no intervention by a healthcare professional is necessary to administer the drug. Oral bioavailability, however, is usually very low. The two main reasons for this failure of uptake are: (i) protein degradation in the gastrointestinal (GI) tract and (ii) poor permeability of the wall of the GI tract in case of a passive transport process (Lee et al., 1991).

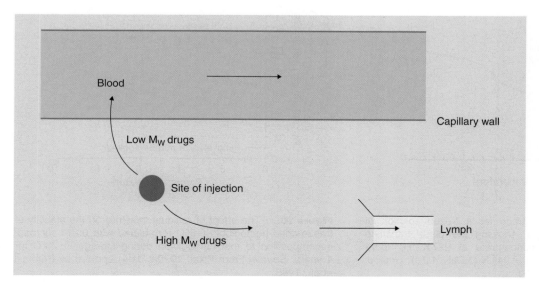

**Figure 11** ■ Routes of uptake of SC or IM injected drugs.

*Regarding point 1*: Protein degradation in the GI tract. The human body has developed a very efficient system to break down proteins in our food to amino acids, or di- or tri-peptides. These building stones for body proteins are actively absorbed for use wherever necessary in the body. In the stomach pepsins, a family of aspartic proteases, are secreted. They are particularly active between pH 3 and 5 and lose activity at higher pH values. Pepsins are endopeptidases capable of cleaving peptide bonds distant from the ends of the peptide chain. They preferentially cleave peptide bonds between two hydrophobic amino acids. Other endopeptidases are active in the GI tract at neutral pH values, e.g., trypsin, chymotrypsin, and elastase. They have different peptide bond cleavage characteristics that more or less complement each other. Exopeptidases, proteases degrading peptide chains from their ends, are present as well. Examples are carboxypeptidase A and B. In the GI lumen the proteins are cut into fragments that effectively further break down to amino acids, di- and tri-peptides by brush border and cytoplasmic proteases of the enterocytes.

*Regarding point 2*: Permeability. High molecular weight molecules do not readily penetrate the intact and mature epithelial barrier if diffusion is the sole driving force for mass transfer. Their diffusion coefficient decreases with increasing molecule size. Proteins are no exception to this rule. Active transport of intact therapeutic recombinant proteins over the GI-epithelium has not been described yet.

The above analysis leads to the conclusion that nature, unfortunately, does not allow us to use the oral route of administration for therapeutic proteins if high (or at least constant) bioavailability is required.

However, for the category of oral vaccines the above-mentioned hurdles of degradation and permeation are not necessarily prohibitive. For oral immunization, only a (small) fraction of the antigen (protein) has to reach its target site to elicit an immune response. The target cells are lymphocytes and antigen presenting accessory cells located in Peyer's patches (Fig. 13). The B-lymphocyte population includes cells that produce secretory IgA antibodies.

These Peyer's patches are macroscopically identifiable follicular structures located in the wall of the GI tract. Peyer's patches are overlaid with microfold (M) cells that separate the luminal contents from the lymphocytes. These M cells have little lysosomal degradation capacity and allow for antigen sampling by the underlying lymphocytes. Moreover, mucus producing goblet cell density is reduced over Peyer's patches. This reduces mucus production and facilitates access to the M cell surface for luminal contents (Jani et al., 1992; Roitt et al., 1993). Attempts to improve antigen delivery via the Peyer's patches and to enhance the immune response are made by using microspheres, liposomes or modified live vectors, such as attenuated bacteria and viruses (Holmgren et al., 1989; Eldridge et al., 1990; Kersten and Hirschberg, 2004, see Chapter 21).

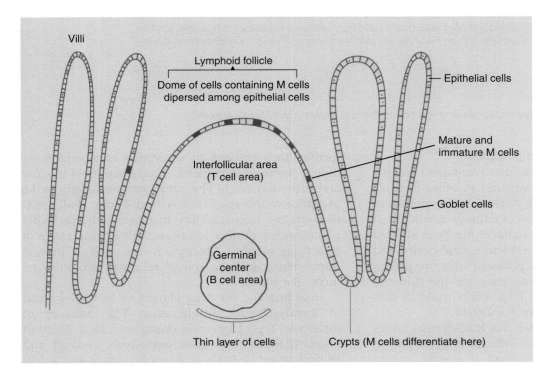

**Figure 13** ■ Schematic diagram of the structure of intestinal Peyer's patches. M cells within the follicle-associated epithelium are enlarged for emphasis. *Source*: Adapted from O'Hagan, 1990.

**Nasal (Edman and Björk, 1992)**

*Advantage*:
Easily accessible, fast uptake, proven track record with a number of "conventional" drugs, probably lower proteolytic activity than in the GI tract, avoidance of first pass effect, spatial containment of absorption enhancers is possible

*Disadvantage*:
Reproducibility (in particular under pathological conditions), safety (e.g., ciliary movement), low bioavailability for proteins

**Pulmonary (Patton and Platz, 1992)**

*Advantage*:
Relatively easy to access, fast uptake, proven track record with "conventional" drugs, substantial fractions of insulin are absorbed, lower proteolytic activity than in the GI tract, avoidance of hepatic first pass effect, spatial containment of absorption enhancers (?)

*Disadvantage*:
Reproducibility (in particular under pathological conditions, smokers/non-smokers), safety (e.g., immunogenicity), presence of macrophages in the lung with high affinity for particulates

**Rectal (Zhou and Li Wan Po, 1991b)**

*Advantage*:
Easily accessible, partial avoidance of hepatic first pass, probably lower proteolytic activity than in the upper parts of the GI tract, spatial containment of absorption enhancers is possible, proven track record with a number of "conventional" drugs

*Disadvantage*:
Low bioavailability for proteins

**Buccal (Zhou and Li Wan Po, 1991b; Ho et al., 1992)**

*Advantage*:
Easily accessible, avoidance of hepatic first pass, probably lower proteolytic activity than in the lower parts of the GI tract, spatial containment of absorption enhancers is possible, option to remove formulation if necessary

*Disadvantage*:
Low bioavailability of proteins, no proven track record yet (?)

**Transdermal (Cullander and Guy, 1992)**

*Advantage*:
Easily accessible, avoidance of hepatic first pass effect, removal of formulation if necessary is possible, spatial containment of absorption enhancers, proven track record with "conventional" drugs, sustained/controlled release possible

*Disadvantage*:
Low bioavailability of proteins

**Table 4** ▓ Alternative routes of administration to the oral route for biopharmaceuticals.

## ■ Alternative Routes of Administration

Parenteral administration has disadvantages (needles, sterility, injection skills) compared to other possible routes. Therefore, systemic delivery of recombinant proteins by alternative routes of administration (apart from the GI tract, discussed above) has been studied extensively. The nose, lungs, rectum, oral cavity, and skin have been selected as potential sites of application. The potential pros and cons for the different relevant routes are listed in Table 4 (Zhou and Li Wan Po, 1991a; Zhou and Li Wan Po, 1991b).

The nasal, buccal, rectal, and transdermal routes all have been shown to be of little clinical relevance if systemic action is required, and if simple protein formulations without an absorption enhancing technology are used. In general, bioavailability is too low and varies too much! The pulmonary route may be the exception to this rule. Table 5 (from Patton et al., 1994) presents the bioavailability in rats of intratracheally administered protein solutions with a wide range of molecular weights. Absorption was strongly protein dependent, with no clear relationship with its molecular weight.

In humans the drug should be inhaled instead of intratracheally adminstered. The delivery of insulin to Type I (juvenile onset) and Type II (adult onset) diabetics has been extensively studied and clinical phase III trials evaluating efficacy and safety

| Molecule | Mw kDa | No. of AA | Absolute bioavailability (%) |
|---|---|---|---|
| α-interferon | 20 | 165 | >56 |
| PTH-84 | 9 | 84 | >20 |
| PTH-34 | 4.2 | 34 | 40 |
| Calcitonin (human) | 3.4 | 32 | 17 |
| Calcitonin (salmon) | 3.4 | 32 | 17 |
| Glucagons | 3.4 | 29 | <1 |
| Somatostatin | 3.1 | 28 | <1 |

*Abbreviations*: AA, number of amino acids; PTH, recombinant human parathyroid hormone.
*Source*: Adapted from Patton et al., 1994.

**Table 5** Absolute bioavailability of a number of proteins (*intratracheal vs. IV*) in rats.

have been performed or are ongoing (Patton et al., 1999). The first pulmonary insulin formulation was approved by FDA in January 2006 (Exubera®). Pulmonary inhalation of insulin is specifically tested for meal time glucose control. Uptake of insulin is faster than after a regular SC insulin injection (peak 5–60 minutes versus 60–180 minutes). The reproducibility of the blood glucose response to inhaled insulin was equivalent to SC injected insulin, but patients preferred inhalation over SC injection. Inhalation technology plays a critical role when considering the prospects of the pulmonary route for the systemic delivery of therapeutic proteins. Dry powder inhalers and nebulizers are being tested. The fraction of insulin that is ultimately absorbed depends on: (*i*) the fraction of the inhaled/nebulized dose that is actually leaving the device, (*ii*) the fraction that is actually deposited in the lung, and (*iii*) the fraction that is being absorbed, i.e., total relative uptake (TO %) = % uptake from device × % deposited in the lungs × % actually absorbed from the lungs. TO % for insulin is estimated to be about 10% (Patton et al., 2004). The fraction of insulin that is absorbed from the lung is estimated to be around 20%. These figures demonstrate that insulin absorption via the lung may be a promising route; but the fraction absorbed is small.

Therefore, different approaches have been evaluated to increase bioavailability of the pulmonary and other non-parenteral routes of administration. The goal is to develop a system that temporarily decreases the absorption barrier resistance with minimum and acceptable safety concerns. The mechanistic background of these approaches is given in Table 6. Until

| Classified according to proposed mechanism of action |
|---|
| ▪ Increase the permeability of the absorption barrier:<br>  ▪ Addition of fatty acids/phospholipids, bile salts, enamine derivatives of phenylglycine, ester and ether type (non)-ionic detergents, saponins, salicylate derivatives, derivatives of fusidic acid or glycyrrhizinic acid, or methylated β cyclodextrins<br>  ▪ Through iontophoresis<br>  ▪ By using liposomes<br>▪ Decrease peptidase activity at the site of absorption and along the "absorption route": aprotinin, bacitracin, soybean tyrosine inhibitor, boroleucin, borovaline<br>▪ Enhance resistance against degradation by modification of the molecular structure<br>▪ Prolongation of exposure time (e.g., bio-adhesion technologies) |

*Source*: Adapted from Zhou and Li Wan Po, 1991a.

**Table 6** Approaches to enhance bioavailability of proteins.

now, no products utilizing one of these approaches have successfully passed clinical test programs. Safety concerns are an important hurdle. Questions center on the specificity and reversibility of the protein permeation enhancing effect and the toxicity.

### ▪ Examples of Absorption Enhancing Effects

The following section deals with the "state of the art" of this important issue: absorption enhancement and non-parenteral administration of recombinant proteins. A number of typical examples are provided.

Table 7 presents an example of the (apparently complex) relationship between nasal bioavailability of some peptide and protein drugs, their molecular weight and the presence of the absorption enhancer glycocholate (Zhou and Li Wan Po, 1991b).

Figure 14 (Björk and Edman, 1988) illustrates another case where degradable starch microspheres loaded with insulin were used and where changes in glucose levels were monitored after nasal administration to rats.

| Molecule | No. of AA | Bioavailability (%) Without glycocholate | Bioavailability (%) With glycocholate |
|---|---|---|---|
| Glucagon | 29 | <1 | 70–90 |
| Calcitonin | 32 | <1 | 15–20 |
| Insulin | 51 | <1 | 10–30 |
| Met-hGH[a] | 191 | <1 | 7–8 |

[a] See Chapter 13, Growth Hormones. *Abbreviation*: AA, amino acids.
*Source*: Adapted from Zhou and Li Wan Po, 1991b.

**Table 7** Effect of glycocholate (absorption enhancer) on nasal bioavailability of some proteins and peptides.

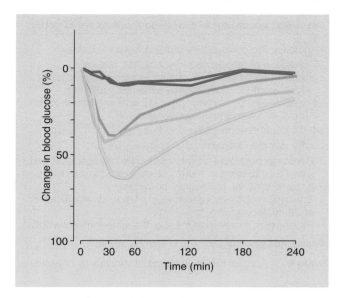

**Figure 14** ▨ Change in blood glucose in rats after intranasal administration of insulin. *Source*: Discussed by Edman and Björk, 1992.
*Key*:
━ Soluble insulin 2.0 IU/kg i.n.
━ Soluble insulin 0.25 IU/kg IV
━ Degradable starch microspheres-insulin 0.75 IU/kg i.n.
━ Degradable starch microspheres-insulin 1.70 IU/kg i.n.
━ Empty degradable starch microspheres 0.5 mg/kg i.n.

In these examples, the effect of the presence of the absorption enhancers is clear. Major issues now being addressed are reproducibility, effect of pathological conditions (e.g., rhinitis) on absorption and safety aspects of chronic use. Interestingly, absorption enhancing effects were shown to be species dependent. Pronounced differences in effect were observed between rats, rabbits, and humans.

With iontophoresis a transdermal electrical current is induced by positioning two electrodes on different places on the skin (Fig. 15). This current induces a migration of (ionized) molecules through the skin. Delivery depends on the current (on/off, pulsed/direct, wave shape), pH, ionic strength, molecular weight, charge on the protein, and temperature. The protein should be charged over the full thickness of the skin (pH of hydrated skin depends on the depth and varies between pH 4 (surface) and pH 7.3), which makes proteins with pI values outside this range prime candidates for iontophoretic transport. It is not clear whether there are size restrictions (protein MW) for iontophoretic transport. However, only potent proteins will be successful candidates. With the present technology the protein flux through the skin is in the $10 \, \mu g/cm^2/hour$ range (Sage et al., 1995).

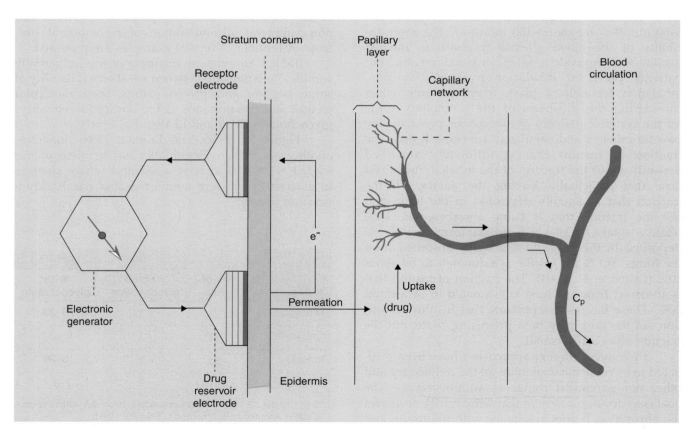

**Figure 15** ▨ Schematic illustration of the transdermal iontophoretic delivery of peptide and protein drugs across the skin. *Source*: Adapted from Chien, 1991.

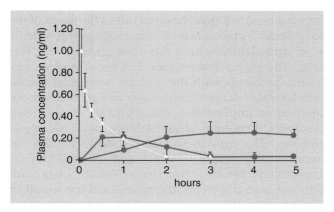

**Figure 16** ▓ Plasma concentration versus time profiles after SC, IV and iontophoretic transdermal administration of GRF (1–44) to hairless guinea pigs. Red, iontophoresis (1 mg/g; 0.17 mA/cm$^2$; 5 cm$^2$ patch). Blue, SC (10 μg/kg; 0.025 mg/ml). Yellow, IV (10 μg/kg; 0.025 mg/ml). *Source*: Adapted from Kumar et al., 1992.

Figure 16 presents the plasma profile of growth hormone releasing factor, GRF (44 amino acids, MW 5 kDa after SC, IV, and iontophoretic transdermal delivery to hairless guinea pigs. A prolonged appearance of GRF in the plasma can be observed. Iontophoretic delivery offers interesting opportunities if pulsed delivery of the protein is required. The device can be worn permanently and only switched on for the desired periods of time, simulating pulsatile secretion of endogenous hormones such as growth hormone and insulin.

## DELIVERY OF PROTEINS: APPROACHES FOR RATE-CONTROLLED AND TARGET SITE-SPECIFIC DELIVERY BY THE PARENTERAL ROUTE

Presently used therapeutic proteins widely differ in their pharmacokinetic characteristics (see Chapter 5). If they are endogenous agents such as insulin, t-PA, growth hormone, erythropoetin, interleukins or factor VIII, it is important to realize why, when and where they are secreted. There are three different ways in which cells can communicate with each other: the endocrine, paracrine, and autocrine pathway (Table 8).

---

▓  *Endocrine hormones*: A hormone secreted by a distant cell to regulate cell functions distributed widely through the body. The blood stream plays an important role in the transport process.
▓  *Paracrine acting mediators*: The mediator is secreted by a cell to influence surrounding cells, short range influence.
▓  *Autocrine acting mediators*: The agent is secreted by a cell and affects the cell by which it is generated, (very) short range influence.

---

**Table 8** ▓ Communication between cells: chemical messengers.

The dose–response relationship of these mediators is often not S-shaped, but, for instance, bell shaped: at high doses the therapeutic effect disappears (see Chapter 5). Moreover, the presence of these mediators may activate a complex cascade of events that needs to be carefully controlled. Therefore, key issues for their therapeutic success are: (*i*) access to target cells, (*ii*) retention at the target site, and (*iii*) proper timing of delivery (Tomlinson, 1987).

In particular, for paracrine and autocrine acting proteins, site-specific delivery can be highly desirable, because otherwise side effects will occur outside the target area. Severe side effects were reported with cytokines, such as tumor necrosis factor and interleukin-2 upon parenteral (IV or SC) administration (see Chapter 11). The occurrence of these side effects limits the therapeutic potential of these compounds. Therefore, the delivery of these proteins at the proper site, rate, and dose is a crucial part in the process of the design and development of these compounds as pharmaceutical entities. The following sections discuss first concepts developed to control the release kinetics and subsequently concepts for site-directed drug delivery.

## APPROACHES FOR RATE-CONTROLLED DELIVERY

Rate control can be achieved by several different technologies similar to those used for "conventional" drugs. Insulin is an excellent example. A spectrum of options is available and accepted: different types of suspensions and continuous infusion systems are marketed (see Chapter 12). Moreover, chemical approaches can be used to change protein characteristics. Polyoxyethylene glycol attachment to proteins changes their circulation half-life in blood dramatically. Figure 17 shows an example of this approach.

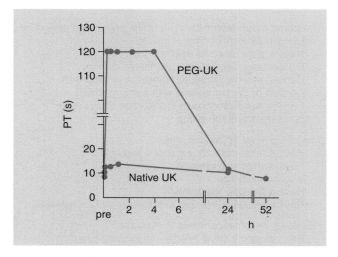

**Figure 17** ▓ Influence of chemical grafting of poly-ethyleneglycol (*PEG*) on the ability of urokinase (*UK*) to affect the prothrombin time (*PT*) in vivo in beagles with time. *Source*: Adapted from Tomlinson, 1987.

*Rate control through open loop type approach*
- Continuous infusion with pumps: mechanically or osmotically driven input: constant/pulsatile/wave form
- Implants: biodegradable polymers, lipids
- Input: limited control

*Rate control through closed loop approach/feed back system*
- Biosensor-pump combination
- Self regulating system
- Encapsulated secretory cells

**Table 9** Controlled release systems for parenteral delivery.

In general, proteins are administered as an aqueous solution. Only recombinant vaccines and most insulin formulations are delivered as (colloidal) dispersions. At the present time, insulin is routinely and clinically applied through some form of controlled release system (see Chapter 12) other than through continuous infusion. As experience with biotech drugs grows, more advanced technologies will definitely be introduced to optimize the therapeutic benefit of the drug. Table 9 lists some of the technologically feasible options. They are briefly touched upon below.

### ■ Open-Loop Systems: Mechanical Pumps
Mechanically driven pumps are common tools to administer drugs intravenously in hospitals (continuous infusion, open-loop type). They are available in different kinds of sizes/prices, portable or not, inside/outside the body, etc. Table 10 presents a checklist of issues to be considered when selecting the proper pump.

Controlled administration of a drug does not necessarily imply a constant input rate. Pulsatile or variable-rate delivery is the desired mode of input for a number of protein drugs, and for these drugs pumps should provide flexible input rate characteristics. Insulin is a prime example of a protein drug, where

*The pump must deliver the drug at the prescribed rate(s) for extended periods of time. It should:*
- Have a wide range of delivery rates
- Ensure accurate, precise and stable delivery
- Contain reliable pump and electrical components
- Contain drugs compatible with pump internals
- Provide simple means to monitor the status and performance of the pump

*The pump must be safe. It should:*
- Have a biocompatible exterior if implanted
- Have overdose protection
- Show no leakage
- Have a fail-safe mechanism
- Have sterilizable interiors and exteriors (if implantable)

*The pump must be convenient. It should:*
- Be reasonably small in size and inconspicuous
- Have a long reservoir life
- Be easy to program

*Source*: Adapted from Banerjee et al., 1991.

**Table 10** Characteristics of the ideal pump.

there is a need to adjust the input rate to the needs of the body. Today by far most experience with pump systems in an ambulatory setting has been gained with this drug. The pump system may fail because of energy failure, problems with the syringe, accidental needle withdrawal, leakage of the catheter and problems at the injection or implantation site (Banerjee et al., 1991). Moreover, long-term drug stability may become a problem. The protein should be stable at 37°C or ambient temperature (internal and external device, respectively) between two refills. Finally, even with high tech pump systems, the patient still has to collect data to adjust the pump rate. This implies invasive sampling from body fluids on a regular basis, followed by calculation of the required input rate. This problem would be solved if the concept of closed-loop systems would be realized (feedback systems, see below).

### ■ Open-Loop Systems: Osmotically Driven Systems
The subcutaneously implantable, osmotic mini-pump developed by ALZA (Alzet minipump, Fig. 18)

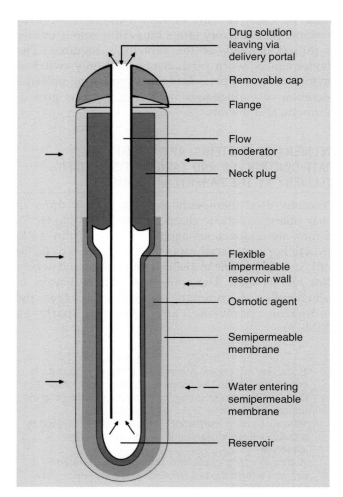

**Figure 18** Cross section of functioning Alza Alzet osmotic minipump. *Source*: Adapted from Banerjee et al., 1991.

(Banerjee et al., 1991)) has proven to be useful in animal experiments where continuous, constant infusion is required over prolonged periods of time. The rate determining process is the influx of water through the rigid, semi-permeable external membrane. The incoming water empties the drug-containing reservoir (solution or dispersion) surrounded by a flexible impermeable membrane. The release rate depends on the characteristics of this semi-permeable membrane and on osmotic pressure differences over this membrane (osmotic agents inside the pump). Zero-order release kinetics exists as long as the osmotic pressure difference over the semi-permeable membrane is maintained constant.

The protein solution (or dispersion) must be physically and chemically stable at body temperature over the full term of the experiment. Moreover, the protein solution must be compatible with the pump parts to which it is exposed. A limitation of the system is the fixed release rate, which is not always desired (see above). These devices have currently not been used on a regular basis in the clinic.

## ■ Open Loop Systems: Biodegradable Microspheres

Polylactic acid–polyglycolic acid (PLGA)-based delivery systems are being used extensively for the delivery of therapeutic peptides, in particular luteinizing hormone-releasing hormone (LHRH) agonists such as leuprolide in the therapy of prostate cancer. The first LHRH agonist controlled release formulations were implants containing leuprolide with dose ranges of 1–3 months. Later, microspheres loaded with leuprolide were introduced and dosing intervals were prolonged to up to 6 months. Critical success factors for the design of these controlled release systems are: (*i*) the drug has to be highly potent (only a small dose is required over the dosing interval), (*ii*) a sustained presence in the body is required, and (*iii*) no adverse reactions at the injection site should occur.

New strategies for controlled release of therapeutic proteins are presently under development. For example, Figures 19 and 20 describe a dextran-based microsphere technology for SC or IM administration that often has an almost 100% protein encapsulation efficiency (Fig. 19). Here, no organic solvents are being

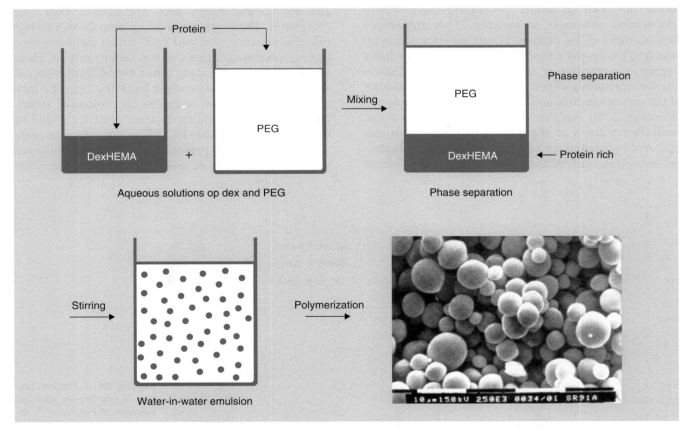

**Figure 19** ■ Schematic representation of the microsphere preparation process for the controlled release of therapeutic proteins from dextran (DexHEMA = modified dextran = dextran hydroxyethylmethacrylate) microspheres. No organic solvents are involved and encapsulation efficiency (percentage of therapeutic protein ending up in the microspheres) is routinely >90%. Polymerization: cross-linking of dextran chains through the HEMA units. *Source*: Adapted from Stenekes, 2000.

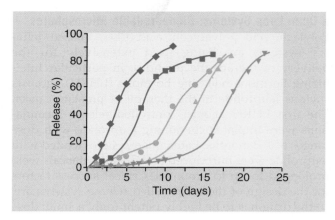

**Figure 20** ■ Cumulative release of IgG from degrading DexHEMA microspheres in time in vitro at pH 7, 37°C. Water content of the dextran microspheres upon swelling: about 60%: DS 3 (■) and water content of about 50%: DS 3 (♦), DS 6 (●), DS 8 (A) and DS 11 (▲). The values are the mean of 2 independent measurements that deviated typically less than 5% from each other. *Abbreviation*: DS, degree of cross-linking. *Source*: Adapted from Stenekes, 2000.

used in the preparation protocol. Thus, a direct interaction of the dissolved protein with an organic phase (as seen in many polymeric microsphere preparation schemes) is avoided. This minimizes denaturation of the protein. Figure 20 shows that by selecting the proper cross-linking conditions one has a degree of control over the release kinetics. Release kinetics are mainly dependent on degradation kinetics of the dextran matrix and size of the protein molecule (Stenekes, 2000). Another approach for prolonged and controlled release of therapeutic proteins is to use microspheres based on another biodegradable hydrogel material. PolyActive™ is a block-copolymer

consisting of polyethylene glycol (PEG) blocks and polybutylene terephthalate blocks (van Dijkhuizen-Radersma et al., 2004). Results of a dose finding study in humans with PolyActive™ microspheres loaded with interferon-α are shown in Figure 21.

### ■ Closed Loop Systems: Biosensor-Pump Combinations

If input rate control is desired to stabilize a certain body function, then this function should be monitored. Via an algorithm and connected pump settings, this data should be converted into a drug-input rate. These systems are called closed-loop systems as compared to the open-loop systems discussed above. If there is a known relationship between plasma level and pharmacological effect, these systems contain (Fig. 22):

(1) a biosensor, measuring the plasma level of the protein;
(2) an algorithm, to calculate the required input rate for the delivery system;
(3) a pump system, able to administer the drug at the required rate over prolonged periods of time.

The concept of a closed-loop delivery of proteins still has to overcome many conceptual and practical problems. A simple relationship between plasma level and therapeutic effect does not always exist (see Chapter 5). There are many exceptions known to this rule, for instance, "hit and run" drugs can have long lasting pharmacological effects after only a short exposure time. Also, drug effect–blood level relationships may be time dependent, as in the case of down regulation of relevant receptors on prolonged stimulation. Finally, if circadian rhythms exist, these will be responsible for variable PK/PD relationships as well.

If the above expressed PK/PD concerns do not apply, as with insulin, technical problems form the

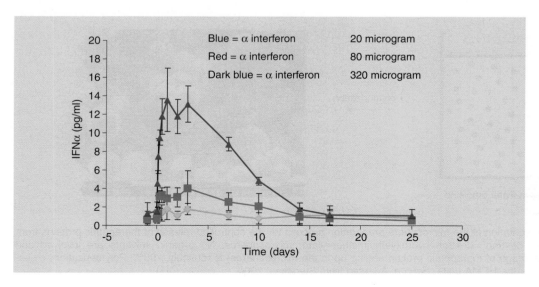

**Figure 21** ■ Plasma profiles of interferon-α after SC injection of PolyActive™ microspheres loaded with interferon-α in volunteers of a dose finding study. The elimination half-life of "free" interferon-α is about 4–16 hours.

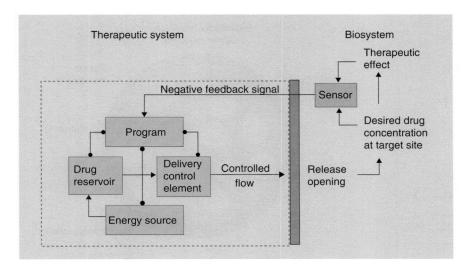

**Figure 22** ■ Therapeutic system with closed control loop. (1) a biosensor, measuring the plasma level of the protein, (2) an algorithm, to calculate the required input rate for the delivery system, and (3) a pump system, able to administer the drug at the required rate over prolonged periods of time. *Source*: Adapted from Heilman, 1984.

second hurdle in the development of closed-loop systems. It has not been possible yet to design biosensors that work reliably in vivo over prolonged periods of time. Biosensor stability, robustness and absence of histological reactions still pose problems.

### ■ Protein Delivery by Self-Regulating Systems

Apart from the design of biosensor-pump combinations, two other developments should be mentioned when discussing closed-loop approaches: self-regulating systems and encapsulated secretory cells. At the present time, both concepts are still under development (Heller, 1993).

In self-regulating systems, drug release is controlled by stimuli in the body. By far most of the research is focused on insulin release as a function of local glucose concentrations in order to stabilize blood glucose levels in diabetics. Two approaches for controlled drug release are being followed: (*i*) competitive desorption and (*ii*) enzyme-substrate reactions. The competitive desorption approach is schematically depicted in Figure 23.

It is based on the competition between glycosylated-insulin and glucose for concanavalin (Con A) binding sites. Con A is a plant lectin with a high affinity for certain sugars. Con A attached to sepharose beads and loaded with glycosylated-insulin (a bioactive form of insulin) is implanted in a pouch with a semipermeable membrane: permeable for insulin and glucose, but impermeable for the sepharose beads carrying the toxic Con A. An example of the performance of a Con A–glycosylated-insulin complex in pancreatectomized dogs is given in Figure 24.

Enzyme-substrate reactions to regulate insulin release from an implanted reservoir are all based on pH drops occurring when glucose is converted to gluconic acid in the presence of the enzyme glucose oxidase. This pH drop then induces changes in the structure of acid-sensitive delivery devices such as acid sensitive polymers, which start releasing insulin, lowering the glucose concentration, and consequently increasing the local pH and "closing the reservoir."

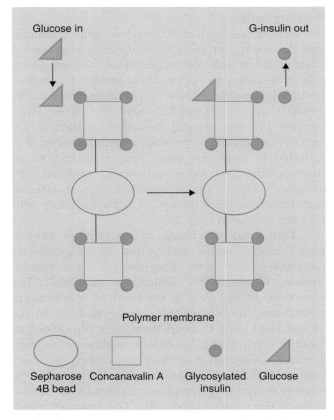

**Figure 23** ■ Schematic design of the Con A immobilized bead/ G (*glycosylated*)-insulin/membrane self-regulating insulin delivery system. *Source*: Adapted from Kim et al., 1990.

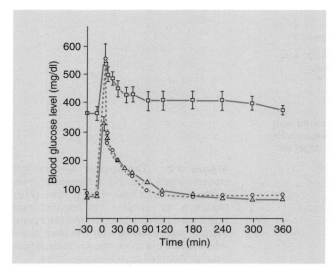

**Figure 24** ■ Peripheral blood glucose profiles of dogs administered bolus dextrose (500 mg/kg) during an IV glucose tolerance test. Normal dogs (○) had an intact pancreas, diabetic dogs (□) had undergone total pancreatectomy; and implant dogs (△) had been intraperitoneally implanted with a cellulose pouch containing a Con A-G-insulin complex. Blood glucose at $t =$ −30 minutes shows the overnight fasting level 30 minutes prior to bolus injection of dextrose. *Source*: Adapted from Heller, 1993.

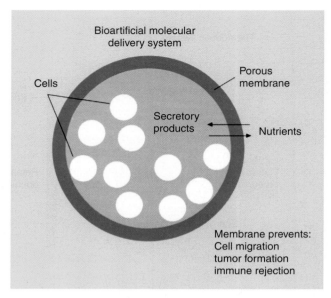

**Figure 25** ■ Schematic illustration of a "bioartificial molecular delivery system." Secretory cells are surrounded by a semi-permeable membrane prior to implantation in host tissue. Nutrients and secretory products passively diffuse through pores in the encapsulating membrane powered by concentration gradients. The use of a membrane that excludes the humoral and cellular components of the host immune system allows immunologically incompatible cells to survive implantation without the need to administer immunosuppressive agents. Extracellular matrix material may be included depending upon the requirements of the encapsulated cells. *Source*: Adapted from Tresco, 1994.

## ■ Protein Delivery by Microencapsulated Secretory Cells

The idea to use implanted, secretory cells to administer therapeutic proteins was launched long ago. A major goal has been the implantation of Langerhans cells in diabetics to restore their insulin production through biofeedback. These implanted secretory cells should be protected from the body environment, since rejection processes would immediately start, if imperfectly matched cell material is used. Besides, it is desirable to keep the cells from migrating in all different directions. When genetically modified cells are used, safety issues would be even stricter. Therefore, (micro)encapsulation of the secretory cells has been proposed (Fig. 25).

Thin (wall thickness in micrometer range), robust, biocompatible and permselective polymeric membranes have been designed for these (micro) capsules (Tresco, 1994; Uludag et al., 1993). The membrane should ensure transport of nutrients (in general low MW) from the outside medium to the encapsulated cells to keep them in a physiological, "healthy" state and to prohibit induction of undesirable immunological responses (rejection processes). Antibodies (MW > 150 kDa) and cells belonging to the immune system (e.g., lymphocytes) should not be able to reach the encapsulated cells. The polymer membrane should have a cut off between 50 and 150 kDa, the exact number still being a matter of debate. In the case of insulin the membrane is permeable for this

relatively small sized hormone (5.4 kDa) and for glucose ("indicator" molecule), which is essential for proper biofeedback processes. Successful studies in diabetic animals were performed. Promising clinical data has been reported with human secretory islet cells encapsulated in alginate-based microspheres (Shoon-Shiong et al., 1994).

## SITE-SPECIFIC DELIVERY (TARGETING) OF PROTEIN DRUGS

Why are we still not able to beat life-threatening diseases such as cancer with our current arsenal of drugs? Causes of failure can be summarized as follows (Crommelin et al., 1992):

(1) The active compound never reaches the target site, because it is rapidly eliminated intact from the body through the kidneys, or it is inactivated through metabolic action (e.g., in the liver).

(2) Only a small fraction of the drug reaches the target site. By far the largest fraction of the drug is distributed over non-target organs, where they exert side effects; in other words, accumulation of the drug at the target site is the exception and not the rule.

(3) Many drug molecules (in particular high MW and hydrophilic molecules, i.e., many therapeutic proteins) do not enter cells easily. This poses a problem if intracellular delivery is required for their therapeutic activity.

Attempts are made to increase the therapeutic index of drugs through drug targeting:

(1) by specific delivery of the active compound to its site of action,
(2) to keep it there until it has been inactivated and detoxified.

Targeted drug delivery should maximize the therapeutic effect and avoid toxic effects elsewhere. The basics of the concept of drug targeting were defined already in the early days of the 20th century by Paul Ehrlich. But only in the last decade substantial progress has been made to implement this site-specific delivery concept. Recent progress can be ascribed to: (*i*) the rapidly growing number of technological options (e.g., safe carriers) for drug delivery; (*ii*) many new insights gained into the pathophysiology of diseases at the cellular and molecular level, including the presence of cell-specific receptors and homing devices to target them (e.g., MAb); and finally, (*iii*) new revelations on the nature of the anatomical and physiological barriers that hinder easy access to target sites. The site-specific delivery systems presently in different stages of development generally consist of three functionally separate units (Table 11).

Nature has provided us with antibodies, which exemplify a class of natural drug targeting devices. In an antibody molecule one can recognize a homing device part (antigen binding site) and "active" parts. These active parts in the molecule are responsible for participating in the complement cascade, or inducing interactions with monocytes when antigen is bound. The rest of the molecule can be considered as carrier.

Most of the drug (protein) targeting work is performed with delivery systems that are designed for parenteral and, more specifically, IV delivery. Only a limited number of papers have dealt with the pharmacokinetics of the drug targeting process (Hunt et al., 1986). From these kinetic models a number of

| 1. | Drugs with high total clearance are good candidates for targeted delivery. |
| 2. | Response sites with a relatively small blood flow require carrier-mediated transport. |
| 3. | Increases in the rate of elimination of free drug from either central or response compartments tend to increase the need for targeted drug delivery; this also implies a higher input rate of the drug-carrier conjugate to maintain the therapeutic effect. |
| 4. | For maximizing the targeting effect, the release of drug from the carrier should be restricted to the response compartment. |

**Table 12** ■ Pharmacokinetic considerations related to protein targeting.

conclusions could be drawn for situations where targeted delivery is, in principle, advantageous (Table 12).

The potential and limitations of carrier-based, targeted drug delivery systems for proteins are briefly discussed. The focus is on concepts where MAb are being used. They can be used as the antibody itself (also in Chapter 15), in modified form when antibodies are conjugated with an active moiety, or attached to drug-laden colloidal carriers such as liposomes.

Two terms are regularly used in the context of targeting: passive and active targeting. With passive targeting the "natural" disposition pattern of the carrier system is utilized for site-specific delivery. For instance, particulate carriers circulating in the blood (see below) are often rapidly taken up by macrophages in contact with the blood circulation and accumulate in liver (Kupffer cells) and spleen. Active targeting is the concept where attempts are made to change the natural disposition of the carrier by some sort of homing device or homing principle to select one particular tissue or cell type.

### ■ Anatomical, Physiological, and Pathological Considerations Relevant for Protein Targeting

Carrier-mediated transport in the body depends on the physicochemical properties of the carrier: its charge, molecular weight/size, surface hydrophobicity, and the presence of ligands for interaction with surface receptors (Crommelin and Storm, 1990). If a drug enters the circulation and the target site is outside the blood circulation, the drug has to pass through the endothelial barrier. Figure 26 gives a schematic picture of the capillary wall structures (under physiological conditions) present at different locations in the body.

Figure 26 shows a diagram of intact endothelium under normal conditions. Under pathological conditions, such as those encountered in tumors and

| 1. An active moiety | For: therapeutic effect |
| 2. A carrier | For: (metabolic) protection, changing the disposition of the drug |
| 3. A homing device | For: specificity, selection of the assigned target site |

**Table 11** ■ Components for targeted drug delivery (carrier based).

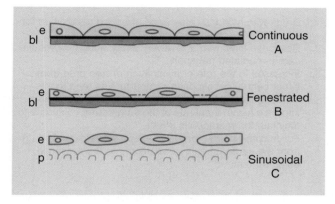

**Figure 26** ■ Schematic illustration of the structure of different classes of blood capillaries. (**A**) Continuous capillary. The endothelium (e) is continuous with tight junctions between adjacent endothelial cells. The subendothelial basement membrane (bl) is also continuous. (**B**) Fenestrated capillary. The endothelium exhibits a series of fenestrae which are sealed by a membranous diaphragm. The subendothelial basement membrane is continuous. (**C**) Discontinuous (sinusoidal) capillary. The overlying endothelium contains numerous gaps of varying size enabling materials in the circulation to gain access to the underlying parenchymal cells (p). The subendothelial basement is either absent (liver) or present as a fragmented interrupted structure (spleen, bone marrow). The fenestrae in the liver are about 0.1 to 0.2 μm; the pores between the endothelial cells and those in the basement membrane outside the liver, spleen, and bone marrow are much smaller. *Source*: Adapted from Poste, 1985.

inflammation sites, endothelium can differ considerably in appearance and endothelial permeability may be widely different from that in "healthy" tissue. Particles with sizes up to about 0.1 μm can enter tumor tissue as was demonstrated with long circulating, colloidal carrier systems (long circulating liposomes). On the other hand, necrotic tissue can also hamper access to tumor tissue (Jain, 1987). In conclusion, the body is highly compartmentalized; it should not be considered as one big pool without internal barriers for transport.

■ **Soluble Carrier Systems for Targeted Delivery of Proteins**

*MAb as Targeted Therapeutic Agents: Human and Humanized Antibodies (see Chapter 15)*

Antibodies are "natural targeting devices." Their homing ability is combined with functional activity (Crommelin and Storm, 1990; Crommelin et al., 1992). MAb can affect the target cell function upon attachment. Complement can be bound via the Fc receptor and subsequently cause lysis of the target cell. Alternatively, certain Fc receptor-bearing killer cells can induce "antibody dependent, cell-mediated cytotoxicity" (ADCC), or contact with macrophages can be established. Moreover, metabolic deficiencies can be

induced in the target cells through a blockade of certain essential cell surface receptors by MAb. Structural aspects and therapeutic potential of MAb is dealt with in detail in Chapter 15.

A problem that occurs when using murine antibodies for therapy is the production of human anti-mouse antibodies (HAMA) after administration. HAMA induction may prohibit further use of these therapeutic MAb by neutralizing the antigen-binding site; anaphylactic reactions are relatively rare. Concurrent administration of immunosuppressive agents is a strategy to minimize side effects. More in depth information regarding immunogenicity of therapeutic proteins is provided in Chapter 6.

There are several other ways to cope with this MAb-induced immunogenicity problem. These are dealt with in more detail in Chapter 15. Here, a brief summary of the options relevant for protein targeting suffices. First of all, the use of F(ab)$_2$ or F(ab) fragments (Fig. 27) avoids raising an immune response against the Fc part, but the development of humanized or human MAb minimizes the induction of HAMA even further. For humanization of MAb several options can be considered. One can build chimeric (partly human, partly murine) molecules consisting of a human Fc part and a murine Fab part, with the antigen binding sites or, alternatively, only the six complementarity determining regions (CDRs) of the murine antibody can be grafted in a human antibody structure. CDR grafting minimizes the exposure to murine material.

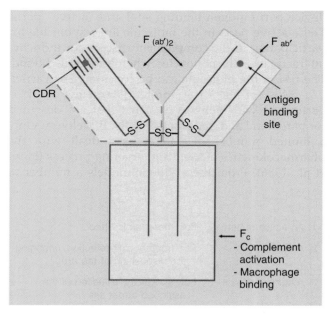

**Figure 27** ■ Highly simplified IgG1 structure. *Abbreviation*: CDR, complementarity determining region.

Completely human MAb can be produced by transfecting human antibody genes into mouse cells, which subsequently produce the human MAb. Alternatively, transgenic mice can be used (see Chapters 7 and 15). These approaches reduce the immunogenicity compared to the existing generation of murine MAb. But even with all these human or humanized MAb, anti-idiotypic immune responses against the binding site structure of the MAb cannot be excluded.

### Bispecific Antibodies (see Chapter 15)

To enhance the therapeutic potential of antibodies, bispecific antibodies have been designed. Bispecific antibodies are manufactured from two separate antibodies to create a molecule with two different binding sites (Fanger and Guyre, 1991). Bispecific MAb bring target cells or tissue (one antigen-binding site) in contact with other structures (second antigen binding site). This second antigen binding site can bind to effector cells via cytotoxicity triggering molecules on T-cells, NK(natural killer) cells, or macrophages, and thus trigger cytotoxicity.

Bispecific antibodies have been used experimentally in the clinic, for instance, to direct intraperitoneally injected autologous T-lymphocytes, stimulated with recombinant interleukin-2, to intraperitoneally located ovarian carcinoma cells. This MAb combines an antigen-binding site for a carcinoma-surface antigen with an antigen-binding site with T-cell affinity. The MAb are in vitro incubated with the stimulated T-lymphocytes prior to IP injection (Crommelin et al., 1992; De Leij et al., 1990).

### Immunoconjugates: Combinations between an Antibody and an Active Compound

In many cases antibodies alone or bispecific antibodies have been shown to lack sufficient therapeutic activity. To enhance their activity, conjugates of MAb and drugs have been designed (Fig. 28). These efforts mainly focus on the treatment of cancer (Crommelin and Storm, 1990). To test the concept of immunoconjugates, a wide range of drugs has been covalently bound to antibodies and has been evaluated in animal tumor models. As only a limited number of antibody molecules can bind to the target cells, only conjugation of highly potent drugs will lead to sufficient therapeutic activity. Gemtuzumab ozogamicin (Mylotarg®) is a conjugate of a monoclonal antibody and calicheamicin (see Chapter 16). The MAb part targets the CD33 surface antigen in CD33-positive acute myeloid leukemia cells (AML). After internalization into the cell the highly cytotoxic calicheamicin is released.

Cytostatics with a high intrinsic cytotoxicity are needed (see above). Because the kinetic behavior

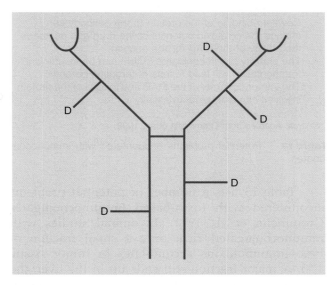

**Figure 28** ■ A schematic view of an immunoconjugate. *Abbreviation*: D, drug molecules covalently attached to antibody (fragments).

of active compounds is strongly affected by the conjugating antibody, not only existing cytostatics, but also active compounds that were never used before as drugs, because of their high toxicity, should now be reconsidered.

Immunoconjugated toxins are now tested as chemotherapeutic agents to treat cancer (immunotoxins). Examples of the toxin family are ricin, abrin, and diphtheria toxin (Fig. 29). These proteins are extremely toxic; they block enzymatically intracellular protein synthesis at the ribosomal level. Ricin (MW 66 kDa) consists of an A and a B chain that are linked through a cystin bridge. The A chain is responsible for blocking protein synthesis at the ribosomes. The B chain is important for cellular uptake of the molecule (endocytosis) and intracellular trafficking.

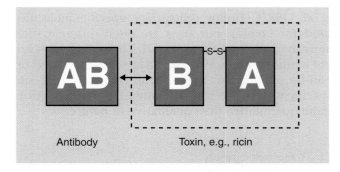

**Figure 29** ■ Immunotoxins are composed of antibody molecules connected to a toxin, e.g., ricin. Both the integral ricin molecule has been used as well as the A-chain alone. *Abbreviations*: AB, antibody; A and B stand for the A and B chain of the ricin toxin, respectively.

- Covalent binding of the protein to the antibody can change the cytotoxic potential of the drug and decrease the affinity of the MAB for the antigen
- The stability of the conjugate in vivo can be insufficient; fragmentation will lead to loss of targeting potential
- The immunogenicity of the MAB and toxicity of the protein involved can change dramatically

*Source*: Adapted from Crommelin et al., 1992.

**Table 13** ▪ Potential problems encountered with immunoconjugates.

Table 13 lists a number of potential problems encountered with toxin-based immunoconjugates (Crommelin et al., 1992). In animal studies with immunoconjugated ricin only a small fraction of these immunotoxins accumulates in tumor tissue (1%). A major fraction still ends up in the liver, the main target organ for "natural" ricin. Moreover, in clinical phase I studies (to assess the safety of the conjugates) the first generation of immunoconjugates turned out to be immunogenic. Now, attempts are being made to adapt the ricin molecule (by genetic engineering) so that liver targeting is being minimized. This can be done by blocking (removing or masking) on the ricin molecule ligands for galactose receptors on hepatocytes. Besides, murine MAb can be replaced by human or humanized MAb (see above) (Ramakrishnan, 1990).

■ **Potential Pitfalls in Tumor Targeting**

Upon IV injection, only a small fraction of the homing device–carrier–drug complex is sequestered at the target site. Apart from the compartmentalization of the body (see above: anatomical and physiological hurdles) and consequently the carrier-dependent barriers that result, several other factors account for this lack of target site accumulation (Table 14).

How successful are MAb in discriminating target cells (tumor cells) from non-target cells? Do all tumor cells expose the tumor-associated antigen? These questions are still difficult to answer (Hellström et al., 1987). Tumor cell-surface specific molecules used for homing purposes are often differentiation antigens on the tumor cell wall. These structures are not unique since they occur in a lower density level on non-target cells as well. Therefore, the target site specificity of MAb raised against these structures is more quantitative than qualitative in nature.

- Tumor heterogeneity
- Antigen shedding
- Antigen modulation

**Table 14** ▪ Factors that interfere with successful targeting of proteins to tumor cells.

Another category of tumor-associated antigens are the clone-specific antigens. They are unique for the clone forming the tumor. However, the practical problem when focusing on clone-specific antibodies for drug targeting is that each patient probably needs a tailor-made MAb.

The surface "make-up" of tumor cells in a tumor or a metastasis is not constant; neither in time nor between cells in the same tumor. There are many subpopulations of tumor cells and they express different surface molecules. This heterogeneity means that not all cells in the tumor will interact with one, single targeted conjugate. Antigen shedding and antigen modulation are two other ways tumor cells can avoid recognition. Shedding of antigens means that antigens are released from the surface. They can then interact with circulating conjugates outside the target area, form an antigen–antibody complex and neutralize the homing potential of the conjugates before the target area has been reached. Finally, antigen modulation can occur upon binding of MAb to the cell surface antigen. Modulation is the phenomenon that upon endocytosis of the (originally exposed) surface antigen–immunoconjugate complex, some of these antigens are not exposed anymore on the surface; there is no replenishment of endocytosed surface antigens.

Four strategies can be implemented to solve problems related to tumor cell heterogeneity, shedding and modulation. (*i*) Cocktails of different MAb attached to the toxin can be used. (*ii*) Another approach is to give up striving for complete target cell specificity and to induce so-called "bystander" effects. Then, the targeted system is designed in such a way that the active part is released from the conjugate after reaching a target cell, but before the antigen-conjugate complex has been taken up (is endocytosed) by the target cell. (*iii*) Not all surface antigens show shedding or modulation. If these phenomena occur, other antigen/MAb combinations should be selected that do not demonstrate these effects. (*iv*) At the present, injection of free MAb prior to injection of the immunoconjugate is under investigation to neutralize "free" circulating antigen; then, the subsequently injected conjugate should not encounter shedded, free antigen.

In conclusion, targeted (modified) MAb and MAb-conjugates are now studied to assess their value in fighting life-threatening diseases such as cancer. During the last decade, technology has evolved quickly; many different new options became available. Lack of detailed pathophysiological and cell biological knowledge about the behavior of tumors, for instance, slows down progress. It is even possible that the whole concept of MAb-(conjugates) will turn out to be only of limited therapeutic value, because of

- Size
- Charge
- Surface hydrophilicity
- Presence of homing devices on their surface
- Exchange of constitutive parts with blood components

**Table 15** ■ Parameters controlling the fate of particulate carriers in vivo.

problems such as tumor cell heterogeneity, poor access to tumors and immunogenicity concerns.

## ■ Colloidal Particulate Carrier Systems for Targeted Delivery of Proteins: Nanotechnology at Work

A wide range of carrier systems in the colloidal size range (diameters up to a few micrometers) has been proposed for protein targeting. Examples are: liposomes, biodegradable polycyanoacrylate nanoparticles, albumin microspheres, polylactic acid microspheres, and low density lipoproteins (LDL). Upon entering the bloodstream after IV injection, it is difficult for many of these particulate systems to pass through epithelial and endothelial membranes in healthy tissue, as the size cut-off for permeation through these multilayered barriers is around 20 nm (excluding the liver, see above and Fig. 26). Parameters that control the fate of particulate carriers in vivo are listed in Table 15.

As a rule, cells of the mononuclear phagocyte system (MPS), such as macrophages, recognize stable, colloidal particulate systems ($< 5 \mu m$) as "foreign body like structures" and phagocytose them. Thus, the liver and spleen, organs rich in blood circulation exposed macrophages, take up the majority of these particulates (Tomlinson, 1987; Crommelin and Storm, 1990). Larger ($> 5 \mu m$) intravenously injected particles tend to form emboli in lung capillaries on their first encounter with this organ.

Liposomes have gained considerable attention among the colloidal particulate systems proposed for site-specific delivery of (or by) proteins. Liposomes are vesicular structures based on (phospho)lipid bilayers surrounding an aqueous core. The main component of the bilayer usually is phosphatidylcholine (Fig. 30).

By selecting their bilayer constituents and one of the many preparation procedures described, liposomes can be made varying in size between 30 nm (e.g., by extrusion or ultrasonication) and 10 μm, and charge (by incorporation negatively or positively charged lipid molecules), and bilayer rigidity (by selecting special phospholipids or adding lipids such as cholesterol). Liposomes can carry their payload (proteins) either in the lipid core of the bilayer through partitioning, attached to the bilayer, or physically entrapped in the aqueous phase. To make liposomes target site specific, except for passive targeting to liver (Kupffer cells) and spleen macrophages, homing devices are covalently coupled to the outside bilayer leaflet (Toonen and Crommelin, 1983). In Table 16 three relative advantages of liposomes over other particulate systems are given.

After injection "standard" liposomes stay in the blood circulation only for a short time. They are taken

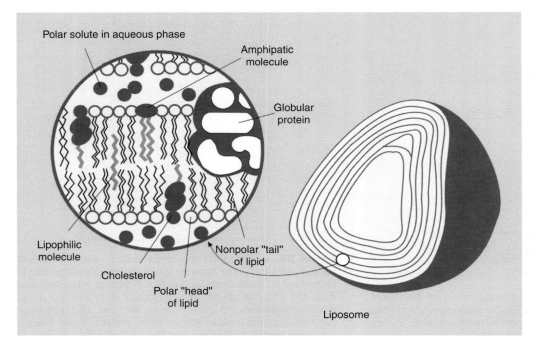

**Figure 30** ■ An artist's interpretation of a multilamellar liposome. The lamellae are bilayers of (*phospho*)lipid molecules with their hydrophobic tails oriented inward and their polar heads directed to, and in contact with, the aqueous medium. The bilayer may accommodate lipophilic drugs inside. Hydrophilic drugs will be found in the aqueous core and in between the bilayers. Depending on their hydrophilic/hydrophobic balance and tertiary structure proteins and peptides will be found in the aqueous phase, at the bilayer–water interface, or inside the lipid bilayer. *Source*: Adapted from Fendler, 1980.

Polar solute in aqueous phase

Amphipatic molecule

Globular protein

Lipophilic molecule

Cholesterol

Nonpolar "tail" of lipid

Polar "head" of lipid

Liposome

**Liposomes stand out among other particulate carrier systems, because:**

- Their relatively low toxicity, existing safety record and experience with marketed, intravenously administered liposome products (e.g., amphotericin B, doxorubicin, daunorubicin) (Storm et al., 1993).
- The presence of a relatively large aqueous core, which is essential to stabilize the structural features of many proteins.
- The possibility to manipulate release characteristics of liposome associated proteins and to control disposition in vivo by changing preparation techniques and bilayer constituents (Crommelin and Schreier, 1994).

**Table 16** ■ Liposomes stand out among other particulate carrier systems.

up by macrophages in liver and spleen, or they degrade by exchange of bilayer constituents with blood constituents. Liposome residence time in the blood circulation can be extended to many hours and even days, if PEG chains are grafted on the surface and stable bilayer structures are used (Fig. 31, see also Fig. 17). These long circulating liposomes apparently are able to escape macrophage uptake for prolonged periods of time and are sequestered in other organs than liver and spleen alone, e.g. tumors and inflamed tissues. In Figure 32 an example is shown of the use of $^{99m}$Tc-labelled liposomes in the detection of inflammation sites in a patient.

The accumulation of protein-laden liposomes in macrophages (passive targeting) offers interesting therapeutic opportunities. Liposome encapsulated lymphokines and "microbial" products, such as interferon-α or muramyl tripeptide phosphatidylethanolamine (MTP-PE), respectively, can activate

macrophages and enable them to kill micrometastases, or help to stimulate immune reactions. Moreover, reaching macrophages may help us to more effectively fight macrophage located microbial, viral or bacterial diseases than with our present approaches (Emmen and Storm, 1987; Crommelin and Schreier, 1994).

Several attempts have been made to sequester immunoliposomes (i.e., antibody (fragment)-liposome combinations) at predetermined sites in the body. Here the aim is active targeting to the desired target site instead of passive targeting to macrophages. The concept is schematically presented in Figure 33.

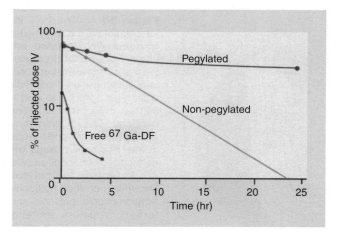

**Figure 31** ■ Comparison of the blood levels of free label, $^{67}$Ga–DF, gallium–desferal with $^{67}$Ga-DF laden pegylated (PEG) and non-pegylated liposomes upon IV administration in rats. *Source*: Adapted from Woodle, et al., 1990.

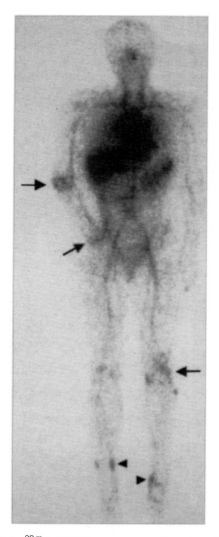

**Figure 32** ■ $^{99m}$Tc-PEG-liposomes scintigraphy of a female patient. Anterior whole body image, 24 h post-injection, shows physiological uptake in the cardiac blood, greater veins, liver, and spleen. Liposome uptake at pathological sites can be noted along synovial lining of the left elbow, left wrist, and right knee (*arrows*) and the medial site of both ankles (*arrow heads*). *Source*: Adapted from Storm and Crommelin, 1998.

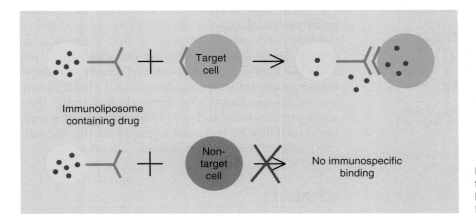

**Figure 33** ■ Schematic representation of the concept of drug targeting with immunoliposomes. *Source*: Adapted from Nässander, et al., 1990.

When designing immunoliposomes, antibodies or antibody-fragments are covalently bound to the surface of liposomes through lipid anchor molecules (Toonen and Crommelin, 1983). Non-PEGylated immunoliposomes have poor access to target sites outside the blood circulation after IV injection. The reason is the high resistance against liposome penetration through the endothelial lining at target sites and their relatively short circulation time (Fig. 26). Therefore, target sites should be sought in the blood circulation (red blood cells, thrombi, lymphocytes, or endothelial cells exposing under stress certain adhesion molecules, e.g. ICAM-1, intercellular cell adhesion molecule) (Vingerhoeds et al., 1994; Crommelin et al., 1995).

Other interesting target sites are those located in cavities, where one can locally administer the drug-carrier combination. The bladder and the peritoneal cavity are such cavities. These cavities can be the sites where the diseased tissue is concentrated. For instance, with ovarian carcinomas the tumors are confined to the peritoneal cavity for most of their lifetime. After IP injection of immunoliposomes directed against human ovarian carcinomas in athymic, nude mice, a specific interaction between immunoliposomes and the human ovarian carcinoma was observed (Nässander and colleagues) (Fig. 34).

A new generation of liposomes is under development that combines PEG coating (long circulation characteristic) and antibody coating (targeting).

Attaching an immunoliposome to target cells usually does not induce a therapeutic effect per se. After establishment of an immunoliposome–cell interaction the protein drug has to exert its action on the cell. To do that, the protein has to be released in its active form. There are several pathways proposed to reach this goal (Fig. 35) (Peeters et al., 1987).

When the immunoliposome–cell complex encounters a macrophage, the cells plus adhering liposome are probably phagocytosed and enter the macrophage (option A). Subsequently, the liposome-associated protein drug can be released. As this will most likely happen in the "hostile" lysosomal environment, little intact protein will become available. In the situation depicted in Figure 35, option B, the drug is released from the adhering immunoliposomes in the close proximity of the target cell. In principle, release rate control is achieved by selecting the proper liposomal bilayers with delayed or sustained drug release characteristics. A third approach is depicted as option C: drug release is induced from liposomal bilayers by external stimuli (local pH change or temperature change). Finally, one can envision that

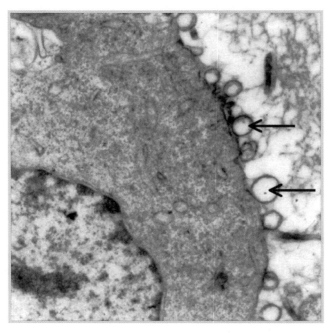

**Figure 34** ■ Electromicrograph showing immunoliposomes (vesicular structures) attached to human ovarian carcinoma cells (see text).

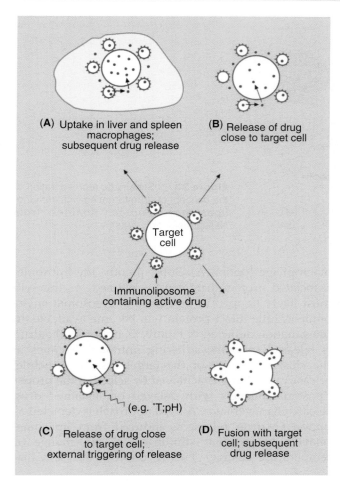

(A) Uptake in liver and spleen macrophages; subsequent drug release

(B) Release of drug close to target cell

Target cell

Immunoliposome containing active drug

(e.g. °T;pH)

(C) Release of drug close to target cell; external triggering of release

(D) Fusion with target cell; subsequent drug release

**Figure 35** ■ Several pathways of drug internalization after immunospecific binding of the immunoliposomes to the appropriate target cell. *Source*: Adapted from Peeters et al., 1987.

immunoliposomes can be built with intrinsic fusogenic potential, which is only activated upon attachment of the carrier to the target cell. This exciting option D, Figure 35, resembles the behavior of certain viruses. Viruses offer interesting pathways as to how to enter target cells and how to deliver their payload successfully in a target organelle (i.e., for viruses the nucleus). This virus-mimicking approach led to the design of artificial viruses for targeted delivery of genetic material, but this can be extended to therapeutic proteins (Mastrobattista et al., 2006).

### ■ Perspectives for Targeted Protein Delivery

Protein targeting strategies have been developing at a rapid pace. A new generation of homing devices (target cell-specific MAb) and a better insight into the anatomy and physiology of the human body under pathological conditions have been critical factors to achieve this success. A much better picture has emerged not only about the potentials, but also the limitations of the different targeting approaches.

Very little attention has been paid to typically pharmaceutical aspects of advanced drug delivery systems such as immunotoxins and immunoliposomes. These systems are now produced on a lab scale and their therapeutic potential is currently under investigation. If therapeutic benefits have been clearly proven in preclinical and early clinical trials, then scaling up, shelf life and quality assurance issues (e.g., reproducibility of technology, purity of the ingredients) will still require considerable attention.

### REFERENCES

Arakawa T, Kita Y, Carpenter JF (1991). Protein–solvent interactions in pharmaceutical formulation. Pharmaceut Res, 8:285–91.

Banerjee PS, Hosny EA and Robinson JR (1991). Parenteral delivery of peptide and protein drugs. In Lee VHL, ed. Peptide and Protein Drug Delivery. New York: Marcel Dekker, 487–543.

Björk E, Edman P (1988). Characterization of degradable starch microspheres as a nasal delivery system for drugs. Int J Pharm, 62:187–92.

Brange J, Langkjaer L (1993). Insulin structure and stability. In: Wang YJ, Pearlman R, eds. Stability and Characterization of Protein and Peptide Drugs. Case Histories. New York: Plenum Press, 315–50.

Chien YW (1991). Transdermal route of peptide and protein drug delivery. In: Lee VHL, ed. Peptide and Protein Drug Delivery. New York: Marcel Dekker, 667–89.

Crommelin DJA, Bergers J, Zuidema J (1992). Antibody-based drug targeting approaches: perspectives and challenges. In: Wermuth CG, Koga N, König H, Metcalf BW, eds. Medicinal Chemistry for the 21st Century. Oxford: Blackwell Scientific Publications, 351–65.

Crommelin DJA, Scherphof G, Storm G (1995). Active targeting with particulate carrier systems in the blood compartment. Adv Drug Deliv Rev, 17:49–60.

Crommelin DJA, Schreier H (1994). Liposomes. In: Kreuter J, ed. Colloidal Drug Delivery Systems. New York: Marcel Dekker, 73–190.

Crommelin DJA, Storm G (1990). Drug Targeting. In: Sammes PG, Taylor JD, eds. Comprehensive Medicinal Chemistry. Oxford: Pergamon Press, 661–701.

Cullander C, Guy RH (1992) Transdermal delivery of peptides and proteins. Adv Drug Deliv Rev, 8:291–329.

De Leij L, De Jonge MWA, Ter Haar J, et al. (1990). Bispecific monoclonal antibody (BIAB) retargeted cellular therapy for local treatment of cancer patients. In: Crommelin DJA, Schellekens H, eds. From Clone to Clinic. Dordrecht: Kluwer Academic, 159–65.

Edman P, Björk E (1992). Nasal delivery of peptide drugs. Adv Drug Deliv Rev 8:165–77.

Eldridge JH, Hammond CJ, Meulbroek, JA, Staas JK, Giley RM, Tice TR (1990). Controlled vaccine release in the gut-associated lymphoid tissues. I. Orally administered biodegradable microspheres target the Peyer's patches. J Control Rel 11:205–14.

Emmen F, Storm G (1987). Liposomes in the treatment of infectious diseases. Pharm Weekblad Sci Ed 9:162–71.

FDA, www.fda.gov/cber/vaccine/thimfaq.htm, 2006

Fanger MW, Guyre PM (1991). Bispecific antibodies for targeted cellular cytotoxicity. TIBTECH 9:375–80.

Fendler JH (1980). Optimizing drug entrapment in liposomes. Chemical and biophysical considerations. In: Gregoriadis G, Allison AC, eds. Liposomes in Biological Systems. Chichester: Wiley, J. & Sons, 87.

Franks F, Hatley RHM, Mathias SF (1991). Materials science and the production of shelf-stable biologicals. Pharmaceut Technol Int, 3.

Groves M (1988). Parenteral Technology Manual. Buffalo Grove, IL: Interpharm Press, Inc.

Halls NA (1994). Achieving Sterility in Medical and Pharmaceutical Products. New York: Marcel Dekker.

Heilmann K (1984). Therapeutic Systems. Rate Controlled Delivery: Concept and Development. Stuttgart: G. Thieme Verlag.

Heller J (1993). Polymers for controlled parenteral delivery of peptides and proteins. Adv Drug Deliv Rev 10:163–204.

Hellström KE, Hellström I, Goodman GE (1987). Antibodies for drug delivery. In: Robinson JR, Lee VHL, eds. Controlled Drug Delivery. New York: Marcel Dekker, 623–53.

Ho NFH, Barsuhn CL, Burton PS, Merkle HP (1992). Mechanistic insights to buccal delivery of proteinaceous substances. Adv Drug Deliv Rev 8:197–235.

Holmgren J, Clemens J, Sack D, Sanchez J, Svennerholm AM (1989). Development of oral vaccines with special reference to cholera. In: Breimer DD, Crommelin DJA, Midha KK, eds. Topics in Pharmaceutical Sciences. The Hague: International Pharmaceutical Federation (FIP), 297–311.

Hunt CA, MacGregor RD, Siegel RA (1986). Engineering targeted in vivo drug delivery. I. The physiological and physicochemical principles governing opportunities and limitations. Pharm Res 3:333–44.

Jain RK (1987). Transport of molecules in the tumor interstitium: A review. Cancer Res 47:3039–51.

Jani PU, Florence AT, McCarthy DE (1992). Further histological evidence of the gastrointestinal absorption of polystyrene nanospheres in the rat. Int J Pharm 84:245–52.

Kersten G, Hirschberg H (2004). Antigen delivery systems. Expert Rev. Vaccin 3:89–99.

Kim SW, Pai CM, Makino K, et al. (1990). Self-regulated glycosylated insulin delivery. J Control Rel 11:193–201.

Klegerman ME, Groves MJ (1992). Pharmaceutical Biotechnology: Fundamentals and Essentials. Buffalo Grove, IL: Interpharm Press.

Kumar S, Char H, Patel S, et al. (1992). In vivo transdermal iontophoretic delivery of growth hormone releasing factor GRF (1–44) in hairless guinea pigs. J Control Rel 18:213–20.

Lee VHL, Dodda-Kashi S, Grass GM, Rubas W (1991). Oral route of peptide and protein drug delivery. In: Lee VHL, ed. Peptide and Protein Drug Delivery. New York: Marcel Dekker, 691–738.

Lee HJ, Riley G, Johnson O, et al. (1997). In vivo characterization of sustained-release formulations of human growth hormone. J Pharmacol Exp Therapeut 281:1431–9.

Maberly GF, Wait GA, Kilpatrick JA, et al. (1982). Evidence for insulin degradation by muscle and fat tissue in an insulin resistant diabetic patient. Diabetologica 23:333–6.

Mastrobattista E, Aa MAEM, van der, Hennink WE, Crommelin DJA (2006). Artificial viruses: A nanotechnological approach to gene delivery. Nat Rev/Drug Dis 5:115–21.

Matthews SJ, McCoy C (2004). Peginterferon Alfa-2a: A review of approved and investigational use. Clin Therapeut 26:991–1024.

Nässander UK, Storm G, Peeters PAM, Crommelin DJA (1990). Liposomes. In: Chasin M, Langer R, eds. Biodegradable Polymers as Drug Delivery Systems. New York: Marcel Dekker, 261–33.

O'Hagan DT (1990). Intestinal translocation of particulates—implications for drug and antigen delivery. Adv Drug Deliv Rev 5:265–85.

Nguyen TH, Ward C (1993). Stability characterization and formulation development of alteplase, a recombinant tissue plasminogen activator. In: Wang YJ, Pearlman R, eds. Stability and Characterization of Protein and Peptide Drugs. Case Histories. New York: Plenum Press, 91–134.

Patton JS, Platz RM (1992). Pulmonary delivery of peptides and proteins for systemic action. Adv Drug Deliv Rev 8:179–96.

Patton JS, Trinchero P, Platz RM (1994). Bioavailability of pulmonary delivered peptides and proteins: Alpha-interferon, calcitonins and parathyroid hormones. J Control Release 28:79–85.

Patton JS, Bukar J, Nagarajan S (1999). Inhaled insulin. Adv Drug Deliv Rev 35:235–47.

Patton JS, Bukar JG, Eldon MA (2004). Clinical pharmacokinetics and pharmacodynamics of inhaled insulin. Clin Pharmacokinet 43:781–801.

Pearlman R, Bewley TA (1993). Stability and characterization of human growth hormone. In: Wang YJ, Pearlman R, eds. Stability and Characterization of Protein and Peptide Drugs. Case Histories. New York: Plenum Press, 1–58.

Peeters PAM, Storm G, Crommelin DJA (1987). Immunoliposomes in vivo: State of the art. Adv Drug Deliv Rev 1:249–66.

Pikal MJ (1990a). Freeze-drying of proteins. Part I: Process Design. BioPharm 3(8):18–27.

Pikal MJ (1990b). Freeze-drying of proteins. Part II: Formulation selection. BioPharm 3:26–30.

Poste G (1985). Drug targeting in cancer therapy. In: Gregoriadis G, Poste G, Senior J, Trouet A, eds. Receptor-Mediated Targeting of Drugs. New York: Plenum Press, 427–74.

Pristoupil TI (1985). Haemoglobin lyophilized with sucrose: Effect of residual moisture on storage. Haematologia 18:45–52.

Ramakrishnan S (1990). Current status of antibody-toxin conjugates for tumor therapy. In: Tyle P, Ram BP, eds.

Targeted Therapeutic Systems. New York: Marcel Dekker, 189–213.

Roitt IM, Brostoff J, Male DK (1993). Immunology. 3rd ed. St. Louis, MO: Mosby.

Sage BH, Bock CR, Denuzzio JD, Hoke RA (1995). Technological and developmental issues of iontophoretic transport of peptide and protein drugs. In: Lee VHL, Hashida M, Mizushima Y, eds. Trends and Future Perspectives in Peptide and Protein Drug Delivery. Chur: Harwood Academic Publishers GmbH, 111–34.

Soon-Shiong P, Heintz RE, Merideth N, et al. (1994). Insulin independence in a type 1 diabetic patient after encapsulated islet transplantation. Lancet 343:950–51.

Stenekes R (2000). Nanoporous dextran microspheres for drug delivery. Thesis, Utrecht University.

Storm G, Oussoren C, Peeters PAM, Barenholz YB (1993). Tolerability of liposomes in vivo. In: Gregoriadis G, ed. Liposome Technology. Boca Raton, FL: CRC Press, 345-83.

Storm G, Nässander U, Vingerhoeds MH, Steerenberg PA, Crommelin DJA (1994). Antibody-targeted liposomes to deliver doxorubicin to ovarian cancer cells. J Liposome Res 4:641–66.

Storm G, Crommelin DJA (1998). Liposomes: Quo vadis? Pharmaceut Sci Technol Today 1:19–31.

Supersaxo A, Hein WR, Steffen H (1990). Effect of molecular weight on the lymphatic absorption of water-soluble compounds following subcutaneous administration. Pharm Res 7:167–9.

Thurow H, Geisen K (1984). Stabilization of dissolved proteins against denaturation at hydrophobic interfaces. Diabetologica 27:212–8.

Tomlinson E (1987). Theory and practice of site-specific drug delivery. Adv Drug Deliv Rev 1:87–198.

Toonen P, Crommelin DJA (1983). Immunogobulins as targeting agents for liposome encapsulated drugs. Pharm Weekblad Sci Ed 16:269–80.

Tresco PA (1994). Encapsulated cells for sustained neurotransmitter delivery to the central nervous system. J Control Rel 28:253–8.

Uludag H, Kharlip L, Sefton MV (1993). Protein delivery by microencapsulated cells. Adv Drug Deliv Rev 10:115–30.

USP 29/NF 24 through second supplement (2006). Rockville, MD: United States Pharmacopeial Convention, Inc.

van Dijkhuizen-Radersma R, Wright SJ, Taylor LM, John BA, de Groot K, Bezemer JM (2004). In vitro/in vivo correlation for $^{14}$C-methylated lysozyme release from poly(ether-ester) microspheres. Pharm Res 21:484–91.

Vemuri S, Yu CT, Roosdorp N (1993a). Formulation and stability of recombinant alpha-antitrypsin. In: Wang YJ, Pearlman R, eds. Stability and Characterization of Protein and Peptide Drugs. Case Histories. New York: Plenum Press, 263–86.

Vemuri S, Yu CT, Roosdorp N (1993b). Formulation and stability of recombinant alpha1-antitrypsin. In: Wang YJ, Pearlman R, eds. Stability and Characterization of Protein and Peptide Drugs. New York: Plenum Press, 263–86.

Vingerhoeds MH, Storm G, Crommelin DJA (1994). Immunoliposomes in vivo. Immunomethods 4:259–72.

Woodle M, Newman M, Collins L, Redemann C, Martin F (1990). Improved long-circulating (Stealth®) liposomes using synthetic lipids. Proc Int Symp Control Rel Bioactive Mater 17:77–8.

Zhou XH, Li Wan Po A (1991a). Peptide and protein drugs: I. Therapeutic applications, absorption and parenteral administration. Int J Pharm 75:97–115.

Zhou XH, Li Wan Po A (1991b). Peptide and protein drugs: II. Non-parenteral routes of delivery. Int J Pharm 75:117–30.

# 5

# Pharmacokinetics and Pharmacodynamics of Peptide and Protein Drugs

*Bernd Meibohm*
University of Tennessee Health Science Center, College of Pharmacy, Department of Pharmaceutical Sciences, Memphis, Tennessee, U.S.A.

*Rene Braeckman*
Reliance Clinical Research Services, Newtown, Pennsylvania, U.S.A.

## INTRODUCTION

The rational use of drugs and the design of effective dosage regimens are facilitated by the appreciation of the central paradigm of clinical pharmacology that there is a defined relationship between the administered dose of a drug, the resulting drug concentrations in various body fluids and tissues, and the intensity of pharmacologic effects caused by these concentrations (Meibohm and Derendorf, 1997). This dose–exposure–response relationship and thus the dose of a drug required to achieve a certain effect are determined by the drug's pharmacokinetic and pharmacodynamic properties (Fig. 1).

Pharmacokinetics describes the time course of the concentration of a drug in a body fluid, preferably plasma or blood, that results from the administration of a certain dosage regimen. It comprises all processes affecting drug absorption, distribution, metabolism, and excretion. Simplified, pharmacokinetics characterizes *what the body does to the drug*. In contrast, pharmacodynamics characterizes the intensity of a drug effect or toxicity resulting from certain drug concentrations in a body fluid, usually at the assumed site of drug action. It can be simplified to *what the drug does to the body* (Fig. 2) (Holford and Sheiner, 1982; Derendorf and Meibohm, 1999).

The understanding of the dose–concentration–effect relationship is crucial to any drug — including peptides and proteins — as it lays the foundation for dosing regimen design and rational clinical application. General pharmacokinetic and pharmacodynamics principles are to a large extent equally applicable to protein and peptide drugs as they are to traditional small molecule-based therapeutics. Deviations from some of these principles and additional challenges with regard to the characterization of the pharmacokinetics and pharmacodynamics of peptide and protein therapeutics, however, arise from some of their specific properties:

a. Their structural similarity to endogenous structural or functional proteins and nutrients.
b. Their intimate involvement in physiologic processes on the molecular level, often including regulatory feedback mechanisms.
c. The analytical challenges to identify and quantify them in the presence of a myriad of similar molecules.
d. Their large molecular weight and macromolecule character (for proteins).

This chapter will highlight some of the major pharmacokinetic properties and processes relevant for the majority of peptide and protein therapeutics and will provide examples of well-characterized pharmacodynamic relationships for peptide and protein drugs. The clinical pharmacology of monoclonal antibodies, including special aspects in their pharmacokinetic and pharmacodynamics, will be discussed in further detail in Chapter 15. For a more general discussion on pharmacokinetic and pharmacodynamic principles, the reader is referred to several textbooks and articles that review the topic in extensive detail (see Further Reading section).

## PHARMACOKINETICS OF PROTEIN THERAPEUTICS

The in vivo disposition of peptide and protein drugs may often be predicted to a large degree from their physiological function (Tang and Meibohm, 2006). Peptides, for example, which frequently have hormone activity, usually have short elimination half-lives, which is desirable for a close regulation of their endogenous levels and thus function. Insulin, for example shows dose-dependent elimination with a relatively short half-life of 26 and 52 minutes at 0.1 and 0.2 U/kg, respectively. Contrary to that, proteins that have transport tasks such as albumin or long-term

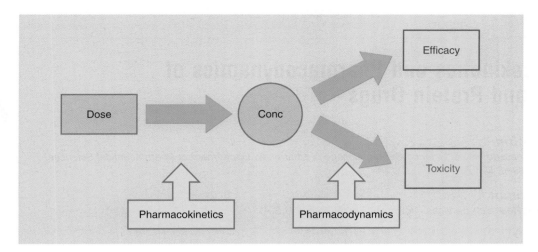

**Figure 1** ■ The central paradigm of clinical pharmacology: The dose–concentration–effect relationship.

immunity functions such as immunoglobulins have elimination half-lives of several days, which enables and ensures the continuous maintenance of physiologically necessary concentrations in the bloodstream (Meibohm and Derendorf, 1994). This is for example reflected by the elimination half-life of antibody drugs such as the anti-epidermal growth factor receptor antibody cetuximab, an IgG1 chimeric antibody for which a half-life of approximately 7 days has been reported (Herbst and Langer, 2002).

■ **Absorption of Protein Therapeutics**

*Enteral Administration*
Peptides and proteins, unlike conventional small molecule drugs, are generally not therapeutically

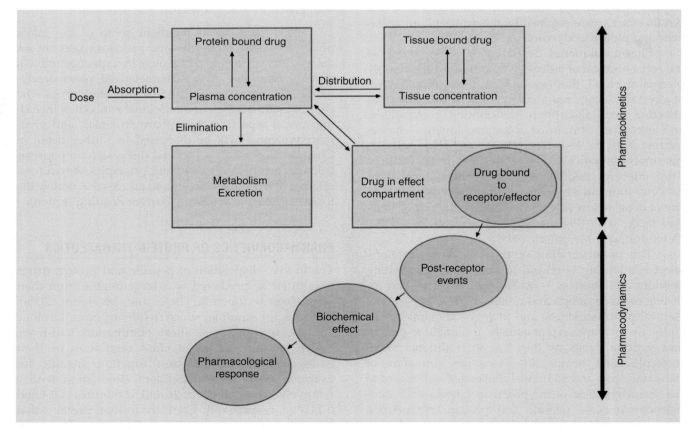

**Figure 2** ■ Physiological scheme of pharmacokinetic and pharmacodynamic processes.

active upon oral administration (Fasano, 1998; Mahato et al., 2003; Tang et al., 2004). The lack of systemic bioavailability is mainly caused by two factors: (1) high gastrointestinal enzyme activity and (2) low permeability through the gastrointestinal mucosa. In fact, the substantial peptidase and protease activity in the gastrointestinal tract makes it the most efficient body compartment for peptide and protein metabolism. Furthermore, the gastrointestinal mucosa presents a major absorption barrier for water-soluble macromolecules such as peptides and proteins (Tang et al., 2004). Thus, although various factors such as permeability, stability and gastrointestinal transit time can affect the rate and extent of absorption of orally administered proteins, molecular size is generally considered the ultimate obstacle (Shen, 2003).

Since oral administration is still a highly desirable route of delivery for protein drugs due to its convenience, cost-effectiveness and painlessness, numerous strategies to overcome the obstacles associated with oral delivery of proteins have recently been an area of intensive research. Suggested approaches to increase the oral bioavailability of protein drugs include encapsulation into micro- or nanoparticles thereby protecting proteins from intestinal degradation (Lee, 2002; Mahato et al., 2003; Shen, 2003). Other strategies are chemical modifications such as amino acid backbone modifications and chemical conjugations to improve the resistance to degradation and the permeability of the protein drug. Coadministration of protease inhibitors has also been suggested for the inhibition of enzymatic degradation (Pauletti et al., 1997; Mahato et al., 2003). More details on approaches for oral delivery of peptide and protein therapeutics are discussed in Chapter 4.

### Parenteral Administration

Most peptide and protein drugs are currently formulated as parenteral formulations because of their poor oral bioavailability. Major routes of administration include intravenous (IV), subcutaneous (SC), and intramuscular (IM) administration. In addition, other non-oral administration pathways are utilized, including nasal, buccal, rectal, vaginal, transdermal, ocular and pulmonary drug delivery (see Chapter 4).

IV administration of peptides and proteins offers the advantage of circumventing presystemic degradation, thereby achieving the highest concentration in the biological system. Protein therapeutics given by the IV route include, among many others, the tissue plasminogen activator (t-PA) analogs alteplase and tenecteplase, the recombinant human erythropoietin epoetin-α, and the granulocyte-colony-stimulating factor filgrastim (Tang and Meibohm, 2006).

IV administration as either a bolus dose or constant rate infusion, however, may not always provide the desired concentration–time profile depending on the biological activity of the product. In these cases, IM or SC injections may be more appropriate alternatives. For example, luteinizing hormone-releasing hormone (LH-RH) in bursts stimulates the release of follicle-stimulating hormone (FSH) and luteinizing hormone (LH), whereas a continuous baseline level will suppress the release of these hormones (Handelsman and Swerdloff, 1986). To avoid the high peaks from an IV administration of leuprorelin, an LH-RH agonist, a long acting monthly depot injection of the drug is approved for the treatment of prostate cancer and endometriosis (Periti et al., 2002). A recent study comparing SC versus IV administration of epoetin-α in patients receiving hemodialysis reports that the SC route can maintain the hematocrit in a desired target range with a lower average weekly dose of epoetin-α compared to IV (Kaufman et al., 1998).

One of the potential limitations of SC and IM administration, however, are the presystemic degradation processes frequently associated with these administration routes, resulting in a reduced bioavailability compared to IV administration. The pharmacokinetically derived apparent absorption rate constant $k_{app}$ for protein drugs administered via these administration routes is thus the combination of absorption into the systemic circulation and presystemic degradation at the absorption site, i.e., the sum of a true first-order absorption rate constant $k_a$ and a first-order degradation rate constant. The true absorption rate constant $k_a$ can then be calculated as

$$k_a = F \cdot k_{app}$$

where $F$ is the bioavailability compared to IV administration. A rapid apparent absorption, i.e., large $k_{app}$, can thus be the result of a slow true absorption and a fast presystemic degradation, i.e., a low systemic bioavailability (Colburn, 1991).

Other potential factors that may limit bioavailability of proteins after SC or IM administration include variable local blood flow, injection trauma, and limitations of uptake into the systemic circulation related to effective capillary pore size and diffusion.

Several peptide and protein therapeutics including anakinra, etanercept, insulin, and pegfilgrastim are administered as SC injections. Following an SC injection, peptide and protein therapeutics may enter the systemic circulation either via blood capillaries or through lymphatic vessels (Porter and Charman, 2000). In general, macromolecules larger than 16 kDa are predominantly absorbed into the lymphatics whereas those under 1 kDa are mostly absorbed into the blood circulation. There appears to be a linear relationship between the molecular weight of the protein and the proportion of the dose absorbed by the lymphatics (see Fig. 12 in Chapter 4) (Supersaxo et al., 1990).

This is of particular importance for those agents whose therapeutic targets are lymphoid cells (i.e., interferons and interleukins). Studies with recombinant human interferon α-2a (rhIFNα2a) indicate that following SC administration, high concentrations of the recombinant protein are found in the lymphatic system, which drains into regional lymph nodes (Supersaxo et al., 1988). Clinical studies show that palliative low-to-intermediate-dose SC recombinant interleukin-2 (rIL-2) in combination with rhIFNα2a can be administered to patients in the ambulatory setting with efficacy and safety profiles comparable to the most aggressive IV rIL-2 protocol against metastatic renal cell cancer (Schomburg et al., 1993; Chen et al., 2000).

## ■ Distribution of Protein Therapeutics

### Distribution Mechanisms and Volumes

The rate and extent of protein distribution is determined largely by their size and molecular weight, physiochemical properties (e.g., charge, lipophilicity), protein binding, and their dependency on active transport processes. Since most therapeutic proteins have high molecular weights and are thus large in size, their apparent volume of distribution is usually small and limited to the volume of the extracellular space due to their limited mobility secondary to impaired passage through biomembranes (Zito, 1997). Active tissue uptake and binding to intra- and extravascular proteins, however, can substantially increase the apparent volume of distribution of protein drugs, as reflected by the relatively large volume of distribution of up to 2.8 L/kg for interferon β-1b (Chiang et al., 1993).

In contrast to small molecule drugs, protein transport from the vascular space into the interstitial space of tissues is largely mediated by convection rather than diffusion, following the unidirectional fluid flux from the vascular space through paracellular pores into the interstitial tissue space. The subsequent removal from the tissues is accomplished by lymph drainage back into the systemic circulation (Flessner et al., 1997). This underlines the unique role the lymphatic system plays in the disposition of protein therapeutics as already discussed in the section on absorption. Another, but much less prominent pathway for the movement of protein molecules from the vascular to the interstitial space is transcellular migration via endocytosis (Baxter et al., 1994; Reddy et al., 2006).

Besides the size-dependent sieving of macromolecules through the capillary walls, charge may

also play an important role in the biodistribution of proteins. It has been suggested that the electrostatic attraction between positively charged proteins and negatively charged cell membranes might increase the rate and extent of tissue distribution. Most cell surfaces are negatively charged because of their abundance of glycoaminoglycans in the extracellular matrix.

After IV administration, peptides and proteins usually follow a biexponential plasma concentration–time profile that can best be described by a two-compartment pharmacokinetic model (Meibohm, 2004). A biexponential concentration–time profile has, for example, been described for clenoliximab, a macaque-human chimeric monoclonal antibody specific to the CD4 molecule on the surface of T-lymphocytes (Mould et al., 1999). Similarly, AJW200, a humanized monoclonal antibody to the von Willebrand factor, exhibited biphasic pharmacokinetics after IV administration (Kageyama et al., 2002). The central compartment in this two-compartment model represents primarily the vascular space and the interstitial space of well-perfused organs with permeable capillary walls, including the liver and the kidneys. The peripheral compartment is more reflective of concentration–time profiles in the interstitial space of slowly equilibrating tissues.

The central compartment in which proteins initially distribute after IV administration has thus typically a volume of distribution equal or slightly larger than the plasma volume, i.e., 3 to 8 L. The total volume of distribution frequently comprises with 14 to 20 L not more than 2 to 3 times the initial volume of distribution (Colburn, 1991; Kageyama et al., 2002). An example for such a distribution pattern is the t-PA analog tenecteplase. Radiolabeled [125]I-tenecteplase was described to have an initial volume of distribution of 4.2 to 6.3 L and a total volume of distribution of 6.1 to 9.9 L with liver as the only organ that had a significant uptake of radioactivity. The authors concluded that the small volume of distribution suggests primarily intravascular distribution for tenecteplase, consistent with the drug's large molecular weight of 65 kDa (Tanswell et al., 2002).

Epoetin-α, for example, has a volume of distribution estimated to be close to the plasma volume at 0.056 L/kg after an IV administration to healthy volunteers (Ramakrishnan et al., 2004). Similarly, volume of distribution for darbepoetin-α has been reported as 0.062 L/kg after IV administration in patients undergoing dialysis (Allon et al., 2002), and distribution of thrombopoietin has also been reported to be limited to the plasma volume (~3 L) (Jin and Krzyzanski, 2004).

It should be stressed that pharmacokinetic calculations of volume of distribution may be problematic for many protein therapeutics (Tang et al., 2004; Straughn, 2006). Non-compartmental determination of volume of distribution at steady state ($V_{ss}$) using statistical moment theory assumes first-order disposition processes with elimination occurring from the rapidly equilibrating or central compartment (Perrier and Mayersohn, 1982; Straughn, 1982; Veng-Pedersen and Gillespie, 1984). These basic assumptions, however, are not fulfilled for numerous protein therapeutics, as proteolysis and receptor-mediated elimination in peripheral tissues may constitute a substantial fraction of the overall elimination process. If protein therapeutics are eliminated from slowly equilibrating tissues at a rate greater than their distribution process, substantial error in the volume of distribution assessment may occur. A recent simulation study could show that if substantial tissue elimination exists, a $V_{ss}$ determined by non-compartmental methods will underestimate the "true" $V_{ss}$, and that the magnitude of error tends to be larger the more extensively the protein is eliminated by tissues routes (Meibohm, 2004; Straughn, 2006; Tang and Meibohm, 2006).

These challenges in characterizing the distribution of protein therapeutics can only be overcome by determining actual protein concentrations in the tissue by biopsy or necropsy, or via biodistribution studies with radiolabeled compound and/or imaging techniques.

Biodistribution studies are imperative for small organic synthetic drugs, since long residence times of the radioactive label in certain tissues may be an indication of tissue accumulation of potentially toxic metabolites. Because of the possible reutilization of amino acids from protein drugs in endogenous proteins, such a safety issue does not exist for protein therapeutics. Therefore, biodistribution studies for protein drugs are usually only performed to assess drug targeting to specific tissues, or to detect the major organs of elimination (usually kidneys and liver).

If the protein contains a suitable amino acid such as tyrosine or lysine, an external label such as [125]I can be chemically coupled to the protein (Ferraiolo and Mohler, 1992). Although this coupling is easily accomplished and a highly specific activity can be obtained, the protein is chemically altered. Therefore, it may be better to label proteins and other biotechnology compounds by introducing radioactive isotopes during their synthesis by which an internal atom becomes the radioactive marker (internal labeling). For recombinant proteins, internal labeling can be accomplished by growing the production cell line in the presence of amino acids labeled with [3]H, [14]C, [35]S, etc. This method is not routinely used because of the prohibition of radioactive contamination of fermentation equipment (Meibohm and Derendorf,

2003). Moreover, internally labeled proteins may be less desirable than iodinated proteins because of the potential reutilization of the radiolabeled amino acid fragments in the synthesis of endogenous proteins and cell structures. Irrespective of the labeling method, but more so for external labeling, the labeled product should have demonstrated physicochemical and biological properties identical to the unlabeled molecule (Bennett and McMartin, 1978).

In addition, as for all types of radiolabeled studies, it needs to be established whether the measured radioactivity represents intact labeled protein, or radiolabeled metabolites, or the liberated label. Trichloro-acetic acid-precipitable radioactivity is often used to distinguish intact protein from free label or low-molecular-weight metabolites, which appear in the supernatant after centrifugation (Meibohm and Derendorf, 2003). Proteins with reutilized labeled amino acids and large protein metabolites can only be distinguished from the original protein by techniques such as polyacrylamide gel electrophoresis (PAGE), high pressure liquid chromatography (HPLC), specific immunoassays, or bioassays (see Chapter 2). This discussion also implies that the results of biodistribution studies with autoradiography can be very misleading. Autoradiography is a technique where tissue samples are brought into contact with X-ray sensitive films to visualize radioactively labeled molecules or fragments of molecules. Although autoradiography is becoming more quantitative, one never knows what is being measured qualitatively (original molecules or its degradation products) without specific assays. It is therefore sometimes better to perform biodistribution studies by the collection of the tissues and the specific measurement of the protein drug in the tissue homogenate.

### Protein Binding of Protein Therapeutics

Another factor that can influence the distribution of therapeutic peptides and proteins is binding to endogenous protein structures. Physiologically active endogenous peptides and proteins frequently interact with specific binding proteins involved in their transport and regulation. Furthermore, interaction with binding proteins may enable or facilitate cellular uptake processes and thus affect the drug's pharmacodynamics. Similarly, therapeutically administered proteins may interact with endogenous binding proteins.

It is a general pharmacokinetic principle, which is also applicable to proteins, that only the free, unbound fraction of a drug substance is accessible to distribution and elimination processes as well as interactions with its target structures at the site of action, for example a receptor or ion channel. Thus, protein binding may affect the pharmacodynamics, but also disposition properties of protein therapeutics. Specific binding proteins have been identified for numerous protein drugs, including recombinant human DNase for use as mucolytic in cystic fibrosis (Mohler et al., 1993), growth hormone (Toon, 1996), and recombinant human vascular endothelial growth factor (rhVEGF) (Eppler et al., 2002).

Protein binding not only affects the unbound fraction of a protein drug and thus the fraction of a drug available to exert pharmacological activity, but many times it also either prolongs protein circulation time by acting as a storage depot or it enhances protein clearance. Recombinant cytokines, for example, may after IV administration encounter various cytokine-binding proteins including soluble cytokine receptors and anti-cytokine antibodies (Piscitelli et al., 1997). In either case, the binding protein may either prolong the cytokine circulation time by acting as a storage depot or it may enhance the cytokine clearance.

Growth hormone, as another example, has at least two binding proteins in plasma (Wills and Ferraiolo, 1992). This protein binding substantially reduces growth hormone elimination with a tenfold smaller clearance of total compared to free growth hormone, but also decreases its activity via reduction of receptor interactions.

Apart from these specific bindings, peptides and proteins may also be non-specifically bound to plasma proteins. For example, metkephamid, a metenkephalin analog, was described to be 44% to 49% bound to albumin (Taki et al., 1998), and octreotide, a somatostatin analog, is up to 65% bound to lipoproteins (Chanson et al., 1993).

*Distribution via Receptor-Mediated Uptake*
Aside from physicochemical properties and protein binding of protein therapeutics, site-specific receptor-mediated uptake can also substantially influence and contribute to the distribution of protein therapeutics,

as well as to elimination and pharmacodynamics (see section on Target mediated-drug disposition).

The generally low volume of distribution should not necessarily be interpreted as low tissue penetration. Receptor-mediated specific uptake into the target organ, as one mechanism, can result in therapeutically effective tissue concentrations despite a relatively small volume of distribution. Nartograstim, a recombinant derivative of the granulocyte-colony-stimulating factor (G-CSF), for example, is characterized by a specific, dose-dependent and saturable tissue uptake into the target organ bone marrow, presumably via receptor-mediated endocytosis (Kuwabara et al., 1995).

### ■ Elimination of Protein Therapeutics
Protein-based therapeutics are generally subject to the same catabolic pathways as endogenous or dietetic proteins. The end products of protein metabolism are thus amino acids that are reutilized in the endogenous amino acid pool for the de novo biosynthesis of structural or functional proteins in the human body (Meibohm, 2004). Detailed investigations on the metabolism of proteins are relatively difficult because of the myriad of potential molecule fragments that may be formed, and are therefore generally not conducted. Non-metabolic elimination pathways such as renal or biliary excretion are negligible for most proteins. If biliary excretion occurs, however, it is generally followed by subsequent metabolic degradation of the compound in the gastrointestinal tract.

*Proteolysis*
The metabolic rate for protein degradation generally increases with decreasing molecular weight from large to small proteins to peptides (Table 1), but is also dependent on other factors such as size, charge,

| Molecular weight | Elimination site | Predominant elimination mechanisms | Major determinant |
|---|---|---|---|
| <500 | Blood, liver | Extracellular hydrolysis<br>Passive lipoid diffusion | Structure, lipophilicity |
| 500–1,000 | Liver | Carrier-mediated uptake<br>Passive lipoid diffusion | Structure, lipophilicity |
| 1,000–50,000 | Kidney | Glomerular filtration and subsequent degradation processes (see Fig. 4) | Molecular weight |
| 50,000–200,000 | Kidney, liver | Receptor-mediated endocytosis | Sugar, charge |
| 200,000–400,000 | | Opsonization | $\alpha_2$-macroglobulin, IgG |
| >400,000 | | Phagocytosis | Particle aggregation |

*Note*: Other determining factors are size, charge, lipophilicity, functional groups, sugar recognition, vulnerability for proteases, aggregation to particles, formation of complexes with opsonization factors, etc. Mechanisms may overlap and endocytosis may occur at any molecular weight range.
*Source*: After Meijer and Ziegler, 1993.

**Table 1** ■ Molecular weight as major determinant of the elimination mechanisms of peptides and proteins.

lipophilicity, functional groups, and glycosylation pattern as well as secondary and tertiary structure.

The clearance of a peptide or protein describes the irreversible removal of active substance from the vascular space, which includes besides metabolism also cellular uptake. Proteolytic degradation of proteins can occur unspecifically nearly everywhere in the body or can be limited to a specific organ or tissue. Due to this unspecific proteolysis of some proteins already in blood as well as potential active cellular uptake, the clearance of protein drugs can exceed cardiac output, i.e., >5 L/min for blood clearance and >3 L/min for plasma clearance (Meibohm, 2004).

Molecular weight determines the major metabolism site as well as the predominant degradation process (Wills, 1991). Proteolytic enzymes such as proteases and peptidases are ubiquitous throughout the body. Sites capable of extensive peptide and protein metabolism are not only limited to the liver, kidneys, and gastrointestinal tissue, but also include blood and vascular endothelium as well as other organs and tissues. As proteases and peptidases are also located within cells, intracellular uptake is per se more an elimination rather than a distribution process (Tang and Meibohm, 2006). While peptidases and proteases in the gastrointestinal tract and in lysosomes are relatively unspecific, soluble peptidases in the interstitial space and exopeptidases on the cell surface have a higher selectivity and determine the specific metabolism pattern of an organ. The proteolytic activity of SC tissue, for example, results in a partial loss of activity of SC compared to IV administrated interferon-γ.

## Gastrointestinal Protein Metabolism

As pointed out earlier, the gastrointestinal tract is a major site of protein metabolism with high proteolytic enzyme activity due to its primary function to digest dietary proteins. Thus, gastrointestinal metabolism of protein drugs is one of the major factors limiting systemic bioavailability of orally administered protein drugs. The metabolic activity of the gastrointestinal tract, however, is not limited to orally administered proteins. Parenterally administered peptides and proteins may also be metabolized in the intestinal mucosa following intestinal secretion. At least 20% of the degradation of endogenous albumin, for example, has been reported to take place in the gastrointestinal tract (Colburn, 1991).

## Renal Protein Metabolism and Excretion

The kidneys are a major site of protein metabolism for smaller sized proteins that undergo glomerular filtration. The size-selective cut-off for glomerular filtration is approximately 60 kD, although the effective molecule radius based on molecular weight and conformation is probably the limiting factor (Edwards et al., 1999). Glomerular filtration is most efficient, however, for proteins smaller than 30 kDa (Kompella and Lee, 1991). Peptides and small proteins (<5 kDa) are filtered very efficiently, and their glomerular filtration clearance approaches the glomerular filtration rate (GFR, ~120 mL/min in humans). For molecular weights exceeding 30 kDa, the filtration rate falls off sharply. In addition to size selectivity, charge selectivity has also been observed for glomerular filtration where anionic macromolecules pass through the capillary wall less readily than neutral macromolecules, which in turn pass through less readily than cationic macromolecules (Deen et al., 2001).

The importance of the kidneys as elimination organ could for example be shown for interleukin-2, macrophage-colony-stimulating factor (M-CSF) and interferon-α (McMartin, 1992; Wills and Ferraiolo, 1992). The relative contributions of renal and hepatic clearances to the total plasma clearance of several proteins are shown in Figure 3.

Renal metabolism of peptides and small proteins is mediated through three highly effective processes (Fig. 4). As a result, only minuscule amounts of intact protein are detectable in urine.

The first mechanism involves glomerular filtration of larger, complex peptides and proteins followed by reabsorption into endocytic vesicles in the proximal tubule and subsequent hydrolysis into small peptide fragments and amino acids (Maack et al., 1985). This mechanism of elimination has been described for IL-2 (Anderson and Sorenson, 1994), IL-11 (Takagi et al., 1995), growth hormone (Johnson and Maack, 1977), and insulin (Rabkin et al., 1984).

The second mechanism entails glomerular filtration followed by intraluminal metabolism, predominantly by exopeptidases in the luminal brush border membrane of the proximal tubule. The resulting peptide fragments and amino acids are reabsorbed into the systemic circulation. This route of disposition applies to small linear peptides such as glucagon and LH-RH (Carone and Peterson, 1980; Carone et al., 1982). Recent studies implicate the proton driven peptide transporters PEPT1 and especially PEPT2 as the main route of cellular uptake of small peptides and peptide-like drugs from the glomerular filtrates (Inui et al., 2000). These high-affinity transport proteins seem to exhibit selective uptake of di- and tripeptides, which implicates their role in renal amino acid homeostasis (Daniel and Herget, 1997).

For both mechanisms, glomerular filtration is the dominant, rate-limiting step as subsequent degradation processes are not saturable under physiologic conditions (Maack et al., 1985; Colburn, 1991). Due to this limitation of renal elimination, the renal contribution to the overall elimination of proteins is

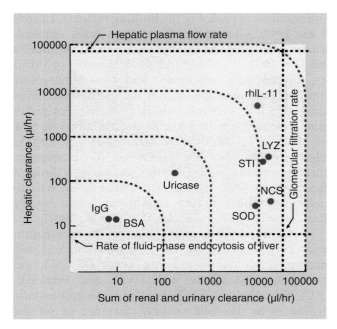

**Figure 3** ■ Hepatic and renal clearances of proteins in mice. *Abbreviations*: LYZ, lysozyme; STI, soy bean trypsin inhibitor; NCS, neocarzinostatin; IgG, immunoglobulin G; BSA, bovine serum albumin; rhIL-11, recombinant human interleukin-11. *Source*: From Takagi et al., 1995.

becomes negligible in the presence of unspecific degradation throughout the body. If the metabolic activity is low in other tissues or if distribution to the extravascular space is limited, however, the renal contribution to total clearance may approach 100%. This is for instance the case for recombinant human interleukin-10 (rhIL-10), for which clearance correlates closely with GFR, making dosage adjustments necessary in patients with impaired renal function (Andersen et al., 1999).

The third mechanism of renal metabolism is peritubular extraction of peptides and proteins from post-glomerular capillaries with subsequent intracellular metabolism. Experiments using radio-iodinated growth hormone ($^{125}$I-rGH) have demonstrated that while reabsorption into endocytic vesicles at the proximal tubule is still the dominant route of disposition, a small percentage of the hormone may be extracted from the peritubular capillaries (Johnson and Maack, 1977; Krogsgaard Thomsen et al., 1994). Peritubular transport of proteins and peptides from the basolateral membrane has also been shown for insulin (Nielsen et al., 1987).

*Hepatic Protein Metabolism*
Aside from renal and gastrointestinal metabolism, the liver may also play a major role in the metabolism of protein therapeutics. Exogenous as well as endogenous proteins undergo proteolytic degradation to dipeptides and amino acids that are reused for endogenous protein

dependent on the proteolytic activity for these proteins in other body regions. If metabolic activity for these proteins is high in other body regions, there is only minor renal contribution to total clearance, and it

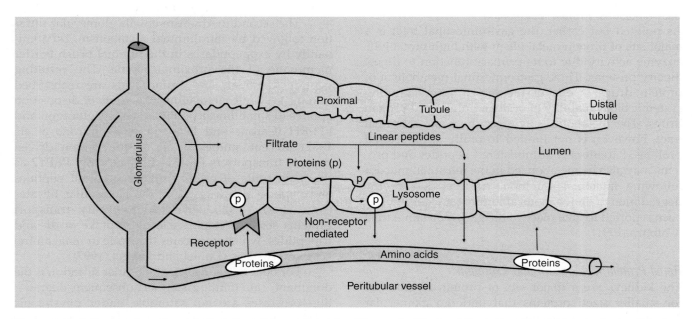

**Figure 4** ■ Pathways of renal metabolism of peptides and proteins: Glomerular filtration followed by either (a) intraluminal metabolism or (b) tubular reabsorption with intracellular lysosomal metabolism, and (c) peritubular extraction with intracellular lysosomal metabolism. *Source*: Modified from Maack et al., 1985.

synthesis. Proteolysis usually starts with endopeptidases that attack in the middle part of the protein, and the resulting oligopeptides are then further degraded by exopeptidases. The rate of hepatic metabolism is largely dependent on the specific amino acid sequence of the protein (Meibohm, 2004).

A prerequisite for hepatic protein metabolism is the uptake of proteins into the hepatocytes. An overview of the different mechanisms of hepatic uptake of proteins is listed in Table 2.

Small peptides may cross the hepatocyte membrane via simple passive diffusion if they have sufficient hydrophobicity. Peptides of this nature include the cyclosporins (cyclic peptides) (Ziegler et al., 1988). Other cyclic and linear peptides of small size (<1.4 kDa) and hydrophobic nature (containing aromatic amino acids), such as cholecystokinin-8 (CCK-8; 8 amino acids), are taken up by the hepatocytes by a carrier-mediated transport (Ziegler et al., 1988), in the case of CCK-8 by the organic anion transporting polypeptide OATP-8 (SLCO1B3) (Ismair et al., 2001). After internalization into the cytosol,

these peptides are usually metabolized by microsomal enzymes (cytochrome P-450 3A for cyclosporin A) or cytosolic peptidases (CCK-8). Substances that enter the liver via carrier-mediated transport are typically excreted into the bile by active export transporters. These hepatic clearance pathways are identical to those known for most small organic hydrophobic drug molecules.

Uptake of larger peptides and proteins is facilitated via various carrier-mediated, energy-dependent transport processes. One of the possibilities is receptor-mediated endocytosis, such as for insulin and epidermal growth factor (Kim et al., 1988; Sugiyama and Hanano, 1989; Burwen and Jones, 1990). In receptor-mediated endocytosis, circulating proteins are recognized by specific hepatic receptor proteins (Kompella and Lee, 1991). The receptors are usually integral membrane glycoproteins with an exposed binding domain on the extracellular side of the cell membrane. After the binding of the circulating protein to the receptor, the complex is already present or moves in coated pit regions, and the membrane

| Cell type | Uptake mechanism | Proteins/peptides transported |
|---|---|---|
| Hepatocytes | Anionic passive diffusion Carrier-mediated transport | Cyclic and linear hydrophobic peptides (<1.4 kDa; e.g., cyclosporins, CCK-8) |
| | RME: Gal/GalNAc receptor (asialoglycoprotein receptor) | N-acetylgalactosamine-terminated glycoproteins, galactose-terminated glycoproteins (e.g., desialylated EPO) |
| | RME: Low density lipo-protein receptor (LDLR) | LDL, apoE- and apoB-containing lipoproteins |
| | RME: LDLR-related protein (LRP receptor) | $\alpha_2$-macroglobulin, apo-E-enriched lipoproteins, lipoprotein lipase (LpL), lactoferrin, t-PA, u-PA, complexes of t-PA and u-PA with plasminogen activator inhibitor type 1 (PAI-1), TFPI, thrombospondin (TSP), TGF-$\beta$ and IL-1$\beta$ bound to $\alpha_2$-macroglobulin |
| | RME: Other receptors | IgA, glycoproteins, lipoproteins, immunoglobulins intestinal and pancreatic peptides, metallo- and hemoproteins, transferrin, insulin, glucagon, GH, EGF |
| | Nonselective pinocytosis (non-receptor-mediated) | Albumin, antigen–antibody complexes, some pancreatic proteins, some glycoproteins |
| Kupffer cells | Endocytosis | Particulates with galactose groups |
| Kupffer and endothelial cells | RME | IgG, N-acetylgalactosamine-terminated glycoproteins |
| | RME: Mannose receptor | Mannose-terminated glycoproteins (e.g., t-PA, renin) |
| | RME: Fucose receptor | Fucose-terminated glycoproteins |
| Endothelial cells | RME: Scavenger receptor | Negatively charged proteins |
| | RME: Other receptors | VEGF, FGF (?) |
| Fat-storing cells | RME: Mannose-6-phosphate receptor | Mannose-6-phosphate-terminated proteins (e.g., IGF-II) |

*Abbreviation*: RME, receptor-mediated endocytosis.
*Source*: From Braeckman, 2000, compiled from several sources (see references in the text), including reviews by Cumming (1991), Kompella and Lee (1991) and Marks et al. (1995).

**Table 2** ■ Hepatic uptake mechanisms for proteins and protein complexes.

invaginates and pinches off to form an endocytotic coated vesicle that contains the receptor and ligand (internalization). The vesicle coat consists of proteins (clathrin, adaptin, and others), which are then removed by an uncoating adenosine triphosphatase (ATPase). The vesicle parts, the receptor, and the ligand dissociate and are targeted to various intracellular locations. Some receptors, such as the low-density lipoprotein (LDL), asialoglycoprotein and transferrin receptors, are known to undergo recycling. Since sometimes several hundred cycles are part of a single receptor's lifetime, the associated receptor-mediated endocytosis is of high capacity. Other receptors, such as the interferon receptor, undergo degradation. This degradation leads to a decrease in the concentration of receptors on the cell surface (receptor down-regulation). Others, such as insulin receptors, for example, undergo both recycling and degradation (Kompella and Lee, 1991).

For glycoproteins, if a critical number of exposed sugar groups (mannose, galactose, fucose, N-acetyl-glucosamine, N-acetylgalactosamine, or glucose) is exceeded, receptor-mediated endocytosis through sugar-recognizing receptors is an efficient hepatic uptake mechanism (Meijer and Ziegler, 1993). Important carbohydrate receptors in the liver are the asialoglycoprotein receptor in hepatocytes and the mannose receptor in Kupffer and liver endothelial cells (Smedsrod and Einarsson, 1990; Bu et al., 1992). The high-mannose glycans in the first kringle domain of t-PA, for example, have been implicated in its hepatic clearance (Cumming, 1991).

Low density lipoprotein receptor-related protein (LRP) is a member of the LDL receptor family responsible for endocytosis of several important lipoproteins, proteases, and protease-inhibitor complexes in the liver and other tissues (Strickland et al., 1995). Examples of proteins and protein complexes for which hepatic uptake is mediated by LRP are listed in Table 2.

Uptake of proteins by liver cells is followed by transport to an intracellular compartment for metabolism. Proteins internalized into vesicles via an endocytotic mechanism undergo intracellular transport towards the lysosomal compartment near the center of the cell. There, the endocytotic vehicles fuse with or mature into lysosomes, which are specialized acidic vesicles that contain a wide variety of hydrolases capable of degrading all biological macromolecules. Proteolysis is started by endopeptidases (mainly cathepsin D) that act on the middle part of the proteins. Oligopeptides—as the result of the first step—are further degraded by exopeptidases. The resulting amino acids and dipeptides reenter the metabolic pool of the cell (Meijer and Ziegler, 1993). The hepatic metabolism of glycoproteins may occur more slowly than the naked protein because

protecting oligosaccharide chains need to be removed first. Metabolized proteins and peptides in lysosomes from hepatocytes, hepatic sinusoidal cells and Kupffer cells may be released into the blood. Degraded proteins in hepatocyte lysosomes can also be delivered to the bile canaliculus and excreted by exocytosis.

A second intracellular pathway for proteins is the direct shuttle or transcytotic pathway (Kompella and Lee, 1991). The endocytotic vesicle formed at the cell surface traverses the cell to the peribiliary space, where it fuses with the bile canalicular membrane, releasing its contents by exocytosis into bile. This pathway, described for polymeric immunoglobulin A, bypasses the lysosomal compartment completely.

### Receptor-Mediated Protein Metabolism

Receptor-mediated metabolism is often a substantial elimination pathway for those protein therapeutics that bind with high affinity to membrane-associated receptors on the cell surface. The interaction of the protein therapeutic with the membrane receptor is frequently part of the pharmacologic effect of the drug, i.e., the receptor is the target structure the protein therapeutic is directed at. This binding can lead to receptor-mediated uptake by endocytosis and subsequent intracellular lysosomal metabolism. Receptor-mediated uptake and metabolism via interaction with these generally high-affinity, low-capacity binding sites is not limited to a specific organ or tissue type. Thus, any tissue, including the therapeutic target cells that express receptors for the drug can contribute to the elimination of the protein therapeutic (Meibohm and Derendorf, 2003).

Since the number of protein drug receptors is limited, receptor-mediated protein metabolism can usually be saturated within therapeutic concentrations, or more specifically at relatively low molar ratios between the protein drug and the receptor. As a consequence, the elimination clearance of these protein drugs is not constant but dose dependent, and decreases with increasing dose. Thus, receptor-mediated elimination constitutes a major source for nonlinear pharmacokinetic behavior of numerous peptide and protein drugs, i.e., systemic exposure to the drug increases more than proportional with increasing dose (Tang et al., 2004).

Recombinant human M-CSF, for example, undergoes besides linear renal elimination a nonlinear elimination pathway that follows Michaelis–Menten kinetics and is linked to a receptor-mediated uptake into macrophages. At low concentrations, M-CSF follows linear pharmacokinetics, while at high concentrations nonrenal elimination pathways are saturated resulting in nonlinear pharmacokinetic behavior (Fig. 5) (Bartocci et al., 1987; Bauer et al., 1994).

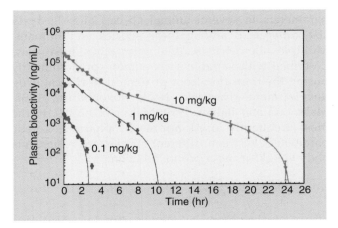

**Figure 5** ▦ Nonlinear pharmacokinetics of M-CSF, presented as measured (*triangles and circles*; mean ± SE) and modeled plasma bioactivity-time curves (*lines*) after IV injection of 0.1 mg/kg ($n = 5$), 1.0 mg/kg ($n = 3$) and 10 mg/kg ($n = 8$) in rats. Bioactivity is used as a substitute for concentration. *Source*: From Bauer et al., 1994.

## ■ Target-Mediated Drug Disposition

Numerous protein therapeutics are characterized by target-mediated drug disposition, which occurs when binding to the pharmacodynamic target structure affects the pharmacokinetics of a drug compound and results in capacity-limited, saturable processes (Levy, 1994). The consequence of these saturable processes caused by the limited availability of enzymes, receptors or other protein structures the drug is interacting with, is nonlinear pharmacokinetic behavior, i.e., plasma concentrations change disproportionately with increasing doses (Mager, 2006).

For conventional small molecule drugs, receptor binding is usually negligible compared to the total amount of drug in the body and rarely affects their pharmacokinetic profile. In contrast, a substantial fraction of a protein therapeutic can be bound to their pharmacologic target structure, for example a receptor. Target-mediated drug disposition can affect distribution as well as elimination processes. Most notably, receptor-mediated protein metabolism is a frequently encountered elimination pathway for many protein therapeutics that is often saturated at therapeutically used dosage regimens (see previous section) (Meibohm, 2004).

Nonlinearity in pharmacokinetics based on target-mediated drug disposition has for example been observed for several monoclonal antibody therapeutics, for instance for the anti-HER2 humanized monoclonal antibody trastuzumab. Trastuzumab is approved for the combination treatment of HER2 protein overexpressing metastatic breast cancer. With increasing dose level, the mean half-life of trastuzumab increases and the clearance decreases, leading to

over-proportional increases in systemic exposure with increasing dose (Tokuda et al., 1999). Since trastuzumab is rapidly internalized via receptor-mediated endocytosis after binding to HER2, its target structure on the cell surface, saturation of this elimination pathway is the likely cause for the observed dose-dependent pharmacokinetics (Kobayashi et al., 2002).

## ■ Immunogenicity and Protein Pharmacokinetics

The antigenic potential of protein therapeutics may lead to antibody formation against the protein therapeutic during chronic therapy. This is especially of concern if animal-derived proteins are applied in human clinical studies, but also if human proteins are used in animal studies. Chapter 6 discusses in detail the phenomenon of immunogenicity and its consequences for the pharmacotherapy with protein therapeutics.

Protein–antibody complexation can not only modulate or even obliterate the biological activity of a protein drug, but may also modify its pharmacokinetic profile. Elimination clearances of protein drugs, for example, may be either increased or decreased by antibody formation and binding (Fig. 6). An increase in clearance is observed if the protein–antibody complex is eliminated more rapidly than the unbound protein (Rosenblum et al., 1985). This increase may occur when high levels of the protein–antibody complex stimulate its clearance by the reticuloendothelial system. In other situations, the serum concentration of a protein can be increased if binding to an antibody slows down its rate of clearance because the protein–antibody complex is eliminated more slowly than the unbound protein (Working and Cossum, 1991). In this case, the complex may act as a depot for the protein and, if the antibody is not neutralizing, a longer duration of the pharmacological

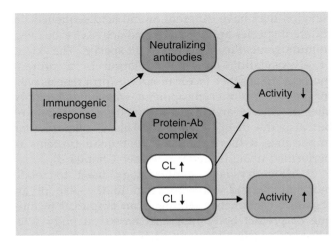

**Figure 6** ▦ Effect of antibody formation on pharmacokinetics and pharmacodynamics of protein drugs.

action may occur. For example, the clearance of rIFNα2a in cancer patients was increased because of an antibody response. In contrast, human leukocyte IFNβ concentration in rats was decreased 15-fold when circulating antibodies were present. A decrease of clearance in the presence of antibody titers was also detected for t-PA in dogs (Working, 1992).

Both an increased and decreased clearance is possible for the same protein, dependent on the dose level administered. At low doses, protein–antibody complexes delay clearance because their elimination is slower than that of the unbound protein. In contrast, at high doses, higher levels of protein–antibody complex result in the formation of aggregates, which are cleared more rapidly than the unbound protein.

The enhancement of the clearance of cytokine interleukin-6 (IL-6) via administration of cocktails of three anti-IL-6 monoclonal antibodies was suggested as a therapeutic approach in cytokine-dependent diseases like multiple myeloma, B-cell lymphoma, and rheumatoid arthritis (Montero-Julian et al., 1995). The authors could show that, while the binding of one or two antibodies to the cytokine led to stabilization of the cytokine, simultaneous binding of three anti-IL-6 antibodies to three distinct epitopes induced rapid uptake of the complex by the liver and thus mediated a rapid elimination of IL-6 from the central compartment.

The immunogenicity of protein therapeutics is also dependent on the route of administration. Extravascular injection is known to stimulate antibody formation more than IV application, which is most likely caused by the increased immunogenicity of protein aggregates and precipitates formed at the injection site (see Chapter 6).

## ■ Species Specificity and Allometric Scaling

Peptides and proteins often exhibit distinct species specificity with regard to structure and activity. Peptides and proteins with identical physiological function may have different amino acid sequences in different species and may have no activity or be even immunogenic if used in a different species. The extent of glycosylation and/or sialylation of a protein molecule is another factor of species differences, e.g., for interferon-α or erythropoietin, which may not only alter its efficacy and immunogenicity (see Chapter 6) but also the drug's clearance. This is of particular importance if the production of human proteins is performed using bacterial cells (see Chapter 3).

Allometry is a methodology used to relate morphology and body function to the size of an organism. Allometric scaling is an empirical technique of predict body functions based on body size. Allometric scaling has found wide application in drug development, especially to predict pharmacokinetic parameters in humans based on the corresponding parameters in several animal species and the body size differences among these species and humans. Multiple allometric scaling approaches have been described with variable success rates, predominantly during the transition from preclinical to clinical drug development (Dedrick, 1973; Boxenbaum, 1982; Mahmood and Balian, 1999; Mahmood, 2002). In the most frequently used approach, pharmacokinetic parameters between different species are related via body weight using a power function:

$$P = a \cdot W^b$$

where $P$ is the pharmacokinetic parameter scaled, $W$ is the body weight in kg, $a$ is the allometric coefficient, and $b$ is the allometric exponent. $a$ and $b$ are specific constants for each parameter of a compound. General tendencies for the allometric exponent are 0.75 for rate constants (i.e., clearance, elimination rate constant), 1 for volumes of distribution, and 0.25 for half-lives.

For most traditional small-molecule drugs, allometric scaling is often imprecise, especially if hepatic metabolism is a major elimination pathway and/or if there are interspecies differences in metabolism. For peptides and proteins, however, allometric scaling has frequently proven to be much more precise and reliable, probably because of the similarity in handling peptides and proteins between different mammalian species (Wills and Ferraiolo, 1992). Clearance and volume of distribution of numerous therapeutically used proteins like growth hormone or t-PA follow a well-defined, weight-dependent physiologic relationship between lab animals and humans. This allows relatively precise quantitative predictions for their pharmacokinetic behavior in humans based on preclinical findings (Mordenti et al., 1991).

Figure 7, for example, shows allometric plots for the clearance and volume of distribution of a P-selectin antagonist, P-selectin glycoprotein ligand-1 (rPSGL-Ig), for the treatment of P-selectin-mediated diseases such as thrombosis, reperfusion injury, and deep vein thrombosis. The protein's human pharmacokinetic parameters could accurately be predicted using allometric power functions based on data from four species, mouse, rat, monkey and pig (Khor et al., 2000).

It needs to be emphasized that allometric scaling techniques are useful tools for predicting a dose that will assist in the planning of dose-ranging studies, including first-in-man studies, but are not a replacement for such studies. The advantage of including such dose prediction in the protocol design of dose-ranging studies is that a smaller number of doses need to be tested before finding the final dose level. Interspecies dose predictions simply narrow the range of doses in the initial pharmacological efficacy

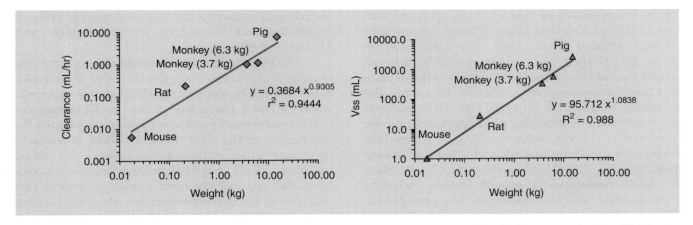

**Figure 7** ■ Allometric plots of the pharmacokinetic parameters clearance and volume of distribution at steady-state ($V_{ss}$) for the P-selectin antagonist P-selectin glycoprotein ligand-1 (rPSGL-Ig). Each data point within the plot represents an averaged value of the respective pharmacokinetic parameter in one of five species: mouse, rat, monkey (3.7 kg), monkey (6.3 kg), and pig, respectively. The solid line is the best fit with a power function to relate pharmacokinetic parameters to body weight. *Source*: From Khor et al., 2000.

studies, the animal toxicology studies, and the human safety and efficacy studies.

## ■ Chemical Modifications for Optimizing the Pharmacokinetics of Protein Therapeutics

In recent years, approaches modifying the molecular structure of protein therapeutics have repeatedly been applied to affect the immunogenicity, pharmacokinetics, and/or pharmacodynamics of protein drugs. These approaches include the addition, deletion or exchange of selected amino acids within the protein's sequence, synthesis of truncated proteins with a reduced amino acid sequence, glycosylation or deglycosylation, and covalent linkage to polymers (Veronese and Caliceti, 2006). The latter approach has been used for several protein therapeutics by linking them to monomethoxy polyethylene glycol (PEG) molecules of various chain lengths in a process called PEGylation (Caliceti and Veronese, 2003).

The conjugation of high polymeric mass to protein drugs is generally aimed at preventing the protein from being recognized by the immune system as well as reducing its elimination via glomerular filtration or proteolytic enzymes, thereby prolonging the oftentimes relatively short elimination half-life of endogenous proteins. Conjugation of protein drugs with PEG chains increases their molecular weight, but because of the attraction of water molecules by PEG even more their hydrodynamic volume, which in turn results in a reduced renal clearance and restricted volume of distribution. PEGylation can also shield antigenic determinants on the protein drug from detection by the immune system through steric hindrance (Walsh et al., 2003). Similarly, amino acid sequences sensitive towards proteolytic degradation may be shielded against protease attack. By adding a large, hydrophilic

molecule to the protein, PEGylation can also increase drug solubility (Molineux, 2003).

PEGylation has been used to improve the therapeutic properties of numerous protein therapeutics including interferon-α, asparaginase, and filgrastim. More details on the general concept of PEGylation and its specific application for protein therapeutics can be found in Chapter 11.

The therapeutic application of L-asparaginase in the treatment of acute lymphoblastic leukemia has been hampered by its strong immunogenicity with allergic reactions occurring in 33% to 75% of treated patients in various studies. The development of pegaspargase, a PEGylated form of L-asparaginase, is a successful example for overcoming this high rate of allergic reactions towards L-asparaginase using PEG conjugation techniques (Graham, 2003). Pegaspargase is well tolerated compared to L-asparaginase, with 3% to 10% of the treated patients experiencing clinical allergic reactions.

Pegfilgrastim is the PEGylated version of the granulocyte-colony-stimulating factor filgrastim, which is administered for the management of chemotherapy-induced neutropenia. PEGylation minimizes filgrastim's renal clearance by glomerular filtration, thereby making neutrophil-mediated clearance the predominant route of elimination. Thus, PEGylation of filgrastim results in so-called "self-regulating pharmacokinetics" since pegfilgrastim has a reduced clearance and thus prolonged half-life and more sustained duration of action in a neutropenic compared to a normal patient because only few mature neutrophils are available to mediate its elimination (Zamboni, 2003).

The hematopoietic growth factor darbepoetin-α is an example of a chemically modified endogenous protein with altered glycosylation pattern. It is a glycosylation analog of human erythropoietin, with two additional N-linked oligosaccharide chains (five in total) (Mould et al., 1999). The additional N-glycosylation sites were made available through substitution of five amino acid residues in the peptide backbone of erythropoietin, thereby increasing the molecular weight from 30 to 37 kDa. Darbepoetin-α has a substantially modified pharmacokinetic profile compared to erythropoietin, resulting in a three-fold longer serum half-life that allows for reduced dosing frequency (Fig. 8) (Macdougall et al., 1999). More details on hematopoietic growth factors, including erythropoietin and darbepoetin-α, are provided in Chapter 10.

## PHARMACODYNAMICS OF PROTEIN THERAPEUTICS

Protein therapeutics are usually highly potent compounds with steep dose–effect curves as they are targeted therapies towards a specific, well-described pharmacologic structure or mechanism. Thus, a careful characterization of the concentration–effect relationship, i.e., the pharmacodynamics, is especially desirable for protein therapeutics (Tabrizi and Roskos, 2006). Combination of pharmacodynamics with pharmacokinetics by integrated pharmacokinetic–pharmacodynamic modeling (PK/PD modeling) adds an additional level of complexity that allows furthermore characterization of the dose–exposure–response relationship of a drug and a continuous description of the time course of effect intensity directly resulting from

the administration of a certain dosage regimen (Fig. 9) (Meibohm and Derendorf, 1997; Derendorf and Meibohm, 1999).

PK/PD modeling is a technique that combines the two classical pharmacologic disciplines of pharmacokinetics and pharmacodynamics. It integrates a pharmacokinetic and a pharmacodynamic model component into one set of mathematical expressions that allows the description of the time course of effect intensity in response to administration of a drug dose. This so-called integrated PK/PD model allows deriving pharmacokinetic and pharmacodynamic model parameters that characterize the dose–concentration–effect relationship for a specific drug based on measured concentration and effect data. In addition, it allows simulation of the time course of effect intensity for dosage regimens of a drug beyond actually measured data, within the constraints of the validity of the model assumptions for the simulated condition. Addition of a statistical model component describing inter- and intraindividual variation in model parameters allows expanding PK/PD models to describe time courses of effect intensity not only for individual subjects, but also for whole populations of subjects.

Integrated PK/PD modeling approaches have widely been applied for the characterization of protein therapeutics (Tabrizi and Roskos, 2006). Embedded in a model-based drug development approach, modeling and simulation based on integrated PK/PD does not only provide a comprehensive summary of the available data, but also enables to test competing hypotheses

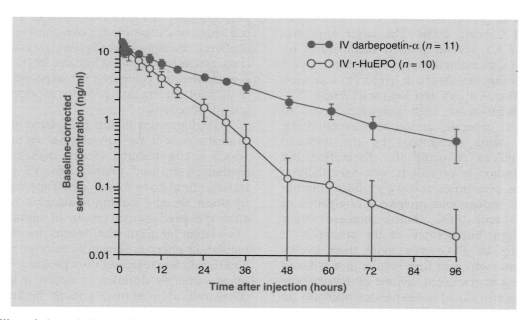

**Figure 8** ■ Effect of glycosylation on pharmacokinetics of erythropoietin: Comparison of the mean (±SD) concentration–time profiles of darbepoetin-α (0.5 μg/kg, *n* = 11) and recombinant human erythropoietin (100 U/kg, *n* = 10) after IV administration in patients with endstage renal disease. Darbepoetin-α is a derivative of erythropoietin with modified glycosylation pattern. Serum concentrations were corrected for endogenous erythropoietin concentrations. *Source*: From Macdougall et al., 1999.

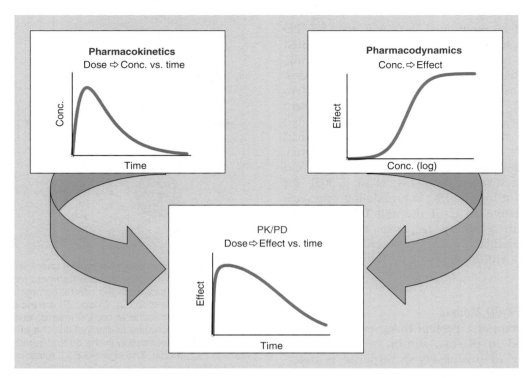

**Figure 9** ▪ General concept of PK/PD modeling. PK/PD modeling combines a pharmacokinetic model component that describes the time course of drug in plasma and a pharmacodynamic model component that relates the plasma concentration to the drug effect in order to describe the time course of the effect intensity resulting from the administration of a certain dosage regimen. *Source*: From Derendorf and Meibohm, 1999.

regarding processes altered by the drug, allows making predictions of drug effects under new conditions, and facilitates to estimate inaccessible system variables (Meibohm and Derendorf, 1997; Mager et al., 2003).

Mechanism-based PK/PD modeling appreciating the physiological events involved in the elaboration of the observed effect has been promoted as superior modeling approach as compared to empirical modeling, especially because it does not only describe observations but also offers some insight into the underlying biological processes involved and thus provides flexibility in extrapolating the model to other clinical situations (Levy, 1994; Derendorf and Meibohm, 1999). Since the molecular mechanism of action of a protein therapeutic is generally well understood, it is often straightforward to transform this available knowledge into a mechanism-based PK/PD modeling approach that appropriately characterizes the real physiological process leading to the drug's therapeutic effect.

The relationship between exposure and response may be either simple or complex, and thus obvious or hidden. However, if no simple relationship is obvious, it would be misleading to conclude a priori that no relationship exists at all rather than that it is not readily apparent (Levy, 1986).

The application of PK/PD modeling is beneficial in all phases of preclinical and clinical drug development and has been endorsed by the pharmaceutical industry, academia and regulatory agencies (Peck et al., 1994; Breimer and Danhof, 1997; Machado et al., 1999; Lesko et al., 2000; Sheiner and Steimer, 2000; Meibohm and Derendorf, 2002), most recently by the Critical Path Initiative of the U.S. Food and Drug Administration (Lesko, 2007). Thus, PK/PD concepts and model-based drug development play a pivotal role especially in the drug development process for biologics, and their widespread application supports a scientifically driven, evidence-based, and focused product development for protein therapeutics.

While a variety of PK/PD modeling approaches has been employed for biologics, we will in the following focus on five classes of approaches to illustrate the challenges and complexities, but also opportunities to characterize the pharmacodynamics of protein therapeutics:

- Direct link PK/PD models
- Indirect link PK/PD models
- Indirect response PK/PD models
- Cell lifespan models
- Complex response models

It should be mentioned, however, that PK/PD models for protein therapeutics are not only limited to continuous responses as shown in the following, but are also used for binary or graded responses. Binary responses are responses with only two outcome levels where a condition is either present or absence, for example, dead versus alive. Graded or categorical responses have a set of predefined outcome levels, which may or may not be ordered, for example the categories "mild," "moderate," and "severe" for a disease state. Lee et al. (2003), for example, used a logistic PK/PD modeling approach to link cumulative AUC of the anti-TNF-α protein etanercept with a binary response, the American College of Rheumatology response criterion of 20% improvement (ARC20) in patients with rheumatoid arthritis.

## ■ Direct Link PK/PD Models

The concentration of a protein therapeutic is usually only quantified in plasma, serum, or blood, while the magnitude of the observed response is determined by the concentration of the protein drug at its effect site, the site of action in the target tissue (Meibohm and Derendorf, 1997). Effect site concentrations, however, are usually not accessible for measurement, and plasma, serum or blood concentrations are usually used as their substitute. The relationship between the drug concentration in plasma and at the effect site may either be constant or undergo time-dependent changes. If equilibrium between both concentrations is rapidly achieved or the site of action is within plasma, serum or blood, there is practically a constant relationship between both concentrations with no temporal delay between plasma and effect site. In this case, measured plasma concentrations can directly serve as input for a pharmacodynamic model (Fig. 10). The most frequently used direct link pharmacodynamic model is a sigmoid $E_{\max}$ model:

$$E = \frac{E_{\max} \cdot C^n}{EC_{50}^n + C^n}$$

with $E_{\max}$ as maximum achievable effect, $C$ as drug concentration in plasma, and $EC_{50}$ the concentration of the drug that produces half of the maximum effect. The Hill coefficient $n$ is a shape factor that allows for an improved fit of the relationship to the observed data. As represented by the equation for the sigmoid $E_{\max}$ model, a direct link model directly connects measured concentration to the observed effect without any temporal delay (Derendorf and Meibohm, 1999).

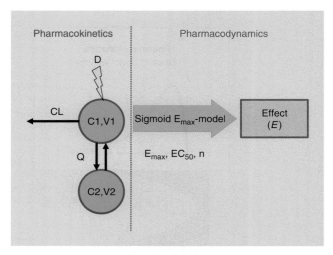

**Figure 10** ■ Schematic of a typical direct link PK/PD model. The PK model is a typical two-compartment model with a linear elimination clearance from the central compartment (CL) and a distributional clearance (Q). $C_1$ and $C_2$ are the concentrations in the central and peripheral compartments, and $V_1$ and $V_2$ are their respective volumes of distribution. The effect ($E$) is directly linked to the concentration in the central compartment $C_1$ via a sigmoid $E_{\max}$ model. The sigmoid $E_{\max}$ relationship is characterized by the pharmacodynamic parameters $E_{\max}$, the maximum achievable effect, $EC_{50}$, the concentration of the drug that produced half of the maximum effect, and the Hill coefficient n as via the sigmoid $E_{\max}$ equation (see text).

A direct link model was, for example, used to relate the serum concentration of the anti-human immunoglobulin E (IgE) antibody CGP 51901 for the treatment of seasonal allergic rhinitis to the reduction of free IgE via an inhibitory $E_{\max}$ model (Fig. 11) (Racine-Poon et al., 1997). It should be noted that the peak and trough concentrations and effects are directly related and thus occur at the same times, respectively, without time delay. Similarly, a direct link model was used to relate the effect of recombinant interleukin-10 (IL-10) on the ex vivo release of the pro-inflammatory cytokines TNF-α and interleukin-1β in LPS-stimulated leukocytes (Radwanski et al., 1998). In the first case, the site of action and the sampling site for concentration measurements of the protein therapeutic were identical, i.e., in plasma, and so the direct link model was mechanistically well justified. In the second case, the effect was dependent on the IL-10 concentration on the cell surface of leukocytes where IL-10 interacts with its target receptor. Again sampling fluid and effect site were in instant equilibrium.

## ■ Indirect Link PK/PD Models

The concentration–effect relationship of many protein drugs, however, cannot be described by direct link PK/PD models, but is characterized by a temporal

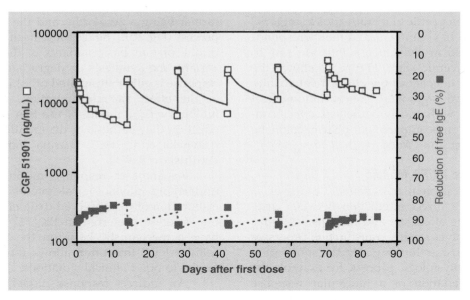

**Figure 11** ■ Observed (□) and model predicted (—) serum concentration of the anti-human IgE antibody CGP 51901 and observed (■) and model predicted (·····) reduction of free IgE in one representative patient, given six IV doses of 60 mg biweekly. The predictions were modeled with a direct link PK/PD model. *Source*: Modified from Racine-Poon et al., 1997.

dissociation between the time courses of plasma concentration and effect. In this case, plasma concentration maxima occur before effect maxima, effect intensity may increase despite decreasing plasma concentrations and may persist beyond the time drug concentrations in plasma are no longer detectable. The relationship between measured concentration and observed effect follows a counter-clockwise hysteresis loop. This phenomenon can either be caused by an indirect response mechanism (see next section) or by a distributional delay between the drug concentrations in plasma and at the effect site.

The latter one can conceptually be described by an indirect link model, which attaches a hypothetical effect-compartment to a pharmacokinetic compartment model (Fig. 12). The effect compartment addition to the pharmacokinetic model does not account for mass balance, i.e., no actual mass transfer is implemented in the pharmacokinetic part of the PK/PD model. Instead, drug transfer with respect to the effect compartment is defined by the time course of the effect itself (Sheiner et al., 1979; Holford and Sheiner, 1982). The effect-compartment approach, however, is necessary, as the effect site can be viewed as a small part of a pharmacokinetic compartment that from a pharmacokinetic point of view cannot be distinguished from other tissues within that compartment. The concentration in the effect compartment represents the active drug concentration at the effect site that is slowly equilibrating with the plasma, and is usually linked to the effect via an $E_{max}$ model.

Although this PK/PD model is constructed with tissue distribution as the reason for the delay of the effect, the distribution clearance to the effect compartment can be interpreted differently, including other reasons of delay, such as transduction processes and secondary post receptor events.

The hypoglycemic effect of insulin has been modeled by this type of PK/PD model (Hooper, 1991; Woodworth et al., 1994). Figure 13 shows the mean

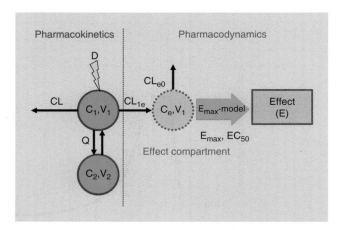

**Figure 12** ■ Schematic of a typical indirect link PK/PD model. A hypothetical effect compartment is linked to the central compartment of a two-compartmental pharmacokinetic model. The concentration in the effect compartment ($C_e$) drives the intensity of the pharmacodynamic effect ($E$) via an $E_{max}$-relationship. $CL_{1e}$ is the transfer clearance from the central to the effect compartment, $CL_{e0}$ the equilibrium clearance for the effect compartment. All other PK and PD parameters are identical to those used in Fig. 10.

serum concentration profile of insulin after a single SC injection of 10 U in 10 volunteers, and the corresponding effect measured as the glucose infusion rate to maintain an euglycemic state. Figure 14 shows the hysteresis in the concentration–effect relationship, and how a typical sigmoidal concentration–effect curve is obtained with the hypothetical effect concentration using a one-compartment pharmacokinetic model with indirect link (Woodworth et al., 1994).

### ■ Indirect Response PK/PD Models

The effect of most protein therapeutics, however, is not mediated via a direct interaction between drug concentration at the effect site and response systems, but frequently involves several transduction processes that include at their rate-limiting step the stimulation or inhibition of a physiologic process, for example the synthesis or degradation of a molecular response mediator like a hormone or cytokine. In these cases, the time courses of plasma concentration and effect are also dissociated resulting in counterclockwise hysteresis for the concentration–effect relationship, but the underlying cause is not a distributional delay as for the indirect link models, but a time-consuming indirect response mechanism (Meibohm and Derendorf, 1997).

Indirect response models generally describe the effect on a representative response parameter via the dynamic equilibrium between increase or synthesis and decrease or degradation of the response, with the former being a zero-order and the latter a first-order process (Fig. 15). The response itself can be modulated in one of four basic variants of the models. In each variant, the synthesis or degradation process of the response is either stimulated or inhibited as a function of the effect site concentration. A stimulatory or inhibitory $E_{max}$ model is used to describe the drug effect on the synthesis or degradation of the response (Dayneka et al., 1993; Sharma and Jusko, 1998; Sun and Jusko, 1999).

As indirect response models appreciate the underlying physiological events involved in the elaboration of the observed drug effect, their application is often preferred in PK/PD modeling as they have a mechanistic basis on the molecular and/or cellular level that often allows for extrapolating the model to other clinical situations.

An indirect response model was for example used in the evaluation of SB-240563, a humanized monoclonal antibody directed towards IL-5 in monkeys (Zia-Amirhosseini et al., 1999). IL-5 appears to play a significant role in the production, activation, and maturation of eosinophils. The delayed effect of SB-240563 on eosinophils is consistent with its mechanism of action via binding to and thus inactivation of IL-5. It was modeled using an indirect response model with inhibition of the production of response (eosinophils count) (Fig. 16). The obtained low $EC_{50}$ value for reduction of circulating eosinophils combined with a long terminal half-life of the

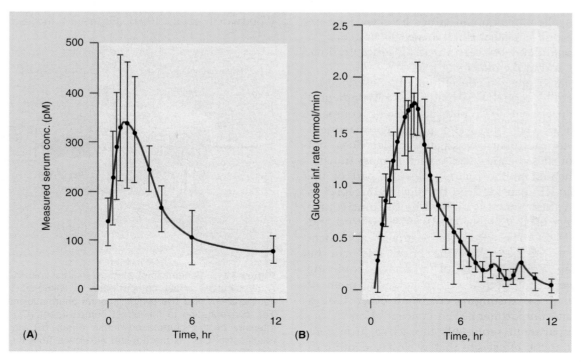

**Figure 13** ■ Mean measured (± SD) serum insulin concentrations after a single 10 U SC dose of regular insulin in 10 volunteers (**A**); corresponding glucose infusion rates needed to maintain euglycemia (**B**). *Source*: From Woodworth et al., 1994.

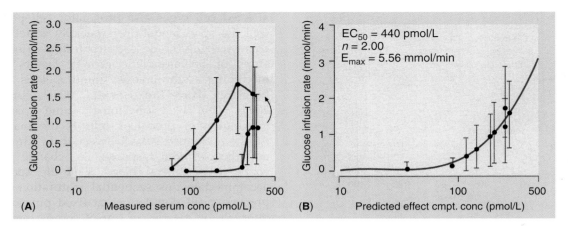

**Figure 14** ▪ Relationship between the glucose infusion rate to maintain euglycemia versus serum insulin concentrations after a single SC dose of 10 U regular insulin in 10 volunteers (**A**). The time-dependent counterclockwise hysteresis, which is an indication of the indirect nature of the concentration–effect relationship, is indicated by the arrow. Panel (**B**) shows the sigmoidal relationship between the effect and the predicted effect compartment concentration ($C_e$), demonstrating the collapse of the hysteresis loop by applying indirect link PK/PD modeling approach with an effect-compartment. *Source*: From Woodworth et al., 1994.

protein therapeutic of 13 days suggests the possibility of an infrequent dosing regimen for SB-240563 in the pharmacotherapy of disorders with increased eosinophil function, such as asthma.

Indirect response models were also used for the effect of growth hormone on endogenous IGF-1 concentration (Sun et al., 1999), as well as the effect of epoetin-α on two response parameters, free ferritin concentration and soluble transferrin receptor concentration (Bressolle et al., 1997). Similarly, a modified indirect response model was used to relate the

concentration of the humanized anti-factor IX antibody SB-249417 to factor IX activity in Cynomolgus monkeys as well as humans (Benincosa et al., 2000; Chow et al., 2002). The drug effect in this model was introduced by interrupting the natural degradation of Factor IX by sequestration of Factor IX by the antibody.

### ▪ Cell Life Span Models
A sizable number of protein therapeutics exerts its pharmacologic effect through direct or indirect modulation of blood and/or immune cell types.

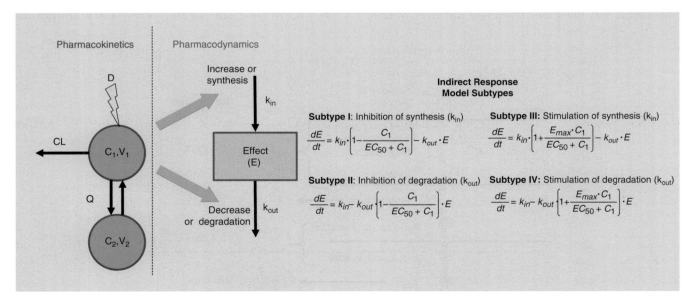

**Figure 15** ▪ Schematic of a typical indirect response PK/PD model. The effect measure ($E$) is maintained by a dynamic equilibrium between an increase or synthesis and a decrease or degradation process. The former is modeled by a zero order process with rate constant $k_{in}$, the latter by a first-order process with rate constant $k_{out}$. Thus, the rate of change in effect ($dE/dt$) is expressed as the difference between synthesis rate ($k_{in}$) and degradation rate ($k_{out}$ times $E$). Drug concentration ($C_1$) can stimulate or inhibit the synthesis or the degradation process for the effect ($E$) via an $E_{max}$ relationship using one of four subtypes (model I, II, III or IV) of the indirect response model. The pharmacokinetic model and all other PK and PD parameters are identical to those used in Fig. 10.

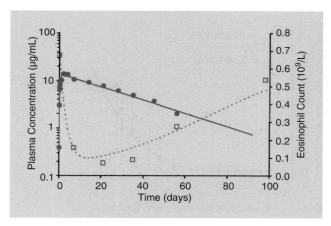

**Figure 16** ■ Model predicted and observed plasma concentration (observed: circles; predicted: solid line) and eosinophil count (observed, squares; predicted, dashed line) following SC administration of 1 mg/kg of the anti-IL-5 humanized monoclonal antibody SB-240563 in a Cynomolgus monkey. A mechanism-based indirect response PK/PD model was used to describe eosinophil count as a function of SB-240563 plasma concentration. The reduction in eosinophil count in peripheral blood (as effect $E$) was modeled as a reduction of the recruitment of eosinophils from the bone, i.e. an inhibition of the production rate $k_{in}$ using the indirect response model of subtype I (see Fig. 15). *Source*: From Zia-Amirhosseini et al., 1999.

For these kinds of therapeutics, cell life span models have been proven useful to capture their exposure-response relationship and describe and predict drug effects (Perez-Ruixo et al., 2005). Cell life span models are mechanism-based, physiologic PK/PD models that are established based on the sequential maturation and lifespan-driven cell turnover of their affected cell types and progenitor cell populations. Cell life span model are especially widely used for characterizing the dose–concentration–effect relationships of hematopoietic growth factors aimed at modifying erythropoiesis, granulopoiesis, or thrombopoiesis (Perez-Ruixo et al., 2005; Agoram et al., 2006). The fixed physiologic time span for the maturation of precursor cells is the major reason for the prolonged delay between drug administration and the observed response, i.e., change in the cell count in peripheral blood. Cell life span models accommodate this sequential maturation of several precursor cell populations at fixed physiologic time intervals by a series of transit compartments linked via first- or zero-order processes with a common transfer rate constant.

A cell life span model was for example used to describe the effect of a multiple dose regimen of recombinant human erythropoietin (rhEPO) 600 IU/kg given once weekly by SC injection (Ramakrishnan et al., 2004). The process of erythropoiesis and the applied PK/PD approach including a cell life span model are depicted in Figures 17 and 18, respectively. rhEPO is known to stimulate the production and release of reticulocytes from the bone marrow. The rhEPO effect was modeled as stimulation of the maturation of two progenitor cell populations (P1 and P2 in Fig. 17), including also a feedback inhibition between erythrocyte count and progenitor proliferation. Development and turn-over of the subsequent populations of reticulocytes and erythrocytes was modeled taking into account their life spans as listed in Figure 17. The hemoglobin concentration as

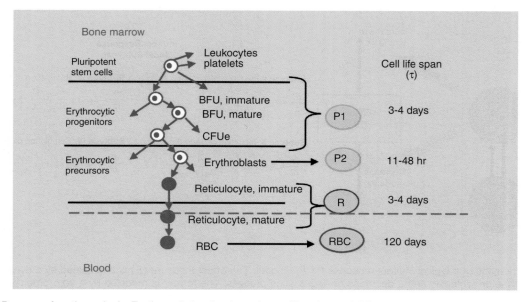

**Figure 17** ■ Process of erythropoiesis. Erythropoietin stimulates the proliferation and differentiation of the erythrocyte progenitors (BFU, burst-forming unit erythroid; CFUe, colony-forming unit erythroid) as well as the erythroblasts in the bone marrow. The life spans ($\tau$) of the various cell populations are indicated at the right. See explanation of $P_1$, $P_2$, and RBC in Figure 18. *Source*: From Ramakrishnan et al., 2004.

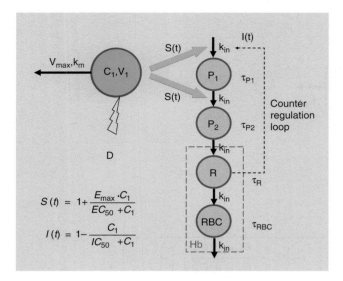

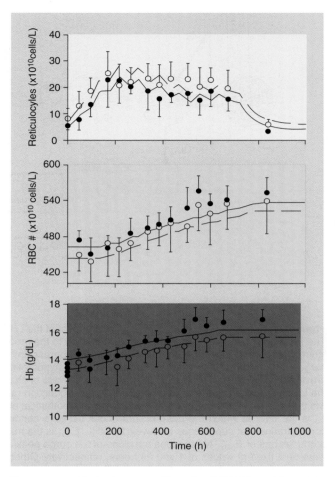

**Figure 18** ▪ A PK/PD model describing the disposition of recombinant human erythropoietin and effects on reticulocyte count, red blood cell count and hemoglobin concentration. The PK model is a one-compartment model with Michaelis–Menten type elimination ($k_m$, $V_{max}$) from the central compartment. The PD model is a cell life span model with four sequential cell compartments, representing erythroid progenitor cells ($P_1$), erythroblasts ($P_2$), reticulocytes (R), and red blood cells (RBC). $\tau_{P1}$, $\tau_{P2}$, $\tau_R$ and $\tau_{RBC}$ are the corresponding cell life spans, $k_{in}$ the common zero-order transfer rate between cell compartments. The target parameter hemoglobin in the blood (Hb) is calculated from the recticulocyte and red blood cell count and the hemoglobin content per cell. The effect of erythropoietin is modeled as a stimulation of the production of both precursor cell populations ($P_1$ and $P_2$) in the bone marrow with the stimulation function $S(t)$. $E_{max}$ is the maximum possible stimulation of reticulocyte production by erythropoietin, $EC_{50}$ the plasma concentration of erythropoietin that produced half maximum stimulation. A counter-regulatory feedback loop represents the feedback inhibition of reticulocytes on their own production by reducing the production rate of cells in the $P_1$ compartment via the inhibitory function $I(t)$. $IC_{50}$ is the reticulocyte count that produced half of complete inhibition. *Source*: Modified from Ramakrishnan et al., 2004.

**Figure 19** ▪ Reticulocyte, red blood cell (RBC), and hemoglobin (Hb) time courses after multiple SC dosing of 600 IU/kg/week recombinant human erythropoietin. Solid and open circles represent data for males and females, whereas the solid and broken lines for the reticulocytes are model fittings. The solid lines in the RBC and Hb panels are the predictions using the model-fitted curves for the reticulocytes and the life span parameters. *Source*: From Ramakrishnan et al., 2004.

pharmacodynamic target parameter was calculated from erythrocyte and reticulocyte counts and hemoglobin content per cell. Figure 19 shows the resulting times courses in reticulocyte count, erythrocyte count and hemoglobin concentration.

■ **Complex Response Models**

Since the effect of most protein therapeutics is mediated via complex regulatory physiologic processes including feedback mechanisms and/or tolerance phenomena, some PK/PD models that have been described for protein drugs are much more sophisticated than the four classes of models previously discussed.

One example of such a complex modeling approach has been developed for the therapeutic

effects of the LH-RH antagonist cetrorelix (Nagaraja et al., 2000; Pechstein et al., 2000; Nagaraja et al., 2003). Cetrorelix is used for the prevention of premature ovulation in women undergoing controlled ovarian stimulation in in vitro fertilization protocols. LH-RH antagonists suppress the LH levels and delay the occurrence of the preovulatory LH surge, and this delay is thought to be responsible for postponing ovulation. The suppression of LH was modeled in the PK/PD approach with an indirect-response model approach directly linked to cetrorelix plasma concentrations (Fig. 20) (Nagaraja et al., 2003). The shift in LH surge was linked to cetrorelix concentration with a simple $E_{max}$-function via a hypothetical effect compartment to account for a delay in response via complex signal transduction steps of unknown mechanism of action. Figure 21 shows the application of

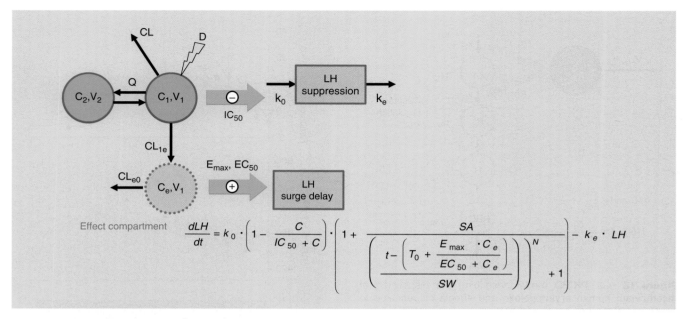

$$\frac{dLH}{dt} = k_0 \cdot \left(1 - \frac{C}{IC_{50} + C}\right) \cdot \left(1 + \frac{SA}{\left(\dfrac{t - \left(T_0 + \dfrac{E_{max} \cdot C_e}{EC_{50} + C_e}\right)}{SW}\right)^N + 1}\right) - k_e \cdot LH$$

**Figure 20** ■ A PK/PD model for the combined effect of the LH-RH antagonist cetrorelix on LH suppression and delay of the LH surge. The PK model is a two-compartment model identical to the model described in Fig. 10. The PD model consists of two components: An indirect response model of subtype I to model the suppression of LH by cetrorelix, and a indirect link model that models the delay in LH surge as a function of the cetrorelix concentration in a hypothetical effect compartment. Both PD model components are combined in the provided mathematical expression that describes the rate of change in LH concentration (dLH/dt) as a function of both processes. LH is the LH concentration, $k_0$ and $k_e$ are the zero-order production rate and first-order elimination rate constant for LH at baseline, $C_1$ and $C_e$ are the cetrorelix concentrations in plasma and a hypothetical effect compartment, respectively, SA is the LH surge amplitude, t is time, $T_0$ is the time at which the peak occurs under baseline conditions, SW is the width of the peak in time units, $IC_{50}$ is the cetrorelix concentration that suppresses LH levels by 50%, $E_{max}$ is the maximum delay in LH surge and $EC_{50}$ is the cetrorelix concentrations that produces half of $E_{max}$. N describes the slope of the surge peak and is an even number. Baseline data analysis indicated that N and SW were best fixed at values of 4 and 24 hours, respectively. Other PK and PD parameters are identical to those used in Fig. 12. *Source*: Modified from Nagaraja et al., 2003.

this PK/PD model to characterize the LH suppression and LH surge delay after SC administration of cetrorelix to groups of 12 women at different dose levels. The analysis revealed a marked dose–response relationship for the LH surge and thus predictability of drug response to cetrorelix (Nagaraja et al., 2000).

Another example for a complex PK/PD model is the cytokinetic model used to describe the effect of pegfilgrastim on the granulocyte count in peripheral blood (Roskos et al., 2006; Yang, 2006). Pegfigrastim is a PEGylated form of the human granulocyte-colony-stimulating factor (G-CSF) analog filgrastim. Pegfilgrastim, like filgrastim and G-CSF, stimulate the activation, proliferation, and differentiation of neutrophil progenitor cells and enhance the functions of mature neutrophils (Roskos et al., 2006). Pegfilgrastim is mainly used as supportive care to ameliorate and enhance recovery from neutropenia secondary to cancer chemotherapy regimens. As already discussed in the section on PEGylation, pegfilgrastim follows target-mediated drug disposition with saturable receptor-mediated endocytosis by neutrophils as major elimination pathway ($CL_N$) and a parallel first-order process as minor elimination pathway ($CL_{lin}$; Fig. 22). The clearance for the receptor-mediated pathway is

determined by the absolute neutrophil count (ANC), the sum of the peripheral blood band cell ($B_p$) and segmented neutrophil ($S_p$) populations.

A maturation-structured cytokinetic model of granulopoiesis was established to describe the relationship between pegfilgrastim serum concentration and neutrophil count (Fig. 22). The starting point is the production of metamyelocytes from mitotic precursors. Subsequent maturation stages are captured as band cells and segmented neutrophils in the bone marrow. Each maturation stage is modeled by three sequential transit compartments. Pegfilgrastim concentrations are assumed to increase ANC by stimulating mitosis and mobilization of band cells and segmented neutrophils from the bone marrow into the systemic circulation. Pegfilgrastim also promotes rapid margination of peripheral blood neutrophils, i.e., adhesion to blood vessels; this effect is modeled as an expansion of neutrophil dilution volume.

Figure 23 shows observed and modeled pegfilgrastim concentration-time and ANC-time profiles after escalating single SC dose administration of pegfilgrastim. The presented PK/PD model for pegfilgrastim allowed determining its $EC_{50}$ for the effect on ANC. Based on this $EC_{50}$ value and the

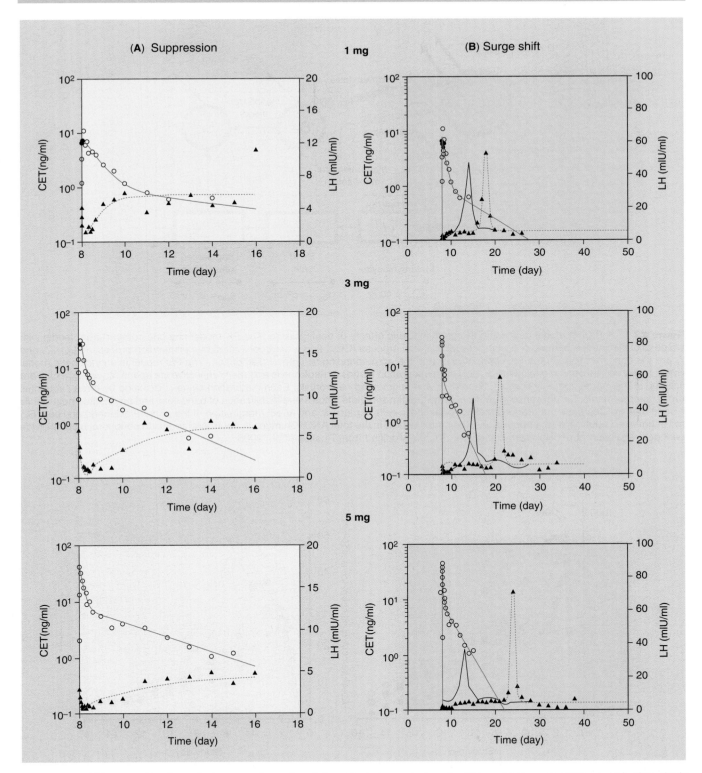

**Figure 21** ▪ Pharmacokinetic and pharmacodynamic relationship between cetrorelix (○) and LH concentrations (▲) after single doses of 1, 3, and 5 mg cetrorelix in representative subjects. Cetrorelix and LH concentrations were modeled using the PK/PD model presented in Fig. 20. (**A**) LH suppression. (**B**) LH suppression and LH surge profiles. The solid red line represents the model fitted cetrorelix concentration, the dashed green line the model fitted LH concentration, and the thin dotted black line in the right panels the pretreatment LH profile (*not fitted*). The cetrorelix-dependent delay in LH surge is visible as the rightward shift of the LH surge profile under cetrorelix therapy compared to the respective pretreatment LH profile. Abbreviation: CET, cetrorelix. *Source*: From Nagaraja et al., 2003.

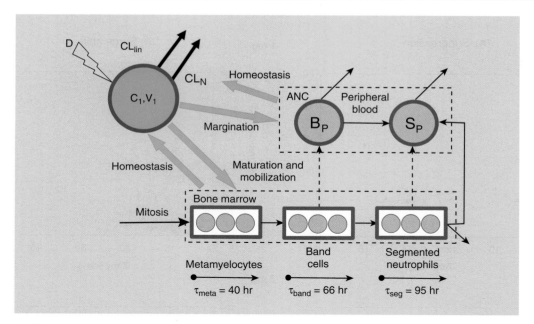

**Figure 22** ■ A PK/PD model describing the granulopoietic effects of pegfilgrastim. The PK model is a one-compartment model with two parallel elimination pathways, a first-order elimination process ($CL_{lin}$) and a neutrophil-mediated elimination process ($CL_N$). $C_1$ and $V_1$ are the concentrations in the PK compartment and the corresponding volume of distribution. The PD model is a cytokinetic model similar to the cell life span model in Fig. 5.18. Three maturation stages of neutrophils and their respective life spans ($t_{meta}$, $t_{band}$, $t_{seg}$) are included in the model, metamyelocytes, band cells and segmented neutrophils. Each maturation stage is modeled by three sequential transit compartments. Serum concentrations of pegfilgrastim stimulate mitosis and mobilization of band cells and segmented neutrophils in bone marrow, decrease maturation times for postmitotic cells in marrow, and affect margination of the peripheral blood band cell ($B_P$) and segmented neutrophil ($S_P$) populations, the sum of which is the total ANC. Changes in neutrophil counts in peripheral blood provide feedback regulation of pegfilgrastim clearance. *Source*: Modified from Roskos et al., 2006.

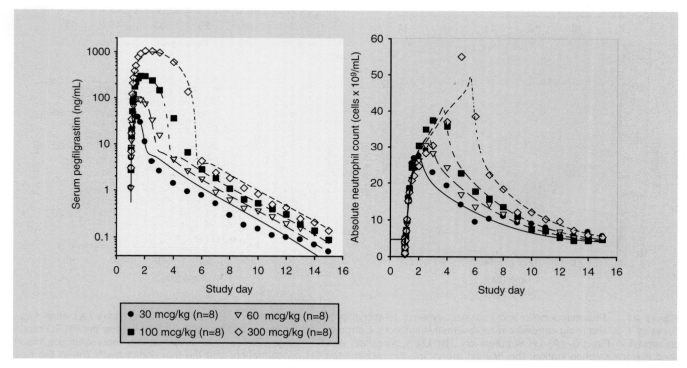

**Figure 23** ■ Pegfilgrastim concentration–time course and absolute neutrophil count (ANC)-time profiles in healthy subjects after a single SC administration of 30, 60, 100, and 300 μg/kg pegfilgrastim ($n = 8$/dose group). Measured data are presented by symbols as mean ± SEM. Lines represent modeled time courses based on the cytokinetic PK/PD model presented in Fig. 5.22. *Source*: From Roskos et al., 2006.

obtained pegfilgrastim plasma concentrations, it was concluded that a 100 µg/kg dose was sufficient to reach the maximum therapeutic effect of pegfilgrastim on ANC (Roskos et al., 2006; Yang, 2006).

## CONCLUSION

The pharmacokinetic and pharmacodynamic characteristics of peptides and proteins form the basis for their therapeutic application. Appreciation of the pharmacokinetic and pharmacodynamic differences between therapeutic biologics and traditional small molecule drugs will empower the drug development scientists as well as the healthcare provider to handle, evaluate and apply these compounds in an optimal fashion during the drug development process as well as during applied pharmacotherapy. Rationale, scientifically-based drug development and pharmacotherapy based on the use of pharmacokinetic and pharmacodynamic concepts will undoubtedly propel the success and future of protein therapeutics, and might ultimately contribute to provide the novel medications that may serve as the key for the aspired 'personalized medicine' in the healthcare systems of the future (Nagle et al., 2003).

## REFERENCES

Agoram B, Heatherington AC, Gastonguay MR (2006). Development and evaluation of a population pharmacokinetic–pharmacodynamic model of darbepoetin alfa in patients with nonmyeloid malignancies undergoing multicycle chemotherapy. Aaps J 8(3): E552–63.

Allon M, Kleinman K, Walczyk M, et al. (2002). Pharmacokinetics and pharmacodynamics of darbepoetin alfa and epoetin in patients undergoing dialysis. Clin Pharmacol Ther 72(5):546–55.

Andersen S, Lambrecht L, Swan S, et al. (1999). Disposition of recombinant human interleukin-10 in subjects with various degrees of renal function. J Clin Pharmacol 39(10):1015–20.

Anderson PM, Sorenson MA (1994). Effects of route and formulation on clinical pharmacokinetics of interleukin-2. Clin Pharmacokinet 27(1):19–31.

Bartocci A, Mastrogiannis DS, Migliorati G, Stockert RJ, Wolkoff AW, Stanley ER (1987). Macrophages specifically regulate the concentration of their own growth factor in the circulation. Proc Natl Acad Sci USA 84(17):6179–83.

Bauer RJ, Gibbons JA, Bell DP, Luo ZP, Young JD (1994). Nonlinear pharmacokinetics of recombinant human macrophage colony-stimulating factor (M-CSF) in rats. J Pharmacol Exp Ther 268(1):152–8.

Baxter LT, Zhu H, Mackensen DG, Jain RK (1994). Physiologically based pharmacokinetic model for specific and nonspecific monoclonal antibodies and

fragments in normal tissues and human tumor xenografts in nude mice. Cancer Res 54(6):1517–28.

Benincosa LJ, Chow FS, Tobia LP, Kwok DC, Davis CB, Jusko WJ (2000). Pharmacokinetics and pharmacodynamics of a humanized monoclonal antibody to factor IX in cynomolgus monkeys. J Pharmacol Exp Ther 292(2):810–6.

Bennett HP, McMartin C (1978). Peptide hormones and their analogues: Distribution, clearance from the circulation, and inactivation in vivo. Pharmacol Rev 30(3):247–92.

Boxenbaum H (1982). Interspecies scaling, allometry, physiological time, and the ground plan of pharmacokinetics. J Pharmacokinet Biopharm 10(2):201–27.

Braeckman RA (2000). Pharmacokinetics and pharmacodynamics of protein therapeutics. In: Reid RE, ed. Peptide and Protein Drug Analysis. New York: Marcel Dekker, 633–69.

Breimer DD, Danhof M (1997). Relevance of the application of pharmacokinetic-pharmacodynamic modelling concepts in drug development. The "wooden shoe" paradigm. Clin Pharmacokinet 32(4):259–67.

Bressolle F, Audran M, Gareau R, Pham TN, Gomeni R (1997). Comparison of a direct and indirect population pharmacodynamic model: Application to recombinant human erythropoietin in athletes. J Pharmacokinet Biopharm 25(3):263–75.

Bu G, Williams S, Strickland DK, Schwartz AL (1992). Low density lipoprotein receptor-related protein/alpha 2-macroglobulin receptor is an hepatic receptor for tissue-type plasminogen activator. Proc Natl Acad Sci USA 89(16):7427–31.

Burwen SJ, Jones AL (1990). Hepatocellular processing of endocytosed proteins. J Electron Microsc Tech 14(2):140–51.

Caliceti P, Veronese FM (2003). Pharmacokinetic and biodistribution properties of poly(ethylene glycol)-protein conjugates. Adv Drug Deliv Rev 55(10):1261–77.

Carone FA, Peterson DR (1980). Hydrolysis and transport of small peptides by the proximal tubule. Am J Physiol 238(3):F151–8.

Carone FA, Peterson DR, Flouret G (1982). Renal tubular processing of small peptide hormones. J Lab Clin Med 100(1):1–14.

Chanson P, Timsit J, Harris AG (1993). Clinical pharmacokinetics of octreotide. Therapeutic applications in patients with pituitary tumours. Clin Pharmacokinet 25(5):375–91.

Chen SA, Sawchuk RJ, Brundage RC, et al. (2000). Plasma and lymph pharmacokinetics of recombinant human interleukin-2 and polyethylene glycol-modified interleukin-2 in pigs. J Pharmacol Exp Ther 2000; 293(1):248–59.

Chiang J, Gloff CA, Yoshizawa CN, Williams GJ (1993). Pharmacokinetics of recombinant human interferon-beta ser in healthy volunteers and its effect on serum neopterin. Pharm Res 10(4):567–72.

Chow FS, Benincosa LJ, Sheth SB, et al. (2002). Pharmacokinetic and pharmacodynamic modeling of humanized anti-factor IX antibody (SB 249417) in humans. Clin Pharmacol Ther 71(4):235–45.

Colburn W (1991). Peptide, peptoid, and protein pharmacokinetics/pharmacodynamics. In: Garzone P, Colburn W, Mokotoff M, eds. Peptides, Peptoids, and Proteins, Vol. 3. Cincinnati, OH, Harvey: Whitney Books, 94–115.

Cumming DA (1991). Glycosylation of recombinant protein therapeutics: Control and functional implications. Glycobiology 1(2):115–30.

Daniel H, Herget M (1997). Cellular and molecular mechanisms of renal peptide transport. Am J Physiol 273(1 Pt 2):F1–8.

Dayneka NL, Garg V, Jusko WJ (1993). Comparison of four basic models of indirect pharmacodynamic responses. J Pharmacokinet Bioharm 21(4):457–78.

Dedrick RL (1973). Animal scale-up. J Pharmacokinet Biopharm 1(5):435–61.

Deen WM, Lazzara MJ, Myers BD (2001). Structural determinants of glomerular permeability. Am J Physiol Renal Physiol 281(4):F579–96.

Derendorf H, Meibohm B (1999). Modeling of pharmacokinetic/pharmacodynamic (PK/PD) relationships: Concepts and perspectives. Pharm Res 16(2):176–85.

Edwards A, Daniels BS, Deen WM (1999). Ultrastructural model for size selectivity in glomerular filtration. Am J Physiol 276(6 Pt 2):F892–902.

Eppler SM, Combs DL, Henry TD, et al. (2002). A target-mediated model to describe the pharmacokinetics and hemodynamic effects of recombinant human vascular endothelial growth factor in humans. Clin Pharmacol Ther 72(1):20–32.

Fasano A (1998). Novel approaches for oral delivery of macromolecules. J Pharm Sci 87(11):1351–6.

Ferraiolo B, Mohler M (1992). Goals and analytical methodologies for protein distribution studies. In: Ferraiolo B, Mohler M, Gloff CA, eds. Protein Pharmacokinetics and Metabolism. New York: Plenum Press.

Flessner MF, Lofthouse J, Zakariael R (1997). In vivo diffusion of immunoglobulin G in muscle: Effects of binding, solute exclusion, and lymphatic removal. Am J Physiol 273(6 Pt 2):H2783–93.

Graham ML (2003). Pegaspargase: A review of clinical studies. Adv Drug Deliv Rev 55(10):1293–302.

Handelsman DJ, Swerdloff RS (1986). Pharmacokinetics of gonadotropin-releasing hormone and its analogs. Endocr Rev 7(1):95–105.

Herbst RS, Langer CJ (2002). Epidermal growth factor receptors as a target for cancer treatment: The emerging role of IMC-C225 in the treatment of lung and head and neck cancers. Semin Oncol 29(1 Suppl 4):27–36.

Holford NH, Sheiner LB (1982). Kinetics of pharmacologic response. Pharmacol Ther 16(2):143–66.

Hooper S (1991). Pharmacokinetics and pharmacodynamics of intravenous regular human insulin. In: Garzone P, Colburn W, Mokotoff M, eds. Petides, Peptoids, and Proteins, Vol. 3. Cincinnati, OH: Harvey Whitney Books, 128–37.

Inui K, Terada T, Masuda S, Saito H (2000). Physiological and pharmacological implications of peptide transporters, PEPT1 and PEPT2. Nephrol Dial Transplant 15(Suppl 6):11–3.

Ismair MG, Stieger B, Cattori V, et al. (2001). Hepatic uptake of cholecystokinin octapeptide by organic anion-transporting polypeptides OATP4 and OATP8 of rat and human liver. Gastroenterology 121(5):1185–90.

Jin F, Krzyzanski W (2004). Pharmacokinetic model of target-mediated disposition of thrombopoietin. AAPS Pharm Sci 6(1):E9.

Johnson V, Maack T (1977). Renal extraction, filtration, absorption, and catabolism of growth hormone. Am J Physiol 233(3):F185–96.

Kageyama S, Yamamoto, H, Nakazawa H, et al. (2002). Pharmacokinetics and pharmacodynamics of AJW200, a humanized monoclonal antibody to von Willebrand factor, in monkeys. Arterioscler Thromb Vasc Biol 22(1):187–92.

Kaufman JS, Reda DJ, Fye CL, et al. (1998). Subcutaneous compared with intravenous epoetin in patients receiving hemodialysis: Department of Veterans Affairs Cooperative Study Group on Erythropoietin in Hemodialysis Patients. N Engl J Med 339(9):578–83.

Khor SP, McCarthy K, DuPont M, Murray K, Timony G (2000). Pharmacokinetics, pharmacodynamics, allometry, and dose selection of rPSGL-Ig for phase I trial. J Pharmacol Exp Ther 293(2):618–24.

Kim DC, Sugiyama Y, Satoh H, Fuwa T, Iga T, Hanano M (1988). Kinetic analysis of in vivo receptor-dependent binding of human epidermal growth factor by rat tissues. J Pharm Sci 77(3):200–7.

Kobayashi H, et al. (2002). Rapid accumulation and internalization of radiolabeled herceptin in an inflammatory breast cancer xenograft with vasculogenic mimicry predicted by the contrast-enhanced dynamic MRI with the macromolecular contrast agent G6-(1B4M-Gd)(256). Cancer Res 62(3):860–6.

Kompella U, Lee V (1991). Pharmacokinetics of peptide and protein drugs. In: Lee V, ed. Peptide and Protein Drug Delivery. New York: Marcel Dekker, 391–484.

Krogsgaard Thomsen M, Friis C, Sehested Hansen B, et al. (1994). Studies on the renal kinetics of growth hormone (GH) and on the GH receptor and related effects in animals. J Pediatr Endocrinol 7(2):93–105.

Kuwabara T, Uchimura T, Kobayashi H, Kobayashi S, Sugiyama Y (1995). Receptor-mediated clearance of G-CSF derivative nartograstim in bone marrow of rats. Am J Physiol 269(1 Pt 1):E1–9.

Lee H, Kimko HC, Rogge M, Wang D, Nestorov I, Peck CC (2003). Population pharmacokinetic and pharmacodynamic modeling of etanercept using logistic regression analysis. Clin Pharmacol Ther 73(4):348–65.

Lee HJ (2002). Protein drug oral delivery: The recent progress. Arch Pharm Res 25(5):572–84.

Lesko LJ (2007). Paving the critical path: How can clinical pharmacology help achieve the vision? Clin Pharmacol Ther 81(2):170–7.

Lesko LJ, Rowland M, Peck CC, Blaschke TF (2000). Optimizing the science of drug development: Opportunities for better candidate selection and accelerated evaluation in humans. J Clin Pharmacol 40(8):803–14.

Levy G (1986). Kinetics of drug action: An overview. J Allergy Clin Immunol 78(4 Pt 2):754–61.

Levy G (1994). Mechanism-based pharmacodynamic modeling. Clin Pharmacol Ther 56(4):356–8.

Maack T, Park C, Camargo M (1985). Renal filtration, transport and metabolism of proteins. In: Seldin D, Giebisch G, ed. The Kidney. New York: Raven Press, 1773–1803.

Macdougall IC, Gray SJ, Elston O et al. (1999). Pharmacokinetics of novel erythropoiesis stimulating protein compared with epoetin alfa in dialysis patients. J Am Soc Nephrol 10(11):2392–5.

Machado SG, Miller R, Hu C (1999). A regulatory perspective on pharmacokinetic/pharmacodynamic modelling. Stat Method Med Res 8(3):217–45.

Mager DE (2006). Target-mediated drug disposition and dynamics. Biochem Pharmacol 72(1):1–10.

Mager DE, Wyska E, Jusko WJ, (2003). Diversity of mechanism-based pharmacodynamic models. Drug Metab Dispos 31(5):510–8.

Mahato RI, Narang AS, Thoma L, Miller DD (2003). Emerging trends in oral delivery of peptide and protein drugs. Crit Rev Ther Drug Carrier Syst 20 (2–3):153–214.

Mahmood I (2002). Interspecies scaling: Predicting oral clearance in humans. Am J Ther 9(1):35–42.

Mahmood I, Balian JD (1999). The pharmacokinetic principles behind scaling from preclinical results to phase I protocols. Clin Pharmacokinet 36(1):1–11.

Marks DL, Gores GJ, LaRusso NF (1995). Hepatic processing of peptides. In: Taylor MD, Amidon GL, eds. Peptide-based Drug Design: Controlling Transport and Metabolism. Washington, DC: American Chemical Society, 221–48.

McMartin C (1992). Pharmacokinetics of peptides and proteins: Opportunities and challenges. Advances in Drug Research 22:39–106.

Meibohm B (2004). Pharmacokinetics of protein- and nucleotide-based drugs. In: Mahato RI, ed. Biomaterials for Delivery and Targeting of Proteins and Nucleic Acids. Boca Raton, FL: CRC Press, 275–94.

Meibohm B, Derendorf H (1994). Pharmacokinetics and pharmacodynamics of biotech drugs. In: Kayser O, Muller R, eds. Pharmaceutical Biotechnology: Drug Discovery and Clinical Applications. Weinheim: Wiley, 141–66.

Meibohm B, Derendorf H (1997). Basic concepts of pharmacokinetic/pharmacodynamic (PK/PD) modelling. Int J Clin Pharmacol Ther 35(10):401–13.

Meibohm B, Derendorf H (2002). Pharmacokinetic/pharmacodynamic studies in drug product development. J Pharm Sci 91(1):18–31.

Meibohm B, Derendorf H (2003). Pharmacokinetics and pharmacodynamics of biotech drugs. In: Muller R, Kayser O, eds. Applications of Pharmaceutical Biotechnology. Weinheim: Wiley-VCH.

Meijer D, Ziegler K (1993). Biological Barriers to Protein Delivery. New York: Plenum Press.

Mohler M, Cook J, Lewis D, et al. (1993). Altered pharmacokinetics of recombinant human deoxyribonuclease in rats due to the presence of a binding protein. Drug Metab Dispos 21(1):71–5.

Molineux G (2003). Pegylation: Engineering improved biopharmaceuticals for oncology. Pharmacotherapy 23(8 Pt 2):3S–8S.

Montero-Julian FA, Klein B, Gautherot E, Brailly H (1995). Pharmacokinetic study of anti-interleukin-6 (IL-6) therapy with monoclonal antibodies: Enhancement of IL-6 clearance by cocktails of anti-IL-6 antibodies. Blood 85(4):917–24.

Mordenti J, Chen SA, Moore JA, Ferraiolo BL, Green JD (1991). Interspecies scaling of clearance and volume of distribution data for five therapeutic proteins. Pharm Res 8(11):1351–9.

Mould DR, Davis CB, Minthorn EA, et al. (1999). A population pharmacokinetic–pharmacodynamic analysis of single doses of clenoliximab in patients with rheumatoid arthritis. Clin Pharmacol Ther 66(3):246–57.

Nagaraja NV, Pechstein B, Erb K, et al. (2003). Pharmacokinetic/pharmacodynamic modeling of luteinizing hormone (LH) suppression and LH surge delay by cetrorelix after single and multiple doses in healthy premenopausal women. J Clin Pharmacol 43 (3):243–51.

Nagaraja NV, Pechstein B, Erb K (2000). Pharmacokinetic and pharmacodynamic modeling of cetrorelix, an LH–RH antagonist, after subcutaneous administration in healthy premenopausal women. Clin Pharmacol Ther 68(6):617–25.

Nagle T, Berg C, Nassr R, Pang K (2003). The further evolution of biotech. Nat Rev Drug Discov 2(1):75–9.

Nielsen S, Nielsen JT, Christensen EI (1987). Luminal and basolateral uptake of insulin in isolated, perfused, proximal tubules. Am J Physiol 253(5 Pt 2):F857–67.

Pauletti GM, Gangwar S, Siahaan TJ, Jeffrey A, Borchardt RT (1997). Improvement of oral peptide bioavailability: Peptidomimetics and prodrug strategies. Adv Drug Deliv Rev 27(2–3):235–56.

Pechstein B, Nagaraja NV Hermann R, Romeis P, Locher M, Derendorf H (2000). Pharmacokinetic–pharmacodynamic modeling of testosterone and luteinizing hormone suppression by cetrorelix in healthy volunteers. J Clin Pharmacol 40(3):266–74.

Peck CC, et al. (1994). Opportunities for integration of pharmacokinetics, pharmacodynamics, and toxicokinetics in rational drug development. J Clin Pharmacol 34(2):111–9.

Perez-Ruixo JJ, Kimko HC, Chow AT, Piotrovsky V, Krzyzanski W, Jusko WJ (2005). Population cell life span models for effects of drugs following indirect mechanisms of action. J Pharmacokinet Pharmacodyn 32(5–6):767–93.

Periti P, Mazzei T, Mini E (2002). Clinical pharmacokinetics of depot leuprorelin. Clin Pharmacokinet 41(7):485–504.

Perrier D, Mayersohn M (1982). Noncompartmental determination of the steady-state volume of distribution for any mode of administration. J Pharm Sci 71(3): 372–3.

Piscitelli SC, Reiss WG, Figg WD, Petros WP(1997). Pharmacokinetic studies with recombinant cytokines. Scientific issues and practical considerations. Clin Pharmacokinet 32(5):368–81.

Porter CJ, Charman SA (2000). Lymphatic transport of proteins after subcutaneous administration. J Pharm Sci 89(3):297–310.

Rabkin R, Ryan MP, Duckworth WC (1984). The renal metabolism of insulin. Diabetologia 27(3):351–7.

Racine-Poon A, Botta L, Chang TW, et al. (1997). Efficacy, pharmacodynamics, and pharmacokinetics of CGP 51901, an anti- immunoglobulin E chimeric monoclonal antibody, in patients with seasonal allergic rhinitis. Clin Pharmacol Ther 62(6):675–90.

Radwanski E, Chakraborty A, Van Wart S, et al. (1998). Pharmacokinetics and leukocyte responses of recombinant human interleukin-10. Pharm Res 15 (12):1895–901.

Ramakrishnan R, Cheung WK, Wacholtz MC, Minton N, Jusko WJ (2004). Pharmacokinetic and pharmacodynamic modeling of recombinant human erythropoietin after single and multiple doses in healthy volunteers. J Clin Pharmacol 44(9):991–1002.

Reddy ST, Berk DA, Jain RK, Swartz MA (2006). A sensitive in vivo model for quantifying interstitial convective transport of injected macromolecules and nanoparticles. J Appl Physiol 101(4):1162–9.

Rosenblum MG, Unger BW, Gutterman JU, Hersh EM, David GS, Frincke JM (1985). Modification of human leukocyte interferon pharmacology with a monoclonal antibody. Cancer Res 45(6):2421–4.

Roskos LK, Lum P, Lockbaum P, Schwab G, Yang BB (2006). Pharmacokinetic/pharmacodynamic modeling of pegfilgrastim in healthy subjects. J Clin Pharmacol 46(7):747–57.

Schomburg A, Kirchner H, Atzpodien J (1993). Renal, metabolic, and hemodynamic side-effects of interleukin-2 and/or interferon alpha: Evidence of a risk/benefit advantage of subcutaneous therapy. J Cancer Res Clin Oncol 119(12):745–55.

Sharma A, Jusko W (1998). Characteristics of indirect pharmacodynamic models and applications to clinical drug responses. Br J Clin Pharmacol 45:229–39.

Sheiner LB, Stanski DR, Vozeh S, Miller RD, Ham J (1979). Simultaneous modeling of pharmacokinetics and pharmacodynamics: Application to d-tubocurarine. Clin Pharmacol Ther 25(3):358–71.

Sheiner LB, Steimer JL (2000). Pharmacokinetic/pharmacodynamic modeling in drug development. Annu Rev Pharmacol Toxicol 40:67–95.

Shen WC (2003). Oral peptide and protein delivery: Unfulfilled promises? Drug Discov Today 8(14):607–8.

Smedsrod B, Einarsson M (1990). Clearance of tissue plasminogen activator by mannose and galactose receptors in the liver. Thromb Haemost 63(1):60–6.

Straughn AB (1982). Model-independent steady-state volume of distribution. J Pharm Sci 71(5):597–8.

Straughn AB (2006). Limitations of noncompartmental pharmacokinetic analysis of biotech drugs. In: Meibohm B, ed. Pharmacokinetics and Pharmacodynamics of Biotech Drugs. Weinheim: Wiley, 181–8.

Strickland DK, Kounnas MZ, Argraves WS (1995). LDL receptor-related protein: A multiligand receptor for lipoprotein and proteinase catabolism. Faseb J 9(10):890–8.

Sugiyama Y, Hanano M (1989). Receptor-mediated transport of peptide hormones and its importance in the overall hormone disposition in the body. Pharm Res 6(3):192–202.

Sun YN, Jusko WJ (1999). Role of baseline parameters in determining indirect pharmacodynamic responses. J Pharm Sci 88(10):987–90.

Sun YN, Lee HJ, Almon RR, Jusko WJ (1999). A pharmacokinetic/pharmacodynamic model for recombinant human growth hormone effects on induction of insulin-like growth factor I in monkeys. J Pharmacol Exp Ther 289(3):1523–32.

Supersaxo A, Hein W Gallati H, Steffen H (1988). Recombinant human interferon alpha-2a: Delivery to lymphoid tissue by selected modes of application. Pharm Res 5(8):472–6.

Supersaxo A, Hein WR, Steffen H (1990). Effect of molecular weight on the lymphatic absorption of water-soluble compounds following subcutaneous administration. Pharm Res 7(2):167–9.

Tabrizi M, Roskos LK (2006). Exposure–reponse relationships for therapeutic biologics. In: Meibohm B, ed. Pharmacokinetics and Pharmacodynamics of Biotech Drugs. Weinheim: Wiley, 295–330.

Takagi A, Masuda H, Takakura Y, Hashida M (1995). Disposition characteristics of recombinant human interleukin-11 after a bolus intravenous administration in mice. J Pharmacol Exp Ther 275(2):537–43.

Taki Y, Sakane T, Nadai T, et al. (1998). First-pass metabolism of peptide drugs in rat perfused liver. J Pharm Pharmacol 50(9):1013–8.

Tang L, Meibohm B (2006). Pharmacokinetics of peptides and proteins. In: Meibohm B, ed. Pharmacokinetics and Pharmacodynamics of Biotech Drugs. Weinheim: Wiley, 17–44.

Tang L, Persky AM, Hochhaus G, Meibohm B (2004). Pharmacokinetic aspects of biotechnology products. J Pharm Sci 93(9):2184–204.

Tanswell P, Modi N, Combs D, Danays T (2002). Pharmacokinetics and pharmacodynamics of tenecteplase in fibrinolytic therapy of acute myocardial infarction. Clin Pharmacokinet 41(15):1229–45.

Tokuda Y, et al. (1999). Dose escalation and pharmacokinetic study of a humanized anti-HER2 monoclonal antibody in patients with HER2/neu-overexpressing metastatic breast cancer. Br J Cancer 81(8):1419–25.

Toon S (1996). The relevance of pharmacokinetics in the development of biotechnology products. Eur J Drug Metab Pharmacokinet 21(2):93–103.

Veng-Pedersen P, Gillespie W (1984). Mean residence time in peripheral tissue: A linear disposition parameter useful for evaluating a drug's tissue distribution. J Pharmacokinet Biopharm 12(5):535–43.

Veronese FM, P. Caliceti (2006). Custom-tailored pharmacokinetics and pharmacodynamics via chemical modifications of biotech drugs. In: Meibohm B, ed. Pharmacokinetics and Pharmacodynamics of Boptech Drugs. Weinheim: Wiley, 271–94.

Walsh S, Shah A, Mond J (2003). Improved pharmacokinetics and reduced antibody reactivity of lysostaphin conjugated to polyethylene glycol. Antimicrob Agents Chemother 47(2):554–8.

Wills R (1991). A kinetic/dynamic perspective of a peptide and protein: GRF and rHuIFN-alpha-2a. In: Garzone P, Colburn W, Mokotoff M, eds. Petides, Peptoids, and Proteins, Vol. 3. Cincinnati, OH: Harvey Whitney Books, 117–27.

Wills RJ, Ferraiolo BL (1992). The role of pharmacokinetics in the development of biotechnologically derived agents. Clin Pharmacokinet 23(6):406-14.

Woodworth JR, Howey DC, Bowsher RR (1994). Establishment of time-action profiles for regular and NPH insulin using pharmacodynamic modeling. Diabetes Care 17(1):64–9.

Working P, Cossum P (1991). Clinical and preclinical studies with recombinant human proteins: Effect of antibody production. In: Garzone P, Colburn W, Mokotoff M, eds. Peptides, Peptoids, and Proteins, Vol. 3. Cincinnati, OH: Harvey Whitney Books, 158–68.

Working PK (1992). Potential effects of antibody induction by protein drugs. In: Ferraiolo BL, Mohler MA, Gloff CA, eds. Portein Pharmacokinetics and Metabolism. New York: Plenum Press, 73–92.

Yang BB (2006). Integration of pharmacokinetics and pharmacodynamics into the drug development of pegfilgrastim, a pegylated protein. In: Meibohm B, ed. Pharmacokinetics and Pharmacodynamics of Biotech Drugs. Weinheim: Wiley, 373–94.

Zamboni WC (2003). Pharmacokinetics of pegfilgrastim. Pharmacotherapy 23(8 Pt 2):9S–14S.

Zia-Amirhosseini P, Minthorn E Benincosa LJ, et al. (1999). Pharmacokinetics and pharmacodynamics of SB-240563, a humanized monoclonal antibody directed to human interleukin-5, in monkeys. J Pharmacol Exp Ther 291(3):1060–7.

Ziegler K, Polzin G, Frimmer M (1988). Hepatocellular uptake of cyclosporin A by simple diffusion. Biochim Biophys Acta 938(1):44–50.

Zito SW (1997). Pharmaceutical biotechnology: A programmed text. Lancaster, PA: Technomic Pub. Co.

## FURTHER READING

### ■ General Pharmacokinetics and Pharmacodynamics

Atkinson A, Abernethy D, Daniels C, Dedrick R, Markey S (2006). Principles of Clinical Pharmacology. San Diego, CA: Academic Press.

Bjornsson TD (1997). Practical uses of individual pharmacokinetic parameters in drug development and clinical practice: Examples and simulations. Eur J Drug Metab Pharmacokinet 22(1):1–14.

Bonate PL (2006). Pharmacokinetic–Pharmacodynamic Modeling and Simulation. New York: Springer.

Derendorf H, Meibohm B (1999). Modeling of pharmacokinetic/pharmacodynamic (PK/PD) relationships: Concepts and perspectives. Pharm Res 16(2):176–85.

Gibaldi M, Perrier D (1982). Pharmacokinetics. New York: Marcel Dekker.

Holford NH, Sheiner LB (1982). Kinetics of pharmacologic response. Pharmacol Ther 16(2):143–66.

Rowland M, Tozer T (1993). Clinical Pharmacokinetics: Concepts and Applications. Media, PA: Williams & Wilkins.

### ■ Pharmacokinetics and Pharmacodynamics of Peptides and Proteins

Baumann A (2006). Early development of therapeutic biologics — pharmacokinetics. Curr Drug Metab 7, 15–21.

Ferraiolo BL, Mohler MA, Gloff CA (1992). Protein Pharmacokinetics and Metabolism. New York: Plenum Press.

Meibohm B (2006). Pharmacokinetics and Pharmacodynamics of Biotech Drugs. Weinheim: Wiley.

Tang L, Persky AM, Hochhaus G, Meibohm B (2004). Pharmacokinetic aspects of biotechnology products. J Pharm Sci 93(9):2184–204.

# 6

# Immunogenicity of Therapeutic Proteins

*Huub Schellekens*
Departments of Pharmaceutical Sciences and Innovation Studies, Utrecht University, Utrecht, The Netherlands

*Wim Jiskoot*
Division of Drug Delivery Technology, Leiden/Amsterdam Center for Drug Research, Leiden University, Leiden, The Netherlands

## INTRODUCTION

The era of the medical application of proteins started at the end of the 19th century when animal sera were introduced for the treatment of serious complications of infections such as diphtheria and tetanus. The high doses used, the general lack of quality controls and a regulatory system, and the impurity of the preparations led to many serious and sometimes even fatal side effects. Many of the problems were caused by the strong immune response these foreign proteins induced, especially when readministered. People who had been treated in general had a warning in their passports or identification cards to alert physicians for a possible anaphylactic reaction after rechallenge with an antiserum. Also serum sickness caused by deposits of antigen–antibody complexes was a common complication of the serum therapy.

Also the porcine and bovine insulins introduced after 1922 induced antibodies in many patients. This was also explained by the animal origin of the products, although over the years the immunogenicity became less because of improvements in the production methods andincreasing purity.

In the second half of the 20th century a number of human proteins from natural sources have introduced such as plasma-derived clotting factors and growth hormone produced from pituitary glands of cadavers. These products were given mainly to children with an innate deficiency who therefore lacked the natural immune tolerance. Therefore, their immune response was also interpreted as a response to foreign proteins. The correlation between the factor VIII gene defect and level of deficiency with the immune response in hemophilia patients confirmed this explanation.

Thus, until the advent of recombinant DNA technology, the immunological response to therapeutic proteins could be explained as a classical immune response comparable to that of a vaccine.

## THE NEW PARADIGM

In 1982, human insulin was marketed as the first recombinant DNA-derived protein for human use. Since then dozens of recombinant proteins have been introduced and some of these products such as the interferons and the epoetins are among the most widely used drugs in the world. And, although these proteins were developed as close copies of human endogenous proteins, nearly all these proteins induce antibodies, sometimes even in a majority of patients (Table 1). In addition, most of these products are used in patients who do not have an innate deficiency and can be assumed to have immune tolerance to the protein.

The initial assumption was that the production by recombinant technology in nonhuman host cells and the downstream processing modified the proteins and the immunological response was the classical response to a foreign protein. However, according to the current opinion the antibody response to human homologues is based on breaking B-cell tolerance. This phenomenon is not yet completely understood but is clearly different from the vaccine type of reaction seen with foreign proteins.

The clinical manifestations of both types of reaction are very different. The vaccine-type response occurs within weeks and sometimes a single injection is sufficient to induce a substantial antibody response. In general high levels of neutralizing antibodies are induced and a rechallenge leads to a booster reaction, indicating a memory response.

However, breaking B-cell tolerance takes in general 6 to 12 months of chronic treatment and often only leads to the production of binding antibodies with no biological effect. The antibodies often disappear shortly after treatment has been stopped and sometimes even during treatment. This response also appears to have no memory, because rechallenging

**Loss of efficacy**
  Insulin
  Factor VIII
  Interferon alpha 2
  Interferon beta
  Interleukin-2
  Human chorionic gonadotropin (HCG)
  Monoclonal antibodies
**Enhancement of efficacy**
  Growth hormone
**Neutralization of endogenous protein**
  Megakaryocyte-derived growth factor (MDGF)
  Epoetin
**General immune effects**
  Allergy
  Anaphylaxis
  Serum sickness, etc.

**Table 1** ■ Nonexhaustive list of recombinant proteins showing immune reactions upon administration.

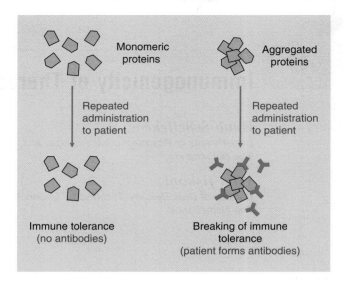

**Figure 1** ■ Dogma: Protein aggregates are immunogenic.

patients in whom the antibody levels have declined does not induce a response.

## THE IMMUNOLOGICAL RESPONSE

The therapeutic proteins currently available cover the whole spectrum, from completely foreign, like bacterial-derived asparaginase to completely human-like interferon α-2a and everything in between. The foreign protein elicits antibodies by the classical pathway which includes ingestion and cleaving of the proteins into peptides by macrophages and dendritic cells, presentation of peptides by the MHC-II system and activation of B-cells and boosting, and affinity maturation and isotype switching of the B-cells by helper T-cells. Furthermore, memory B-cells are induced (see Chapter 21 for details)

It is much less clear how B-cell tolerance is broken. There are always autoreactive B-cells present. When the receptor on these B-cells meets its epitope on the protein in solution, this interaction does not lead to activation. When these B-cells meet their epitope in a regularly repeated form, then the B-cell receptor oligomerizes and the cell is activated, and starts to divide and produce antibodies. So, B-cells can recognize three-dimensional repeated protein structures as has been shown experimentally in a number of studies. The explanation why is based on evolution. The only naturally occurring, narrowly spaced repeated protein structures are found on the surface of viruses and some bacterial structures (Bachmann et al., 1993). Apparently, the B-cell system was also selected for its potential to respond to microbial structures independent of the system which discriminates self from nonself.

This explanation of nonself-independent response by repeated protein structures fits nicely with aggregates being recognized as the main driver of an autoreactive response by human therapeutic proteins, because in protein aggregates certain structures are also presented in a repeated form (Fig. 1) (Moore and Leppert, 1980).

Thus, the initial activation of B-cells by aggregates can be explained and also how these cells start with producing IgM. It is not known how the isotype switching from IgM to IgG occurs. Some studies suggest that aggregates after reacting with the B-cell receptor are internalized. And by internalizing, the B-cells become helper cells and start to produce cytokines which will activate other B-cells. Others claim that helper T-cells are involved. However, studies to show the presence of specific T-cell activity in patients producing antibodies to human therapeutic proteins have failed. In addition, a T-cell independent mechanism is suggested by the lack of any association with HLA-type and the absence of memory.

## FACTORS INFLUENCING ANTIBODY FORMATION TO THERAPEUTIC PROTEINS

Figure 2 depicts the different factors that influence immunogenicity (Schellekens, 2002; Hermeling et al., 2004).

### ■ Structural Factors

The degree of nonself and presence of aggregates are the initial triggers of an antibody response to a therapeutic protein. The degree of nonself necessary to induce a vaccine-type response is highly dependent on the protein involved and the site of the divergence from the natural sequence of the endogenous protein. For insulin there are single mutations which lead to a new epitope and an antibody response while other

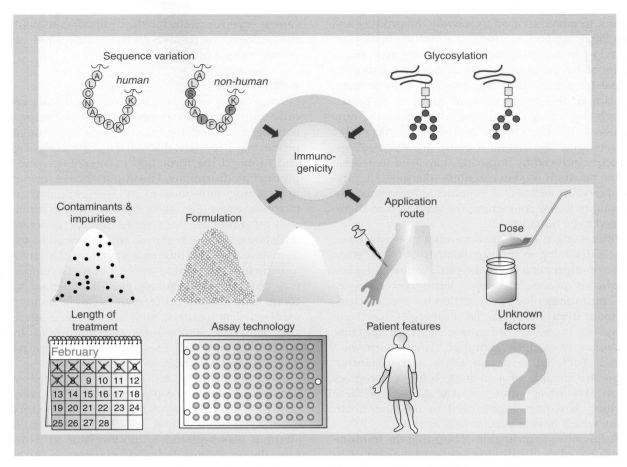

**Figure 2** ▨ Factors relevant in immunogenicity. *Source*: From Schellekens, 2002.

mutations have no influence at all. Consensus interferon α in which more than 10% of the amino acids diverge from the nearest naturally occurring interferon α subtype shows not more immunogenicity than the interferon α-2 homologue.

Glycosylation is another important structural factor for the immunogenicity of therapeutic proteins. There is little evidence that modified glycosylation, e. g., by expressing human glycoproteins in plant cells or other nonhuman eukaryotic hosts, may induce an immunogenic response. However, the level of glycosylation has a clear effect. Interferon β produced in *Escherichia coli* is much more immunogenic than the same product produced in mammalian cells. The explanation is the lower solubility causing aggregation in the nonglycosylated *E. coli* product. Glycosylation is also reported to influence antigenicity by antibody binding. Nonglycosylated epoetin was reported to have a higher affinity to antibodies than epoetin with a normal level of glycosylation; the opposite has been shown for epoetin engineered to have extra glycosylation. However, such data should

be interpreted with caution. Antigenicity does not equal immunogenicity (Fig. 3). A protein or peptide with a high affinity for antibodies may not be able to induce antibodies at all.

### ▪ Impurities

Impurities are apparently important factors in the immunogenicity of therapeutic proteins. Substances like host cell components, resins from chromatographic

---

**The difference between antigenicity and immunogenicity**

– **Antigenicity:** the capability of a substance to interact with (pre-existing) components of the immune system

– **Immunogenicity:** the capability of a substance to elicit an immune response

**Figure 3** ▨ Immunogenicity versus antigenicity.

columns, or enzymes used to activate the product and monoclonal antibodies used for affinity purification may end up in the final product. Impurities may also be introduced by the components of the formulation or may leak from the container and sealing of the product. These impurities may boost an immune response, although they are not capable of initiating an immune response to the therapeutic protein. However, these products may be immunogenic by themselves. Antibodies induced by impurities may lead to general immune reactions as skin reactions, allergies, anaphylaxis, and serum sickness. Antibodies to impurities also raise quality issues concerning the product and therefore need to be monitored.

Interestingly, there are a number of examples of products declining in immunogenicity over the years because of improvements in the purification and other downstream processing steps. Impurities may enhance immunogenicity via different mechanisms. Endotoxin from the bacterial host cells has been reported to cause the immunogenicity of the first recombinant DNA-derived human growth hormones. G-C rich bacterial host cell DNA and denatured proteins are capable of activating Toll-like receptors and can also act as adjuvants. The activity of these impurities, however, is restricted to the nonhuman proteins which have a vaccine-like activity.

Adjuvants are incapable of boosting the immune response based on T-cell independent breaking of B-cell tolerance. However, impurities that are modified human proteins such as clipped and oxidized variants which can be present in therapeutic protein products could indirectly induce antibodies which react with the unmodified protein. This immunological mimicry has been described in dogs treated with human epoetin. The degree of nonself of this protein for dogs is sufficient to induce an immune response. But there is still enough homology between the human and canine erythropoietin for the antibodies to neutralize the endogenous, canine erythropoietin, and causing severe anemia.

### ■ Formulation

Human therapeutic proteins are often highly biologically active and the doses may be at the μg level, making it a technological challenge to formulate the product to keep it stable with a reasonable shelf-life and to avoid the formation of aggregates and other product modifications. The importance of formulation in avoiding immunogenicity is highlighted in two historical cases (Fig. 4). In the case of interferon α-2a, a large difference was noted among different formulations. A freeze-dried formulation, containing human serum albumin as a stabilizer that according to its instructions could be kept at room temperature was particularly immunogenic. It appeared that at room temperature interferon α-2a became partly oxidized. The oxidized molecules formed aggregates also with the unmodified interferon and human serum albumin, and these aggregates were responsible for the immune response.

More recently an antibody-mediated severe form of anemia (pure red cell aplasia; PRCA) occurred after the formulation of an epoetin-α product was changed (Casadevall et al., 2002). Human serum albumin was replaced by polysorbate 80. How this formulation change induced immunogenicity is still not certain. However, the most likely explanation is a less stable new formulation resulting in aggregate formation when not appropriately handled.

### ■ Route of Administration

There is a clear effect of route of administration on the immunogenicity. The subcutaneous route is the most immunogenic and the intravenous the least immunogenic one. However, immunogenicity can be seen

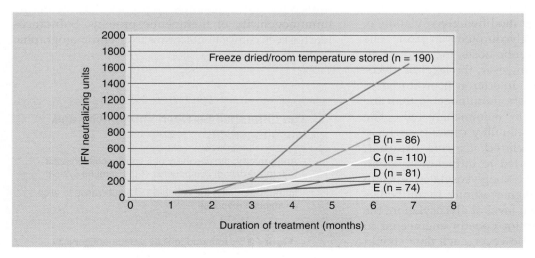

**Figure 4** ■ Immunogenicity differences between interferon (IFN) α formulations in patients. *Source*: From Ryff, 1997.

after any route of application including the mucosal and the intrapulmonary route.

## ■ Dose

The effect of the dose is not quite clear. There are studies with the lowest incidence of antibody formation in the highest dose group. However, such data should be interpreted with caution. In the highest dose group there may be more product in the circulation interfering with the assay or the antibody level maybe lower by increased immune complex formation.

## ■ Patient Features

There are also a number of patient-related factors which influence the incidence of antibody formation. The biological effect of the product can either enhance or inhibit the antibody formation as can the concomitant treatment of patients. Sometimes the concomitant treatment is administered to inhibit antibody formation, e.g., methotrexate treatment to inhibit antibody formation to etanercept (Enbrel®).

The underlying disease for which the patients are being treated is also important. Patients treated with interferon α-2 for chronic hepatitis are more likely to produce antibodies than patients with solid tumors. The upsurge of epoetin-α induced PRCA after the formulation change was only seen in patients with chronic kidney disease and not in patients with cancer.

As discussed before there are many indications that breaking B-cell tolerance is T-cell independent and thereby independent of HLA-type. Indeed a number of clinical studies have failed to show an association between antibody response and HLA-type.

## ■ ASSAYS FOR ANTIBODIES

Assays are probably an important factor influencing the reported incidence of antibody induction by therapeutic proteins. In the published studies with interferon α-2 in patients with viral infections the incidence of antibody induction varied from 0% to more than 60% positive patients. This variation must be assay related. Evaluations of the performance of different test laboratories with blind panel testing showed a more than 50-fold difference in titers found in the same sera. Thus, any reliable comparison between different groups of patients when looking for a clinical effect of antibodies or studying factors influencing immunogenicity can only be done if the antibody quantification is done with in a well-validated assay in the same laboratory.

There is obviously a lack of standardization of assay methodology. There are also only a few reference and/or standard antibody preparations available. Recently, a number of white papers have appeared mainly authored by representatives of the biotechnology industry in the United States (Mire-Sluis et al., 2004). Although the area of biotechnology-derived therapeutics is still too much in development to formulate a definite assay methodology, there is a growing consensus on the general principles.

There is agreement that a single assay is not sufficient to evaluate the immunogenicity of a new protein drug, but a number of assays need to be used in conjunction. Most antibody assay strategies are based on a two-tier approach: a screening assay to identify the antibody positive sera followed by further characterization such as whether the antibodies are neutralizing and what is the titer, affinity and isotype.

In general, the screening assay is a binding assay, mostly an ELISA type of assay (see Chapter 2) with the radioimmune-precipitation methodology as an alternative. Binding antibodies have mostly no biological consequences. However, assays for the more biologically important neutralizing antibodies are in general cumbersome and expensive. Thus, screening with a binding assay to select the positive sera for the neutralizing assay saves time and money.

Screening assays are designed for optimal sensitivity to avoid false negatives. For new proteins defining an absolute sensitivity is impossible because of the lack of positive sera. An alternative approach is to set the cut-point for the assay at a 5% false-positive level using a panel of normal human sera and/or untreated patient sera representative of the groups to be treated.

The assay for neutralizing antibodies is in general a modification of the potency assay for the therapeutic protein product. The potency assay is in most cases an in vitro cell-based assay. A predefined amount of product is added to the serum and a reduction of activity evaluated in the bioassay.

An important caveat in interpreting the neutralization assay results is the possible presence of inhibitors of the products other than antibodies (e.g., soluble receptors) in human serum, or factors stimulating the bioassay which may compensate for the neutralizing activity. To overcome these problems, patient serum should also be tested as control. IgG-depleted serum should also be tested for neutralizing activity to identify neutralizing factors other than antibodies. Further characterization of the antibodies may include evaluation of Ig isotype and affinity.

## ISSUES SPECIFICALLY RELATED TO MONOCLONAL ANTIBODIES

The thinking about the immunogenicity of monoclonal antibodies went through the same paradigm shift as occurred with therapeutic proteins in general. The first generation of monoclonal antibodies was of murine origin. They induced an immune response in the majority of patients as foreign proteins should trigger a classical vaccine-type immune response. This so-called human antimurine antibodies (HAMA) response was a major restriction in the clinical success of these murine antibodies. Over the years, however, methods were introduced to humanize monoclonal antibodies in different stages (see Chapter 15). Recombinant DNA technology was used to exchange the murine constant parts of the immune globulin chains with their human counterparts resulting in chimeric monoclonal antibodies. The next step was to graft murine complementarity determining regions (CDRs), which determine the specificity, into a human immune globulin backbone creating humanized monoclonal antibodies. And the final step was the development of transgenic animals, phage display technologies, and other developments allowing the production of human monoclonal antibodies.

However, the assumption that human monoclonal antibodies would have no immunogenicity proved to be wrong. Although humanization has reduced the immunogenicity, even completely human monoclonal antibodies have been shown to induce antibodies. The introduction of chimeric antibodies by the exchange of the murine constant regions with their human counterparts has resulted in a substantial reduction of the induction of antibodies. Whether further humanization has resulted in an additional decrease is less clear. As discussed, the presence of aggregates has been identified as a major cause of immunogenicity of human therapeutic proteins. It is likely that with human monoclonal antibodies aggregates are also responsible for antibody induction. In fact in the classical studies of B-cell tolerance done more than 40 years ago aggregated immunoglobulin preparations were used to break tolerance (Weigle, 1971).

Monoclonal antibodies have properties, which may contribute to their immunogenicity. They can activate T-cells by themselves and may boost the immune response by their Fc functions such as macrophage activation and complement activation. Indeed removal of N-linked glycosyl chains from the Fc part of the immunoglobulin may reduce Fc function and lead to a diminished immunogenicity.

What the antibodies are binding is also influencing their immunogenicity. Monoclonal antibodies targeting cell-bound antigens induce a higher level of antibody formation than those with circulating targets. Monoclonal antibodies directed to antigens on immune cells with the purpose of inducing immune suppression also suppress an immunogenic response.

Although more injections and higher doses are associated with a higher immune response, in some cases chronic treatment and higher doses were reported to be less immunogenic than episodic treatment and lower doses. The interpretation of these data is difficult because under these treatment conditions the level of circulating product is higher and more persistent and the presence of circulating monoclonal antibodies during the time of blood sampling may mask the detection of induced antibodies. Only a few studies were performed in which the subcutaneous and intravenous route of administration of monoclonal antibodies were compared showing little difference in immunogenicity.

The immune status of the patients influences the antibody response as with other protein therapeutics. Many of the patients receiving monoclonal antibodies are immune compromised by diseases such as cancer or by immune suppressive treatment and are less likely to produce antibodies than patients with a normal immune status. Sometimes immune suppressive agents such as methotrexate are given to patients with the purpose of inhibiting an antibody response.

Another important aspect when studying the immunogenicity of monoclonal antibodies is timing of the blood sampling of patients. These products have a relative long half-life (several weeks) and the circulating product may interfere with the detection of induced antibodies and may lead to false-negative results. Sampling sera up to 20 weeks after the patient has received the last injection may be necessary to avoid the interference of circulating monoclonal antibodies. Also natural antibodies, soluble receptors, and immune complexes may interfere with assays and lead to either false-positive or false-negative results (as explained above).

## CLINICAL EFFECTS OF INDUCED ANTIBODIES

Despite the methodological drawbacks, the list of protein products with clinically relevant immunogenic side effects is growing. The most common consequence is loss of efficacy. Sometimes this loss can be overcome by increasing the dose or changing to another product.

The most dramatic and undisputed complication occurs when the antibodies to the product cross neutralize an endogenous factor with an important biological function. This has been described for a megakaryocyte growth and differentiation factor which induced antibodies cross reacting with endogenous thrombopoietin (Table 1). Volunteers and patients in a clinical trial developed severe thrombocytopenia and needed platelet transfusions. Because of this complication the product was withdrawn from further development.

More recently the upsurge of PRCA (see above) associated with a formulation change of epoetin-α marketed outside the United States occurred. The antibodies induced by the product neutralized the residual endogenous erythropoietin in these patients resulting in a severe anemia which could only be treated with blood transfusions.

Antibodies can also influence the side effects of therapeutic proteins. The consequences are dependent on the cause of the side effects. If the adverse effects are the results of the intrinsic activity of the products antibodies may reduce the side effects, as it is the case with interferon α-2. Sometimes the mitigation of the side effects is even the first clinical sign of the induction of antibodies.

With some products the side effects are caused by the antibody formation. This is in general the case when the product is administered in relatively high doses, like with some monoclonal antibodies. Symptoms caused by immune complexes like delayed-type hypersensitivity and serum sickness are related to the level of antibodies induced.

The general effects caused by an immune reaction to a therapeutic protein such as acute anaphylaxis, hypersensitivity, skin reaction, serum sickness, etc. are relatively common when large amounts of nonhuman proteins are administered. These effects are relatively rare for modern biotechnology-derived products which are highly purified human proteins administered in relatively low amounts. However, these side effects caused by an immune response are currently still relatively common during treatment with high doses of monoclonal antibodies.

## PREDICTING AND REDUCING IMMUNOGENICITY

As discussed the mechanisms leading to antibody induction by therapeutic proteins are still not completely understood. As a consequence it is impossible based on our current knowledge to fully predict the immunogenicity of a new product in patients. For nonhuman proteins which induce the classical immune response, the level of nonself is a relative predictor of an immune response. However, it is not an absolute predictor. Sometimes a single amino acid change is sufficient to make a self protein highly immunogenic. With other proteins substantial divergence from the natural sequence has no effect. For foreign proteins a number of in vitro stimulation and binding tests and computational models are advertised as predictors of immunogenicity. However, all these tests have their limitations. T-cell proliferation assays, for example, have the drawback that many antibodies are capable of inducing some level of T-cell activation or inhibit cell proliferation. The computational algorithms which predict binding of antigens to HLA class II only give limited information on the interaction of the proteins with the immune system and also under-detect epitopes (Stevanovic, 2005). These limitations are also evident when these assays or algorithms are used to reduce immunogenicity: there is hardly any convincing evidence of a clinically relevant reduction of antibody induction.

For human homologues the best predictor of immunogenicity is the presence of aggregates and to a minor degree the presence of impurities. Thus, the quality of the therapeutic protein and its formulation are important factors. There is also evidence about immunogenicity introduced by a change in formulation and a reduction in immunogenicity by avoiding aggregation and improving purification and formulation (see above).

Although animal studies are helpful in obtaining control sera and may provide insight in the possible clinical effects of immunogenicity, they are not very good predictors of immunogenicity in patients. All proteins, including the human homologues, will be in principle immunogenic in animals. Sometimes animal studies may help to study the relative immunogenicity of different products or formulations, although their predictive value for the clinic is questionable. Even monkeys studies do not completely predict immunogenicity in patients. Some products which are immunogenic in nonhuman primates do not induce antibodies in humans and vice versa.

The animal model to study the factors important for the breaking of tolerance are transgenic mice carrying the gene for the human protein (Hermeling et al., 2005). These animals have an immune tolerance comparable to the immune tolerance in patients. These animals have also been successfully used to identify new epitopes in modified products. Although transgenic animals have been proven to be important scientific tools, the experience is still too limited to claim they can serve to completely predict the human response.

### ■ Reducing Immunogenicity

Several strategies are being applied to reduce immunogenicity besides changing the amino acid sequence of the product. Linking proteins to polymers such as polyethylene glycol (see Chapter 5) and low-molecular-weight dextran reduces immunogenicity. However, these modifications also make the molecules less active, necessitating higher doses. This and their increased half-life extend their exposure to the immune system, which can increase the immunogenic potential. Another approach is to reduce the immunogenic response by immunosuppressive treatments. In addition, tolerance induction is being applied, e.g., in hemophilia patients with antibodies to factor VIII.

## CONCLUSIONS

The most important points of this chapter are summarized as follows:

- The immunogenicity of therapeutic proteins is a generally occurring phenomenon
- The clinical consequences can vary
- Validated detection systems are essential to study the immunogenicity of therapeutic proteins
- The prediction of immunogenicity in patients based on physicochemical characterization and animal studies is not easy
- The regulatory process for new therapeutic proteins now includes the evaluation of immunogenicity
- There is still a lot to be learned about why and how patients produce antibodies to therapeutic proteins

## REFERENCES

Bachmann MF, Rohrer UH, Kundig TM, Burki K, Hengartner H and Zinkernagel RM. (1993). The influence of antigen organization on B-cell responsiveness. Science 262:1448–51.

Casadevall N, Nataf J, Viron B, et al. (2002). Pure red-cell aplasia and antierythropoietin antibodies in patients treated with recombinant erythropoietin. N Engl J Med 346:469–75.

Hermeling S, Crommelin DJA, Schellekens H, Jiskoot W. (2004) Structure-immunogenicity relationships of therapeutic proteins. Pharm Res 21:897–903.

Hermeling S, Jiskoot W, Crommelin DJA, Bornaes C, Schellekens H. (2005). Development of a transgenic mouse model immune tolerant for human interferon β. Pharm Res 22:847–51.

Mire-Sluis AR, Barrett YC, Devanarayan V, et al. (2004). Recommendations for the design and optimization of immunoassays used in the detection of host antibodies against biotechnology products. J Immunol Methods 289:1–16.

Moore WV, Leppert P. (1980) Role of aggregated human growth hormone (hGH) in development of antibodies to hGH. J Clin Endocrinol Metab 51:691–97.

Ryff J-C. (1997). Clinical investigation of the immunogenicity of interferon-α2a. J Interferon Cytokine Res 17:529–533.

Schellekens H. (2002). Bioequivalence and the immunogenicity of biopharmaceuticals. Nat Rev Drug Discov 1:1–7.

Stevanovic S. (2005). Antigen processing is predictable: From genes to T cell epitopes. Transpl Immunol 14:171–4.

Weigle WO. (1971) Recent observations and concepts in immunological unresponsiveness and autoimmunity. Clin Exp Immunol 9:437–47.

## FURTHER READING

Hermeling S, Crommelin DJA, Schellekens H, Jiskoot W. (2007). Immunogenicity of therapeutic proteins. In: Gad SC, ed. Handbook of Pharmaceutical Biotechnology. Hoboken, NJ: John Wiley & Sons, 911–31.

Schellekens H, Crommelin D, Jiskoot W (2007). Immunogenicity of antibody therapeutics. In: Dübel S, ed. Handbook of Therapeutic Antibodies. Weinheim, Germany: Wiley-VCH, 267–76.

# 7

# Genomics, Other "Omics" Technologies, Personalized Medicine, and Additional Biotechnology-Related Techniques

*Robert D. Sindelar*
*The University of British Columbia, Vancouver, British Columbia, Canada*

## PHARMACOTHERAPY INFORMATION

Further information on the applied pharmacotherapy related to "omics" technologies and/or personalized medicine can be found in the following frequently used textbooks:

- **Applied Therapeutics: The Clinical Use of Drugs** (Koda-Kimble, MA, et al., Eds.), 8th edition, Williams & Wilkins, Baltimore 2005: Chapter 5.
- **Pharmacotherapy: A Pathophysiologic Approach** (DiPiro, JT, et al., Eds.), 6th edition, McGraw-Hill, New York 2005: Chapters 6, 10.
- **Textbook of Therapeutics: Drug and Disease Management** (Helms, RA, et al., Eds.), 8th edition, Lippincott Williams & Wilkins, Baltimore 2006: Chapters 2, 4, 7.

## INTRODUCTION

Pharmaceutical biotechnology and the products resulting for biotechnologies continue to grow at an exponential rate. Note that 2005 was a record setting year with the U.S. Food and Drug Administration (FDA) approval of 21 biopharmaceutical products. There were 15 FDA approvals in 2004, 20 in 2003, and 13 in 2002 since the last edition of this textbook (Rader 2006; Staff, 2006). Early 2006 saw approvals of several unique new biopharmaceutical entities including a recombinant vaccine widely hailed as the first vaccine for the prevention of an oncogenic virus-associated cancer. However, until recently, the techniques made available by advances in molecular biology and biotechnology that have provided currently approved therapeutic agents generally fell into two broad areas: recombinant DNA (rDNA) technology and hybridoma techniques (to produce monoclonal antibodies). The technology that is fueling our ever-widening understanding of human cellular function and disease processes is undergoing an explosive evolution. A wealth of additional and innovative biotechnologies, have been, and will continue to be, developed in order to harvest the information found in the human genome. These technological advances will provide a better understanding of the relationship between genetics and biological function, unravel the underlying causes of disease, explore the association of genomic variation and drug response, enhance pharmaceutical research, and fuel the discovery and development of new and novel biopharmaceuticals. These revolutionary technologies and additional biotechnology-related techniques are improving the very competitive and costly process of drug development of new medicinal agents, diagnostics and medical devices. Some of the technologies and techniques described in this chapter are both well established and commonly used applications of biotechnology producing potential therapeutic products now in development including clinical trials. Still more applications are evolving as you read this text. Their full impact on the future of molecular medicine has yet to be imagined.

No meaningful discussion of pharmaceutical biotechnology and 21st century healthcare can occur without mention of "omics" technologies. Research in genomics and proteomics is heralded as the next important supply source of innovative future drug design targets. With the Human Genome Project (HGP) rapidly approaching closure, researchers are turning increasingly to the task of converting the DNA sequence data into information that will potentially improve, and perhaps even revolutionize, drug discovery (Fig. 1) and pharmaceutical care. Pharmaceutical scientists are poised to take advantage of this scientific breakthrough by incorporating state-of-the-art genomics and proteomics techniques along with the associated technologies utilized in bioinformatics, metabonomics/metabolomics, systems biology, pharmacogenomics, toxicogenomics, glycomics, and chemical genomics into a new drug discovery, development, and clinical translation paradigm.

Techniques such as genetically engineered animals (including transgenic animals, transgenic plants, and knockout mice), protein engineering, peptide chemistry and peptidomimetics, cell therapy and

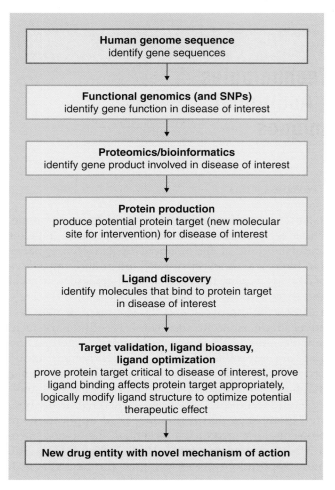

```
┌─────────────────────────────────────┐
│         Human genome sequence        │
│        identify gene sequences       │
└─────────────────────────────────────┘
                   │
                   ▼
┌─────────────────────────────────────┐
│      Functional genomics (and SNPs)  │
│  identify gene function in disease   │
│            of interest               │
└─────────────────────────────────────┘
                   │
                   ▼
┌─────────────────────────────────────┐
│       Proteomics/bioinformatics      │
│  identify gene product involved in   │
│         disease of interest          │
└─────────────────────────────────────┘
                   │
                   ▼
┌─────────────────────────────────────┐
│          Protein production          │
│  produce potential protein target    │
│  (new molecular site for             │
│  intervention) for disease of        │
│  interest                            │
└─────────────────────────────────────┘
                   │
                   ▼
┌─────────────────────────────────────┐
│            Ligand discovery          │
│  identify molecules that bind to     │
│  protein target in disease of        │
│  interest                            │
└─────────────────────────────────────┘
                   │
                   ▼
┌─────────────────────────────────────┐
│  Target validation, ligand bioassay, │
│        ligand optimization           │
│  prove protein target critical to    │
│  disease of interest, prove ligand   │
│  binding affects protein target      │
│  appropriately, logically modify     │
│  ligand structure to optimize        │
│  potential therapeutic effect        │
└─────────────────────────────────────┘
                   │
                   ▼
┌─────────────────────────────────────┐
│ New drug entity with novel mechanism │
│            of action                 │
└─────────────────────────────────────┘
```

**Figure 1** ▪ The genomics strategy for new drug discovery.

regenerative medicine are directly influencing the pharmaceutical sciences and are well positioned to impact significantly modern medical and pharmaceutical care. These additional techniques in biotechnology and molecular biology are being rapidly exploited to bring new drugs to market.

It is not the intention of this author to detail each and every biotechnology technique exhaustively, since numerous specialized resources already meet that need. Rather, this chapter will illustrate and enumerate various biotechnologies that should be of key interest to pharmacy students, practicing pharmacists, and pharmaceutical scientists because of their effect on many aspects of pharmacy.

## AN INTRODUCTION TO "OMICS" TECHNOLOGIES

Since the discovery of DNA's overall structure in 1953, the world's scientific community has continued to gain a better understanding of the genetic information encoded by DNA and the genetic information carried by a cell or organism. In the 1980s and 1990s,

biotechnology techniques produced novel therapeutics and a wealth of information about the mechanisms of various diseases such as cancer. Yet the etiology of many other diseases, including obesity and heart disease, remained unknown at the genetic and the molecular level, presenting no obvious target to attack with a small molecule drug or biotechnology-produced therapeutic agent. The answers were hidden in what was unknown about the human genome. Despite the increasing knowledge of DNA structure and function in the 1990s, the genome, the entire collection of genes and all other functional and non-functional DNA sequences in the nucleus of an organism, had yet to be sequenced. DNA may well be the largest, naturally occurring molecule known. Successfully meeting the challenge of sequencing the entire human genome is one of history's great milestones and heralds enormous potential (Venter et al., 2001; The Genome International Sequencing Consortium, 2001). While the genetic code for transcription and translation has been known for years, sequencing the human genome provides a blueprint for all human proteins and the sequences of all regulatory elements that govern the developmental interpretation of the genome. The potential significance includes identifying genetic determinants of common and rare diseases, providing a methodology for their diagnosis, suggesting interesting new molecular sites for intervention (Fig. 1), and the development of new biotechnologies to bring about their eradication. Unlocking the secrets of the human genome may lead to a paradigm shift in clinical practice toward true targeted molecular medicine and patient-specific therapy.

## ▪ Genomics

Sequencing the human genome and the genomes of other organisms has lead to an enhanced understanding of human biology and disease. Many industry analysts predicted a tripling of pharmaceutical R&D productivity due to the sequencing of the human genome (Williams, 2007). Success to date has been limited and there is significant debate as to the impact of genomics on successful drug discovery and development (Nirmala, 2006; Caldwell et al., 2007). Validation of viable drug targets identified by genomics has been challenging (Bagowski, 2005). An interesting concept is that of the "druggable" genome (Hopkins and Groom, 2002). This is an estimate at 600 to 1,500 valid molecular targets for drug discovery, as assessed as the intersection of the number of human genes identified linked to disease with the subset of the human genome products that could be modulated by small-molecule targets. However, the genomics revolution has been the foundation for an explosion in "omics" technologies that find application in research to address neglected diseases.

## Structural Genomics and the Human Genome Project

Genomics is the comparative study of the complete genome sequence and its function from different organisms (Caldwell et al., 2007). Initially, genetic analysis focused on structural genomics, basically the characterization of the structure of the genome. Structural genomics intersects the techniques of DNA sequencing, cloning, PCR, protein expression, crystallography, and data analysis. It focuses on the physical aspects of the genome through the construction and analysis of gene sequences and gene maps. Proposed in the late 1980s, the publicly funded HGP or Human Genome Initiative (HGI) was officially sanctioned in October 1990 to map the structure and to sequence human DNA (Collins and Galas, 1993; Cantor and Smith, 1999). As described in Table 1, HGP structural genomics was envisioned to proceed through increasing levels of genetic resolution: detailed human genetic linkage maps [approximately 2 megabase pairs (Mb = million base pairs) resolution], complete physical maps (0.1 Mb resolution), and ultimately complete DNA sequencing of the approximately 3.5 billion base pairs (2, 3 pairs of chromosomes) in a human cell nucleus [1 base pair (bp) resolution] (Griffiths et al., 2000). Projected for completion in 2003, the goal of the project was to learn not only what was contained in the genetic code, but also how to "mine" the genomic information to cure or help prevent the estimated 4,000 genetic diseases afflicting humankind. In May 1999, 700 million base pairs of the human genome were deposited in public archives. After merely fifteen months of additional studies, the figure had increased to greater than 4 billion base pairs (Pennisi, 2000). Two years earlier than projected, a milestone in genomic science was reached on June 26, 2000, when researchers at the privately funded Celera Genomics and the publicly funded Genome International Sequencing Consortium (the international collaboration associated with the HGP) jointly announced that they had completed sequencing 97% to 99% of the human genome. The journal *Science* rates the mapping of the human genome as its "breakthrough of the year" in its December 22, 2000 issue. The two groups published their results in 2001 (Venter et al., 2001; The Genome International Sequencing Consortium, 2001).

The genome sequencing strategies of the HGP and Celera Genomics differed (Brown, 2000). HGP utilized a "nested shotgun" approach. The human DNA sequence was "chopped" into segments of ever decreasing size and the segments put into rough order. Each segment was further "blasted" into small fragments. Each small fragment was sequenced and the sequenced fragments assembled according to their known relative order. The Celera researchers employed a "whole shotgun" approach where they "blasted" the whole genome into small fragments. Each fragment was sequenced and assembled in order by identifying where they overlapped. Each approach required unprecedented computer resources (the field of bioinformatics is described later in this chapter).

Regardless of genome sequencing strategies, the collective results are impressive. More than 27 million high quality sequence reads provided five-fold coverage of the entire human genome. Genomic studies have identified over 1 million single nucleotide polymorphisms (SNPs), binary elements of genetic variability (SNPs are described later in this chapter). While original estimates of the number of human genes in the genome varied consistently between 80,000 to 120,000, the genome researchers unveiled a number far short of biologist's predictions; 32,000 (Venter et al., 2001; The Genome International

| Human genome project goals | Base pair resolution |
|---|---|
| **Detailed genetic linkage map** <br> *Comments*: Poorest resolution; depicts relative chromosomal locations of DNA markers, genes, or other markers and the spacing between them on each chromosome. | 2 Mb[a] |
| **Complete physical map** <br> *Comments*: Instead of relative distances between markers, maps actual physical distance in base pairs between markers; lower resolution = actual observance of chromosomal banding under microscope; higher resolution is "restriction map" generated in presence of restriction enzymes. | 0.1 Mb |
| **Complete DNA sequence** <br> *Comments*: The ultimate goal; determine the base sequence of the genes and markers found in mapping techniques along with the other segments of the entire genome; techniques commonly used include DNA amplification methods such as cloning, PCR and other techniques described in Chapter 1 along with novel sequencing and bioinformatics techniques. | 1 bp[b] |

[a] Mb = megabase = 1 million base pairs; [b] bp = base pair.

**Table 1**    The increasing levels of genetic resolution obtained from structural genomic studies of the HGP.

Sequencing Consortium, 2001). Within months, others suggested that the human genome possesses between 65,000 and 75,000 genes (Wright et al., 2001). Approximately 25,000 genes is now most often cited number (Lee et al., 2006).

Newer structural genomics projects focus on lowering the average costs of structure determination while quantifying novel structures by direct sequence comparison (Chondonia and Brenner, 2006). The move toward low cost, high throughput sequencing is essential for the implementation of genomics in the individualized medicine clinical laboratory. The $1000 (U.S.) genome remains the target.

### Functional and Comparative Genomics

Now that the sequencing of the entire genome is a reality, the chore of sorting through human, pathogen and other organism diversity factors and correlating them with genomic data to provide real pharmaceutical benefits is an active area of research (Kramer and Cohen, 2005). Pharmaceutical company drug pipelines are loaded with promising therapeutic agent leads, due in large part to the application of biotechnology to the discovery process. Early supporters of the human genome project characterized it as a potential medical panacea that would rapidly add to the pipeline. However, attempts to translate genomic sequence data from structural genomics toward biological function has been predicted to fuel discoveries from the bench top to the patient's bedside. This requires a through understanding of what genes do, how they are regulated, and the direct relationship between genes and their activity. The DNA sequence information itself rarely provides definitive information about the function and regulation of that particular gene. Yet there was hope that completing the human genome sequence would dramatically alter prevention, treatment, and even our definition of disease (Temple et al., 2001). The study of functional genomics is hoped to play a key role in new drug target identification and validation (Caldwell et al., 2007). After genome sequencing, this approach is the next step in the knowledge chain to identify functional gene products that are potential biotech drug leads and new drug discovery targets (Fig. 1). Functional genomics focuses on genome-wide patterns of gene expression, the mechanisms by which gene expression is coordinated, and the interrelationships of gene expression when a cellular environmental change occurs.

To relate functional genomics to therapeutic clinical outcomes, the human genome sequence must reveal the thousands of genetic variations among individuals that will become associated with diseases in the patient's lifetime. Sequencing alone is not the end, simply the end of the beginning of the genomic

medicine era. Determining gene functionality in any organism opens the door for linking a disease to specific genes or proteins, which become targets for new drugs, methods to detect organisms (i.e., new diagnostic agents), and or biomarkers (the presence or change in gene expression profile that correlates with the risk, progression or susceptibility of a disease).

The face of biology has changed forever with the sequencing of the genomes of numerous organisms. Biotechnologies applied to the sequencing of the human genome are also being utilized to sequence the genomes of comparatively simple organisms as well as other mammals. Often, the proteins encoded by the genomes of lesser organisms and the regulation of those genes closely resemble the proteins and gene regulation in humans. Since model organisms are much easier to maintain in a laboratory setting, researchers are actively pursuing "comparative" genomics studies (Clark, 1999; Hardison, 2003). Unlocking genomic data for each of these organisms provides valuable insight into the molecular basis of inherited human disease (Karow, 2000). *S. cerevisiae* is a good model for studying cancer and is a common organism used in rDNA methodology. For example, it has become well known that women who inherit a gene mutation of the *BRCA1* gene have a high risk, perhaps as high as 85%, of developing breast cancer before the age of 50 (source: www.ncbi.nlm.nih.gov). The first diagnostic product generated from genomic data was the *BRCA1* test for breast cancer predisposition. The gene product of *BRCA1* is a well-characterized protein implicated in both breast and ovarian cancer. Evidence has accumulated suggesting that the Rad9 protein of *S. cerevisiae* is distantly, but significantly, related to the *BRCA1* protein. The fruit fly possesses a gene similar to *p53*, the human tumor suppressor gene. Studying *C. elegans* has provided much of our early knowledge of apoptosis, the normal biological process of programmed cell death. Greater than 90% of the proteins identified thus far from a common laboratory animal, the mouse, have structural similarities to known human proteins. Mapping the whole of a human cancer cell genome will pinpoint the genes involved in cancer and aid in the understanding of cell changes and treatment of human malignancies (Collins and Barker, 2007). The consensus coding sequences of human breast and colorectal cancers have been elucidated. The U.S. National Institutes of Health (NIH) Cancer Genome Atlas is one such project.

Not all comparative genomic studies are looking for similarities to the human genome. For example, some may provide the basis for creating new and novel potential antibiotic and antiviral targets for drug design (Guild, 1999). Comparative genomics is being used to provide a compilation of genes that code for proteins that are essential to the growth or viability of a pathogenic organism, yet differ from any human protein. The worldwide effort to sequence the severe acute respiratory syndrome (SARS) associated coronavirus genome is one such example that will aid diagnosis, antiviral discovery, and vaccine development (Marra et al., 2003). Assuring selective toxicity to the organism, not the human patient, this genomic mining of new targets for drug design may aid the quest for new antibiotics in a clinical environment of increasing incidence of antibiotic resistance.

DNA banking, the collection, storage, and analysis of hundreds of thousands of specimens containing analyzable DNA, is proving to be a valuable tool for genetics research (Thornton et al., 2005). All nucleated cells, including cells from blood, hair follicles, buccal swabs, cancer biopsies, and urine specimens, are suitable specimens for DNA analysis in the present or at a later date. These banks have become valuable resources for the discovery of new and improved medical treatments in several disease states, especially cancer.

## Epigenomics

Using a whole-genome approach, epigenomics is the study of environmental or developmental genetic effects such as DNA methylation, on gene function. Thus, epigenomics focuses on those genes whose function is determined by external factors. Epidemiological evidence increasingly suggests that external factors including environmental exposures early in development have a role in disease susceptibility (Jirtle and Skinner, 2007).

## ■ "Omics" Enabling Technology: Bioinformatics

Structural genomics, functional genomics, proteomics, and other "omic" technologies have generated an enormous volume of genetic and biochemical data to store. The entire encoded human DNA sequence alone requires computer storage of approximately $10^9$ bits of information: the equivalent of a thousand 500-page books! GenBank (managed by the National Center for Biotechnology Information, NCBI, of the National Institutes of Health), the European Molecular Biology Laboratory (EMBL), and the DNA Data Bank of Japan (DDBJ) are three of the many centers worldwide that collaborate on collecting DNA sequences. These databanks, (both public and private) store tens of millions of sequences (Martin et al., 2007). Metabolic databases and other collections of biochemical and bioactivity data add to the complexity and wealth of information (Olah and Oprea, 2007). Once stored, analyzing the volumes of data, (i.e., comparing and relating information from various sources) to identify useful and/or predictive characteristics or trends, such as selecting a group of drug targets from all proteins in the human body,

presents a Herculean task. This approach has the potential of changing the fundamental way in which basic science is conducted and valid biological conclusions are reached (Baxevanis, 2001).

Scientists have applied advances in information technology, innovative software algorithms and massive parallel computing to the on-going research in genetics, genomics, proteomics, and related areas to give birth to the fast growing field of bioinformatics (Emmett, 2000; Felton, 2001; Watkins, 2001; Lengauer and Hartman, 2007). Bioinformatics is the application of computer technologies to the biological sciences with the object of discovering knowledge. With bioinformatics, a researcher can now better exploit the tremendous flood of genomic and proteomic data, more cost-effectively data mining for a drug discovery "needle" in that massive data "haystack." In this case, data mining refers to the bioinformatics approach to "sifting" through volumes of raw data, identifying and extracting relevant information, and developing useful relationships among them. Modern drug discovery will utilize bioinformatics techniques to gather information from multiple sources (such as the HGP, functional genomic studies, proteomics, phenotyping, patient medical records, and bioassay results including toxicology studies), integrate the data, apply life science developed algorithms, and generate useful target identification and drug lead identification data. Another goal of bioinformatics is to be able to study the molecules and processes discovered by genomics and proteomics research *in silico*: that is, to be able to predict chemical and physical structure and properties by computer (Rashidi and Buehler, 2000).

Bioinformatics in its multi-faceted implementations may be thought of as a technique of "electronic biology" (eBiology), conceptual biology, *in silico* biology, or computational biology (Blagosklonny and Pardee, 2002). A data-driven tool, the integration of bioinformatics with functional knowledge of the complex biological system under study remains the critical of any of the omic technologies described above and to follow. As seen in Figure 2, the hierarchy of information collection goes well beyond the biodata contained in the genetic code that is transcribed and translated.

## ■ Transcriptomics

This technology examines the complexity of messenger RNA transcripts of an organism (i.e., transcriptome), under a variety of internal and external conditions reflecting the genes that are being actively expressed at any given time (with the exception of mRNA degradation phenomena such as transcriptional attenuation) (Subramanian et al., 2005). Therefore, the transcriptome can vary with external environmental conditions while the genome is roughly fixed for a given cell line (excluding

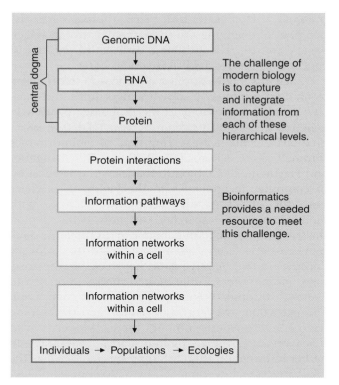

Figure 2 ■ The information challenge of systems biology in the genomics era. *Source*: Aderem and Hood, 2001.

mutations). The transcriptomes of stem cells and cancer cells are of particular interest to better understand the processes of cellular differentiation and carcinogenesis. High-throughput techniques based on microarray technology are used to examine the expression level of mRNAs in a given cell population.

### ■ Proteomics, Structural Proteomics, and Functional Proteomics

Functional genomics research will provide an unprecedented information resource for the study of biochemical pathways at the molecular level. Certainly a large number of the ~25,000 genes identified in sequencing the human genome will be shown to be functionally important in various disease states (see druggable genome discussion above). This will result in the identification of a vast array of proteins implicated as playing pivotal roles in disease processes (Evans, 2003). These key identified proteins will serve as potential new sites for therapeutic intervention (Fig. 1). The research area called proteomics seeks to define the function and correlate that with expression profiles of all proteins encoded within an organism's genome or "proteome" (Edwards et al., 2000; Kreider, 2001; Voshol et al., 2007). The ~25,000 human genes can produce 100,000 proteins. The number, type and concentration may vary depending on cell or tissue type, disease state, and other factors. The proteins' function(s) are dependent on the primary, secondary, and tertiary structure of the protein and the molecules they interact with. Less than 20 years old, the concept of proteomics requires determination of the structural, biochemical and physiological repertoire of all proteins. Proteomics is a greater scientific challenge than genomics due to the intricacy of protein expression and the complexity of 3-D protein structure (structural proteomics) as it relates to biological activity (functional proteomics) (Saeks, 2001). Protein expression, isolation, purification, identification, and characterization are among the key procedures utilized in proteomics research. To perform these procedures, technology platforms such as 2-D gel electrophoresis, mass spectrometry, chip-based microarrays (discussed later in this chapter), X-ray crystallography (discussed later in this chapter), protein nuclear magnetic resonance (NMR) (also discussed later in this chapter), and phage displays are employed. Initiated in 2002, the Human Proteome Organization (HUPO) recently completed the first large-scale study to characterize the human serum and plasma proteins, i.e., the human serum and plasma proteome (States et al., 2006). Pharmaceutical scientists anticipate that many of the proteins identified by proteomic research will be entirely novel, possessing unknown functions. This scenario offers not only a unique opportunity to identify previously unknown molecular targets, but also to develop new ultrasensitive diagnostics to address unmet clinical needs (Petricoin et al., 2002). Today's methodology does not allow us to identify valid drug targets and new diagnostic methodologies simply by examining gene sequence information. However, "*in silico* proteomics", the computer-based prediction of 3-D protein structure, intermolecular interactions, and functionality is currently a very active area of research (Roberts and Swinton, 2001; Voshol et al., 2007).

Often, multiple genes and their protein products are involved in a single disease process. Since few proteins act alone, studying protein interactions will be paramount to a full understanding of functionality. Also, many abnormalities in cell function may result from over-expression of a gene and/or protein, under-expression of a gene and/or protein, a gene mutation causing a malformed protein, and post-translation modification changes that alter a protein's function. Therefore, the real value of human genome sequence data will only be realized after every protein coded by the 25,000 genes has a function assigned to it.

### ■ "Omics" Enabling Technology: Microarrays

The biochips known as DNA microarrays and oligonucleotide microarrays are a surface collection of hundreds to thousands of immobilized DNA sequences or oligo-nucleotides in a grid created with specialized equipment that can be simultaneously examined to conduct expression analysis (Khan et al., 1999; Southern, 2001; Amaratunga et al., 2007). Biochips may contain representatives of a particular set of gene sequences (i.e., sequences coding for all human cytochrome P450 isozymes) or may contain sequences representing all genes of an organism. They can produce massive amounts of genetic information (Butte, 2002; Vaince et al., 2006). While the in vitro diagnostics market has been difficult to enter, Roche Diagnostics AmpliChip CYP 450 is a FDA-approved diagnostic tool able to determine a patient's genotype with respect to two genes that govern drug metabolism. This information obtained may be useful by a physician to select the appropriate drug and/or dosage for a given patient in the areas of cardiovascular disease, high blood pressure, depression, and others (according to the company).

Commonly, arrays are prepared on non-porous supports such as glass microscope slides. DNA microarrays generally contain high-density microspotted cDNA sequences approximately 1 Kb in length representing thousands of genes. The field was advanced significantly when technology was developed to synthesize closely spaced oligo-nucleotides on glass wafers using semiconductory industry photolithographic masking techniques (Fig. 3). Oligonucleotide microarrays (often called oligonucleotide arrays or DNA chips) contain closely spaced synthetic gene-specific oligonucleotides representing thousands of gene sequences. Microarrays can provide expression analysis for mRNAs. Screening of DNA variation is also possible. Thus, biochips can provide polymorphism detection and genotyping as well as hybridization-based expression monitoring.

Microarray analysis has gained increasing significance as a direct result of the genome sequencing studies. Array technology is a logical tool for studying functional genomics since the results obtained may link function to expression. Microarray technology's potential to study key areas of molecular medicine and drug discovery is unlimited at this stage of development. For example, gene expression levels of thousands of mRNA species may be studied simultaneously in normal versus cancer cells, each incubated with potential anticancer drug candidates. Related microarray technologies include protein microarrays, tissue microarrays, cell microarrays (also called transfection microarrays), chemical compound microarrays, and antibody microarrays. The principles are he same, while the immobilized collections differ accordingly.

## "Omics" Enabled Technology: Brief Introduction to Biomarkers

Biomarkers are clinically relevant substances used as indicators of a biologic state (Shaffer, 2006; DePrimo, 2007). Detection or concentration change of a biomarker may indicate a particular disease state (e.g., the presence of an antibody may indicate an infection), physiology, or toxicity. A change in expression or state of a protein biomarker may correlate with the risk or progression of a disease, with the susceptibility of the disease to a given treatment, or the drug's safety profile. Implemented in the form of a medical device, a measured biomarker becomes an in vitro diagnostic tool (Williams et al., 2006). While it is well beyond this chapter to provide a detailed discussion of biomarkers, it is important to note that omics technologies including omics-enabled technologies such as microarrays are being developed as clinical measuring devices for biomarkers. Biomarkers enable characterization of patient population undergoing clinical trials or drug therapy, and accelerate drug development. Modern drug discovery often simultaneously involves biomarker discovery and diagnostic development (Frank and Hargreaves, 2003; Pien et al., 2005).

A "Theranostic" is a rapid diagnostic, possibly a microarray, measuring a clinically significant biomarker, which may identify patients most likely to benefit or be harmed by a new medication (Warner, 2004). Bundled with a new drug (and likely developed in parallel with that drug), the theranostic's diagnosis of the requisite biomarker (e.g., the over-expression of the HER2 gene product in certain breast cancer patients) influences the physician's therapeutic decisions [i.e., prescribing the drug trastuzumab (Herceptin) for HER2 receptor positive breast cancer patients]. Thus, the diagnostic and the therapy are distinctly coupled = theranostic. The theranostic predicts clinical success of the drug. This example used to introduce the concept of a theranostic, is possibly the best example of personalized medicine (see later in this chapter), achieving the best medical outcomes by choosing treatments that work well with a person's genomic profile, or with certain characteristics.

## Metabonomics and Metabolomics

The vast information revealed with the sequencing of the human genome has yet to produce the advances in personalized medicine expected. However, the techniques and processes of identifying clinically significant biomarkers of human disease and drug safety have fostered the systematic study of the unique chemical fingerprints that specific cellular processes leave behind, specifically, their small-molecule metabolite profiles (Nicholson and Wilson, 2003; Fernie et al., 2004; Delnomdedieu and Schneider, 2005; Lindon et al., 2005; Weckwerth and Morgenthal, 2005) The human "metabolome" represents the collection of all metabolites in a biological organism, which are the end products of its gene expression and

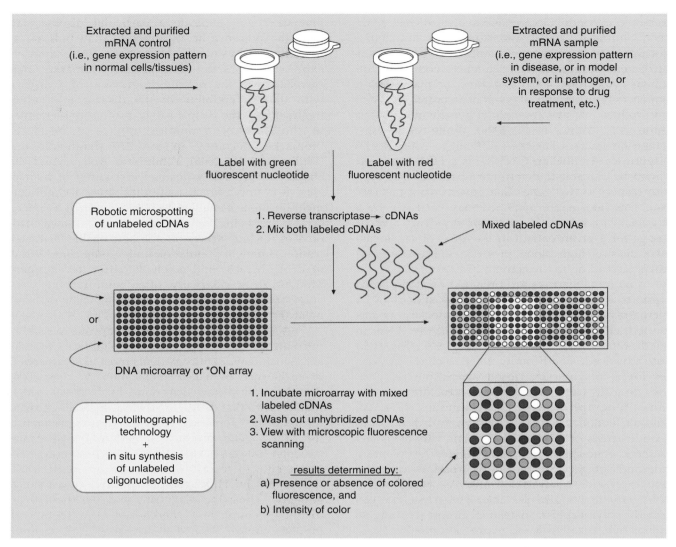

**Figure 3** ■ Principle of operation of a representative DNA microarray or oligonucleotide (*ON) microarray.

gene product function. Thus, while genomics and proteomics do not tell the whole story of what might be happening within a cell, metabolic profiling can give an instantaneous snapshot of the physiology of that cell.

High performance liquid chromatography coupled with sophisticated NMR and mass spectrometry (MS) techniques are used to separate and quantify complex metabolite mixtures found in biological fluids to get a picture of the metabolic continuum of an organism influenced by an internal and external environment. The field of metabonomics is the holistic study of the metabolic continuum at the equivalent level to the study of genomics and proteomics. However, unlike genomics and proteomics, microarray technology is little used since the molecules assayed in metabonomics are small molecule end products of gene expression and resulting

protein function. The term metabolomics has arisen as the metabolic composition of a cell at a specified time whereas metabonomics includes both the static metabolite composition and concentrations as well as the full time course fluctuations. Coupling the information being collected in biobanks, large collections of patient's biological samples and medical records, with metabonomic and metabolomic studies will not only detect why a given metabolite level is increasing or decreasing, but may reliably predict the onset of disease. Also, the techniques are finding use in drug safety screening, identification of clinical biomarkers, and systems biology studies (see below).

■ **Pharmacogenetics and Pharmacogenomics**

It has been noted for decades that patient response to the administration of a drug was highly variable within a diverse patient population. Efficacy as determined in clinical trials is based upon a standard dose range derived from the large population studies. Better understanding of the molecular interactions occurring within the pharmacokinetics phase of a drug's action, coupled with new genetics knowledge and then genomics knowledge of the human have advanced us closer to a rational means to optimize drug therapy. Optimization with respect to the patients' genotype, to ensure maximum efficacy with minimal adverse effects is the goal. Environment, diet, age, lifestyle, and state of health all can influence a person's response to medicines, but understanding an individual's genetic makeup is thought to be the key to creating personalized drugs with greater efficacy and safety. Approaches such as the related pharmacogenetics and pharmacogenomics promise the advent of "personalized medicine", in which drugs and drug combinations are optimized for each individual's unique genetic makeup (Silber, 2001; Huang and Lesko, 2005).

## Single Nucleotide Polymorphisms (SNPs)

While comparing the base sequences in the DNA of two individuals reveals them to be approximately 99.9 per cent identical, base differences, or polymorphisms, are scattered throughout the genome. The best-characterized human polymorphisms are SNPs occurring approximately once every 1000 bases in the 3.5 billion base pair human genome (Cargill et al., 1999; Silber, 2001; Kassam et al., 2005). The DNA sequence variation is a single nucleotide — A, T, C, or G — in the genome difference between members of a species (or between paired chromosomes in an individual). For example, two sequenced DNA fragments from different individuals, AAGTTCCTA to AAGTTCTTA, contain a difference in a single nucleotide. Commonly referred to as "snips," these subtle sequence variations account for most of the genetic differences observed among humans. Thus, they can be utilized to determine inheritance of genes in successive generations. Technologies available from several companies allow for genotyping hundreds of thousands of SNPs for typically under $1,000 in a couple of days.

Research suggests that, in general, humans tolerate SNPs as a probable survival mechanism. This tolerance may result because most SNPs occur in non-coding regions of the genome. Identifying SNPs occurring in gene coding regions (cSNPs) and/or regulatory sequences may hold the key for elucidating complex, polygenic diseases such as cancer, heart disease, and diabetes, and understanding the differences in response to drug therapy observed in individual patients (Grant and Phillips, 2001; also see SNP Consortium website, *http://snp.cshl.org/*). Some cSNPs do not result in amino acid substitutions

in their gene's protein product(s) due to the degeneracy of the genetic code. These cSNPs are referred to as synonymous cSNPs. Other cSNPs, known as nonsynonymous, can produce conservative amino acid changes, such as similarity in sidechain charge or size, or more significant amino acid substitutions.

SNPs, when associated with epidemiological and pathological data, can be used to track susceptibilities to common diseases such as cancer, heart disease, and diabetes (Davidson and McInerney, 2004). Biomedical researchers have recognized that discovering SNPs linked to diseases will lead potentially to the identification of new drug targets and diagnostic tests. The identification and mapping of hundreds of thousands of SNPs for use in large-scale association studies may turn the SNPs into biomarkers of disease and/or drug response (McCarthy, 2005). The projected impact of SNPs on our understanding of human disease led to the formation of the SNP Consortium in 1999, an international research collaboration involving pharmaceutical companies, academic laboratories, and private support. Visit the following sites for extensive information on SNPs discovered to date: *http://www.snps.com/*, *http://www.ncbi.nlm.nih.gov/LocusLink/*, and *http://dir.niehs.nih.gov/egsnp/status/*.

## Pharmacogenetics Versus Pharmacogenomics

In simplest terms, pharmacogenomics is the whole genome application of pharmacogenetics, which examines the single gene interactions with drugs. Tremendous advances in biotechnology are causing a dramatic shift in the way new pharmaceuticals are discovered, developed, and monitored during patient use. Pharmacists will utilize the knowledge gained from genomics and proteomics to tailor drug therapy to meet the needs of their individual patients employing the fields of pharmacogenetics and pharmacogenomics (Evans and Relling, 1999; Lau and Sakul, 2000; Kalow, 2004; Weinshilboum and Wang, 2004; Lindpaintner, 2007).

Pharmacogenetics is the study of how an individual's genetic differences influence drug action, usage, and dosing. A detailed knowledge of a patient's pharmacogenetics in relation to a particular drug therapy may lead to enhanced efficacy and greater safety. Pharmacogenetics analysis may identify the responsive patient population prior to administration.

The field of pharmacogenetics is almost 50 years old, but is undergoing renewed, exponential growth at this time. Of particular interest in the field of pharmacogenetics is our understanding of the genetic influences on drug pharmacokinetic profiles such as genetic variations affecting liver enzymes (i.e., cytochrome P450 group) and drug transporter proteins, and the genetic influences on drug pharmacodynamic profiles such as the variation in receptor protein expression (Kalow, 2004; Weinshilboum and Wang, 2004; Lindpaintner, 2007).

In contrast, pharmacogenomics is linked to the whole genome, not a SNP in a single gene (Weinshilboum and Wang, 2004; Lindpaintner, 2007). It is the study of the entirety of the genome of an organism (i.e., human patient), both the expressed and the non-expressed genes in any given physiologic state. Pharmacogenomics combines traditional pharmaceutical sciences with annotated knowledge of genes, proteins, and SNPs. It might be viewed as a logical convergence of the step-wise advances in genomics with the growing field of pharmacogenetics. Incorrectly, the definitions of pharmacogenetics and pharmacogenomics are often used interchangeably. Whatever the definitions, they share the challenge of clinical translation, moving from benchtop research to bedside application for patient care.

## ■ On the Path to Personalized Medicine: A Brief Introduction

The hopes and realities of personalized medicine (sometimes referred to as part of "molecular medicine"), pharmacotherapy informed by a patient's individual genomics and proteomics information, is dependent on the successful implementation of multiple omics technologies (Knoell and Sadee, 2004; Gurwitz and Manolopoulos, 2007). Our limited discussion here will focus on pharmacogenomics and pharmacogenetics, however other technologies including proteomics, metabolomics, and nanobiotechnologies will be crucial for the successful implementation of personalized medicine. This information-based medicine approach is being driven by the explosion of research in the fields of pharmacogenetics and pharmacogenomics. The hope is that omic science will bring predictability to the optimization of drug selection and drug dosage to assure safe and effective pharmacotherapy (Fig. 4).

For our discussion, it is again important to recognize that pharmacogenetics pharmacogenomics are subtly different (Kalow, 2001). Pharmacogenomics introduces the additional element of our present technical ability to pinpoint patient-specific DNA variation using genomics techniques. The area looks at the genetic composition or genetic variations of an organism and their connection to drug response. Variations in target pathways are studied to understand how the variations are manifested and how they influence response. While overlapping fields of study, pharmacogenomics is a much newer term that

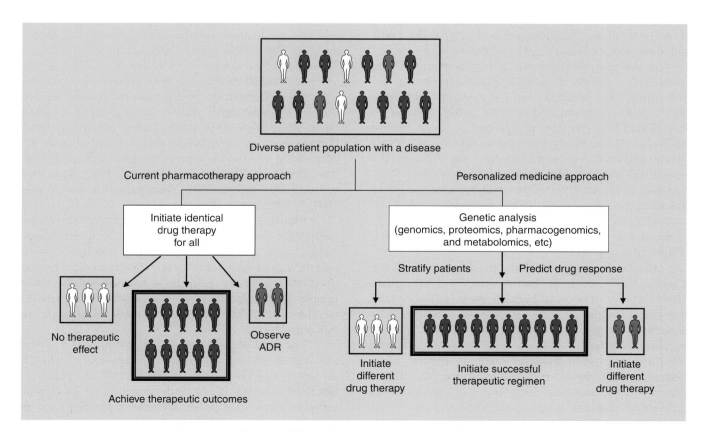

**Figure 4** ■ The role of "omics" technologies in personalized medicine.

correlates an individual patient's DNA variation (SNP level of variation knowledge rather than gene level of variation knowledge) with his or her response to pharmacotherapy. Personalized medicine will employ both technologies.

Optimized personalized medicine utilizing pharmacogenomic knowledge would not only spot disease before it occurs in a patient, increase drug efficacy upon pharmacotherapy, and reduce drug toxicity, it would also facilitate the drug development process (Fig. 1) including improving clinical development outcomes, reducing overall cost of drug development, leading to development of new diagnostic tests that impact on therapeutic decisions, etc. (Valgus, 2004). Individualized optimized pharmacotherapy would first require a detailed genetic analysis of a patient, assembling a comprehensive list of SNPs. Pharmacogenomic tests most likely in the form of microarray technology and based upon clinically validated biomarkers would be administered to pre-identify responsive patients before dosing with a specific agent. Examples of such microarray-based diagnostics are the FDA approved AmpliChip P450 from Roche to screen a patient for the presence of any of 27 SNPs in CYP2D6 and CYP2C19, and investigational assays DrugMEt (tests for 29 SNPs in 8 CYP 450 enzymes) and MegAllele DME-T (tests for approximately 170 SNPs across 29 metabolic genes). The impact of the patient's SNPs on the use of new or existing drugs would thus be predicted, and individualized drug therapy would be identified that assures maximal efficacy and minimal toxicity.

It is well understood that beyond genomics and proteomics, a patient's behavioral and environmental factors influence clinical outcomes and susceptibility to disease. Emerging fields of nutrigenomics and envirogenomics are studying these additional layers of complexity. Personalized medicine will become especially important in cases where the cost of testing is either less than the cost of the drug, or the cost of correcting adverse drug reactions (ADRs) caused by the drug. Pharmaceutical care would begin by identifying a patient's susceptibility to a disease, then administering the right drug to the right patient at the right time. For example, the monoclonal antibody trastuzumab (Herceptin) is a personalized breast cancer therapy specifically targeted to the HER2 gene product (25–30% of human breast cancers overexpress the human epidermal growth factor receptor, HER2 protein) (Gutjahr and Reinhardt, 2005). Exhibiting reduced side effects as compared to standard chemotherapy due to this protein target specificity, trastuzumab is not prescribed to treat a breast cancer patient unless the patient has first tested positive for HER2 over-expression. While currently an immuno-histochemical assay, not a sophisticated DNA microarray assay, the example shows the power of such future tests.

The concept of targeted therapy for personalized medicine has fostered the concept that the era of the blockbuster drug may be over and will be replaced by the "niche buster" drug, a highly effective medicine individualized for a small group of responding patients identified by genomic and proteomic techniques. Also, while numerous articles predicted that pharmacogenomics would revolutionize medicine, the initial predictions have not been lived up to the hype due to statistical, scientific, and commercial hurdles. With more than 11 million SNP positions believed to be present in the human population, large-scale detection of genetic variation holds the key to successful personalized medicine (Geistlinger and Ahnert, 2005). Correlation of environmental factors, behavioral factors, genomic and proteomic factors (including pharmacogenomic and metabolomic factors), and phenotypical observables across large populations remains a daunting data-intensive challenge. Yet, pharmacogenetics and pharmacogenomics are having an impact on modern medicine.

## Human Genomic Variation Affecting Drug Pharmacokinetics

Genetic variation associated with drug metabolism and drug transport, processes resulting from products of gene expression (metabolic enzymes and transport proteins, respectively) play a critical role in determining the concentration of a drug in its active form at the site of its action and also at the site of its possible toxic action(s). Thus having significant clinical consequences, extensive pharmacogenetic an pharmacogenomic analysis of drug metabolism and drug transport is finding value in understanding and predicting the affect of genetic variation on drug effectiveness and safety (Frye, 2004; Kroetz and Nguyen, 2004; Gurwitz and Manolopoulis, 2007).

It is well recognized that specific drug metabolizer phenotypes may cause adverse drug reactions. For instance, some patients lack an enzymatically active form, have a diminished level, or possess a modified version of CYP2D6 (a cytochrome P450 allele) and will metabolize certain classes of pharmaceutical agents differently to other patients expressing the native active enzyme. All pharmacogenetic polymorphisms examined to date differ in frequency among racial and ethnic groups. For example, CYP2D6 enzyme deficiencies may occur in $\leq 2\%$ Asian patients, $\leq 5\%$ black patients and $\leq 11\%$ white patients (Freeman, 2001). A diagnostic test to detect CYP2D6 deficiency could be used to identify patients that should not be administered drugs metabolized predominantly by CYP2D6. Also, pharmacogenetics represents one of many genetic responses to environmental impacts affecting human biochemistry and drug action. Table 2 provides some selected examples of common drug metabolism polymorphisms and their pharmacokinetic consequences.

With the burgeoning understanding of the genetics of warfarin metabolism, warfarin anticoagulation therapy is becoming a leader in pharmacogenetic analysis for pharmacokinetic prediction (Cavallari, 2004). ADRs for warfarin account for 15% of all ADRs in the United States, second only to digoxin. Warfarin dose is adjusted with the goal of achieving an INR (International Normalized ratio = ratio of patient's prothrombin time as compared to that of a normal control) of 2.0 to 3.0. The clinical challenge is to limit hemorrhage, the primary ADR, while achieving the optimal degree of protection against thromboembolism. Deviation in the INR has been shown to be the strongest risk factor for bleeding complications. The major routes of metabolism of warfarin are by CYP2C9 and CYP3A4. Some of the compounds, which have been identified to influence positively or negatively, warfarin's INR include: cimetidine, clofibrate, propranolol, celecoxib (a competitive inhibition of CYP2C9), fluvoxamine (an inhibitor of several CYP enzymes), various antifungals and antibiotics (e.g., miconazole, fluconazole, erythromycin), omeprazole, alcohol, ginseng, and garlic. Researchers have determined that the majority of individual patient variation observed clinically in response to warfarin therapy is genetic in nature, influenced by the genetic variability of metabolizing enzymes, vitamin K cycle enzymes, and possibly transporter proteins. The CYP2C9 genotype polymorphisms alone explain about 10% of the variability observed in the warfarin maintenance dose.

Many studies at both the basic research and clinical level involve the effect of drug transport proteins on the pharmacokinetic profile of a drug (Kroetz and Nguyen, 2004; Gurwitz and Manolopoulis, 2007). Some areas of active study of the effect of genetic variation on clinical effectiveness include efflux transporter proteins (for bioavailability, CNS exposure, and tumor resistance) and neurotransmitter uptake transporters (as valid drug targets). Novel transporter proteins are still being identified as a result of the HGP and subsequent proteomics research. More study is needed on the characterization of expression, regulation, and functional properties of known and new transporter proteins to better assess the potential for prediction of altered drug response based on transporter genotypes.

| Enzyme | Common variant | Potential consequence |
|---|---|---|
| CYP1A2 | CYP1A2*1F | Increased inducibility |
| CYP1A2 | CYP1A2*1K | Decreased metabolism |
| CYP2A6 | CYP2A6*2 | Decreased metabolism |
| CYP2B6 | CYP2B6*5 | No effect |
| CYP2B6 | CYP2B6*6 | Increased metabolism |
| CYP2B6 | CYP2B6*7 | Increased metabolism |
| CYP2C8 | CYP2C8*2 | Decreased metabolism |
| CYP2C9 | CYP2C9*2 | Altered affinity |
| CYP2C9 | CYP2C9*3 | Decreased metabolism |
| CYP2D6 | CYP2D6*10 | Decreased metabolism |
| CYP2D6 | CYP2D6*17 | Decreased metabolism |
| CYP2E1 | CYP2E1*2 | Decreased metabolism |
| CYP3A7 | CYP3A7*1C | Increased metabolism |
| Flavin-containing monooxygenase-3 | FMO3*2 | Decreased metabolism |
| Flavin-containing monooxygenase-3 | FMO3*4 | Decreased metabolism |

**Table 2** ■ Some selected examples of common drug metabolism polymorphisms and their pharmacokinetic consequences.

### Human Genomic Variation Affecting Drug Pharmacodynamics

Genomic variation affects not only the pharmacokinetic profile of drugs, it also strongly influences the pharmacodynamic profile of drugs via the drug target. To understand the complexity of most drug responses, factors influencing the expression of the protein target directly with which the drug interacts must be studied. Targets include the drug receptor involved in the response as well as the proteins associated with disease risk, pathogenesis, and/or toxicity (Johnson, 2004; Gurwitz and Manolopoulis, 2007). There are increasing numbers of prominent examples of inherited polymorphisms influencing drug pharmacodynamics. To follow on the warfarin example above, the majority of individual patient variation observed clinically in response to anticoagulant therapy is genetic in nature. However, the CYP2C9 genotype polymorphisms alone only explain about 10% of the variability observed in the warfarin maintenance dose. Warfarin effectiveness is influenced by the genetic variability of vitamin K cycle enzymes also. The drug receptor for warfarin is generally recognized as vitamin K epoxide reductase, the enzyme that recycles vitamin K in the coagulation cascade. Vitamin K epoxide reductase complex1 (VKORC1) has been determined to be highly variant with as much as 50% of the clinical variability observed for warfarin resulting from polymorphisms of this enzyme.

Associations have been implicated between drug response and in genetic variations targets for a variety of drugs including: antidepressants (G-protein beta3), antipsychotics (dopamine D2, D3, D4; serotonin 5HT2A, 5HT2C), sulfonylureas (sulfonylurea receptor protein), and anesthetics (ryanodine receptor) (Johnson, 2004). In addition, similar association have been studied for drug toxicity and disease polymorphisms including: abacavir (major histocompatability proteins; risk of hypersensitivity), cisapride and terfenadine (HERG, KvLQT1, Mink, MiRP1; increased risk of drug-induced torsade de pointes), and oral contraceptives (prothombin and Factor V; increased deep vein thrombosis) (Johnson, 2004). Likewise, similar associations for efficacy are known such as: statins (apolipoprotein E; enhanced survival prolongation with simvastatin) and tacrine (apolipoprotein E; clinical improvement of Alzheimer's symptoms) (Johnson, 2004).

### Value of Personalized Medicine in Disease

Due to the intimate role of genetics in carcinogenesis, personalized medicine is rapidly becoming a success story in oncology based on genetic profiling using proteomic analyses of tumor biopsies. As described above, targeted cancer therapies such as trastuzumab (Herceptin) are successful and are viewed as the way of the future. Also, clinically important polymorphisms predict increased toxicity in patients with cancer being treated with the chemotherapeutic drugs, for example 6-mercaptopurine (thiopurine methyltransferase (TPMT) *2, *3A, and *3C variants), 5-fluorouracil (5-FU) (dihydropyrimidine dehydrogenase *2A variant), and irinotecan (UGT1A1*28 allele; FDA approved Invader UGT1A1 Molecular Assay diagnostic available to screen for presence of this allele associated with irinotecan toxicity) (Kolesar, 2004). Likewise, clinically important pharmcogenetics predicts efficacy in oncology patients treated with 5-FU (thymidylate synthase *2 and *3C variants).

A classic application of pharmacogenetics is our present understanding of the potentially fatal hematopoietic toxicity that occurs in some patients administered standard doses of the antileukemic agents azathioprine, mercaptopurine and thioguanine (Zhou, 2006). These drugs are metabolized by the enzyme TPMT to the inactive S-methylated products. Gene mutations (polymorphisms) may occur in as many as 11% of patients resulting in decreased TPMT-mediated metabolism of the thiopurine drugs. A diagnostic test for TPMT is now available and used clinically. Identified patients with poor TPMT metabolism may need their drug dose lowered 10- to 15-fold. Mechanisms of multidrug resistance to cancer drugs are influenced by genetic differences. A number of polymorphisms in the MDR-1 gene coding for P-glycoprotein, the transmembrane protein drug efflux pump responsible for multidrug resistance, have been identified. One, known as the T/T genotype and correlated with decreased intestinal expression of P-glycoprotein and increased drug bioavailability, has an allele frequency of 88% in African-American populations, yet only approximately 50% in Caucasian-American populations (Kolesar, 2004).

Pharmacogenetic and pharmacogenomic analysis of patients is being actively studied in many disease states. However, a detailed discussion goes beyond what this introduction may provide. The reader is encouraged to read further in the suggested readings listed at the end of this chapter. Some examples include infectious disease (genetic predisposition to infection to infection in the host; Rogers, 2004), cardiovascular disease (genes linked to heart failure and treating hypertension, warfarin anticoagulant therapy, lipid lowering drugs; Cavallari, 2004), psychiatry (the roles of drug metabolism and receptor expression in drug response rates for antidepressants and antipsychotic drugs, weight gain from antipsychotics; Ellingrod and Bishop, 2004), asthma (leukotriene inhibitors and beta-agonists; Lima and Wang, 2004), and transplantation (cyclosporine metabolism and multidrug resistance efflux meahanisms; Zheng and Burckart, 2004).

### Challenges in Personalized Medicine

There are many keys to success for personalized medicine that hinge on continued scientific advancement. There are also economic, societal, and ethical issues that must be addressed to successfully implement genetic testing-based individualized pharmacotherapy. It is fair to state that most drugs will not be effective in all patients all of the time. Thus the pressure of payers to move from a "payment for product" to a "payment for clinically significant health outcomes" model is reasonable. The use of omic health technologies and health informatics approaches to stratify patient populations for drug effectiveness and drug safety are laudable goals. However, the technologies are currently quite expensive and the resulting drug response predictability is now just being validated clinically. Cost-effectiveness and cost–benefit analyses are limited at this date.

Also, the resulting environment created by these technologies in the context of outcomes expectations and new drug access/reimbursement models will give rise to a new pharmaceutical business paradigm that is still evolving and not well understood.

In 2005, the FDA approved what some referred to as the "first racially targeted drug," BiDil (isosorbide/hydralzaine; from NitroMed) (Branca, 2005). Omic technologies were not generally involved in the development and approval process. Based on the analysis of health statistics suggesting that the rate of mortality in blacks with heart disease is twice as high in whites in the 45 to 64 age group, a clinical trial of this older drug combination in 1,050 African-Americans was conducted and the 43% improvement in survival in the treatment arm resulted in FDA approval of the drug exclusively in African Americans. Yet, modern anthropology and genetics have shown that while race does exist as a real social construct, there are no genetically distinguishable human racial groups (Ossorio, 2004). Thus, attributing observed differences in biomedical outcomes and phenotypical observations to genetic differences among races is problematic and ethically challenging. Race is likely just a surrogate marker for the environmental and genetic causes of disease and response to pharmacotherapy. Now, factor in the introduction of omic technologies broadly into healthcare in a manner to segregate patient populations based on genomic and proteomic characteristics. It is obvious that these modern technologies pose provocative consequences for public policy (including data protection, insurability and access to care) and these challenges must be addressed by decision makers, scientists, healthcare providers and the public for personalized medicine to be successful (see Rothstein, 2003 in Further Reading).

## ■ Toxicogenomics

Toxicogenomics is related to pharmacogenomics, combining toxicology, genetics, molecular biology, and environmental health to elucidate the response of living organisms to stressful environments or toxic agents (Rockett, 2003; Waring et al., 2004). Likewise, new drug candidates can be screened through a combination of gene expression profiling and toxicology to understand gene response and possibly predict safety (Furness, 2002). Genomic techniques utilized include gene expression level profiling and single-nucleotide polymorphism analysis of the genetic variation of individuals generally employing microarray technology. Toxicogenomic studies are correlated to adverse toxicological effects in clinical trials so that suitable biomarkers for these adverse effects can be developed. Using such methods, it would then theoretically possible to test an individual patient for his or her susceptibility to these adverse effects before administering a drug. Patients that would show the marker for an adverse effect would be switched to a different drug. At this time however, the field is in its infancy.

## ■ Glycomics and Glycobiology

The novel scientific field of glycomics, or glycobiology, may be defined most simply as the study of the structure, synthesis and biological function of all glycans (may be referred to as oligosaccharides or polysaccharides, depending on size) and glycoconjugates in simple and complex systems (Varkin et al., 1999; Fukuda and Hindsgauld, 2000; Alper, 2001). The application of glycomics or glycobiology is sometimes called glycotechnology to distinguish it from biotechnology (referring to glycans rather than proteins and nucleic acids). However, many in the biotech arena consider glycobiology one of the research fields encompassed by the term biotechnology. In the postgenomic era, the intricacies of protein glycosylation, the mechanisms of genetic control, and the internal and external factors influencing the extent and patterns of glycosylation are important to understanding protein function and proteomics. Like proteins and nucleic acids, glycans are biopolymers. While once referred to as the last frontier of pharmaceutical discovery, recent advances in the biotechnology of discovering, cloning, and harnessing sugar cleaving and synthesizing enzymes have enabled glycobiologists to analyze and manipulate complex carbohydrates more easily (Walsh and Jefferis, 2006).

Many of the proteins produced by animal cells contain attached sugar moieties, making them glycoproteins). The majority of protein-based medicinal agents contain some form of post-translational modification that can profoundly affect the biological activity of that protein. Bacterial hosts for recombinant DNA could produce the animal proteins with identical or nearly identical amino acid sequences. The bacteria, however, lacked the "machinery" to attach sugar moieties to proteins (a process called glycosylation). Many of the non-glycosylated proteins differed in their biological activity as compared to the native glycoprotein. The production of animal proteins that lacked glycosylation provided an unexpected opportunity to study the functional role of sugar molecules on glycoproteins. There has been extensive progress in glycoengineering of yeast to humanize N-glycosylation pathways resulting in therapeutic glycoprotein expression in yeasts (Wildt and Gerngross, 2005).

The complexity of the field can best be illustrated by reviewing the building blocks of glycans, the simple carbohydrates called saccharides or sugars and their derivatives (i.e., amino sugars). Simple carbohydrates can be attached to other types of biological molecules to form glycoconjugates including glycoproteins (predominantly protein), glycolipids and proteoglycans (about 95% polysaccharide and 5% protein). While carbohydrate chemistry and biology have been active areas of research for centuries, advances in biotechnology have provided techniques and added energy to the study of glycans. Oligosaccharides found conjugated to proteins (glycoproteins) and lipids (glycolipids) display a tremendous structural diversity. The linkages of the monomeric units in proteins and in nucleic acids are generally consistent in all such molecules. Glycans, however, exhibit far greater variability in the linkage between monomeric units than that found in the other biopolymers. As an example, Figure 5 illustrates the common linkage sites to create polymers of glucose. Glucose can be linked at four positions: C-2, C-3, C-4, and C-6 and also can take one of two possible anomeric configurations at C-2 ($\alpha$ and $\beta$). The effect of multiple linkage arrangements is seen in the estimate of Kobata (Kobata, 1996). He has estimated that for a 10-mer (oligomer of length 10) the number of structurally distinct linear oligomers for each of the biopolymers is: DNA (with 4 possible bases), $1.04 \times 10^6$; protein (with 20 possible amino acids), $1.28 \times 10^{13}$; and oligosaccharide (with eight monosaccharide types), $1.34 \times 10^{18}$.

### Glycosylation and Medicine

Patterns of glycosylation affect significantly the biological activity of proteins (McAuliffe and Hindsgaud, 2000; Wildt and Gerngross, 2005; Walsh and Jefferis, 2006). Many of the therapeutically used recombinant DNA-produced proteins are glycosylated including erythropoietin, glucocerebrosidase and tissue plasminogen activator. Without the appropriate carbohydrates attached, none of these proteins will function therapeutically as does the parent glycoprotein. Glycoforms (variations of the glycosylation pattern of a glycoprotein) of the same protein may differ in physicochemical and biochemical properties. For example, erythropoietin has one O-linked and three N-linked glycosylation sites. The removal of the terminal sugars at each site destroys in vivo activity and removing all sugars results in a more rapid clearance of the molecule and a shorter circulatory half-life (Takeuchi et al., 1990). Yet, the opposite effect is observed for the deglycosylation of the hematopoietic cytokine granulocyte-macrophage colony-stimulating factor (GM-CSF) (Cebon et al., 1990). In that case, removing the carbohydrate residues increases the specific activity sixfold. The sugars of glycoproteins are known to play a role in the recognition and binding of biomolecules to other molecules in disease states such as asthma, rheumatoid arthritis, cancer, HIV-infection, the flu and other infectious diseases.

### ■ "Omics" Integrating Technology: Systems Biology

The massive scientific effort embodied in the HGP and the development of bioinformatics technologies have catalyzed fundamental changes in the practice of modern biology (Aderem and Hood, 2001). Biology has become an information science defining all the elements in a complex biological system and placing them in a database for comparative interpretation. As seen in Figure 2, the hierarchy of information collection goes well beyond the biodata contained in the genetic code that is transcribed and translated. It involves a complex interactive system. Systems biology is often described as a non-competitive technology by the pharmaceutical industry (a foundational technology that must be developed to better succeed at the competitive technology of drug discovery and development). It is the study of the interactions between the components of a biological system, and how these interactions give rise to the function and behavior of that system. The biological system may involve enzymes and metabolites in a metabolic pathway or other interacting biological molecules affecting a biological process. Characterized by a cycle of theory, computational modeling and experiment to quantitatively describe cells or cell processes, systems biology is a data intensive endeavor (Klipp et al., 2005; Rothberg et al., 2005). Since the objective is a model of all the interactions in a system, the experimental techniques that most suit systems biology are those that are system-wide and attempt to be as complete as possible. High-throughput omics technologies such as proteomics, pharmacogenomics, transcriptomics, metabolomics, and toxicogenomics are used to collect quantitative data for the construction and validation of systems models.

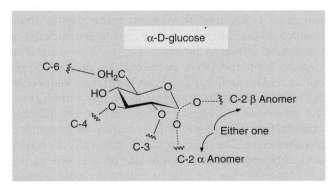

**Figure 5** ▉ Illustration of the common linkage sites to create biopolymers of glucose. Linkages at four positions: C-2, C-3, C-4 and C-6 and also can take one of two possible anomeric configurations at C-2 ($\alpha$ and $\beta$).

## ■ Other "Omics" Technologies

The burgeoning fields of genomics, proteomics, etc. have spawned an ever increasing number of sub-disciplines and related specialty areas of study. The complexity in terminology for "omic" technologies has amplified even further with the introduction of terms such as interactomics, proteogenomics, nutri-genomics, etc. Interactomics is the data intensive broad system study of the interactome, which is the interaction among proteins and other molecules within a cell. Proteogenomics has been used as a broadly encompassing term to describe the merging of genomics, proteomics, small molecules, and informatics. Nutrigenomics is a new field evaluating the response of living organisms to the presence or absence of important nutrients. Lipidomics is obviously the large-scale study of all non-water-soluble lipid metabolites in an organism. The "omics" explosion will continue.

## TRANSGENIC ANIMALS AND PLANTS

For thousands of years, man has selectively bred animals and plants either to enhance or to create desirable traits in numerous species. The explosive development of recombinant DNA technology and other molecular biology techniques have made it possible to engineer species possessing particular unique and distinguishing genetic characteristics. The genetic material of an animal or plant can be manipulated so that extra genes may be inserted (transgenes), replaced (i.e., human gene homologs coding for related human proteins), or deleted (knockout). Theoretically, these approaches enable the introduction of virtually any gene into any organism. A greater understanding of specific gene regulation and expression will contribute to important new discoveries made in relevant animal models. Such genetically altered species have found utility in a myriad of research and potential commercial applications including the generation of models of human disease, protein drug production, creation of organs and tissues for xenotransplantation, a host of agricultural uses, and drug discovery (Dunn et al., 2005).

## ■ Transgenic Animals

Gordon and Ruddle first used the term "transgenic" in 1981 to describe an animal in which a foreign DNA segment (a transgene) was incorporated into their genome. Later, the term was extended to also include animals in which their endogenous genomic DNA has had its molecular structure manipulated (Gordon and Ruddle, 1981; Isola and Gordon, 1991). While there are some similarities between transgenic technology and

gene therapy (see Chapter 8), it is important to distinguish clearly between them. Technically speaking, the introduction of foreign DNA sequences into a living cell is called gene transfer. Thus, one method to create a transgenic animal involves gene transfer (transgene incorporated into the genome). Gene therapy is also a gene transfer procedure and, in a sense, produces a transgenic human. In transgenic animals, however, the foreign gene is transferred indiscriminately into all cells, including germ line cells. The process of gene therapy differs generally from transgenesis since it involves a transfer of the desired gene in such a way that involves only specific somatic and hematopoietic cells, and not germ cells. Thus unlike in gene therapy, the genetic changes in transgenic organisms are conserved in any offspring according to the general rules of Mendelian inheritance.

The production of transgenic animals is not a new technology (Dunn et al., 2005). They have been produced since the 1970s. However, modern biotechnology has greatly improved the methods of inducing the genetic transformation. While the mouse has been the most studied animal species, transgenic technology has been applied to cattle, fish (especially Zebrafish), goats, poultry, rabbits, rats, sheep, swine, and various lower animal forms. Transgenic animals have already made valuable research contributions to studies involving regulation of gene expression, the function of the immune system, genetic diseases, viral diseases, cardiovascular disease, and the genes responsible for the development of cancer. Transgenic animals have proven to be indispensable in drug lead identification, lead optimization, preclinical drug development, and disease modeling.

### Production of Transgenic Animals by DNA Microinjection and Random Gene Addition

The production of transgenic animals has most commonly involved the microinjection (also called gene transfer) of 100 to 200 copies of exogenous transgene DNA into the larger, more visible male pronucleus (as compared to the female pronucleus) of a recipient fertilized embryo (Fig. 6). The transgene contains both the DNA encoding the desired target amino acid sequence along with regulatory sequences that will mediate the expression of the added gene. The microinjected eggs are then implanted into the reproductive tract of a female and allowed to develop into embryos. The foreign DNA generally becomes randomly inserted at a single site on just one of the host chromosomes (i.e., the founder transgenic animal is heterozygous). Thus each transgenic founder animal (positive transgene incorporated animals) is a unique species. Interbreeding of founder transgenic animals where the transgene has been incorporated into germ cells may result in the birth of a homozygous progeny provided the transgene incorporation did not induce a mutation of an essential endogenous gene. All cells of the transgenic animal will contain the transgene if DNA insertion occurs prior to the first cell division. However, usually only 20% to 25% of the offspring contain detectable levels of the transgene. Selection of neonatal animals possessing an incorporated transgene can readily be accomplished either by the direct identification of specific DNA or mRNA sequences or by the observation of gross phenotypic characteristics.

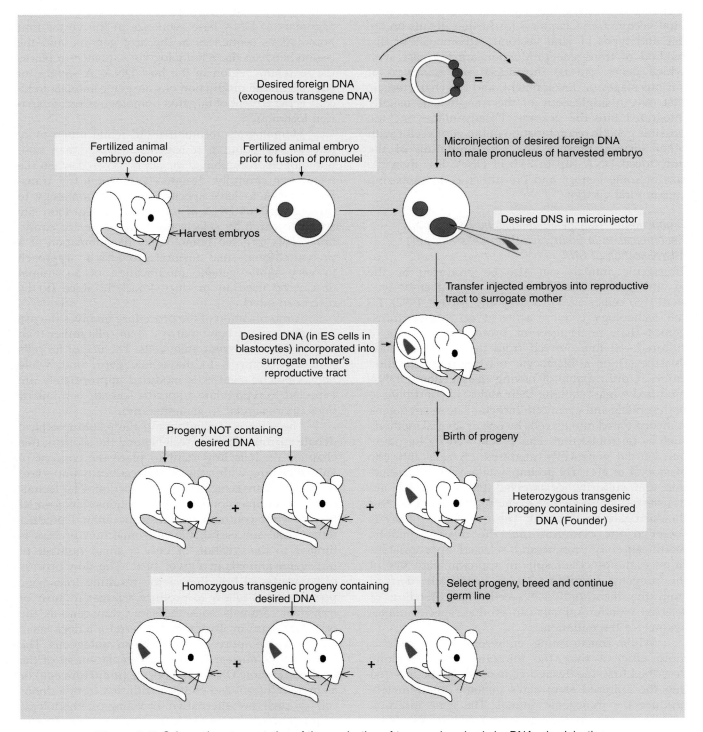

**Figure 6** ■ Schematic representation of the production of transgenic animals by DNA microinjection.

## Production of Transgenic Animals by Retroviral Infection

The production of the first genetically altered laboratory mouse embryos was by insertion of a transgene via a modified retroviral vector. The non-replicating viral vector binds to the embryonic host cells, allowing subsequent transfer and insertion of the transgene into the host genome. Many of the experimental human gene therapy trials employ the same viral vectors (see Chapter 8 for further details on the use and types of viral vectors). Advantages of this method of transgene production are the ease with which genes can be introduced into embryos at various stages of development, and the characteristic that only a single copy of the transgene is usually integrated into the genome. Disadvantages include possible genetic recombination of the viral vector with other viruses present, the size limitation of the introduced DNA (up to 7 kb of DNA, less than the size of some genes), and the difficulty in preparing certain viral vectors.

## Production of Transgenic Animals by Homologous Recombination in Embryonic Stem Cells following Microinjection of DNA

Transgenic animals can also be produced by the in vitro genetic alteration of pluripotent embryonic stem (ES) cells (Fig. 7) (Sedivy and Joyner, 1992). ES cell technology is more efficient at creating transgenics than microinjection protocols. ES cells, a cultured cell line derived from the inner cell mass (blastocyst) of a blastocyte (early preimplantation embryo), are capable of having their genomic DNA modified while retaining their ability to contribute to both somatic and germ cell lineages. The desired gene is incorporated into ES cells by one of several methods such as microinjection. This is followed by introduction of the genetically modified ES cells into the blastocyst of an early preimplantation embryo, selection and culturing of targeted ES cells which are transferred subsequently to the reproductive tract of the surrogate host animal. The resulting progeny is screened for evidence that the desired genetic modification is present and selected appropriately. In mice, the process results in approximately 30% of the progeny containing tissue genetically derived from the incorporated ES cells. Interbreeding of selected founder animals can produce species homozygous for the mutation.

While transforming embryonic stem cells is more efficient than the microinjection technique described first, the desired gene must still be inserted into the cultured stem cell's genome to ultimately produce the transgenic animal. The gene insertion could occur in a random or in a targeted process. Non-homologous recombination, a random process, readily occurs if the desired DNA is introduced into the ES cell genome by a gene recombination process that does not require any sequence homology between genomic DNA and the foreign DNA. While most ES cells fail to insert the foreign DNA, some do. Those that do are selected and injected into the inner cell mass of the animal blastocyst and thus eventually lead to a transgenic species. In still far fewer ES cells, homologous recombination occurs by chance. Segments of DNA base sequence in the vector find homologous sequences in the host genome and the region between these homologous sequences replaces the matching region in the host DNA. A significant advance in the production of transgenic animals in ES cells is the advent of targeted homologous recombination techniques.

Homologous recombination, while much more rare to this point in transgenic research than non-homologous recombination, can be favored when the researcher carefully designs (engineers) the transferred DNA to have specific sequence homology to the endogenous DNA at the desired integration site and also carefully selects the transfer vector conditions. This targeted homologous recombination at a precise chromosomal position provides an approach to very subtle genetic modification of an animal or can be used to produce knockout mice (to be discussed later).

A modification of the procedure involves the use of hematopoietic bone marrow stem cells rather than pluripotent embryonic stem cells. The use of ES cells results in changes to the whole germ line, while hematopoietic stem cells modified appropriately are expected to repopulate a specific somatic cell line or lines (more similar to gene therapy).

The science of cloning and the resulting ethical debate surrounding it is well beyond the scope of this chapter. Yet it is important to place the concept of animal cloning within the pharmaceutically important context of transgenic animal production. The technique of microinjection (and its variations) has formed the basis for commercial transgenic animal production. While successful, the microinjection process is limited to the creation of only a small number of transgenic animals in a given birth. The slow process of conventional breeding of the resulting transgenic progeny must follow to produce a larger number of transgenic animals with the same transgene as the original organism. To generate a herd (or a flock, etc.), an alternative approach would be advantageous. The technique of nuclear transfer, the replacement of the nuclear genomic DNA of an oocyte (immature egg) or a single-cell fertilized embryo with that from a donor cell is such an alternative breeding methodology. Animal "cloning" can result from this nuclear transfer technology. Judged Science's most important

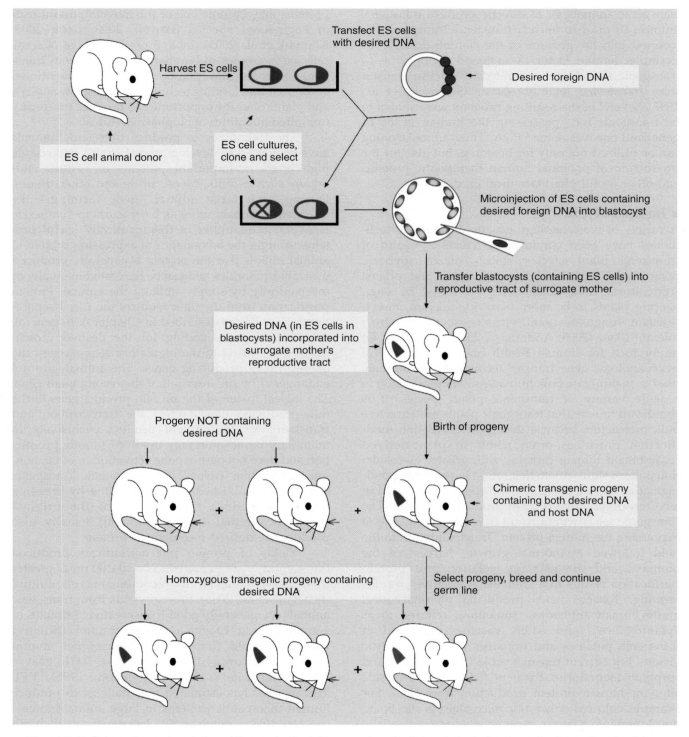

**Figure 7** ■ Schematic representation of the production of transgenic animals by pluripotent embryonic stem cell methodology.

breakthrough of 1997 (Sailor, 1997), creating the sheep Dolly, the first cloned mammal, from a single cell of a 6-year old ewe was a feat many had thought impossible. Dolly was born after nuclear transfer of the genome from an adult mammary gland cell. Since this announcement, commercial and exploratory development of nuclear transfer technology has progressed rapidly with various species cloned. It is important to note that the cloned sheep Dolly was NOT a transgenic animal. While Dolly was a clone of an adult ewe, she did not possess a transgene. However, cloning could be used to breed clones of transgenic animals, or to directly produce transgenic animals (if prior to nuclear transfer, a transgene was inserted into the genome of the cloning donor). For example, human factor IX (a blood factor protein) transgenic sheep were generated by nuclear transfer from transfected fetal fibroblasts (Schniecke et al., 1997). Several of the resulting progeny were shown to be transgenic (i.e., possessing the human factor IX gene) and one was named Polly. Thus, animal cloning can be utilized not only for breeding, but also for the production of potential human therapeutic proteins and other useful pharmaceutical products.

■ **Transgenic Plants**

A variety of biotechnology genetic engineering techniques have been employed to create a wealth of transgenic plant species: cotton, maize, soybean, potato, petunia, tobacco, papaya, rose and others. Agricultural enhancements have resulted by engineering plants to be more herbicide-tolerant, insect-resistant, fungus-resistant, virus resistant, and stress tolerant (Baez, 2005; Andrawiss, 2006; Fox, 2006). Of importance for human health and pharmaceutical biotechnology, gene transfer technology is routinely used to manipulate bulk human protein production in a wide variety of transgenic plant species. It is significant to note that transgenic plants are attractive bulk bioreactors because their post-translation modification processes often result in plant-derived recombinant human proteins with greater glycosylation pattern similarity to that found in the corresponding native human proteins than would be observed in a corresponding mammalian production system. The transgenic seeds would result in seedlings capable of expressing the human protein. Transplantation to the field followed by normal growth, harvest of the biomass, and downstream isolation and protein purification results in a valuable alternative crop for farming. Tobacco fields producing pharmaceutical grade human antibodies (sometimes referred to as "plantibodies") and edible vaccines contained in transgenic potatoes and tomatoes are not futuristic visions, but current research projects in academic and corporate laboratories. Farmers' fields are not the sole sites for human protein production from flora. For example, cultured eukaryotic mico-algea is also being developed into a useful expression system, especially for human and humanized antibodies (Mayfield and Franklin, 2005). With antibody-based targeted therapeutics becoming increasingly important, the use of transgenic plants will continue to expand.

*Biopharmaceutical Protein Production in Transgenic Animals and Plants: "Biopharming"*

The use of transgenic animals and plants as bioreactors for the production of pharmaceutically important proteins may become one of the most important uses of engineered species (Powell, 2003; Baez, 2005; Klimyuk et al., 2005). Table 3 provides a list of some selected examples of biopharmaceuticals from transgenic animals and plants. Utilizing conventional agronomic and farming techniques, transgenic animals and plants offer the opportunity to produce practically unlimited quantities of biopharmaceuticals.

The techniques to produce transgenic animals have been used to develop animal strains that secrete high levels of important proteins in various end-organs such as milk, blood, urine and other tissues. During such large animal "gene farming," the transgenic animals serve as bioreactors to synthesize recoverable quantities of therapeutically useful proteins. Among the advantages of expressing protein in animal milk is that the protein is generally produced in sizable quantities and can be harvested manually or mechanically by simply milking the animal. Protein purification from the milk requires the usual separation techniques as described in Chapter 3. In general, recombinant genes coding for the desired protein product are fused to the regulatory sequences of the animal's milk-producing genes. The animals are not endangered by the insertion of the recombinant gene. The logical fusion of the protein product gene to the milk-producing gene targets the transcription and translation of the protein product exclusively in mammary tissues normally involved in milk production and does not permit gene activation in other, non-milk producing tissues in the animal. Transgenic strains are established and perpetuated by breeding the animals since the progeny of the original transgenic animal (founder animal) usually also produce the desired recombinant protein.

Yields of protein pharmaceuticals produced transgenically are expected to be 10–100 times greater than those achieved in recombinant cell culture (Echelard et al., 2005). Protein yields from transgenic animals are generally good [conservative estimates of 1 gram/Liter (g/L) with a 30% purification efficiency] with milk yield from various species per annum estimated at: cow = 10,000 L; sheep = 500 L; goat = 400 L; and pig = 250 L (Rudolph, 1995). PPL Therapeutics has estimated that the cost to produce human therapeutic proteins in large animal bioreactors could be as much as 75% less expensive than cell culture. In addition, should the desired target protein require post-translational modification, the large mammals used in milk production of pharmaceuticals would be a bioreactor capable of adding those groups (unlike a recombinant bacterial culture).

Some examples of human long peptides and proteins under development in the milk of transgenic animals include growth hormone, interleukin-2, calcitonin, insulin-like growth factor, alpha 1 antitrypsin, clotting Factor VIII, clotting Factor IX, tissue plasminogen activator (tPA), lactoferrin, gastric lipase, vaccine derived from Escherichia coli LtB toxin subunit, protein C and various human monoclonal antibodies (MAbs) (such as those from the Xenomouse) (Garner and Colman, 1998; Rudolph, 2000). The first approved biopharmaceutical from transgenic animals is recombinant human antithrombin (tradename ATryn, see Echelard et al., 2005). Produced in a herd of transgenic dairy goats, rhAT is expressed in high level in he milk. The human AT transgene was assembled by linking the AT cDNA to a normal milk protein sequence (XhoI site of the goat beta casein vector). See Table 3 for additional examples.

Using genetic engineering techniques to create transgenic plants, "pharming" for pharmaceuticals is producing an ever-expanding list of drugs and diagnostic agents derived from human genes (Baez, 2005; Andrawiss, 2006; Fox, 2006). Some examples of human peptides and proteins under development in transgenic plants include TGF-beta, virtonectin, thyroid-stimulating hormone receptor, insulin, glucocerebrosidase, and apoplipoprotein A-1. See Table 3 for additional examples.

## ■ Xenotransplantation: Transplantable Transgenic Animal Organs

An innovative use of transgenics for the production of useful proteins is the generation of clinically transplantable transgenic animal organs. The success of human-to-human transplantation of heart, kidney, liver, and other vascularized organs (allotransplantation) created the significant expectation and need for donor organs. Primate-to-human transplantation (xenotransplantation was successful, but ethical issues and limited number of donor animals were significant barriers. Transplant surgeons recognized early on that organs from the pig were a rational choice for xenotransplantation (due to physiological, anatomical, ethical, and supply reasons) if the serious hyperacute rejection could be overcome. Several research groups in academia and industry have pioneered the transgenic engineering of pigs expressing both human complement inhibitory proteins as well as key human blood group proteins (antigens) (Makowka, 1993; Fodor et al., 1994; McCurry et al., 1995; Saadi and Platt, 1997; Dunn et al., 2005). Cloning has now produced transgenic pigs for xenotransplantation. Cells, tissues and organs from these double transgenic animals appear to be very resistant to the humoral immune system mediated reactions of both primates and likely humans. These findings begin to pave the way for potential xenograft transplantation of animal components into humans with a lessened chance of acute rejection.

## ■ Knockout Mice

While many species including mice, zebra fish, nemotodes, etc. have been transformed to lose genetic function for the study of drug discovery and disease modeling, mice have proven to be the most useful. Mice are the laboratory animal species most closely related to humans in which the knockout technique can be easily performed, so they are a favorite subject for knockout experiments, While a mouse carrying an introduced transgene is called a transgenic mouse, transgenic technologies can also produce a knockout animal (mice are the most studied animal species). A knockout mouse, also called a gene knockout mouse or a gene-targeted knockout mouse, is an animal in which an endogenous gene (genomic wild-type allele) has been specifically inactivated by replacing it with a null allele (Mak et al., 2001; Lesney, 2003; Sharpless and DePinho, 2006). A null allele is a nonfunctional allele of a gene generated by either deletion of the entire gene or mutation of the gene resulting in the synthesis of an inactive protein. Recent advances in intranuclear gene targeting and embryonic stem cell technologies as described above are expanding the capabilities to produce knockout mice routinely for studying certain human genetic diseases or elucidating the function of a specific gene product.

The procedure for producing knockout mice basically involves a four-step process. A null allele (i.e., knockout allele) is incorporated into one allele of murine ES cells. Incorporation is generally quite low; approximately one cell in a million has the required gene replacement. However, the process is designed to impart neomycin and ganciclovir resistance only to those ES cells in which homologous gene integration has resulted. This facilitates the selection and propagation of the correctly engineered ES cells. The resulting ES cells are then injected into early mouse embryos creating chimeric mice (heterozygous for the knockout allele) containing tissues derived from both host cells and ES cells. The chimeric mice are mated to confirm that the null allele is incorporated into the germ line. The confirmed heterozygous chimeric mice are bred to homogeneity producing progeny that are homozygous knockout mice. Worldwide, three major mouse knockout programs are proceeding in collaboration to create a mutation in each of the approximately 20,000 protein-coding genes in the mouse genome using a combination of gene trapping and gene targeting in mouse embryonic stem (ES) cells (Staff, 2007). These include: (1) KOMP (KnockOut Mouse Project, http://www.knockoutmouse.org), funded by the NIH; (2) EUCOMM (EUropean COnditional Mouse Mutagenesis

| Species | Protein product | Potential indication(s) |
|---------|-----------------|-------------------------|
| Cow | Collagen | Burns, bone fracture |
| Cow | Human fertility hormones | Infertility |
| Cow | Human serum albumin | Surgery, burns, shock, trauma |
| Cow | Lactoferrin | Bacterial GI infection |
| Goat | α-1-anti-protease inhibitor | Inherited deficiency |
| Goat | α-1-antitrypsin | Anti-inflammatory |
| Goat | Anti-thrombin III (ATryn) | Associated complications from genetic or acquired deficiency |
| Goat | Growth hormone | Pituitary dwarfism |
| Goat | Human fertility hormones | Infertility |
| Goat | Human serum albumin | Surgery, burns, shock, trauma |
| Goat | LAtPA2 | Venous status ulcers |
| Goat | Monoclonal antibodies | Colon cancer |
| Goat | tPA2 | Myocardial infarct, pulmonary embolism |
| Pig | Factor IX | Hemophilia |
| Pig | Factor VIII | Hemophilia |
| Pig | Fibrinogen | Burns, surgery |
| Pig | Human hemoglobin | Blood replacement for transfusion |
| Pig | Protein C | Deficiency, adjunct to tPA |
| Rabbit | Insulin-like growth factor | Wound healing |
| Rabbit | Interleukin-2 | Renal cell carcinoma |
| Rabbit | Protein C | Deficiency, adjunct to tPA |
| Sheep | α–1-antitrypsin | Antiinflammatory |
| Sheep | Factor VIII | Hemophilia |
| Sheep | Factor IX | Hemophilia |
| Sheep | Fibrinogen | Burns |
| Sheep | Protein C | Deficiency, adjunct to tPA |
| Tobacco | IgG | Systemic therapy (rabies virus, hepatitis B virus) |
| Tobacco | TGF-β2 | Ovarian cancer |
| Tobacco | Virtonectin | Protease |
| Tobacco | RhinoR | Fusion of human adhesion protein and human IgA for common cold |
| Safflower | Insulin | Diabetes |
| Corn | Meripase | Cystic fibrosis |
| Duckweed | Lacteron | Controlled release of α-interferon for hepatitis B and C |
| Potato | Poultry vaccine | Avian influenza (H5N1) |

*Abbreviations*: tPA, tissue plasminogen activator; LAtPA, long acting tissue plasminogen activator; TGF-β[3], tissue growth factor-beta.

**Table 3** ▓ Some examples of human proteins under development in transgenic animals and plants.

Program, http://www.eucomm.org), funded by the FP6 program of the EC; and (3) NorCOMM (North American COnditional Mouse Mutagenesis Project, http://norcomm.phenogenomics.ca/index.htm) is a Canadian project, funded by Genome Canada and partners. To date, nearly 4000 targeted knockouts of genes have been accomplished. This comprehensive and publicly available resource will aid researchers examining the role of each gene in normal physiology and development, and shed light on the pathogenesis of abnormal physiology and disease. RNA silencing and interference techniques (siRNA and RNAi) are impacting knockout mice production and are discussed in Chapter 9.

Extensive previous research has generated and the continuing discoveries of the three worldwide mouse knockout consortia will further create better models of human monogenic and polygenic diseases such as cancer, diabetes, obesity, cardiovascular disease, and psychiatric and neurodegenerative diseases. For example, knockout mice have been engineered that have extremely elevated cholesterol levels while being maintained on normal chow diets due to their inability to produce apolipoprotein E (apoprotein E) (Zhang et al., 1992; Breslow, 1994). Apoprotein E is the major lipoprotein component of very low-density lipoprotein (VLDL) responsible for liver clearance of VLDL. These engineered mice are being examined as animal models of atherosclerosis useful in cardiovascular drug discovery and development. Table 4 provides a list of some additional selected examples of knockout mouse disease models.

The knockout mouse is becoming the basic tool for researchers to determine gene function in vivo in numerous biological systems. For example, knockout mouse technology has helped transform our understanding of the immune response (Mak et al., 2001). The study of single and multiple gene knockout animals have provided new perspectives on T-cell development, co-stimulation and activation. "Humanized mice," transgenic Severe Combined Immunodeficient (SCID) mice grafted with human cells and tissues enable research in regenerative medicine, infectious disease, cancer, and human hematopoiesis. In addition, high-throughput DNA sequencing efforts, positional cloning programs, and novel embryonic stem cell-based gene discovery research areas all exploit the knockout mouse as their laboratory.

Engineered animal models are proving invaluable to pharmaceutical research since small animal models of disease may be created and validated to mimic a disease in human patients. Mouse, rat, and Zebrafish are the most common models explored and used. Genetic engineering can predispose an animal to a particular disease under scrutiny and the insertion of human genes into the animal can initiate the development of a more clinically relevant disease condition. In human clinical studies, assessments of efficacy and safety often rely on measured effects for surrogate biomarkers and adverse event reporting. Validated transgenic animal models of human disease allow for parallel study and possible predictability prior to entering clinical trials. Also, it is possible to screen potential drug candidates in vivo against a

| Genetic engineering | Gene (a) | Disease model |
|---|---|---|
| Knockout | BRCA1, BRCA2 | Breast cancer |
| Knockout | Apolipoprotein E | Atherosclerosis |
| Knockout | Glucocerebrosidase | Gaucher's disease |
| Knockout | HPRT | Lesch-Nyhan syndrome |
| Knockout | Hexokinase A | Tay-Sachs disease |
| Knockout | Human CFTR | Cystic fibrosis |
| Knockout | P53 | Cancer suppressor gene deletion |
| Knockout | P-glycoprotein | Multidrug resistance (MDR) |
| Knockout | $\alpha$-globin and $\beta$-globin | Sickle cell anemia |
| Knockout | Urate oxidase | Gout |
| Knockout | Retinoblastoma-1 | Familial retinoblastoma |
| Transgene | c-neu oncogene | Cancer |
| Transgene | c-myc oncogene | Cancer |
| Transgene | Growth hormone | Dwarfism |
| Transgene | H-ras oncogene | Cancer |
| Transgene | Histocompatibility antigens | Autoimmunity |
| Transgene | HIV tat | Kaposi's sarcoma |
| Transgene | Human APP | Alzheimer's disease |
| Transgene | Human $\beta$-globin | Thalassemia |
| Transgene | Human CD4 expression | HIV infection |
| Transgene | Human $\beta$-globin mutant | Sickle cell anemia |
| Transgene | Human CETP | Atherosclerosis |
| Transgene | LDL acceptor | Hypercholesterolemia |

**Table 4**    Some selected examples of genetically engineered animal disease models.

human receptor target inserted into an animal model. The number of examples of transgenic animal models of human disease useful in drug discovery and development efforts is growing rapidly (Sharpless and DePinho, 2006; Schultz et al., 2007). Such models have potential to increase the efficiency and decrease the cost of drug discovery and development by reducing the time it takes to move a medicinal agent from discovery into clinical trials. Table 4 provides a list of some selected examples of genetically engineered animal models of human disease.

## TECHNIQUES TO MODIFY AND STUDY PROTEINS AND PRODUCTS OF BIOTECHNOLOGY

### ■ Protein Engineering

Many early biotechnology-produced protein drug candidates failed in clinical trials due to their short biological half-life, low affinity for their receptor, or immunogenicity (McCafferty and Glover, 2000). Recombinant DNA technology has made it possible to engineer specifically altered or new and novel protein molecules possessing tailored chemical and biological characteristics. Termed protein engineering, the deliberate design and construction of unique proteins with enhanced or novel molecular properties is a result of specifying the exact amino acid sequence (protein primary structure) of that protein (Narang, 1990; Richardson and Richardson, 1990; Cleland and Craik, 1996). When applied to enzymes, the process is often called enzyme engineering.

As described in Chapter 2, the primary structure affects the protein's conformation. The conformation of each and every amino acid component present in the protein influences the protein's complex three-dimensional (3-D) structure. The conformational preference of the protein chain residues determines the protein's secondary structure including α-helices and β-sheets or reverse turns. The local secondary structures are folded into 3-D tertiary structures made up of domains. The domains are not only structural units, but are also functional units often containing intact ligand binding (in a receptor) or enzyme catalytic sites. Thus, protein engineering provides an approach to modify a native protein's structure specifically or to create a unique, new protein with a particular structure. Protein engineering has numerous powerful theoretical and practical implications for examining and modifying protein structure and function, probing enzyme mechanisms, investigating protein folding and conformation, enhancing protein stability, introducing detectable groups into proteins as an analytical tool, producing improved second generation tailored biopharmaceuticals, and in the case of enzymes, improving catalytic function (Fothergill-Gilmore, 1993; Nixon et al., 1998).

Engineered proteins have been prepared by many different approaches. Direct chemical synthetic routes for small proteins with modified amino acid sequences have been devised using either solution chemistry or solid supports (chemistry occurring while reactants are attached to resin beads) techniques. Peptide synthesizers have been designed to automate the process. Dugas provides a useful overview of the chemistry of protein engineering (including site-directed mutagenesis) (Dugas, 1999). The synthesis of gene fragments coding for the mutation(s) is another approach to produce engineered proteins (Johnson and Reitz, 1998). Completely synthetic genes of as many as 100 nucleotides coding for the desired mutation can be inserted into a gene of a prokaryotic (such as Phage M13) or eukaryotic expression vector. The resulting mutant gene (hybrid gene) is then cloned and expressed producing the engineered protein. The genetic route to engineered proteins is limited to the repertoire of the 20 natural amino acids, yet new technologies appear to be moving toward an expanded repertoire including moieties that would result in peptidomimetics. The purely chemical route allows for the introduction of alternative structures (e.g., non-natural amino acids) in the peptide chain (see section "Peptide Chemistry and Peptidomimetics").

### Site-Directed Mutagenesis

Site-directed mutagenesis (also called site-specific mutagenesis) is a protein engineering technique allowing specific amino acid residue (site-directed) alteration (mutation) to create new protein entities (Johnson and Reitz, 1998). Mutagenesis at a single amino acid position in an engineered protein is called a point mutation. Therefore, site-directed mutagenesis techniques can aid in the examination at the molecular level of the relationship between 3-D structure and function of interesting proteins.

Figure 8 suggests an excellent example of possible theoretical mutations of the active site of a model serine protease enzyme that could be engineered to probe the mechanism of action of the enzyme. Structures B and C of Figure 8 represent a theoretical mutation to illustrate the technique. Craik and co-workers have actually tested the role of the aspartic acid residue in the serine protease catalytic triad Asp, His, and Ser. They replaced Asp[102] (carboxylate anion side chain) of trypsin with Asn (neutral amide side chain) by site-directed mutagenesis and observed a pH dependent change in the catalytic activity compared to the wild-type parent serine protease (Fig. 8, structure D) (Craik et al., 1987). Site-directed mutagenesis studies also provide invaluable insight into the nature of intermolecular interactions of ligands with their receptors. For example, studies of the effect of the site-directed mutagenesis of various key amino acid residues on the binding of neurotransmitters to G-protein coupled receptors has helped define more accurate models for alpha-adrenergic, D2-dopaminergic, 5HT2a-serotonergic and both M1 and M3 muscarinic receptors (Bikker, et al., 1998).

### Directed Evolution

Today, many of the techniques to engineer proteins with improved properties such as enhanced biological activity, improved catalytic specificity, metabolic

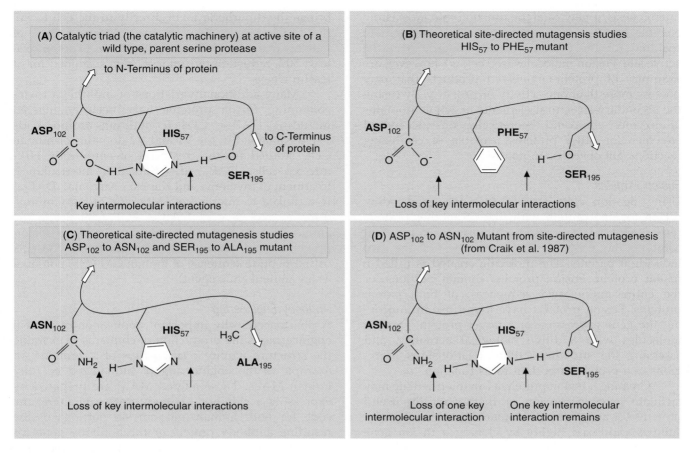

**Figure 8** ▪ Some possible site-directed mutations of the amino acids composing the catalytic triad of a serine protease: influence on key hydrogen bonding.

stability, etc. are often referred to as "directed evolution" (Oelschlaeger and Mayo, 2005; Pelletier, 2007 and references contained therein). Studying the relationship between a protein's sequence and the resulting protein's property allows for a prediction of the optimal structure-property relationship and thus the "evolved" protein to be synthesized by standard techniques of biotechnology. Enzyme engineering to evolve a protein is achieved typically by reasoned direct experimental manipulation of protein structure, computationally, or more recently, a combination of both (Fox et al., 2007). The variations resulting from all the possible protein sequences to be explored (referred to as "sequence space") to guide the directed evolution of even an average-sized protein are astronomically large. Thus, while the approach holds great promise to engineer new protein products, directed evolution on a practical scale is still limited at this time.

*Enzyme Engineering*
Enzyme engineering is the application of protein engineering techniques to enzymatic molecules.

Enzyme engineering can optimize catalytic reactions, improve an enzyme's function under abnormal conditions, and enhance or change the catalytic reaction of unnatural substrates (Nixon, et al., 1998). An exciting application of protein engineering is the preparation of enzymes that have improved catalytic activity and stability in organic solvents, rather than requiring an aqueous environment. In that case, site-directed mutagenesis replaces hydrophilic, charged amino acids and hydrogen bonding residues at the surface of the enzyme with amino acids that stabilize the conformational stability of the protein at the organic solvent–protein surface interface.

The generation of enzyme hybrids, enzymes composed of elements of more than one enzyme, is an exciting area of current study using enzyme engineering techniques. Some examples include the hybridization of the enzyme trypsin to hydrolyze either trypsin and chymotrypsin substrates, and the modification of the substrate specificity of lactate dehydrogenase (pyruvate) to include also oxaloacetate (Nixon, et al., 1998). While enzyme engineering is a powerful technique, it is difficult to engineer, via site-directed mutagenesis, a new catalytic function into an existing enzyme because of the precise spatial arrangement required for the catalytic functional groups at the active site. Fusion molecules (see below), however, are examples of protein-engineered products that may possess more than one activity or property. By fusing the secondary-structural elements or whole domains of enzymes, one could theoretically construct hybrid enzymes (or other proteins) capable of catalyzing reactions not observed in nature.

*Fusion Proteins*
Using ligation chemistry to fuse the gene-coding region for one protein with that of another protein, researchers have created chimeric proteins that combine the properties and activities of the two individual parents. The molecule created is called a fusion protein. Fusion proteins contain portions, or the entire amino acid sequences, of both parent proteins. Fusion proteins have found use in improving the gene expression of a target protein, creating molecules with additive biological activities, and assessing the structure-activity relationships of regions in a protein important to its function.

Creating a fusion protein as an intermediate may facilitate gene expression of therapeutically useful proteins (or any protein). Human recombinant proinsulin is expressed highly by cloning a fusion gene consisting of the codes for both proinsulin and the enzyme galactosidase. After recovering the fusion protein from *E. coli* culture, cleavage of the methionine peptide bond linking the two proteins with the chemical cyanogen bromide yields the free proinsulin.

Ligation chemistry can create DNA coding for fusion molecules with additive properties in comparison to the individual parent proteins. Numerous fusion proteins have been created that contain a toxin fused to another protein. Cutaneous T-cell lymphoma (CTCL) is a general term for a group of low-grade non-Hodgkin's lymphomas affecting approximately 1000 new patients/year. For many patients, CTCL is a persistent, disfiguring and debilitating disease that requires multiple treatments over time. Malignant CTCL cells express one or more of the components of the IL-2 receptor. Thus, the IL-2 receptor may be a homing device to attract a "killer." The IL-2 fusion protein $DAB_{389}$ IL-2 (also called IL-2 fusion toxin) is a recombinant protein consisting of amino acid residues 2–133 of human IL-2 (the IL-2 residues replace the amino acids of the receptor-binding domain of the native diphtheria toxin) "fused" to the first 389 amino acid residues of diphtheria toxin (catalytic and lipophilic domains) (VanderSpek et al., 1993). Denileukin diftitox (Ontak) is such a FDA-approved rDNA-derived cytotoxic IL-2 "fusion" protein. The drug targets IL-2 receptors (the IL-2 portion), and

brings the diphtheria toxin directly to the cell to kill the CTCL targets. Studies have observed 30% of patients treated with Denileukin diftitox experience at least 50% reduction of tumor burden sustained for at least 6 weeks.

Many additional variations of diphtheria toxin-containing fusion proteins have been engineered including $DAB_{389}$ CD4 (containing amino acids 1–178 contained in the V1 and V2 domains of human CD4; studied for the treatment of chronically HIV-infected cells), $DAB_{389}$ IL-4 (linked to interleukin 4; treatment of myeloma and Kaposi's sarcoma), $DAB_{389}$ IL-6 (linked to interleukin 6; therapy of autoimmune diseases and cancer), $DAB_{389}$ EGF (containing the amino acid sequence of epidermal growth factor; prevention of restenosis), and $DAB_{389}$ hGM-CSF (fused peptide sequence of human GM-CSF; potential as an antileukemic agent).

*Antibody Engineering*
A pharmaceutically important application of protein engineering is the production of chimeras to examine the structure-activity relationships of a protein. An example is the engineering of humanized or fully human MAbs. These altered MAbs are prepared by expressing a chimeric antibody gene containing the code for both human and murine portions of the resulting antibody protein or the antibody gene for the fully human protein, respectively. The differences between species in the structure-activity relationships and the structure-function relationships of these chimeric or human antibodies can be examined by studying properties such as antigen specificity, affinity, and avidity (see Chapters 15–18) (Pluckthun, 1992; Andersen and Reilly, 2004; Hoogenboom, 2005; Chowdhury and Wu, 2005). MAbs (chimeric, humanized, fully human) and improved antibody fragments are necessary to support research and pharmacotherapy. The application of protein engineering to the synthesis of new antibodies or improved antibody fragments is called antibody engineering. A significant effort is also invested in modifying glycosylation patterns and simplifying production methods.

Designed, potent antibody therapeutics constitutes one of the most rapidly growing class of human therapeutics (Carter, 2006). Immunoadhesins are antibody engineered fusion proteins containing the immunoglobulin Fc effector domain and a molecule that will adhere specifically to other target molecules. Examples include the replacement of the variable region of an antibody with either the helper T-cell CD4 surface protein or tumor necrosis factor receptor (Fig. 9). These immunoadhesins would retain the antibody's Fc effector region (see Chapter 15), but would display specificity for HIV or tumor necrosis

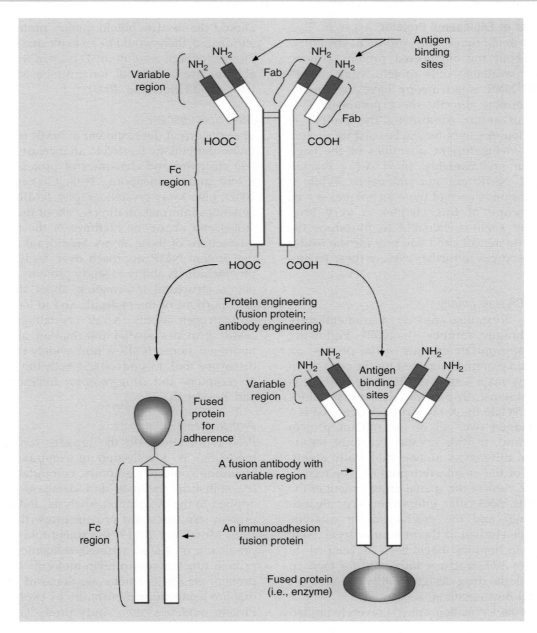

**Figure 9** ▪ Protein engineering (antibody engineering) to produce fusion antibodies.

factor, respectively. Tumor necrosis factor-alpha is a proinflammatory cytokine released during various immune challenges. A soluble TNF-alpha receptor could bind to circulating TNF and remove the proinflammatory protein. The biopharmaceutical Etanercept (Enbrel) was approved for the reduction of signs and symptoms in rheumatoid arthritis patients refractory to disease-modifying antirheumatic drugs. It is a fusion protein combining a rDNA, soluble P75 TNF receptor (this portion acts as natural antagonist to TNF) fused with a human IgG Fc region. Thus, the drug binds excess circulating TNF preventing it from binding to its membrane receptor.

Alternatively, a fused protein can be produced that consists of an antibody with an intact variable region to recognize and bind a specific target (i.e., an antifibrin antibody) along with an enzyme (i.e., tissue plasminogen activator, tPA) resulting in a more specific and potent agent (i.e., a fibrin specific thrombolytic agent). In other words, the antibody first attaches the enzyme (tPA) specifically to fibrin clots. The enzyme tPA will activate circulating plasminogen by converting it from plasminogen into plasmin. This plasmin locally attacks fibrin clots and dissolves them. The concept is called antibody-directed enzyme prodrug therapy, ADEPT.

## ■ 3D Structures of Engineered Proteins

A variety of techniques can produce structural information about the engineered protein. Among the techniques available, only protein X-ray crystallography and NMR spectroscopy have the routine ability to determine directly the experimental 3-D arrangement of atoms comprising the protein at atomic resolution. A computer can be used for protein modeling, when insufficient quantities of the engineered protein are available, or if X-ray crystallography and NMR are not amenable. While a detailed discussion of each of these techniques is well beyond the scope of this chapter, a very brief introduction of each is valuable to introduce the concepts. The references cited will provide the reader with useful resources to further explore these techniques in detail.

### Protein X-Ray Crystallography

Protein X-ray crystallography is a tremendously powerful technique (Stubbs II, 2007). Following formation of appropriate crystals of the protein, an X-ray diffraction pattern is obtained for the crystal. An electron density map is derived from the diffraction data, which subsequently provides the atom positions in the protein. While the X-ray structure obtained is a structure averaged over all of the mutant protein molecules found in the crystal (various subtle conformational differences among chemically identical molecules of the engineered protein), the technique provides a view of the spatial arrangement of the protein's atoms. Molecular interactions (i.e., ligand-protein binding) and the mechanism of catalytic reactions can be studied at the molecular level. New and exciting techniques have been developed to validate protein 3-D structure; important for modern methods of rational drug design (Joosten, et al., 2007; Laskowski and Swaminathan, 2007).

Protein X-ray crystallography is severely limited by the availability of appropriate crystals for analysis. While sufficient quantities used to be a problem, biotechnology techniques have addressed this difficulty (Bauer and Schnapp, 2007). Other limitations include the inability to get most hydrogen positional information and the fact that the X-ray structure represents a crystal structure, which is not necessarily equal to a solution structure (Schulz, 2007). An exciting advance that may overcome the serious handicap of the necessity for growing quality protein crystals to solve a 3D structure is the use of high-resolution single molecule diffraction images (Miao, et al., 2001). This new methodology utilizes a powerful X-ray free electron laser (X-FEL) and an algorithm that can solve protein structures from the X-FEL-produced diffraction patterns from single biomolecules rather than multiple molecules held in a specific crystal lattice.

Should the need to obtain quality protein crystals be eliminated, there would be an explosive increase in the number of high-resolution 3D protein structures available for use in rational, structure-based drug design (Hogg and Hilgenfeld, 2007).

### NMR Spectroscopy

The concurrent development of NMR techniques and molecular biology has led to an increased study of the 3-D structure and dynamics of proteins in solution (Clore and Gronenborn, 1998; Carlomagno, et al., 2007). Like X-ray crystallography, NMR spectroscopy generates information directly about the proximity of atoms and about the lifetimes of the through-space interactions of those atoms. Significant advantages of the protein NMR approach over X-ray crystallography include its ability to study proteins in solution, to obtain structural information about dynamic (flexible) portions of the molecule and to look specifically at hydrogen atoms. X-ray crystallography, unlike NMR, provides spatial information about all non-hydrogen atoms. NMR is now widely used as a drug discovery tool, to understand both the 3-D structure of receptors and drug-receptor interactions (Klages and Kessler, 2007).

### Protein Modeling

Protein modeling (in the broader sense, molecular modeling) is a collection of computer techniques, including computer graphics, computational chemistry, statistical methods and database management, applied to the description, analysis, and prediction of protein structures and protein properties (Charifson, 1997; Murcko et al., 1999). Protein folding (including prediction of 3-D structures), dynamics simulations, protein function and protein-molecule (ligand, DNA, protein, etc.) interactions are some of the problems that are being studied currently by protein modeling. Protein modelers often study products from protein engineering. The 3-D protein structures used in modeling are frequently derived from X-ray crystallography and NMR analyses. When structures are not available from these structural techniques, either de novo methods or homology modeling approaches must be used (Charifson, 1997; Laskowski and Swaminathan, 2007). De novo methods involve the prediction of secondary protein structure from an analysis of the amino acid sequence. Homology modeling uses the known structures of homologous or similar proteins as 3-D templates on which one constructs the framework of the protein being studied. Validation of the computer model resulting from either of these methods with experimental observations is necessary. The limited success rate for homology modeling approaches to accurately predict a protein's 3-D structure (ascertained by comparing a protein's homology modeling predicted structure with its experimentally determined X-ray crystallographic structure) has limited their broader use (Baker and Sali, 2001).

## ■ Peptide Chemistry and Peptidomimetics

Peptide chemistry and biology have become very popular fields of study since the discovery that a large number of hormones, neurotransmitters and other endogenous chemical mediators are peptides (some examples are listed in Table 5). Peptide receptors are attractive targets in drug discovery and design efforts. Thus, both peptides and proteins have the potential to be developed into useful therapeutic agents. Peptides, like the larger proteins, may be produced by various genetic methods (as described for proteins in Chapters 1, 3 and earlier in this chapter). As smaller molecules, however, chemical synthesis is quite viable. Both classical solution methods and newer solid phase approaches based on the technique originally developed by Merrifield (the chemistry occurs while the growing peptide chain is anchored

| Peptide | No. of amino acids |
|---------|---------------------|
| Angiotensin II | 8 |
| β-endorphin | 31 |
| Bradykinin | 9 |
| Cholecystokinin | 33 |
| Corticotropin | 39 |
| Dynorphin B | 17 |
| Endothelin-1 | 21 |
| Gastrin | 17 |
| Glucagon | 29 |
| Insulin | 51 (two chains) |
| Leu-enkephalin | 5 |
| Met-enkephalin | 5 |
| Neuropeptide Y | 36 |
| Neurotensin | 13 |
| Oxytocin | 9 |
| Somatostatin | 14 |
| Substance P | 11 |
| Thyrotropin releasing factor | 3 |
| Tuftsin | 4 |

**Table 5** ■ Some endogenous peptide hormones, neurotransmitters and chemical mediators.

onto a polymeric bead) have been applied to the synthesis of thousands of peptides of diverse structure (Seneci, 2000; Mitscher and Dutta, 2003; Seneci, 2007; Ashton and Moloney, 2007). Peptides of 50 amino acids or greater are synthesized by automated solid phase peptide synthesizers.

Despite their achievable synthesis, peptides suffer from a number of characteristics that make them less suitable as drugs than the classical small organic molecule agents. In most cases, peptide pharmaceuticals are characterized by low oral bioavailability, poor passage through the blood-brain barrier (for CNS targeted peptides), metabolic instability catalyzed by endogenous peptidases (hydrolysis of the amide bond), and rapid urinary and biliary excretion (Luthman and Hacksell, 1996). Also, the inherent flexibility of peptide molecules allows them to adopt multiple, low energy conformations or shapes. This property permits a peptide drug to interact with several different similar peptide receptors. Side effects and low affinity can result from this lack of selectivity at target receptor sites. Numerous peptide modifications have been studied to overcome the limitations that make peptides poorly suited as drugs (Goodman and Ro, 1995; Luthman and Hacksell, 1996; Nakanishi and Kahn, 1996; Abell, 1999; Estiarte and Rich, 2003).

### Peptidomimetics

The isolation and structure elucidation of two endogenous morphine-like pentapeptides, leu-enkephalin and metenkephalin, formally introduced the study of peptidomimetics. Morphine, a narcotic alkaloid, and the enkephalins were conclusively demonstrated to elicit their analgesia by binding to the same opioid receptor (Fig. 10). Therefore, morphine acts as a narcotic analgesic because it is a nature-synthesized mimic of the endogenous pentapeptides. Peptidomimetics (sometimes called peptide mimetics and nonpeptide mimetics) are substitutes for peptides that possess not only the peptide's affinity for interactions with receptors and/or enzymes, but also efficacy. Numerous reviews on the topic are available (Giannis and Rubsam, 1997; Ripka and Rich, 1998; Estiarte and Rich, 2003).

There are a number of approaches to the discovery of peptidomimetics that interact with specific peptide receptors (Obrecht et al., 1999). An empirical approach to peptidomimetic discovery is the screening of pure compound libraries and complex mixtures (from natural product extracts, microbial fermentations or combinatorial chemistry) (Giannis and Rubsam, 1997; Gron and HydeDeRuyscher, 2000). A screening success was the discovery of the potent cholecystokinin (CCK) receptor antagonist asperlicin (Fig. 10) from a fermentation and the subsequent

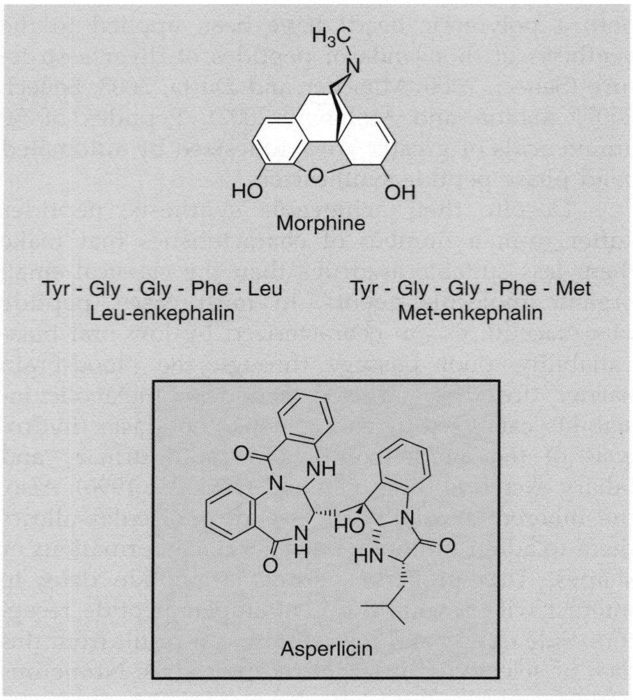

**Figure 10** ■ Discovery of peptidomimetics: opioid pentapeptides and the CCK antagonist asperlicin.

medicinal chemistry development of additional agents (Wiley and Rich, 1993). This nonpeptide natural product containing a 1,4-benzodiazepine moiety acts as a peptidomimetic antagonist at a receptor for a neuroactive peptide ligand (CCK). Computer-aided molecular modeling is often used to design better analogs (exhibiting improved affinity and selectivity) of the lead molecule discovered via such an empirical approach.

*Peptidomimetic Approaches*

The peptidomimetic approach known as "pseudopeptides" is an attempt to improve the biostability of peptides (Hirschmann et al., 1995). Numerous pseudopeptides (also called amide bond surrogates) have been prepared that substitute an amide bond bioisostere for the amide peptide bond. A bioisostere is a replacement of an atom or groups of atoms while retaining a broadly similar bioactivity. Examples of some bioisosteric peptide bond replacements are shown in Figure 11 (Luthman and Hacksell, 1996). This type of substitution changes the backbone of the peptide and may alter its conformation. Bioisosteric pseudopeptides do exhibit decreased endogenous peptidase-mediated hydrolysis, however, many still suffer from insufficient oral bioavailability. An interesting amide bond bioisostere is the tetrazole analog (a five-membered ring with four nitrogens, see Fig. 11) that also serves to restrict the backbone conformation of the peptide amide bond to the *cis*-orientation (see Chapter 2).

# CELL THERAPY AND REGENERATIVE MEDICINE

Certainly among the most exciting, yet controversial areas of biotechnology are cell therapy and regenerative medicine. The FDA defines cell therapy as, "The prevention, treatment, cure or mitigation of disease or injuries in humans by the administration of autologous, allogeneic or xenogeneic cells that have been manipulated or altered ex vivo." Thus, the goal of cell therapy, is to repair, replace or restore damaged tissues or organs. Stem cell technology is thought to hold the most potential for cell therapy. Regenerative medicine is broadly overlapping with cell therapy. It is a broad definition for innovative medical therapies that will enable the body to repair, replace, restore and regenerate damaged or diseased cells, tissues and organs. These research emphases include a variety of research areas such as stem cells, tissue engineering, biomaterials engineering, growth factors and transplantation science. The U.S. Department of Health and Human Safety report "2020—A New Vision: A Future for Regenerative Medicine" suggests that the field has the potential to exceed $500 billion within the next 20 years (Flannagan, 2007).

■ **Stem Cells**

Stem cell research is advancing at a rapid pace and is the subject of significant scientific, ethical, and political discussion (Ho and Gibaldi, 2003). A timely, informative discussion of totipotent and pluripotent stem cells, and their potential for repair of tissues and organs is well beyond the scope of this chapter. For general information about stem cells, the reader is encouraged to research the topic in any biology textbook and a plethora of websites. Specialized stem cell topics can be studied using readily available online databases (journal and abstract) and website search engines. The U.S. National Institutes of Health (NIH) has a valuable resource on stem cells that can be found at www.nih.gov/news/stemcell/index.htm. A brief introduction follows solely to provide the reader with insights into the unproven potential of pluripotent stem cell research in advancing tissue engineering capabilities.

During normal human development, a single cell is produced from the joining of a sperm cell and an egg cell (please see source for this introduction at NIH *Stem Cell Primer*, www.nih.gov/news/stemcell/primer.htm). This single cell, capable of forming an entire human, initially undergoes division into two identical daughter cells. These are totipotent cells. Each totipotent cell has the capability to differentiate into the embryo, extraembryonic membranes and tissues, and all postembryonic tissues and organs. Placing one of the identical cells (or both for identical twins) in a woman's uterus has the potential to develop into a fetus. Several cycles of cell

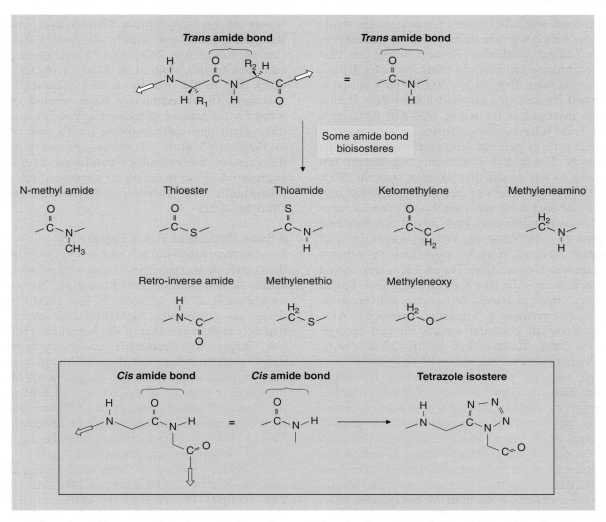

**Figure 11** ▪ Pseudopeptides: examples of some bioisosteric peptide bond replacements. *Source*: Adapted from Goodman and Ro 1995 and Luthman and Hacksell 1996.

division cause the beginning of cell specialization and the formation of a blastocyst, a hollow sphere of cells. The placenta and other supporting tissues needed for fetal development in the uterus is formed from the outer layer of cells of the blastocyst while the inner cell layer can become virtually every cell type found in the human body; "virtually" every cell type. The inner cell mass is pluripotent, that is, they are capable of giving rise to many types of cells, but not all cells and not an embryo. Their potential is not total (totipotent). Further cell divisions and specializations result in cells that are committed to give rise to cells that perform specialized functions. These multipotent stem cells are extremely important to the process of cell proliferation and differentiation occurring during early human development. Types are also found in children and adults. They may be multipotent or pluripotent.

Stem cells are cells that possess the ability to divide into daughter cells and multiply for infinite periods in culture giving rise to daughter cells with identical developmental potential and/or a cell with less potential. A totipotent stem cell can give rise to daughter totipotent stem cells and/or pluripotent stem cells. Likewise, a pluripotent stem cell can give rise to daughter pluripotent stem cells and/or multipotent stem cells, etc. For example, hematopoietic stem cells are multi-potent stem cells that give rise to multipotent hematopoietic stem cells and/or white blood cells, red blood cells and platelets (see Chapter 10). Cord (blood) stem cells are found in umbilical cords (multipotent mesenchymal stem cells) at birth. Adult stem cells are present in some fully formed organs (such as bone marrow, brain, and skin) in which they produce new cells that are damaged and/or destroyed. Therefore, pluripotent stem cells are of real potential value to tissue engineering and regenerative medicine because of their pluripotent capabilities.

Fundamental discoveries remain to be made before this bench top research can be translated into bedside clinical medicine. Results from the first controlled human cell therapy trials for heart disease are now in (Chien, 2006; Shaw, 2006). The Reinfusion of Enriched Progenitor Cells and Infarct Remodeling in Acute myocardial Infarction (REPAIR-AMI) trial studied direct intracoronary infusion of bone marrow progenitor cells in patients who had successful acute MI therapy. Small, but statistically significant improvement to left ventricular ejection fraction (5.5% vs. 3% LVEF) was observed in a double-blinded trial in those patients who received bone marrow stem cells. However, results have been mixed. Another trial attempted to repopulate injured myocardium with autologous skeletal muscle myoblasts to achieve cardiac muscle regeneration. The trial was terminated due to a lack of sufficient therapeutic effect. Spinal cord injury, stroke, diabetes, depression, autism, sickle cell anemia, Parkinson's, muscular dystrophy, ALS, and aging are all potential targets for cell therapy (Enserink, 2006; Madsen and Serup, 2006; Everts, 2007). Predicting what the future of cell therapy and stem cell research will hold is fraught with risk. However, biotechnology has experienced exponential advances in capabilities since the first edition of this text was written. If the natural requisite growth factors and appropriate differentiation/proliferation conditions can be identified and mimicked reproducibly, tissue engineering with pluripotent stem cells may give rise to repairing virtually all cells, tissues and organs including bone marrow, nerve cells, heart muscle, breast replacements, pancreatic islet cells, skin, a liver, etc. Researchers are also attempting to determine if there are conditions in which multipotent stem cells that are already more differentiated and committed to particular cell types can be converted to pluripotent capabilities.

## ■ Tissue Engineering

Tissue engineering, the multidisciplinary field of varied strategies to regenerate natural or grow new human tissues and organs, has burgeoned over the past 15 years (Mooney and Mikos, 1999; Brownlee, 2001; Petit-Zeman, 2001; Stock and Vacanti, 2001; Willis, 2004). Recently, a popular news magazine predicted that tissue engineering would be the hottest employment opportunity of the 21st century. Sometimes referred to as the more general term "regenerative medicine," tissue engineering has integrated biotechnology, clinical medicine, cell biology, developmental biology, and biomaterials engineering into an effort to overcome the challenges associated with conventional surgical approaches to tissue and organ repair or replacement. Each year, over eight million surgeries are performed in the U.S. alone to repair or replace human tissues and organs at staggering costs and significant patient discomfort (Vunjak-Novakovic, 2006). Only a fraction of patients admitted to the hospital in need of organs receive them due to the dearth of transplantable organs. Advances in biotechnology have created opportunities for the science of tissue engineering to address these challenges and improve health care. Another exciting application of tissue engineering is the delivery of biotechnology-produced drugs using engineered tissue materials as controlled-release and microfluidic drug delivery vehicles (Saltzman and Olbricht, 2002).

## ■ Some Products of Tissue Engineering

Regenerative medicine has had success in stimulating the body's own repair mechanisms by mimicking the action of endogenous growth factors. For example, recombinant DNA technology has produced such drugs as epoetin alfa, filgrastim, and sargramostim that accomplish just that in the hematopoietic system (see Chapter 10). Research is underway to test new tissue growth factors for their ability to regenerate human tissue. Active research programs are studying the effect of growth factors on wound healing, bone repair, blood vessel generation, and nerve regeneration. Successes in genomics and proteomics should have a major impact on tissue engineering as new growth factor genes are discovered.

Several products of tissue engineering are now available for use as replacement skin and cartilage. The leading skin product is graftskin (Apligraf), approved by the FDA in 1998. It is a living skin equivalent indicated for the treatment of foot and leg ulcers. Generated in tissue culture and started from cells of human foreskin removed during infants' circumcisions, graftskin possesses a dermis, epidermis and structural matrix like normal human skin tissue. In addition to skin replacement, tissue engineering has created cartilage replacements. Autologous cultured chondrocytes (Carticel) is an approved product/procedure to repair clinically significant, symptomatic painful knee cartilage damage (medial, lateral, or trochlear) caused by acute or repetitive trauma. The patient's orthopedic surgeon sends the manufacturer a biopsy of the patient's own cartilage, which is then cultured for reinjection into the knee.

Tissue engineers are actively exploring ways to create specialized tissues and vital organs. An exciting approach is the use of a scaffold made from a biodegradable polymer matrix shaped to fit the need (e.g., in the shape of a nose or an ear, etc.). An important pharmaceutical area of study is the use of hydrogels for scaffold development (Lee and Mooney, 2001). The patient's own cells, donor cells or engineered cells are used to seed the scaffold. The cell-seeded scaffold is treated with requisite growth factors and placed in an appropriate growth environment so that the cells can multiply and differentiate into the appropriate different cell types. The biopolymer degrades after transplantation providing functioning tissue or organ.

Currently, there are several clinical trials underway testing novel technologies to replace damaged bone. Transgenic pigs and other animals are being engineered to provide organs for xenotransplantation to human patients that do not cause the immune system to initiate rejection mechanisms. Methodologies to introduce genes into patients to repair tissues "on-site" are being studied. Another area of active investigation is the development of technologies that can rejuvenate old tissues by manipulation of the cell's own aging mechanisms.

## BIOTECHNOLOGY AND DRUG DISCOVERY

Pharmaceutical scientists have taken advantage of every opportunity or technique available to aid in the long, costly, and unpredictable drug discovery process. In essence, Chapter 7 is an overview of some of the many applications of biotechnology and related techniques useful in drug discovery or design, lead optimization, and development. In addition to recombinant DNA and hybridoma technology, the techniques described throughout Chapter 7 have changed the way drug research is conducted, refining the process that optimizes the useful pharmacological properties of an identified novel chemical lead and minimizing the unwanted properties. The promise of genomics, proteomics, metabolomics, pharmacogenomics/pharmacogenetics, toxicogenomics, and bioinformatics to radically change the drug discovery paradigm is eagerly anticipated (Beeley et al., 2000; Ohlstein et al., 2000; Wierenga 2002; Basu and Oyelere, 2003; Loging et al., 2007). Figure 12 shows schematically the interaction of three key elements that are essential for modern drug discovery: new targets identified by genomics, proteomics, and related technologies; validation of the identified targets; rapid, sensitive bioassays utilizing high-throughput screening methods; and new molecule creation and optimization employing a host of approaches. The key elements are underpinned at each point by bioinformatics. Several of the technologies, methods and approaches listed in Figure 12 have been described previously in this chapter. Others will be described below.

### ■ Screening and Synthesis

Traditionally, drug discovery programs relied heavily upon random screening followed by analog synthesis and lead optimization via structure-activity relationship studies. Discovery of novel, efficacious, and safer small molecule medicinal agents with appropriate drug-like characteristics is an increasingly costly and complex process (Arlington, 2000, Williams, 2007). Therefore, any method allowing for a reduction in time and money is extremely valuable. Advances in biotechnology have contributed to a greater understanding of the cause and progression of disease and have identified new therapeutic targets forming the basis of novel drug screens. New technical discoveries in the fields of proteomics for target discovery and validation, and systems biology are expected to facilitate the discovery of new agents with novel mechanisms of action for diseases that were previously difficult or impossible to treat. In an effort to decrease the cost of identifying and optimizing useful, quality drug leads against a pharmaceutically important target; researchers have developed newer approaches including high-throughput screening and high-throughput synthesis methods.

### Advances in Screening: High Throughput Screening (HTS)

Recombinant DNA technology has provided the ability to clone, express, isolate and purify receptor enzymes, membrane bound proteins, and other binding proteins in larger quantities than ever before. Instead of using receptors present in animal tissues or partially purified enzymes for screening, in vitro bioassays now utilize the exact human protein target. Applications of biotechnology to in vitro screening include the improved preparation of: (1) cloned membrane-bound receptors expressed in cell-lines carrying few endogenous receptors; (2) immobilized preparations of receptors, antibodies and other ligand-binding proteins; and (3) soluble enzymes and extracellular cell-surface expressed protein receptors. In most cases today, biotechnology contributes directly to the understanding, identification and/or the generation of the drug target being screened (e.g., radioligand binding displacement from a cloned protein receptor).

Previously, libraries of synthetic compounds along with natural products from microbial fermentation, plant extracts, marine organisms and invertebrates provide a diversity of molecular structures that were screened randomly. Screening can be made more directed if the compounds to be investigated are selected on the basis of structural information about the receptor or natural ligand. The development of sensitive radioligand binding assays and the access to fully automated, robotic screening techniques have accelerated the screening process.

High-throughput screening (HTS) provides for the bioassay of thousands of compounds in multiple assays at the same time (Houston and Banks, 2003;

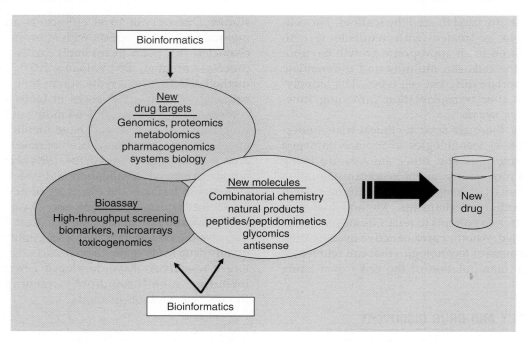

**Figure 12** ▦ Elements of modern drug discovery: impact of biotechnology.

Cik and Jurzak, 2007). The process is automated with robots and utilizes multi-well microtiter plates. While 96-well microtiter plates are a versatile standard in HTS, the development of 1536-and 3456-well nanoplate formats and enhanced robotics brings greater miniaturization and speed to cell based and biochemical assays. Now, companies can conduct 100,000 bioassays a day. In addition, modern drug discovery and lead optimization with DNA microarrays allows researchers to track hundreds to thousands of genes.

Enzyme inhibition assays and radioligand binding assays are the most common biochemical tests employed. The technology has become so sophisticated and the interactive nature of biochemical events so much better understood (through approaches such as system biology) that HT whole cell assays have become commonplace. Reporter gene assays are routinely utilized in HTS (Ullmann, 2007). Typically, a reporter gene, that is a reporter that indicates the presence or absence of a particular gene product that in tern reflects the changes in a biological process or pathway, is transfected into a desired cell. When the gene product is expressed in the living cell, the reporter gene is transcribed and the reporter is translated to yield a protein that is measured biochemically. A common reporter gene codes for the enzyme luciferase, and the intensity of the resulting green fluorescent protein (i.e., a quantitative measure of concentration) is a direct function of the assayed molecule's ability to stimulate or inhibit the biologic process or signaling pathway under

study. A further advance in HT screening technologies for lead optimization is rapid, high content pharmacology. This HT screening approach can be used to evaluate solubility, adsorption, toxicity, metabolism, etc. (Brown et al., 2003).

### High-Throughput Chemistry: Combinatorial Chemistry and Multiple Parallel Synthesis

Traditionally, small drug molecules were synthesized by joining together structural pieces in a set sequence to prepare one product. One of the most powerful tools to optimize drug discovery is automated high-throughput synthesis. When conducted in a combinatorial approach, high-throughput synthesis provides for the simultaneous preparation of hundreds or thousands of related drug candidates (Fenniri, 2000; Sucholeiki, 2001; Mason and Pickett, 2003; Pirrung, 2004). The molecular libraries generated are screened in high-throughput screening assays for the desired activity, and the most active molecules are identified and isolated for further development.

There are two overall approaches to high-throughput synthesis (Bunin et al., 2003; Mitscher and Dutta, 2003; Seneci, 2007; Ashton and Moloney, 2007). True combinatorial chemistry applies methods to substantially reduce the number of synthetic operations or steps needed to synthesize large numbers of compounds. Combichem, as it is sometimes referred to, is conducted on solid supports (resins) to facilitate the manipulations required to reduce labor. Differing from combinatorial chemistry, multiple parallel synthesis procedures apply automation to the synthetic process, but the number of operations needed to carry out a synthesis is practically the same as the conventional approach. Thus, the potential productivity of multiple parallel methods is not as high as combinatorial chemistries. Parallel chemistries can be conducted on solid-phase supports or in solution. Figure 13 provides an illustration of a combinatorial mix-and-match process in which a simple building block (a starting material such as an amino acid, peptide, heterocycle, other small molecule, etc.) is joined to one or more other simple building blocks in every possible combination.

Assigning the task to automated synthesizing equipment results in the rapid creation of large collections or libraries (as large as 10,000 compounds) of diverse molecules. Ingenious methods have been devised to direct the molecules to be synthesized, to identify the structure of the products, to purify the products via automation, and to isolate compounds. When coupled with high-throughput screening, thousands of compounds can be generated, screened, and evaluated for further development in a matter of weeks.

Building blocks include amino acids, peptides, nucleotides, carbohydrates, lipids, and a diversity of small molecule scaffolds or templates (Mason and

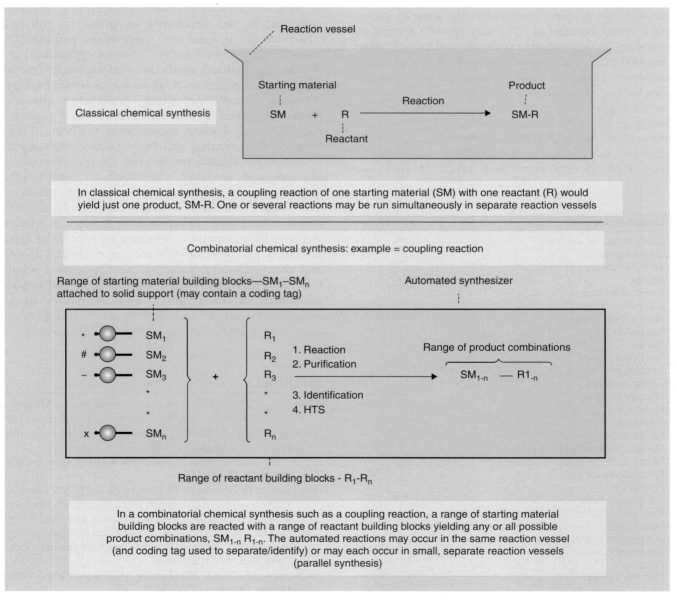

**Figure 13** ■ A schematic representation of a coupling reaction: difference between classical chemical synthesis and combinatorial chemistry.

Pickett, 2003). A selection of reaction types used in combinatorial chemistry to produce compound libraries is found in Table 6.

### ■ Chemical Genomics

Chemical genomics is an emerging "omics" technology not discussed above. The development of high-throughput screening and combinatorial chemistry coupled with omic technologies has changed the drug discovery paradigm and the approach for the investigation of target pharmacology (Bleicher, 2002; Kubinyl, 2007; Flaumenhaft, 2007). In modern drug discovery, chemical genomics (sometimes called chemogenomics or more generally included as a subset of chemical biology) involves the screening of large chemical libraries (typically combinatorially-derived "druggable" small molecule libraries covering a broad expanse of "diversity space") against all genes or gene products, such as proteins or other targets (i.e., chemical universe screened against target universe). Drug candidates are expected from the correlations observed during functional analysis of the molecule — gene product interactions. Genomic profiling by the chemical library may also yield relevant new targets and mechanisms. Chemical genomics is expected to be a critical component of drug lead identification and proof of principle

| Compound types |
| --- |
| α,β-unsaturated ketones |
| α-hydroxy acids |
| Acyl piperidines |
| Azotes |
| β-mercaptoketones |
| β-turn mimetics |
| Benzisothiazolones |
| Benzodiazepines |
| Biaryls |
| Cyclopentenones |
| Dihydropyridines |
| γ-butyrolactones |
| Glycosylamines |
| Hydantoins |
| Isoxazoles |
| Isoxazolines |
| Modified oligonucleotides |
| Peptoids |
| Piperazinediones |
| Porphyrins |
| 1,3-propanediols |
| Protease inhibitors |
| Pyrrolidines |
| Sulfamoylbenzamides |
| Tetrahydrofurans |
| Thiazole |
| Thiazolidinones |

**Table 6** ■ A sample of the diversity of compounds capable of being synthesized by combinatorial chemistry methods.

determination for selective modulators of complex enzyme systems including proteases, kinases, G-protein coupled receptors, and nuclear receptors.

### CONCLUSION

Tremendous advances have occurred in biotechnology since Watson and Crick determined the structure of DNA. Improved pharmaceuticals, novel therapeutic agents, unique diagnostic products, and new drug design tools have resulted from the escalating achievements of pharmaceutical biotechnology. While recombinant DNA technology and hybridoma techniques received most of the press in the late 1980s and early 1990s, a wealth of additional and innovative biotechnologies and approaches have been, and will continue to be, developed in order to enhance pharmaceutical research. Genomics, proteomics, transcriptomics, microarrays, pharmacogenomics/genetics, personalized medicine, metabonomics/metabolomics, toxicogenomics, glycomics, systems biology, chemical biology, genetically engineered animals, protein engineering, peptide chemistry and peptidomimetics, cell therapy, regenerative medicine, high-throughput screening and high-speed combinatorial synthesis are directly influencing the pharmaceutical sciences and are well positioned to significantly impact modern pharmaceutical care. Application of these and yet to be discovered biotechnologies will continue to reshape effective drug therapy as well as improve the competitive, challenging process of drug discovery and development of new medicinal agents and diagnostics. Pharmacists, pharmaceutical scientists and pharmacy students should be poised to take advantage of the products and techniques made available by the unprecedented scope and pace of discovery in biotechnology in the 21st century.

### REFERENCES

Abell A (1999). Advances in Amino Acid Mimetics and Peptidomimetics, Vol. 2. Stamford, Connecticut: JAI.

Aderem A, Hood L (2001). Immunology in the post-genomic era. Nature Immunol 2:373–5.

Alper J (2001). Searching for medicine's sweet spot. Science 291:2338–43.

Amaratunga D, Gohlmann H, Peeters PJ (2007). Microarrays. In: Kubinyi H, ed. Comprehensive Medicinal Chemistry II, Vol. 3. Amsterdam, The Netherlands: Elsevier, 87–106.

Andersen DC, Reilly DE (2004). Production technologies for monoclonal antibodies and their fragments. Curr Opin Biotech 15(5):456–62.

Andrawiss M (2006). Plant-made pharmaceuticals. Drug Discov Develop (3):40–50.

Arlington S (2000). The challenge of developing new drugs. Pharmaceut Execut 20:74–84.

Ashton M, Maloney B (2007). Solution phase parallel chemistry. In: Kubinyi H, ed. Comprehensive Medicinal Chemistry II, Vol. 3. Amsterdam, The Netherlands: Elsevier, 761–90.

Baez J (2005). Biopharmaceuticals derived from transgenic plants and animals. In: Knablein J, ed. Modern Biopharmaceuticals, Vol. 3. Weinheim, Germany: Wiley–VCH, 833–92.

Bagowski CP (2005). Target validation: An important early step in the development of novel biopharmaceuticals in the post-genomic era. In: Knablein J, ed. Modern Biopharmaceuticals, Vol. 2. Weinheim, Germany: Wiley–VCH, 621–47.

Baker D, Sali A (2001). Protein structure prediction and structural genomics. Science 294:93–6.

Basu S, Oyelere AK (2003). Application of recombinant DNA technology in medicinal chemistry and drug discovery. In: Abraham DJ, ed. Burger's Medicinal Chemistry and Drug Discovery, 6th ed., Vol. 2. NY: John Wiley & Sons, 81–114.

Bauer MMT, Schnapp G (2007). Protein production for three-dimensional structural analysis. In: Kubinyi H, ed. Comprehensive Medicinal Chemistry II, Vol. 3. Amsterdam, The Netherlands: Elsevier, 411–32.

Baxevanis AD (2001). Bioinformatics and the internet. In: Baxevanis AD, Ouellette BFF, eds. Bioinformatics: A Practical Guide to the Analysis of Genes and Proteins, 2nd ed. NY: John Wiley & Sons, 1–11.

Beeley L.J, Duckworth DM, Southan C (2000). The impact of genomics on drug discovery. Prog Med Chem 37:1–43.

Bikker JA, Trumpp-Kallmeyer S, Humblet C (1998). G-Protein coupled receptors: Models, mutagenesis, and drug design. J Med Chem 41:2911–27.

Blagosklonny MV, Pardee AB (2002). Conceptual biology: Unearthing the gems. Nature 416:373

Bleicher KH (2002). Chemogenomics: bridging a drug discovery gap. Curr Med Chem 9:2077–84.

Branca MA (2005). BiDil raises questions about race as a marker. Nature Rev Drug Discov 4(8):615–6.

Breslow J (1994). Lipoprotein and heart disease: Transgenic mice models helping in the search for new therapies. Bio/Technology 12:365–70.

Brown K (2000). The human genome business today. Sci Am 283:50–5.

Brown SJ, Clark IB, Pandi B (2003). Rapid, high content pharmacology. In: Abraham DJ, ed. Burger's Medicinal Chemistry and Drug Discovery, 6th ed., Vol. 2. NY: John Wiley & Sons, 71–80.

Brownlee C (2001). The mechanics of tissue engineering. Mod Drug Discov 4:35–8.

Bunin BA, Dener JM, Livingston DA (1999). Applications of combinatorial and parallel synthesis to medicinal chemistry. Ann Rep Med Chem 34:267–86.

Butte A (2002). The Use and analysis of microarray data. Nature Rev Drug Discov 1:951–60.

Caldwell JS, Chanda SK, Irelan J, Koenig R (2007). Genomics. In: Kubinyi H, ed. Comprehensive Medicinal Chemistry II, Vol. 3. Amsterdam, The Netherlands: Elsevier, 1–26.

Cantor CR, Smith CL (1999). Genomics — The Science and Technology Behind the Human Genome Project. NY: John Wiley & Sons.

Cargill M, Altshuler A, Ireland J, et al. (1999). Characterization of single-nucleotide polymorphisms in coding regions of human genes. Nature Genet 22:231–8.

Carlomagno T, Baldus M, Griesinger C (2007). Bio-nuclear magnetic resonance. In: Kubinyi H, ed. Comprehensive Medicinal Chemistry II, Vol. 3. Amsterdam, The Netherlands: Elsevier, 473–506.

Carter PJ (2006). Potent antibody therapeutics by design. Nature Rev Immunol 6:343–57.

Cavallari LH (2004). Cardiovascular diseases. In: Allen WL, Johnson JA, Knoell DL, Kolesar, JM, McInerney JD, McLeod HL, Spencer HT, Tami JA, eds. Pharmacogenomics: Applications to Patient Care. Kansas City, Missouri: American College of Clinical Pharmacy, 495–532.

Cebon J, Nicola N, Ward M, et al. (1990). Granulocyte-macrophage colony stimulating factor from human lymphocytes. J Biol Chem 265:4483–91.

Charifson PS (1997). Practical Application of Computer-Aided Drug Design. NY: Marcel Dekker.

Chien K (2006). Making a play at regrowing hearts. The Scientist 20(8):34–8.

Chondonia J-M, Brenner SE (2006). The impact of structural genomics. Science 311:347–51.

Chowdhury PS, Wu H (2005). Tailor-made antibody therapeutics. Methods 36(1):11–24.

Cik M, Jurzak (2007). High-throughput and high-content screening. In: Kubinyi H, ed. Comprehensive Medicinal Chemistry II, Vol. 3. Amsterdam, The Netherlands: Elsevier, 679–96.

Clark MS (1999). Comparative genomics: The key to understanding the human genome project. Bioessays 21:121–30.

Cleland JL, Craik CS (1996). Protein Engineering Principles and Practice. NY: Wiley–Liss.

Clore GM, Gronenborn AM (1998). Determining the structures of large proteins and protein complexes by NMR. TIBECH 16:22–34.

Collins FS, Barker AD (2007). Mapping the cancer genome. Sci Am 296(3):50–7.

Collins F, Galas D (1993). A new five-year plan for the U.S. human genome. Science 262:43–6.

Craik CS, Roczniak S, Largman C, Rutter WJ (1987). The catalytic role of the active site aspartic acid in serine proteases. Science 237:909–13.

Davidson RG, McInerney JD (2004). Principles of genetic medicine. In: Allen WL, Johnson JA, Knoell DL, Kolesar JM, McInerney JD, McLeod HL, Spencer HT, Tami JA, eds. Pharmacogenomics: Applications to Patient Care. Kansas City, Missouri: American College of Clinical Pharmacy, 1–52.

Delnomdedieu M, Schneider RP (2005). The utility of metabonomics for drug safety assessment. Ann Rep Med Chem 40:387–402.

DePrimo SE (2007). Biomarkers. In: Kubinyi H, ed. Comprehensive Medicinal Chemistry II, Vol. 3. Amsterdam, The Netherlands: Elsevier, 69–85.

Dugas H (1999). Bioorganic Chemistry: A Chemical Approach to Enzyme Action, 3rd ed. NY: Springer–Verlag.

Dunn DA, Kooyman DL, Pinkert CA (2005). Transgenic animals and their impact on the drug discovery industry. Drug Discov Today 10(11):757–67.

Echelard Y, Meade HM, Ziomek CA (2005). The first biopharmaceutical from transgenic animals: Atryn. In: Knablein J, ed. Modern Biopharmaceuticals, Vol. 3. Weinheim, Germany: Wiley–VCH, 995–1020.

Edwards AM, Arrowsmith CH, Pallieres B (2000). Proteomics: new tools for a new era. Mod Drug Discov September 3:34–44.

Ellingrod VL, Bishop J (2004). Central nervous system/psychiatry. In: Allen WL, Johnson JA, Knoell DL, Kolesar JM, McInerney JD, McLeod HL, Spencer HT, Tami JA, eds. Pharmacogenomics: Applications to Patient Care. Kansas City, Missouri: American College of Clinical Pharmacy, 533–70.

Emmett A (2000). The state of bioinformatics. The Scientist 14(23):1, 10, 12, 19.

Enserink M (2006). Selling the stem cell dream. Science 313:160–3.

Evans L (2003). Proteomic: A new force in drug discovery. Current Drug Discov (3):15–9.

Evans WE, Relling MV (1999). Pharmacogenomics: Translating functional genomics into rational therapies. Science 286:487–91.

Everts S (2007). Taming stem cells. Chem Eng News 85(Jan 15):19–26.

Felton MJ (2001). Bioinformatics: The child of success. Mod Drug Discov 4:25–8.

Fenniri H (2000). Combinatorial Chemistry: A Practical Approach. Oxford, UK: Oxford University Press.

Fernie AR, Trethewey RN, Krotzky AJ, Willmitzer L (2004) Metabolite profiling: From diagnostics to systems biology. Nature Rev Cancer 4:638–44.

Flanagan N (2007) Regenerative medicine enters the realm of reality. Genet Eng Biotech News 27(7):1, 52–4.

Flaumenhaft R (2007). Chemical biology. In: Kubinyi H, ed. Comprehensive Medicinal Chemistry II, Vol. 3. Amsterdam, The Netherlands: Elsevier, 129–49.

Fodor WL, William BL, Matis LA, et al. (1994). Expression of a functional human complement inhibitor in a transgenic pig as a model for the prevention of xenogeneic hyperacute organ rejection. Proc Natl Acad Sci USA 91:11153–7.

Fothergill-Gilmore LA (1993). Recombinant protein technology. In: Franks F, ed. Protein Biotechnology. Totowa, NJ: Humana Press, 467–87.

Fox JL (2006). Turning plants into protein factories. Nature Biotech 24(10):1191–3.

Fox RJ, Davis SC, Mundorff EC, et al. (2007). Improving catalytic function by ProSAR-driven enzyme evolution. Nature Biotech 25:338–44.

Frank R, Hargreaves R (2003). Clinical biomarkers in drug discovery and development. Nature Rev Drug Discov 2:564–5.

Freeman TR (2001). Pharmacogenomics: Opening new vistas in pharmacotherapy. J Am Pharmaceut Assoc 41:629–30.

Frye RF (2004). Pharmacogenetics of oxidative drug metabolism and its clinical applications. In: Allen WL, Johnson JA, Knoell DL, Kolesar JM, McInerney JD, McLeod HL, Spencer HT, Tami JA, eds. Pharmacogenomics: Applications to Patient Care. Kansas City, Missouri: American College of Clinical Pharmacy, 273–307.

Fukuda M, Hindsgaul O (2000). Molecular and Cellular Glycobiology. Oxford, UK: Oxford University Press.

Furness LM (2002). Genomics applications that facilitate the understanding of drug action and toxicity. In: Licinio J, Wong M-L, eds. Pharmacogenomics, The Search for Individualized Therapies. Weinheim, Germany: Wiley–BCH Verlag GmbH & Co., 83–125.

Garner I, Colman A (1998). Therapeutic proteins form livestock. In: Clark AJ, ed. Animal Breeding-Technology for the 21st Century. Amsterdam: Harwood Academic Publishers, 215–27.

Geistlinger J, Ahnert P (2005). Large-scale detection of genetic variation: The key to personalized medicine. In: Knablein J, ed. Modern Biopharmaceuticals, Vol. 2. Weinheim, Germany: Wiley–VCH, 71–98.

Giannis A, Rubsam F (1997). Peptidomimetics in drug design. Adv. Drug Res 29:1–78.

Goodman M, Ro S (1995). Peptidomimetics for drug design. In: Wolff ME, ed. Burger's Medicinal Chemistry, 5th ed., Vol. 1. NY: John Wiley & Sons, 803–61.

Gordon JW, Ruddle FH (1981). Integration and stable germ line transmission of genes injected into mouse pronuclei. Science 214:1244–6.

Grant DM, Phillips MS (2001). Technologies for analysis of single-nucleotide polymorphisms. In: Kalow W, Meyer UA, Tyndale RF, eds. Pharmacogenomics. NY: Marcel Dekker, 183–9.

Gron H, Hyde-DeRuyscher R (2000). Peptides as tools in drug discovery. Curr Opin Drug Discovery Dev 3:636–45.

Griffiths AJF, Miller JH, Suzuki DT, Lewontin RC, Gelbart WM (2000). An Introduction to Genetic Analysis, 7th ed. NY: W.H. Freeman and Company.

Guild BC (1999). Genomics, target selection, validation, and assay considerations in the development of antibacterial screens. Ann Rep Med Chem 34:227–36.

Gurwitz D, Manolopoulos VG (2007). Personalized medicine. In: Kennewell PD, ed. Comprehensive Medicinal Chemistry II, Vol. 2. Amsterdam, The Netherlands: Elsevier, 279–95.

Gutjahr TS, Reinhardt C (2005). The development of herceptin: Paving the way for individualized cancer therapy. In: Knablein J, ed. Modern Biopharmaceuticals, Vol. 2. Weinheim, Germany: Wiley–VCH, 127–50.

Hardison RC (2003). Comparative genomics. Pub Lib Sci (Biol) 1(2):e58.

Hirschmann R, Smith III AB, Sprengeler PA (1995). Some interactions of macromolecules with low molecular weight ligands: Recent advances in peptidomimetic research. In: Dean, PM, Jolles G, Newton CG, eds. New Perspectives in Drug Design. San Diego, CA: Academic Press, 1–14.

Ho RJY, Gibaldi M (2003). Gene and cell therapy. In: Ho RJY, Gibaldi M, eds. Biotechnology and Biopharmaceuticals. Hoboken, NJ: Wiley–Liss, 401–26.

Hogg T, Hilgenfeld H (2007). Protein crystallography in drug discovery. In: Kubinyi H, ed. Comprehensive

Medicinal Chemistry II, Vol. 3. Amsterdam, The Netherlands: Elsevier, 875–900.

Hoogenboom HR (2005). Selecting and screening recombinant antibody libraries. Nature Biotech 23(9):1105–16.

Hopkins AL, Groom CR (2002). The druggable genome. Nature Drug Discov 1:727–30.

Houston JG, Banks MN (2003). High-throughput screening for lead discovery. In: Abraham DJ, ed. Burger's Medicinal Chemistry and Drug Discovery, 6th ed., Vol. 2. NY: John Wiley & Sons, 37–69.

Huang S-M, Lesko LJ (2005). The role of pharmacogenetics/pharmacogenomics in drug development and regulatory review: Current status. In: Knablein J, ed. Modern Biopharmaceuticals. Weinheim, Germany: Wiley–BCH Verlag GmbH & Co. KgaA, 49–70.

Isola LM, Gordon JW (1991). Transgenic animals: a new era in developmental biology and medicine. In: First NL, Haseltine FP, eds. Transgenic Animals. Boston, MA: Butterworth–Heinemann, 3–20.

Jirtle RL, Skinner MK (2007). Environmental epigenomics and disease susceptibility. Nature Rev Genet 8(4): 253–62.

Johnson AC, Reitz M (1998). Site-directed mutagenesis. In: Greene JJ, Rao VB, eds. Recombinant DNA Principles and Methodologies. NY: Marcel Dekker, 699–719.

Johnson JA (2004). Drug target pharmacogenetics. In: Allen WL, Johnson JA, Knoell DL, Kolesar JM, McInerney JD, McLeod HL, Spencer HT, Tami JA, eds. Pharmacogenomics: Applications to Patient Care. Kansas City, Missouri: American College of Clinical Pharmacy, 337–75.

Joosten RP, Chinea G, Kleywegt GJ, Vriend G (2007). Protein three-dimensional structure validation. In: Kubinyi H, ed. Comprehensive Medicinal Chemistry II, Vol. 3. Amsterdam, The Netherlands: Elsevier, 507–30.

Kalow W (2001). Historical aspects of pharmacogenetics. In: Kalow W, Meyer UA, Tyndale RF, eds. Pharmacogenomics. NY: Marcel Dekker, 1–9.

Kalow W (2004). Pharmacogenetics: A historical perspective. In: Allen WL, Johnson JA, Knoell DL, Kolesar JM, McInerney JD, McLeod HL, Spencer HT, Tami JA, eds. Pharmacogenomics: Applications to Patient Care. Kansas City, Missouri: American College of Clinical Pharmacy, 251–72.

Karow J (2000). The "Other" Genomes. Sci Am 283:53.

Kassam S, Meyer P, Corfield A, Mikuz G, Sergi C (2005) Single nucleotide polymorphisms (SNPs): History, biotechnological outlook and practical applications. Current Pharmacogenomics 3(3):237–45.

Khan J, Bittner ML, Chen Y, Meltzer PS, Trent JM (1999). DNA microarray technology: The anticipated impact on the study of human disease. Biochim Biophys Acta 1423:M17–28.

Klages J, Kessler H (2007). Nuclear magnetic resonance in drug discovery. In: Kubinyi H, ed. Comprehensive Medicinal Chemistry II, Vol. 3. Amsterdam, The Netherlands: Elsevier, 901–20.

Klimyuk V, Marillonnet S, Knablein J, McCaman M, Gleba Y (2005). Biopharmaceuticals derived from transgenic plants and animals. In: Knablein J, ed. Modern Biopharmaceuticals, Vol. 3. Weinheim, Germany: Wiley–VCH, 893–917.

Klipp E, Herwig R, Kowald A, Wierling C, Lehrach H (2005). Basic principles. In: Klipp E, Herwig R, Kowald A, Wierling C, Lehrach H, eds. Systems Biology in Practice. Weinheim, Germany: Wiley–BCH Verlag GmbH & Co. KgaA, 3–17.

Knoell DL, Sadee W (2004). Applications of genomics in human health and complex disease. In: Allen WL, Johnson JA, Knoell DL, Kolesar JM, McInerney JD, McLeod HL, Spencer HT, Tami JA, eds. Pharmacogenomics: Applications to Patient Care. Kansas City, Missouri: American College of Clinical Pharmacy, 193–224.

Kobata A (1996). Function and pathology of the sugar chains of human immunoglobulin G. Glycobiology 1:5–8.

Kolesar JM (2004). Oncology and hematology. In: Allen WL, Johnson JA, Knoell DL, Kolesar JM, McInerney JD, McLeod HL, Spencer HT, Tami JA, eds. Pharmacogenomics: Applications to Patient Care. Kansas City, Missouri: American College of Clinical Pharmacy, 443–72.

Kramer R, Cohen D (2005). Functional genomics to new drug targets. Nature Rev Drug Discov 4:965–72.

Kreider BL (2001). Proteomics:defining protein function in the post genomics Era. Ann Rep Med Chem 36:227–34.

Kroetz DL, Nguyen TD (2004). Drug transporter pharmacogenetics. In: Allen WL, Johnson, JA, Knoell DL, Kolesar JM, McInerney, JD, McLeod HL, Spencer HT, Tami JA, eds. Pharmacogenomics: Applications to Patient Care. Kansas City, Missouri: American College of Clinical Pharmacy, 309–36.

Kubinyi H (2007). Chemogenomics. In: Kubinyi H, ed. Comprehensive Medicinal Chemistry II, Vol. 3. Amsterdam, The Netherlands: Elsevier, 921–37.

Laskowski RA, Swaminathan GJ (2007). Problems of protein three-dimensional structures. In: Kubinyi H, ed. Comprehensive Medicinal Chemistry II, Vol. 3. Amsterdam, The Netherlands: Elsevier, 531–50.

Lau KF, Sakul H (2000). Pharmacogenomics. Ann Rep Med Chem 36:261–9.

Lee KY, Mooney DJ (2001). Hydrogels for tissue engineering. Chem Rev: 101:1869–1879.

Lee LJ, Hughes TR, Frey BJ (2006). How many new genes are there? Science 311:1709.

Lengauer T, Hartmann C (2007). Bioinformatics. In: Kubinyi H, Comprehensive Medicinal Chemistry II, Vol. 3. Amsterdam, The Netherlands: Elsevier, 315–48.

Lesney MS (2003). A dnockouts tale. Modern drug discov., 6 (6):26–31.

Lima JJ, Wang J (2004). Respiratory Diseases. In: Allen WL, Johnson JA, Knoell, DL, Kolesar, JM, McInerney, JD, McLeod HL, Spencer HT, Tami JA, eds. Pharmacogenomics: Applications to Patient Care., Kansas City, Missouri: American College of Clinical Pharmacy, 571–615.

Lindon JC, Holmes E, Nicholson JK (2005). An overview of metabonomics. In: Robertson, DG, Lindon J, Nicholson, JK, Holmes E, eds. Metabonomics in Toxicity. Boca Raton, Florida: Taylor & Francis Group, 1–26.

Lindpainter K (2007). Pharmacogenomics. In: Kubinyi H, ed. Comprehensive Medicinal Chemistry II, Vol. 3. Amsterdam, The Netherlands: Elsevier, 51–68.

Liskamp RMJ (1994). Conformationally restricted amino acids and dipeptides, (non)peptidomimetics and secondary structure mimetics. Recl Trav Chim Pays–Bas 113:1–19.

Loging W, Harland L, Williams–Jones B (2007). High-throughput electronic biology: mining information for drug discovery. Nature Rev Drug Discov 6(3):220–30.

Luthman K, Hacksell U (1996). Peptides and peptidomimetics. In: Krogsgaard-Larsen P, Liljefors T, Madsen U, eds. A Textbook of Drug Design and Development, 2nd ed. Amsterdam, The Netherlands: Harwood Academic Publishers GmbH, 386–406.

Madsen OD, Serup P (2006). Towards cell therapy for diabetes. Nature Biotech 24(12):1481–3.

Mak TW, Penninger JM, Ohashi PS (2001). Knockout mice: A paradigm shift in modern immunology. NatureRev Immunol 1:11–9.

Marra MA et al. (2003). The genome Sequence of the SARS-Associated Coronavirus. Science 300:1399–404.

Martin M-J, Kulikova T, Pruess M, Apeeiler R (2007). Gene and protein sequence databases. In: Kubinyi H, ed. Comprehensive Medicinal Chemistry II, Vol. 3. Amsterdam, The Netherlands: Elsevier, 349–72.

Mason JS, Pickett SD (2003). Combinatorial library design, molecular similarity, and diversity applications. In: Abraham DJ, ed. Burger's Medicinal Chemistry and Drug Discovery, 6th ed., Vol. 1. NY: John Wiley & Sons, 187–242.

Makowka L (1993). Pig liver xenografts as a temporary bridge for human allografting. Xenotransplant 1:27–9.

Mayfield SP, Franklin SE (2005). Expression of human antibodies in eukaryotic micro-algea. Vaccine 23(15):1828–32.

McAuliffe JC, Hindsgaul JC (2000). Carbohydrates in medicine. In: Fukuda M, Hindsgaul O, eds. Molecular and Cellular Glycobiology. Oxford, UK: Oxford University Press, 249–85.

McCafferty J, Glover DR (2000). Engineering therapeutic proteins. Curr Opin Struct Biol 10:417–20.

McCarthy JJ (2005). Turning SNPs into useful markers of drug response. In: Licinio J, Wong M-L, eds. Pharmacogenomics: The Search for Individualized Therapies. Weinheim, Germany: Wiley–BCH Verlag GmbH & Co. KgaA, 35–55.

McCurry KR, Kooyman DL, Alvarado CG, et al. (1995). Human complement regulatory proteins protect swine-to-primate cardiac xenografts from humoral injury. Nature Med 1:423–7.

Miao J, Hodgson KO, Sayre D (2001). An approach to three-dimensional structures of biomolecules by using single-molecule diffraction images. Proc Natl Acad Sci USA 98:6641–5.

Mitscher LA, Dutta A (2003). Combinatorial chemistry and multiple parallel synthesis. In: Abraham DJ, ed. Burger's Medicinal Chemistry and Drug Discovery, 6th ed., Vol. 2. NY: John Wiley & Sons, 1–35.

Mooney DJ, Mikos AG (1999). Growing new organs. Sci Amer, 281:60–5.

Murcko MA, Caron PR, Charifson PS (1999). Structure-based drug design. Ann Rep Med Chem 34:297–306.

Nakanishi H, Kahn M (1996). Design of peptidomimetics. In: Wemuth CG, ed. The Practice of Medicinal Chemistry. San Diego, California: Academic Press, 570–90.

Narang SA (1990). Protein Engineering, Approaches to the Manipulation of Protein Folding. Stoneham, Massachusetts: Butterworth Publishers.

Nicholson JK, Wilson ID (2003). Understanding 'Global' systems biology: Metabonomics and the continuum of metabolism. Nature Rev Drug Discov 2:668–76.

Nirmala NR (2006). Genomic data mining and its impact on drug discovery. Ann Rep Med Chem 41:319–30.

Nixon AE, Ostermeier M, Benkovic SJ (1998). Hybrid enzymes: Manipulating enzyme design. TIBECH 16:258–64.

Obrecht D, Altorfer M, Robinson JA (1999). Novel peptide mimetic building blocks and strategies for efficient lead finding. Adv MedChem 4:1–68.

Oelschlaeger P, Mayo SL (2005). Hydroxyl groups in the (beta)beta sandwich of metallo-beta-lactamases favor enzyme activity: A computational protein design study. J Mol Biol 350(3):395–401.

Ohlstein EH, Ruffolo Jr RR, Elliott JD (2000). Drug discovery in the next millennium. Annu Rev Pharmacol Toxicol 40:177–91.

Olah M, Oprea TI (2007). Bioactivity databases. In: Kubinyi H, ed. Comprehensive Medicinal Chemistry II, Vol. 3. Amsterdam, The Netherlands: Elsevier, 293–314.

Ossorio P (2004). Societal and ethical issues in pharmacogenomics. In: Allen WL, Johnson JA, Knoell DL, Kolesar JM, McInerney JD, McLeod HL, Spencer HT, Tami JA, eds. Pharmacogenomics: Applications to Patient Care. Kansas City, Missouri: American College of Clinical Pharmacy, 399–442.

Pelletier JN (2007). Sequence-activity relationships guide directed evolution. Nature Biotech 25(3):297–8.

Pennisi E (2000). Genomics comes of age. Science 290:2220–1.

Petit-Zeman S (2001). Regenerative medicine. Nature Biotech 19:201–6.

Petricoin EF, Zoon KC, Kohn EC, Barrett JC, Liotta LA (2002). Clinical Proteomics: Translating benchside promise into bedside reality. Nature Rev Drug Discov 1:683–709.

Pien HH, Fischman AJ, Thrall JH, Sorensen AG (2005). Using imaging biomarkers to accelerate drug development and clinical trials. Drug Discov Today 10(4):259–66.

Pirrung MC (2004). Molecular Diversity and Combinatorial Chemistry. Amsterdam, The Netherlands: Elsevier.

Pluckthun A (1992). Mono- and bivalent antibody fragments produced in Escherichia coli: engineering, folding and antigen binding. Immunol Rev 130:151–8.

Powell K (2003). Barnyard biotech — lame duck or golden goose? Nature Biotech 21(9):965–7.

Rader RA (2006). Biopharmaceutical approvals review. Genet Eng News 26(8):70–4.

Rashidi HH, Buehler LK (2000). Bioinformatics Basics — Applications in Biological Science and Medicine. Boca Raton, Florida: CRC Press, 1–32.

Richardson JS, Richardson DC (1990). The de novo synthesis of proteins. In: Bradshaw RA, Purton M, eds. Proteins: Form and Function. Cambridge, England: Elsevier Trends Journal, 173–82.

Ripka AS, Rich DH (1998). Peptidomimetic design. Curr Opin Chem Biol 2:441–52.

Roberts GW, Swinton J (2001). In silico proteomics: Playing by the rules. Curr Drug Discov August:30–3.

Rockett JC (2003). The future of toxicogenomics. In: Burczynski ME, ed. An Introduction to Toxicogenomics. Boca Raton, Florida: CRC Press LLC, 299–317.

Rogers PD (2004). Infectious diseases. In: Allen WL, Johnson JA, Knoell DL, Kolesar JM, McInerney JD, McLeod HL, Spencer HT, Tami JA, eds. Pharmacogenomics: Applications to Patient Care. Kansas City, Missouri: American College of Clinical Pharmacy, 473–93.

Rothberg BEG, Pena CEA, Rothberg JM (2005). A systems biology approach to target identification and validation for human chronic disease drug discovery. In: Knablein J, ed. Modern Biopharmaceuticals, Design, Development and Optimization Vol. 1. Weinheim, Germany: Wiley–BCH Verlag GmbH & Co. KgaA, 99–125.

Rudolph NS (1995). Advances continue in production of proteins in transgenic animal milk. Genet Eng News October 15:8–9.

Rudolph NS (2000). Biopharmaceutical production in transgenic livestock. TIBTECH, 17:367–74.

Saadi S, Platt JL (1997). Immunology of xenotransplantation. Life Sci 62:365–87.

Saeks J (2001). Towards a proteomic future. Curr Drug Discov August:9–10.

Sailor MJ (1997). The Lamb That Roared. Science 278:2038–9.

Saltzman WM, Olbricht WL (2002). Building drug delivery into tissue engineering. Nature Rev drug Discov 1:177–86.

Schniecke AE, Kind AJ, Ritchie WA, et al. (1997). Human factor IX transgenic sheep produced by transfer of nuclei from transfected fetal fibroblasts. Science 278:2130–3.

Shultz LD, Ishikawa F, Greiner DL (2007). Humanized mice in translational biomedical research. Nature Rev Immunol 7(2):118–30.

Schulz GE (2007). Protein crystallization. In: Kubinyi H, ed. Comprehensive Medicinal Chemistry II, Vol. 3. Amsterdam, The Netherlands: Elsevier, 433–48.

Sedivy JM, Joyner AL (1992). Gene Targeting. NY: W.H. Freeman & Co.

Seneci P (2000). Solid–Phase Synthesis and Combinatorial Technologies. NY: Wiley-Interscience.

Seneci P (2007). Combinatorial chemistry. In: Kubinyi H, ed. Comprehensive Medicinal Chemistry II, Vol. 3. Amsterdam, The Netherlands: Elsevier, 315–48.

Shaffer, C (2006). Taking biomarkers into the clinic. Drug Discov Develop 9 (6):60–4.

Shaw G (2006). Can stem cells repair a broken heart. Drug Discov Develop November: 20–6.

Silber BM (2001). Pharmacogenomics, biomarkers, and the promise of personalized medicine. In: Kalow W, Meyer UA, Tyndale RF, eds. Pharmacogenomics. NY: Marcel Dekker, 11–31.

Sharpless NE, DePinho RA (2006). The mighty mouse: genetically engineered mouse models in cancer drug development. Nature Rev Drug Discov 5, 9, 741–754.

Sjoblom T et al. (2006). The consensus coding sequences of human breast and colorectal cancers. Science 314:268–74.

Staff (2006). Biopharmaceutical benchmarks. Nature Biotech 24(7), table inset.

Staff (2007). A mouse for all reasons — The international mouse knockout consortium. Cell 128:9–13.

States DJ, Omenn GS, Blackwell TW, et al. (2006). Challenges in deriving high-confidence protein identifications from data gathered by HUPO plasma proteome collaborative study. Nature Biotech 24:333–8.

Stock UA, Vacanti JP (2001). Tissue engineering: current state and prospects. Ann Rev Med 52:443–51.

Stubbs II MT (2007). Protein crystallization. In: Kubinyi H, ed. Comprehensive Medicinal Chemistry II, Vol. 3. Amsterdam, The Netherlands: Elsevier, 449–72.

Subramanian A, Tamayo P, Mootha VK, et al. (2005). Gene set enrichment analysis: A knowledge-based approach for interpreting genome-wide expression profiles. Proc Natl Acad Sci USA 102(43):15545–50.

Sucholeiki I (2001). High–Throughput Synthesis: Principles and Practices. NY: Marcel Dekker.

Takeuchi M, Takasaki S, Shimada M, Kobata A (1990). Role of sugar chains in the in vitro biological activity in human erythropoietin produced in recombinant Chinese hamster ovary cells. J Biol Chem 265:12127–30.

Temple LKF, McLeod RS, Gallinger S, Wright JG (2001). Defining disease in the genomics era. Science 293:807–8.

The Genome International Sequencing Consortium. (2001). Initial sequencing and analysis of the human genome. Nature 409:860–921.

Thorton M, Gladwin A, Payne R, et al. (2005). Automation and validation of DNA–banking systems. Drug Discov Today 10(20):1369–75.

Ullmann D (2007). Fluorescence screening assays. In: Kubinyi H, ed. Comprehensive Medicinal Chemistry II, Vol. 3. Amsterdam, The Netherlands: Elsevier, 599–615.

Vaince F, Bona J, Fathallah-Shaykh HM (2006). Microarray data analysis: current practices and future directions. Curr Pharmacogenom 4:209–18.

Valgus (2004). Pharmacogenomics in drug discovery and drug development. In: Allen WL, Johnson JA, Knoell DL, Kolesar JM, McInerney JD, McLeod HL, Spencer HT, Tami JA, eds. Pharmacogenomics: Applications to Patient Care. Kansas City, Missouri: American College of Clinical Pharmacy, 377–97.

VanderSpek JC, Mindell JA, Finkelstein A, Murphy JR (1993). Structure/function analysis of the transmemberane domain of $DAB_{389}$-interleukin-2, an interleukin-2 receptor-targeted fusion toxin. The amphipathic helical region of the transmembrane domain is essential for the efficient delivery of the catalytic domain to the cytosol of target cells. J Biol Chem 268:12077–82.

Varkin A, Cummings R, Esko J, Freeze H, Hart G, Marth J (1999). Essentials of Glycobiology. LaJolla, CA: Cold Spring Harbor Laboratory Press.

Venter JC, et al. (2001). The sequence of the human genome. Science 291:1304–51.

Voshol H, Hoving S, van Oostrum J (2007). Proteomics. In: Kubinyi H, ed. Comprehensive Medicinal Chemistry II, Vol. 3. Amsterdam, The Netherlands: Elsevier, 28–50.

Vunjak-Novakovic G (2006). Transplants made to order. The Scientist 20:35–41.

Walsh G, Jefferis R (2006). Post-translational modifications in the context of therapeutic proteins. Nature Biotech 24(10):1241–52.

Warner S (2004). Diagnostics + Therapy = Theranostics. The Scientist 18(16):38–9.

Watkins KJ (2001). Bioinformatics: Making sense of information mined from the human genome is a massive undertaking for a fledgling industry. Chem Eng News 79(Feb 19):29–45.

Weckwerth W, Morgenthal K (2005). Metabolomics: From pattern recognition to biological interpretation. Drug Discov Today 10(22):1551–8.

Weinshilboum R, Wang L (2004) Pharmacogenomics: Bench to bedside. Nature Rev Drug Discov 3:739–48.

Wierenga W (2002). The Motivation: A Top-Down View. In: Mei H-Y, Czarnik AW, eds. Integrated Drug Discovery Technologies. NY: Marcel Dekker, 1–17.

Wildt S, Gerngross TU (2005). The humanization of N-glycosylation pathways in yeast. Nature Rev Microbiol 3(2):119–26.

Wiley RA, Rich DH (1993). Peptidomimetics derived from natural products. Med Res Rev 13:327–84.

Williams M (2007). Enabling technologies in drug discovery: The technical and cultural integration of the new with the old. In: Moos WH, ed. Comprehensive Medicinal Chemistry II, Vol. 2. Amsterdam, The Netherlands: Elsevier, 265–88.

Williams SA, Slavin DE, Wagner JA, Webster CJ (2006). A cost effectiveness approach to the qualification and acceptance of biomarkers. Nature Rev Drug Discov 5:897–902.

Willis RC (2004). Piece by Piece. Modern Drug Discov 7 (9):34–9.

Wright FA, et al. (2001). A draft annotation and overview of the human genome. Genome Biol 2:1–18.

Zhang SH, Reddick RL, Piedrahita JA, Maeda N (1992). Spontaneous hypercholesterolemia and arterial lesions in mice lacking apolipoprotein E. Science 258:468.

Zheng HX, Burckart GJ (2004). Transplantation. In: Allen WL, Johnson JA, Knoell DL, Kolesar JM, McInerney JD, McLeod HL, Spencer HT, Tami JA, eds. Pharmacogenomics: Applications to Patient Care. Kansas City, Missouri: American College of Clinical Pharmacy, 617–48.

Zhou S (2006). Clinical pharmacogenomics of thiopurine S-methyltransferase. Curr Clin Pharmacol 1:119–28.

## FURTHER READING

Allen WL, Johnson JA, Knoell DL, Kolesar JM, McInerney JD, McLeod HL, Spencer HT, Tami JA, eds. (2004). Pharmacogenomics: Applications to Patient Care. Kansas City, Missouri: American College of Clinical Pharmacy.

Baxevanis AD, Ouellette BFF (2001). Bioinformatics: A Practical Guide to the Analysis of Genes and Proteins. NY: John Wiley and Sons.

Bolon B (2007). Genetically engineered animals. In: Kubinyi H, ed. Comprehensive Medicinal Chemistry II, Vol. 3. Amsterdam, The Netherlands: Elsevier, 151–70.

Dunn MJ (2000). From Genome to Proteome: Advances in the Practice and Application of Proteomics. Weinheim, Federal Republic of Germany: Wiley–VCH.

Ghose AK, Viswanadhan VN, eds. (2001). Combinatorial Library Design and Evaluation. NY: Marcel Dekker.

Hartl DL, Jones EW (2001). Genetics: Analysis of Genes and Genomes. Sudbury, MA: Jones and Bartlett Publishers.

Ho RJY, Gibaldi M (2003). Biotechnology and biopharmaceuticals. Hoboken, NJ: John Wiley & Sons.

Houdebine LM (1997). Transgenic animals—generation and use. Amsterdam: Harwood Academic Publishers.

Hunt SP, Livesey FJ (2000). Functional genomics: approaches and methodologies. In: Functional Genomics Oxford England: Oxford University Press,1–7.

Kalow W Meyer UA, Tyndale RF (2001). Pharmacogenomics. NY: Marcel Dekker.

Kayser O, Muller RH (2004). Pharmaceutical Biotechnology — Drug Discovery and Clinical Applications. Weinheim, Germany: Wiley–VCH.

Kubinyi H, Muller G, eds. (2004). Chemogenomics in Drug Discovery Vol. 22. Weinheim, Germany: Wiley–BCH Verlag GmbH & Co. KgaA.

Mei H-Y, Czarnik AW (2002). Integrated Drug Discovery Technologies. NY: Marcel Dekker.

Patrick Jr CW, Mikos AG, McIntire LV (1998). Frontiers in Tissue Engineering. Oxford, UK: Pergamon Press.

Pennington SR, Dunn MJ (2001). Proteomics: From protein sequence to function. NY: Bios Scientific Publishers Limited.

Rothstein MA, ed. (2003). Pharmacogenomics: Social, Ethical, and Clinical Dimensions. Hoboken, NJ: John Wiley & Sons.

Southern EM (2001). DNA microarrays. In: Rampal JB, ed. DNA Arrays: Methods and Protocols. Totowa, NJ: Humana Press 1–13.

Tsurushita N, Hinton PR, Kumar S (2005). Design of humanized antibodies: From anti-Tac to zenapax. Methods 36(1):69–83.

Walsh G (2003). Biopharmaceuticals — Biochemistry and Biotechnology, 2nd ed. Chichester, England: John Wiley & Sons.

Wobus AM, Boheler KR (2005). Embryonic stem cells: prospectives for developmental biology and cell therapy. Physiol Rev 85(2):635–73.

# 8

# Gene Therapy

*Maria A. Croyle*
*College of Pharmacy, The University of Texas at Austin, Austin, Texas, U.S.A.*

## INTRODUCTION

The pioneering report of James Watson and Francis Crick describing the helical structure of DNA spurred an upsurge of biomedical research focusing on the composition of DNA, RNA and proteins and their role in health and disease that continues today. This "molecular revolution" has markedly influenced understanding of the pathophysiology of a diverse collection of disease states ranging from cystic fibrosis (CF), inborn errors of metabolism and immunodeficiencies to cancer, cardiovascular disease and diabetes. Rapid development of recombinant DNA technology prompted sequencing of the human genome and identifying genotype–phenotype relationships in human disease. Although these efforts have produced highly sophisticated, extremely sensitive diagnostic tests, the development of successful molecular therapies based upon this expanded knowledge of disease pathogenesis is still in progress.

Gene therapy is the use of nucleic acids as therapeutic medicinal compounds. The most straightforward gene therapy strategy is to compensate for abnormal gene expression. Gene medicines can also be engineered to reconstitute a diseased organ, either by directing regeneration of specific tissues through expression of embryonic genes to induce cell growth and development or, in the case of cell-based therapies, by using natural or genetically corrected stem cells to produce healthy tissues. The field of gene therapy is still in its infancy with the first testing of this concept in the clinic occurring in 1990. This landmark trial, for adenosine deaminase (ADA) deficiency, involved the use of peripheral blood lymphocytes treated with a retrovirus expressing ADA in ADA-deficient patients (Anonymous, 1990). Ten years after treatment, lymphocytes from one patient continued to express the recombinant transgene, indicating that the effects of gene transfer can be long lasting (Muul, 2003). Another patient developed an immune response to the gene transfer system and, as a result, did not express the therapeutic gene, illustrating the promises and problems that afflict this innovative area of medicine. This chapter will discuss the current state of gene therapy and common approaches to gene transfer. Diseases currently subject to gene transfer applications will also be reviewed. The biology and utility of several gene transfer systems will be discussed, highlighting areas in which the pharmacist and pharmaceutical scientist can play a significant role in their development as viable medicinal products.

## EX VIVO VERSUS IN VIVO GENE THERAPY

Gene therapy is a means of treatment for diseases that have limited or no therapeutic options. Once a disease has been identified as a possible candidate, the gene necessary for treatment must be identified and cloned. Enough must be understood about the disease and the gene product in order to ensure that the therapeutic component is delivered to the appropriate cellular compartment responsible for its processing and subsequent biological activity. The necessity for long-term gene expression or requirements that expression be timed with other biological processes will influence the design of the vector component of the therapy. The target tissue/organ must be readily accessible and a defined, measurable endpoint must be identified for assessment of therapeutic efficacy. Several strategies can be used for gene transfer. Direct injection of vector/DNA complexes into the bloodstream is often characterized by low levels of gene expression, making large amounts of vector necessary for therapeutic efficacy. Broad distribution of the vector may adversely affect the function and health of normal tissues and cause adverse reactions. This method also has limited utility for the treatment of tissues with restricted blood supplies such as muscle and tumors. Other delivery methods employed for in vivo gene transfer include intratumoral, intraperitoneal subcutaneous, and intramuscular injection. These are crude, invasive and, in some cases, require specialized surgical skills, making efficient tissue-targeted delivery systems essential for successful gene transfer.

Ex vivo gene transfer strategies involve isolation and culture of cellular targets. Gene transfer is achieved by direct application of the vector (virus, plasmid) for efficient gene expression (Fig. 1). Cells are then studied after treatment and only healthy cells expressing the therapeutic gene collected and given to the patient. Initially, this approach was limited to disorders in which the relevant cell population (i.e., bone marrow, hepatocytes) could be removed from the affected individual, modified and then replaced. Today, cells can be administered by local or systemic injection, delivered in encapsulated form or as tissues comprised of cells seeded on scaffolds. Patient safety is often improved with ex vivo gene transfer since the host immune response to the vector or toxic effects associated with transfection reagents are eliminated.

## GENE THERAPY IN THE CLINIC: DISEASE TARGETS

There are currently 1,260 active gene therapy clinical trials worldwide (Anonymous, 2006). Approximately 67% of these trials are for cancer. Treatment of monogenetic diseases, the premise of early gene transfer experiments, is the goal of only ~8% of active clinical trials. General indications for all gene therapy trials in the clinic are summarized in Table 1. Currently, gene therapy trials are primarily held in the United States (65% of all trials), the United Kingdom (12%) and Germany (5.9%). The geographical distribution of gene therapy clinical trials is summarized in Table 2.

| Disease | Gene therapy clinical trials | |
|---|---|---|
| | Number | Percentage |
| Cancer | 842 | 67.0 |
| Vascular diseases | 113 | 9.0 |
| Monogenetic diseases | 104 | 8.6 |
| Infectious disease | 81 | 6.4 |
| Gene marking | 50 | 4.2 |
| Healthy volunteers | 21 | 1.7 |
| Other diseases[a] | 47 | 3.7 |

[a]Grouped in this category are treatments for: inflammatory bowel disease, rheumatoid arthritis, chronic renal disease, carpal tunnel syndrome, Alzheimer's disease, diabetic neuropathy, Parkinson's disease, erectile dysfunction, retinitis pigmentosa and glaucoma. *Source*: From Anonymous, 2006 and Edelstein, 2004.

**Table 1** ▪ Summary of current gene therapy clinical trials by indication.

### ▪ Gene Therapy for Cancer

The objective of cancer gene therapy is to destroy tumor cells and preserve normal tissue. Strategies to achieve this goal include: (*a*) correction of genetic mutations contributing to the malignant phenotype, (*b*) stimulation of a T-cell-mediated immune response against the tumor (immunotherapy), (*c*) use of oncolytic viruses that replicate in and destroy tumor cells (virotherapy), and (*d*) use of enzyme pro-drug systems that destroy tumor cells by converting a

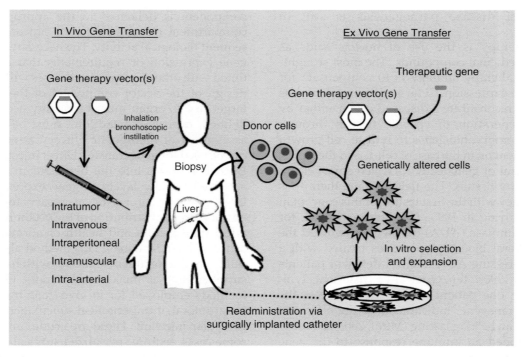

**Figure 1** ▪ Methods of administration of gene therapy vectors. In vivo gene transfer involves direct administration of the vector in the tissue of interest. Ex vivo gene transfer requires collection of cellular targets from the patient. The cells are treated in culture with the vector. Cells expressing the therapeutic transgene are harvested and given back to the patient.

| Country | Gene therapy clinical trials | |
| --- | --- | --- |
| | Number | Percentage |
| United States | 815 | 65.0 |
| United Kingdom | 150 | 12.0 |
| Germany | 74 | 5.9 |
| Switzerland | 42 | 3.3 |
| France | 20 | 1.6 |
| Belgium | 19 | 1.5 |
| Australia | 17 | 1.3 |
| Japan | 16 | 1.3 |
| Canada | 17 | 1.3 |
| Italy | 15 | 1.2 |
| Other countries[a] | 75 | 5.9 |

[a] Countries included in this category are: Austria, China, Czech Republic, Denmark, Egypt, Finland, Israel, Mexico, The Netherlands, New Zealand, Norway, Poland, Russia, Singapore, South Korea, Spain, Sweden and Taiwan. Trials held in each of these countries represent less than 1% of all clinical trials held worldwide. *Source*: From Anonymous, 2006 and Edelstein, 2004.

**Table 2** ▪ International status of gene therapy clinical trials.

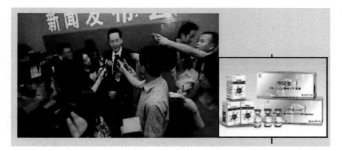

**Figure 2** ▪ The first gene therapy product is approved. On October 16, 2003, China's SFDA approved an adenovirus-based product, Gendicine, for treatment of head and neck cancer. The product was commercially available in January 2004 through the company SiBiono GeneTech. *Source*: SiBiono GeneTech press release.

non-toxic medicinal compound to cytotoxic metabolites. Enzyme pro-drug therapies are further discussed in the Drug Metabolism and Gene Therapy section later in this chapter.

### Correction of Genetic Mutations

Understanding cancer at the molecular level is the platform for gene correction in cancer therapy. Although the complex process of tumor development and growth limits the utility of this strategy, approximately 12% of cancer gene therapy clinical trials involve over-expression of tumor suppressor genes such as p53, MDA-7 and ARF (Majhen, 2006). The p53 tumor suppressor gene is one of the most studied candidates for cancer gene therapy (Bouchet, 2006) which led to the approval of a recombinant adenovirus expressing this transgene, Gencidine, by China's State Food and Drug Administration (SFDA) making it the first gene therapy product available for worldwide clinical use (Fig. 2). Early attempts at gene transfer for cancer have been promising, but have also been pivotal in identifying the challenges of gene delivery. Efficient delivery of genes deep within tumors is difficult and restriction of gene expression to malignant tissue challenging. Gene silencing has also limited success of this approach especially when continuous expression is required. Despite this, prostate, lung, and pancreatic tumors have been successfully treated in the clinic with a variety of genes and transfer methods.

### Immunotherapy

Strategies for inducing the immune system to target and destroy malignant cells has had limited success due to limited expression and low avidity of tumor-associated antigen-specific cytotoxic T-cells and the inherent ability of tumor cells to evade immune detection. Expression of either pro-inflammatory cytokines (interleukin (IL)-2, IL-4 and IL-12), co-stimulatory molecules (HLA-B7, and lymphocyte function-associated antigen 3 (LFA-3)) or tumor-specific antigens such as mucin-1 and human carcino-embryonic antigen to stimulate anti-tumor immune responses has been tested clinically (Majhen, 2006). The vector expressing the transgene is often placed directly in the tumor to stimulate immune responses within lesions to induce long-lasting protective immunity (Fig. 3A). Tumor cells isolated from the patient or cancer cell lines can also be induced to express one or more immunostimulatory genes ex vivo (Fig. 3B). Culturing the patient's T-cells or bone marrow in the presence of a tumor antigen or transducing them with a stimulatory gene, priming them to recognize and remove cancer cells after readministration, has also been tested (Fig. 3C). These strategies are showing great promise for the treatment of many cancers unresponsive to conventional therapy.

### Oncolytic Viruses (Virotherapy)

Oncolytic viruses induce cell death through replication, expression of cytotoxic proteins and cell lysis in malignant cells while remaining innocuous in the rest of the body. Vaccinia, herpes simplex type I (HSV), reovirus, Newcastle disease virus, poliovirus and adenovirus are often selected for this application because they naturally target cancers and contain genomes that can be easily manipulated (Aghi, 2005). A problem with this tactic is that many people naturally have antibodies that clear the virus before it can successfully replicate. Significant safety

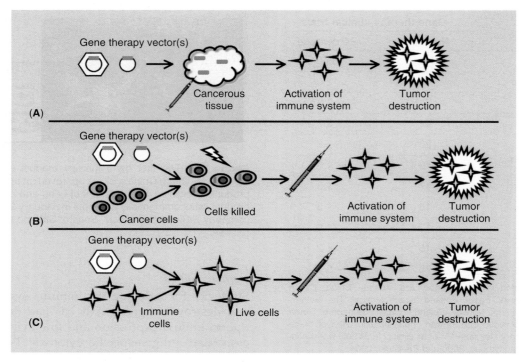

**Figure 3** ▪ Gene-based immunotherapy for cancer. Efficient removal of malignant tissue by the immune system can be achieved by: (**A**) Direct injection of a vector expressing immunostimulatory molecules or tumor-specific antigens in a tumor. As the transgene product is released, macrophages, dendritic cells, natural killer cells and T-cells are activated and migrate to the tumor where they destroy cells expressing the transgene. (**B**) Cells isolated from the patient or cancerous cell lines are treated with the vector in culture, killed by irradiation and given back to the patient. Epitopes on the cells prompt the immune system to attack and remove malignant cells. (**C**) T-cells or bone marrow cells from the patient are cultured with a vector and/or tumor antigens. Live cells that attack and remove malignant cells are given back to the patient.

precautions must also be taken, making clinical trials with these viruses extremely expensive and cumbersome. Despite this, oncolytic virotherapy has had some clinical success (Markert, 2000; Varghese, 2002; Argnani, 2005). Gene therapy for cancer is a rapidly progressing field and will undoubtedly be implemented into more chemotherapeutic protocols in the future. Many trials have shown that a gene-based approach can improve currently available treatment options and that more than one therapeutic modality may be necessary for clinical success.

## ▪ Gene Therapy for Vascular Disease

The current understanding of molecular mechanisms of cardiovascular disease has uncovered a large number of genes that could serve as potential targets for molecular therapies. Over-expression of genes involved in vasodilation such as endothelial nitric oxide synthase (eNOS) and heme oxygenase-1 (HO-1) or inhibition of molecules involved in vasoconstriction (angiotensin converting enzyme (ACE), angiotensinogen (AGT)) have reduced blood pressure in animal models of hypertension (Melo, 2006). This approach has not yet been clinically tested due to the availability of highly effective, conventional medications with

similar pharmacology. However, long-term control of blood pressure by gene transfer could overcome problems with non-compliance with traditional medications in hypertensive patients.

Most clinical trials for cardiovascular disease are designed for the treatment of coronary and peripheral ischemia. Over-expression of pro-angiogenic factors such as vascular endothelial growth factor (VEGF), fibroblast growth factor (FGF), and hepatocyte growth factor (HGF) have been effective in myocardial and peripheral ischemia (Springer, 2006). Over-expression of endothelial and inducible NOS has been shown to reduce the failure rate of coronary artery bypass grafting procedures due to restenosis and atherosclerosis. Over-expression of genes that can reduce cholesterol such as apoproteins ApoA-1 and ApoE and the low density lipoprotein (LDL) and very low density lipoprotein (VLDL) receptors have been used for the treatment of inherited disorders of lipid metabolism such as familial homozygotic hypercholesterolemia (FHH) and ApoE deficiency (Grossman, 1995; Vahakangas, 2005). Although each of these approaches have been shown to be well tolerated in the clinic (Losordo, 1998; Mann, 1999; Fortuin, 2003; Springer, 2006), none have demonstrated unequivocal therapeutic efficacy (Alexander, 2005; Conte, 2006). Larger, highly controlled, multi-center trials are needed to minimize the potential for placebo effects suspected to occur in some trials. Stringent criteria for patient selection is needed as many with cardiovascular disease often have underlying conditions that may cloud results. Endpoints for assessing efficacy and measures to assess potential short- and long-term complications must also be standardized. The efficacy of gene therapy for cardiovascular disease will most likely be enhanced by strategies that incorporate multiple gene targets with cell-based approaches.

## ■ Gene Therapy for Mongenetic Inherited Disorders

Of the 25,000 genes that comprise the human genome, mutations in over 1,800 have been identified as the cause of a variety of hereditary disorders. The ultimate therapeutic goal of gene therapy for mono-genetic disorders is to permanently replace a gene with its functioning counterpart in stem cells to restore normal function and permanently reverse disease processes. To date, clinical trails have not met this objective. They have shown, however, that gene transfer is feasible and phenotypic correction possible. Of the 102 active clinical gene therapy trials for monogenetic diseases, approximately 33% focus on CF, the most common inherited genetic disease in Europe and the United States (Wiley, 2006). To date, the severe combined immunodeficiency syndromes, comprising 20% of trials for inherited disorders, is the only group of diseases in which gene therapy has shown lasting, clinically meaningful therapeutic benefit. Other monogenetic diseases currently in clinical trials are listed in Table 3.

Issues which have prevented successful gene transfer for monogenetic diseases to date include: (*a*) lack of suitable gene delivery technologies, (*b*) unfavorable interactions between the host and gene transfer vector, (*c*) complex biology and pathology of monogenetic diseases and target organs, and (*d*) lack of relevant measures to assess the clinical efficacy of gene transfer. The greatest challenges that remain in the treatment of monogenetic disease are inducing gene expression sufficient to correct the clinical phenotype without precipitation of host immune responses and minimizing the risk of insertional mutagenesis for integrating vectors in dividing cellular targets. Improvements in vector technology and advancements in the understanding of cellular processes will vastly improve methods for correction of genetic disease.

## ■ Gene Therapy for Infectious Disease

Seventy-eight gene therapy trials for the treatment of infectious disease have been initiated (Wiley, 2006). Gene transfer for acquired immunodeficiency

- Cystic fibrosis
- Hurler syndrome
- Hunter syndrome
- Huntington's chorea
- Canavan disease
- Gaucher disease
- Wiskott-Aldrich syndrome
- Leber congenital amaurosis
- Severe combined immunodeficiency (SCID)
- Duchenne muscular dystrophy
- Chronic granulomatous disease
- Familial hypocholesterolemia
- Purine nucleoside phosphorylase deficiency
- Ornithine transcarbamylase (OTC) deficiency
- Leukocyte adherence deficiency
- Amyotrophic lateral sclerosis
- Junctional epidermolysis bullosa
- Hemophilia A and B
- Fanconi's anemia
- Gyrate atrophy
- RPE 65 defects
- Fabry disease
- Mucopolysaccharidosis type IV
- Lipoprotein-lipase deficiency
- Late infantile neuronal ceroid lipofuscinosis

*Source*: From O'Connor, 2006 and Edelstein, 2004.

**Table 3** ■ Monogenetic diseases treated by gene transfer in the clinic.

syndrome (AIDS) is the main application in this category. Many gene therapy trials for AIDS involve ex vivo transfer of genetic material to autologous T-cells using murine leukemia virus, or, more recently, lentivirus (Manilla, 2005; Levine, 2006). Over-expression of proteins that interfere with human immuno-deficiency virus (HIV) replication such as RevM10 to block nuclear export of HIV RNA and virus assembly has markedly increased CD4$^{+}$ T-cell survival in HIV-infected individuals (Ranga, 1998; Morgan, 2005). RNA-based strategies such as ribozymes, RNA decoys and antisense oligonucleotides that bind multiple sequences on the HIV genome attack different stages of virus replication and minimize the risk of viral resistance (Flotte, 2006 Macpherson, 2005; Dropulic, 2006).

## VECTORS FOR GENE TRANSFER

### ■ General Considerations

Preparations for gene delivery are colloidal suspensions consisting of complex molecules with average hydrodynamic radii ranging from 40 to 1,000 nm. Particles of this size are readily taken up by organs of the reticuloendothelial system (RES) such as the liver, spleen, bone marrow and adrenal glands and efficiently cleared from the circulation. They are also highly susceptible to opsonization, where they are coated with serum proteins such as complement and taken up by macrophages in the liver and spleen within minutes after intravenous administration (Dash, 1999; Read, 2005). Conjugation of vectors with biodegradable polymers has been shown to successfully prevent interaction with the RES and serum components (Oupicky, 2002; Demeneix, 2004; Kommareddy, 2005), however, this effect is often avoided by instillation of the vector directly into the target organ or tissue.

Even though a vector is administered by direct injection, it still must overcome certain epithelial barriers designed to restrict entry of macromolecules into the target tissue/organ. Cells lining the organ surface are often covered with a thick mucous layer that physically prevents contact with cellular targets and contains enzymes capable of rapidly degrading the vector. Cells under this layer are often ciliated and form tight junctions, which restrict entry. Many vectors carry a negative charge on their surface, making interaction with the cell, also negatively charged, difficult. Use of cationic compounds and mucolytic reagents to facilitate cellular interactions and hypotonic formulations to disrupt tight junctions and enhance cellular penetration has successfully enhanced gene transfer (Weiss, 2002; Tiera, 2006).

Once a vector enters a cell, it must next escape the endosomal/lysosomal environment. Some vectors have been administered with compounds that swell within the acidic endosomal environment and protect the genetic material from exposure to significant changes in pH and enzymatic digestion and promote vector release (Alexander, 2006). Others have used inactivated virus as well as specific components from bacteria, viruses and toxins that promote endosomal escape (Wagner, 2005). Once in the cytoplasm, the vector must successfully reach the nucleus where it can use the cells endogenous transcriptional machinery to express the therapeutic transgene. To accomplish this, non-viral and viral gene transfer vectors are used.

### ■ General Anatomy and Production of a Gene Transfer Vector

A gene-based medicine typically consists of an expression cassette made of cDNA flanked by a promoter on the 5′ side and a transcription stop and polyadenylation site on the 3′ side (Fig. 4A). This is incorporated into a DNA plasmid or a recombinant virus, based upon therapeutic requirements (Tables 4 and 5). The genes responsible for the pathogenicity of viral vectors are removed and replaced with the expression cassette in order to limit virus reproduction and fulminant disease. In many vectors, all that remains of the original virus genome are long terminal repeats (LTRs), 5 and 3 terminal regions of the virus that control transcription for RNA viruses or inverted terminal repeats (ITRs), identical but oppositely oriented sequences that drive DNA replication and stabilize the genome of DNA viruses. The packaging signal ($\psi$), responsible for virus assembly, is also kept intact. Genes for replication are supplied *in trans* by a producer/packaging cell line for large-scale production (Fig. 4B). Virus biology will dictate the manner in which the recombinant vector is produced. Careful thought must go into the design of a packaging cell line in order to minimize overlap between sequences in the virus genome and the cell that dictate replication and/or pathogenesis. If substantial overlap exists, these sequences can inadvertently be incorporated in the recombinant virus by homologous recombination. Replication competent (pathogenic) virus particles will then be produced with replication deficient particles. Preparations are often screened for replication competent virus (RCV) prior to clinical use. After production and harvest from a packaging cell line, recombinant vectors are purified, quantified and/or titered. Traditionally, purification strategies have relied upon density gradient ultracentrifugation to separate the vector from cellular proteins. This process is laborious, difficult to scale up and can reduce the effective titer of stock preparations by disrupting vector structure (Shamlou, 2003; Burova, 2005). Advances in column chromatography have mitigated these issues for many vectors, allowing them to be grown and purified to high concentrations needed for human use.

Given the diversity of diseases suitable for gene therapy, it is apparent that there can be no single vector that is appropriate for all gene transfer applications. Thus, selection of an appropriate vector for gene delivery requires careful consideration of a number of factors including: (*a*) size limitations for transgene cassettes, (*b*) transduction efficiency in therapeutic target (ability to infect dividing and/or non-dividing cells, appropriate receptors present on target cells), (*c*) duration of gene expression required for treatment (long-term vs. transient expression, integrating vs. non-integrating vectors), (*d*) necessity of temporal gene expression (inducible expression vs. constitutive expression), (*e*) maximum threshold of vector-induced immune response and toxicity

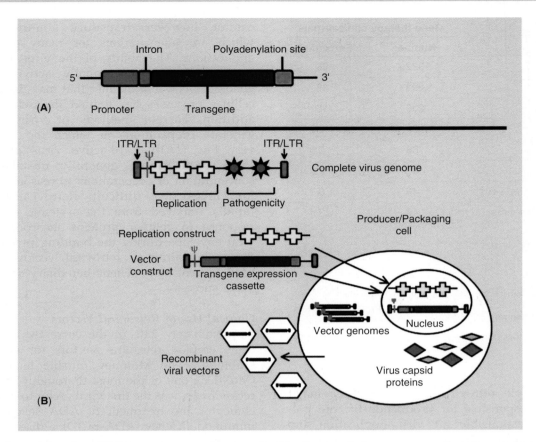

**Figure 4** ■ General overview: **(A)** Transgene expression cassette. The therapeutic transgene cassette is bounded by a promoter at the 5′ end and a polyadenylation site at the 3′ end. This can be cloned in a plasmid and used directly for gene transfer or it can be cloned in a plasmid containing viral elements to produce a recombinant virus with the help of a producer/packaging cell line. **(B)** Producer/packaging cell line. A packaging cell line is created by stably transfecting cells with a plasmid containing genes needed for virus replication. The vector construct often contains only the packaging signal (ψ) and the transgene cassette flanked by the viral ITR/LTR sequences. Genes responsible for fulminant virus infection are removed from the vector construct. The vector construct is introduced to the cell by transfection. Many copies of the vector genome are produced in the presence of replication genes supplied by the cell. These are exported from the nucleus and interact with viral proteins also supplied by the cell. The packaging signal dictates virus assembly. Complete virus particles are released from the cell according to vector-specific mechanisms (budding, lysis, etc.).

acceptable for the host, (*f*) purity requirements for the vector and ease of large scale production, (*g*) route and ease of administration, (*h*) ability of the vector to protect the genetic material, and (*i*) robustness and physical stability of the vector system.

### ■ Viral Vectors for Gene Transfer

Viruses, natural parasites that efficiently enter cellular targets and hijack cellular machinery for propagation, are currently the most effective vectors for gene therapy. Approximately 70% of all gene therapy clinical trials employ viral vectors (Table 4). Many viruses with divergent properties have been developed for gene transfer. Retroviruses, adenoviruses and adeno-associated viruses (AAVs) are the most extensively studied to date. Characteristics of each are summarized in Table 5.

### *Retroviral Vectors*

#### *Biology*

Retroviruses are 80 to 100 nm in diameter and contain two copies of a single-stranded RNA genome, 7 to 11 killobases (kb) in length. Within the capsid, the RNA is in close association with reverse transcriptase (RT), integrase (IN), and protease (PR) enzymes, necessary for virus replication (Fig. 5A). These elements are surrounded by a shell of nucleocapsid (NC) proteins enclosed in the capsid matrix (MA), which forms the core of the retroviral particle. The protein capsid is surrounded by a protein-lipid envelope derived from the host cell membrane. Embedded within this lipid bilayer are transmembrane (TM) and surface (SU) glycoproteins.

Retroviruses are commonly divided into two categories based upon the complexity of their

**Table 4** — Vectors currently in clinical trials for gene therapy.

| Vector | Gene therapy clinical trials | |
|---|---|---|
| | Number | Percentage |
| Adenovirus | 322 | 26 |
| Retrovirus | 293 | 23 |
| Plasmid DNA | 230 | 18 |
| Lipofection | 99 | 7.9 |
| Vaccinia virus | 88 | 7.0 |
| Poxvirus | 85 | 6.8 |
| Adeno-associated virus | 46 | 3.7 |
| Herpes simplex virus | 43 | 3.4 |
| RNA transfer | 16 | 1.3 |
| Others[a] | 31 | 2.4 |
| Unknown[a] | 36 | 2.9 |

[a]Information about the vectors employed in these trials was not reported.
Source: From Anonymous, 2006.

genome. Simple retroviruses possess three major genes: gag (responsible for production of core proteins), pol (responsible for virus replication and integration) and env (responsible for production of envelope proteins), while complex retroviruses like the lentivirus, contain genes for virus replication and evasion of the host immune response (Fig. 5B). During replication, RT converts the viral RNA to linear double-stranded DNA that integrates into the host genome with the help of the viral IN. The integrated construct, the provirus, will later undergo transcription and translation as cellular genes do to produce viral genomic RNA and mRNA encoding viral proteins. Virus particles then assemble in the cytoplasm and bud from the host cell to infect other cells (Fig. 6).

### Suitability of Retroviruses as Vectors for Gene Transfer

Retroviruses have many attributes that make them attractive for gene transfer applications (Table 5). They can accommodate transgene cassettes of 8 kb. They are capable of producing stable, long-term transgene expression in dividing cells, due to their ability to integrate into the host genome. "Pseudotyping," a process in which the SU glycoproteins are replaced with those from unrelated viruses such as vesicular stomatitis virus or Ebola virus, has significantly expanded the number of cell types capable of being transduced by these vectors (Cronin, 2005). This also improves the physical stability of the retrovirus particle. Retroviruses

cannot, however, transduce non-dividing cells, which are often targets for many gene transfer applications. The ability of the virus to randomly integrate in transcriptionally active regions of genomic DNA in a manner that may disrupt normal cellular processes has limited their clinical use. In addition, current methods of virus production generate preparations in which the virus titer is very low ($1 \times 10^5$–$1 \times 10^7$ active virus particles/mL). Virus particles are generally unstable, making concentration of preparations to reasonable volumes for clinical use difficult. Retroviruses are also rapidly removed from the systemic circulation in response to cellular proteins incorporated in the viral envelope during the budding process. Despite these shortcomings, retroviral vectors have been used to treat monogenetic hereditary disorders with some success.

### Clinical Use of Retroviral Vectors

Approximately 23% of the currently active clinical trials employ retroviral vectors for gene transfer (Table 4). The Moloney murine leukemia virus (MoMLV), one of the most thoroughly characterized retroviruses, was the first viral vector to be used in the clinic for the treatment of ADA severe combined immunodeficiency (ADA–SCID), a disease caused by abnormal purine catabolism, which prohibits the expansion of lymphocytes (1990; Blackburn, 2005). MoMLV expressing recombinant ADA was used to transduce mature T-cells ex vivo. Sustained engraftment of cells has been documented 10 years after the last infusion and no severe adverse effects from this therapy have been reported.

One of the most promising clinical trials employing retroviruses was for the treatment of a rare form of X-linked severe combined immunodeficiency (SCID-X1) (Cavazzana-Calvo, 2000; Hacein-Bey-Abina, 2002). MoMLV expressing the γ-interleukin receptor was used to transduce hematopoietic stem cells ex vivo. This treatment could reconstitute the immune systems of each patient such that they are no longer living in isolated environments. However, an uncontrolled T-cell lymphoproliferative syndrome was reported in 3 of 10 patients enrolled in the trial (Hacein-Bey-Abina, 2003). Although chemotherapy was initiated at the time of diagnosis, one of these patients died. In 2 of the 3 cases, the retrovirus integrated in cellular DNA near the LIM domain only 2 (LMO2) promoter, an oncogenic promoter in T-cells (Nam, 2006), during a time when the children contracted chicken pox, which initiated T-cell proliferation that did not subside (Hacein-Bey-Abina, 2003). As a result, the U.S. Food and Drug Administration (FDA), the Gene Therapy Advisory Committee (GTAC) and Committee of Safety of

| | Retrovirus | Lentivirus | Adenovirus | Adeno-associated virus |
|---|---|---|---|---|
| Genetic material | RNA | RNA | dsDNA | ssDNA |
| Genome size | 7–11 kb | 8 kb | 36 kb | 4.7 kb |
| Cloning capacity | 8 kb | 8 kb | 7 kb[a]<br>35 kb[c] | <5 kb |
| Genome forms | Integrated | Integrated | Episomal | Stable/episomal |
| Diameter (nm) | 100–145 | 80–120 | 80–100 | 20–22 |
| Tropism | Dividing cells only | Broad, dividing and non-dividing cells | Broad, dividing and non-dividing cells | Broad, not suitable for hematopoietic cells |
| Virus protein expression | No | Yes/no | Yes[a]/no[b] | No |
| Transgene expression | Slow, constitutive | Slow, constitutive | Rapid, transient | Moderate, constitutive, transient |
| Large-scale production | Simple | Complex | Simple[a]<br>Complex[b] | Moderate |
| Delivery method | Ex vivo | Ex vivo | Ex/in vivo | Ex/in vivo |
| Typical yield (virus particle/ml) | $<10^8$ | $<10^7$ | $<10^{14}$ | $<10^{13}$ |
| Pre-existing immunity | Unlikely | Perhaps, post-entry | Yes | Yes |
| Immunogenicity | Low | Low | High | Moderate |
| Potential pathogenicity | Low | High | Low | None |
| Safety | Insertional mutagenesis | Insertional mutagenesis | Potent inflammatory response | None to date but long-term not clear |
| Physical stability | Poor | Poor | Fair | High |

[a] First generation, replication defective adenovirus.
[b] Helper-dependent adenovirus.
*Source*: From Edelstein, 2004; Weber, 2006; Wang and Yuan, 2006; Mangeat and Trono, 2005.

**Table 5** ▪ Characteristics of viral vectors for gene transfer.

Medicine in the United Kingdom have declared that this approach should not be first line therapy for SCID-X1, but should be considered in the absence of other therapeutic options (Kaiser, 2005; Secretariat, 2005).

### Suitability of Lentiviruses as Vectors for Gene Transfer

Lentiviruses, like HIV, are specialized retroviruses that can infect non-dividing cells. The ability to efficiently infect neurons, hepatocytes, macrophages and hematopoietic stem cells has increased the popularity of this virus as a gene transfer vector. Although lentiviruses can integrate in the host genome, their integration sites are significantly more restricted than for other retroviruses. While this minimizes the risk of insertional mutagenesis, a primary concern for the clinical use of lentiviruses is the potential for recombination and production of replication-competent viruses. Development of self-inactivating vectors that contain deletions within the 3′ LTR, eliminating transcription of the packaging signal to prevent virus assembly has significantly improved the safety profile of lentiviruses.

### Clinical Use of Lentiviral Vectors

Because of the perceived risks associated with use of lentivirises, clinical trials with these vectors were not initiated until 2003. Most are for treatment of HIV infection in HIV positive subjects (Dropulic, 2006). In each of these trials, the lentivirus is delivered to autologous peripheral blood mononuclear cells ex vivo. One of the lessons learned from the clinic is that limited transduction efficiency of the virus stems from the low concentration of the final purified product. Long-term gene expression of the virus is compromised by the immune response to serum and other cell culture reagents used during virus production as well as cellular proteins incorporated during

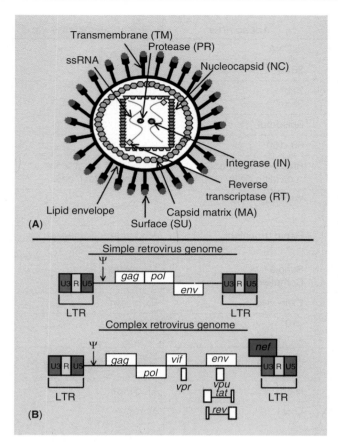

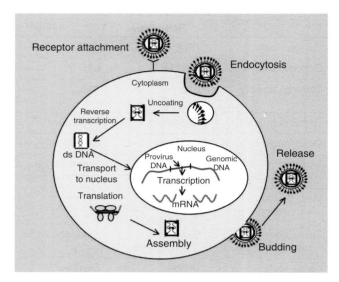

**Figure 6** ■ The retrovirus replication cycle. Retroviruses enter cells by receptor-mediated endocytosis. In the endosome, the lipid envelope and capsid matrix proteins are degraded. Once in the cytoplasm, the viral RT converts the viral RNA into double-stranded DNA which is shuttled to the nucleus. In the nucleus, the double-stranded viral DNA is inserted into genomic DNA as a provirus. RNA polymerase in the cell copies the viral RNA in the nucleus. These molecules are shuttled out of the nucleus and serve as templates for making additional copies of viral RNA and mRNA that is translated into viral proteins that form the envelope. New virus particles are assembled in the cytoplasm and bud from the cell membrane.

**Figure 5** ■ The retrovirus. (**A**) General structure. Two copies of the single stranded RNA genome are surrounded by NC proteins with RT, IN and PR. This is enclosed in the capsid matrix (MA), which is surrounded by a lipid envelope decorated with TM glycoproteins and SU proteins. (**B**) Retrovirus genomes. Retrovirus genomes contain *gag, pol* and *env* sequences flanked by viral LTRs, which contain U3 (red boxes), R (yellow boxes), and U5 (blue boxes) sequences. Some retroviruses like the lentivirus contain additional sequences and are quite complex. *Tat* and *rev* products are RNA binding proteins. *Nef* (green box) and *vpu* are responsible for down-regulation of cell SU expression of CD4 molecules and stimulation of HIV infection. *Vpr* and *vif* both facilitate HIV replication.

budding from producer cell lines. Thus, large-scale production processes capable of generating highly purified, concentrated retroviral preparations are needed.

### Production and Processing of Recombinant Retroviruses

Replication defective recombinant retroviruses are propagated in genetically engineered packaging cell lines created by transfection with plasmids that contain *gag* and *pol* genes (Zhang, 2006). These cells are transfected with a second plasmid that contains viral LTRs, packaging sequences and the transgene cassette. In pseudotyping strategies, *env* genes are not expressed in packaging cells. Instead, sequences for SU proteins of unrelated viruses are cloned in a

separate plasmid that does not share sequence homology with *gag* and *pol* genes, making production of a panel of vectors with different tissue specificities easy. Retrovirus packaging cell lines have been derived from either NIH-3T3 mouse fibroblasts or 293T human embryonic kidney cells. Use of non-human cell lines provokes immune recognition of cellular components incorporated in the virus envelope during budding. Thus, several other human-derived packaging cell lines such as AM12, ψ-CRIM and PG13 have also been used (Merten, 2004). Under optimized conditions, packaging cell lines can be maintained in a functional state for approximately 4 weeks.

Retroviral vectors have been routinely produced in adherent cell monolayers grown in T flasks or roller bottles. Culture media is collected and directly added to cells ex vivo. The quantity of active virus produced in this manner is extremely low, as indicated by the large volumes of supernatant used for clinical trials (200–800 mL/patient) (Rodrigues, 2006). Retrovirus particles are unstable at 37°C ($t_{1/2} \sim$ 5–8 hours), the temperature at which the producer cells are maintained. The presence of free cellular glycoproteins also inhibits transduction (Le Doux, 1998). Optimization of culture conditions and use of continuous feed bioreactors that permit removal of toxic materials and collection of culture supernatants over time has greatly improved the quality of retroviral preparations (see Chapter 3). To date, purification of retrovirus preparations for phase I clinical trials has been minimal at best and concentration of culture supernatants insufficient to meet the stringent quality standards required for in vivo therapy (Rodrigues, 2006). Centrifugation and microfiltration techniques are extremely useful for clarification of culture supernatants and removal of cellular debris (Segura, 2006). Ion-exchange, size exclusion and affinity chromatography techniques have also been employed to remove excess salt, serum and low molecular weight contaminants also concentrated with the virus (Rodrigues, 2006).

Retrovirus preparations are commonly stored at $-80\,^\circ$C as culture supernatants prior to clinical use. Since the virus particles are fragile, consideration must be given to the formulation and storage conditions for highly purified, concentrated preparations. Stability of the virus at all stages of the purification process must also be assessed to maximize yield and performance. The impact of temperature, pH and salt concentration on the physical stability of retroviral vectors has been described (Cruz, 2006; Rodrigues, 2006). Others have shown that the stability of retroviral vectors is also dictated by the type of packaging cell line, the cholesterol content in the virus envelope and proteins selected for pseudotyping (Beer, 2003; Merten, 2004; Cronin, 2005; Rodrigues, 2006). To date, very little work has been done in the area of formulation development and stability of retroviral vectors with additives that are suitable and approved for human use, making this an exciting area of research for the pharmaceutical scientist that is crucial to the development of these viruses as viable medicinal agents.

### Adenoviral Vectors

#### Biology

Adenoviruses are non-enveloped, lytic, DNA viruses with a linear double-stranded genome and icosahedral symmetry. Since the isolation of the first human adenovirus in 1953 from tonsils and adenoid tissue (Rowe, 1953), 50 additional serotypes have been identified and grouped into six species (A–F) based on genome size, composition and homology, hemagglutinating properties and oncogenicity in rodents. Because the subgroup C adenoviruses 2 and 5 have been studied extensively, they were the first to be adapted as vectors for gene therapy. The virus genome, 36 kb in length, is divided into early and late transcription units, based upon the kinetics of viral infection. There are five early (E1A, E1B, E2, E3, and E4) and four intermediate (IVa2, IX, VAI, and VAII)

transcriptional units (Nevins, 1987). The E1A transcription unit activates other early transcription units, optimizing the environment for virus replication by inducing the cell to enter the S phase of division (Berk, 2005). E1B proteins prevent apoptosis and promote cell survival. E2A encodes for DNA polymerase, preterminal and single-stranded DNA binding proteins, involved in virus replication (de Jong, 2003). E3 is responsible for elusion of the host immune response and promoting the survival of infected cells while products of the E4 transcription unit influence the cell cycle and cell transformation (Lichtenstein, 2004; Weitzman, 2005). Late region genes are transcribed as one long precursor transcript from the major late promoter and processed into five mRNA molecules (L1–L5) that encode capsid structural proteins (McConnell, 2004). The essential E1 region of viral genome was deleted in the first adenoviruses developed for gene therapy applications to prevent replication. The E3 region was also often removed to accommodate transgene expression cassettes.

Adenovirus particles are approximately 70 to 90 nm in size (Fig. 7B). The protein capsid consists of 252 protein subunits. There are 240 copies of the trimeric hexon protein (Fig. 7A). Five copies of the penton protein are located at each of the 12 vertices of the capsid and are responsible for holding fiber proteins in place. The twelve fiber proteins are asymmetrical and consist of a thin shaft protein topped by a globular knob. While it is ultimately the elements of the viral genome and the capacity of the cell to support virus infection that determine the efficiency of transgene expression, adenoviral capsid proteins also facilitate binding, entry and translocation of the genome into the cell (Medina-Kauwe, 2003).

Adenovirus infection begins with binding of the knob domain of the fiber capsid protein to the Coxsackievirus and Adenovirus receptor (CAR) (Fig. 8) (Bergelson, 1997). Adenovirus also can bind to the $\alpha_2$ domain of the human major histocompatibility complex class I (MHC I) molecule and heparan sulfate glycosaminoglycans (HS GAGs) to initiate infection (Hong, 1997; Dechecchi, 2001). After initial binding, an Arg-Gly-Asp (RGD) motif within the penton base interacts with $\alpha_V\beta_3$ and $\alpha_V\beta_5$ integrin receptors (Nemerow, 1999). Engagement of integrins initiates a series of cell signaling processes associated with virus infection and facilitates efficient internalization of adenovirus particles, escape from the endosomal compartment and nuclear targeting of the adenovirus genome (Medina-Kauwe, 2003). Adenovirus particles enter the nucleus as early as 30 minutes after initial cellular contact. Early mRNA and viral proteins can be detected within an hour after the virus binds to cellular receptors. Viral DNA replication and particle

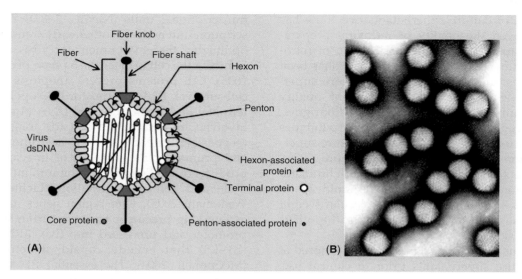

**Figure 7** ■ The adenovirus. **(A)** Cross section of an adenovirus particle. The virus consists of a double-stranded DNA genome encased in a protein capsid. The capsid is primarily made up of hexon proteins. Penton proteins are positioned at each of the vertices of the icosahedral capsid and serve as the base for each fiber protein. Hexon-associated and penton-associated proteins are the glue that holds these proteins together within and across the facets of the capsid. Core proteins bind to penton proteins and serve as a bridge between the virus core and the capsid. Terminal proteins, located at each end of the viral genome, serve as primers for DNA replication and mediate attachment of the viral genome to the nuclear matrix. **(B)** Electron micrograph of intact adenovirus serotype 5 particles.

assembly in the nucleus starts 8 hours after infection and culminates in the release of $10^4$ to $10^5$ mature virus particles per cell 30–40 hours post-infection by cell lysis (Majhen, 2006).

### Suitability of Adenoviruses for Gene Transfer

Adenoviruses have several characteristics that make them attractive for gene transfer (Table 5). Biology of the virus is well understood, making adenovirus-

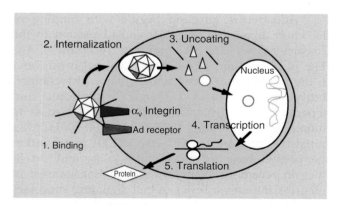

**Figure 8** ■ The adenovirus infection cycle. Adenovirus infection begins with the attachment of fiber proteins to cellular receptors. Binding of capsid penton proteins to integrin receptors facilitates the internalization process. Once the virus enters the endosome, the pH inside the vesicle drops and degraded capsid proteins and the virus genome release into the cytoplasm. Viral DNA is transported to the nucleus where it is transcribed to RNA. Messenger RNA is transported out of the nucleus and into the cytoplasm where it is translated to therapeutic protein molecules. This entire process is complete within 2 hours.

based vectors relatively easy to construct. High quality, purified preparations can be easily produced at titers of $1 \times 10^{13}$ virus particles/ml in well-defined cell systems. Transgene expression from these vectors is rapid and robust and is enhanced with strong heterologous promoters. Unlike some viruses, adenoviruses are physically stable, allowing them to survive stringent purification protocols and long-term storage. Adenoviruses can infect a wide range of dividing and non-dividing cells. Use of animal-specific adenovirus serotypes for human gene transfer and retargeting strategies at the molecular and macromolecular levels are under development to limit transduction to target tissues (Mizuguchi, 2004; Bangari, 2006). Adenoviruses do not integrate into the host genome. While this minimizes the risk of insertional mutagenesis, gene expression is transient, making them unsuitable for long-term correction of genetic defects. Because the adenovirus genome can accommodate large transgene cassettes, hybrid adenovirus–adeno-associated virus vectors have been designed for region-specific chromosomal integration and prolonged transgene expression (Lundstrom, 2004).

A significant drawback to the use of recombinant adenoviruses is the ability of the virus to elicit a strong immune response. The host response to adenovirus has been well documented and occurs in three phases in animal models and humans (Nazir, 2005). The first phase occurs within an hour after systemic administration, lasts for 4 days and is characterized by thrombocytopenia and elevated liver enzymes, the severity of which is dose dependent. The second phase, occurring 5 to 7 days after administration, is highlighted by removal of transduced cells by activated lymphocytes in the target tissue and localized, self-limited inflammation (Muruve, 2004). During the third phase, CD4$^+$ T-cell-dependent humoral immunity develops and neutralizing antibodies clear the virus from the circulation and prevent effective readministration (Xu, 2005). Successful readministration of adenoviral vectors is difficult since ~50% to 90% of the world's population has high levels of anti-adenovirus serotype 5 antibodies (Nwanegbo, 2004) which have been shown to significantly reduce the efficacy of these vectors in mice, primates and humans in a phase I clinical trial (Ertl, 2005; Kresge, 2005).

The significance of the immune response generated by adenoviral vectors has been illustrated in the clinic. Intra-hepatic administration of an E1/E4 deleted adenovirus failed to produce a therapeutic effect in patients enrolled in a clinical trial designed to correct ornithine transcarbamylase (OTC) deficiency (Raper, 2002). This was associated with a mild immune response to the virus and rapid clearance of vector and transgene. One patient in the highest dose cohort (6×10$^{11}$ virus particles/kg) experienced a severe immune response syndrome characterized by multiorgan failure and sepsis and died soon after treatment (Raper, 2003). This was the first reported death ascribed to gene therapy (Raper, 2002). Likewise, a trial for hemophilia A using intravascular delivery of an adenoviral vector was stopped because of transient thrombocytopenia and transaminase elevation in patients (High, 2003). As a result, it is now recognized that recombinant adenoviruses can be safely administered directly to target organs at doses of up to 1×10$^{11}$ virus particles (O'Connor, 2006).

### Averting the Immune Response Against Adenovirus

A significant effort has been put forth to address the problem of the adenovirus-mediated immune response. Coadministration of immunosuppressive agents such as cyclophosphamide, FK506, and cyclosporin A extended the duration of transgene expression, but did not prevent development of neutralizing antibodies (Xu, 2005). Virus-induced toxicity was also reduced through modification of the viral genome. Second generation vectors, attenuated in regions E1–E4, have reduced the inflammatory response and extended the duration of transgene expression (Fig. 9) (McConnell, 2004). Deletion of all early and late genes in the helper-dependent adenovirus, has improved toxicity and transgene expression. Neutralizing antibodies, however, are still detected after treatment with any of these vectors.

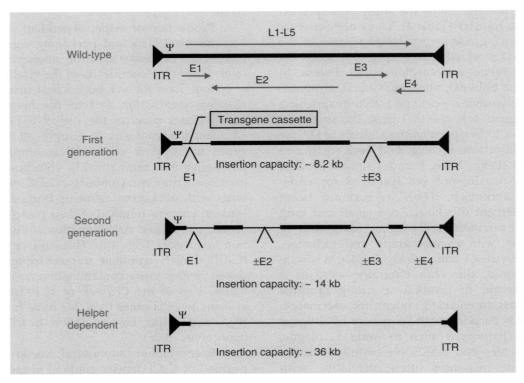

**Figure 9** ■ Genome structure and composition of recombinant adenovirus vectors. Arrows indicate the direction of transcription and translation of adenovirus early (E) and late (L) gene products in the wild-type adenovirus genome (thick black line at top of figure). Regions that have been removed and replaced by non-viral sequences are represented by thin black lines. The maximal insert capacity accommodated by each vector is indicated. *Abbreviations*: ITR, inverted terminal repeat; ψ, packaging signal.

"Seroswitching," the use of either non-human or rare human adenovirus serotypes, is one approach to address the problem of pre-exiting immunity to adenovirus serotype 5 (Bangari, 2006). Recombinant adenoviruses derived from human serotypes 35 and 11 with low exposure rates in the general population can induce high levels of transgene expression and are minimally affected by pre-existing immunity to adenovirus 5. Since antibodies capable of neutralizing virus particles are directed primarily against hexon proteins (Sumida, 2005), hexon-chimeric viruses have also been developed (Roberts, 2006). Although they avoid neutralization, they are very difficult to produce. Covalent attachment of polyethylene glycol or incorporation into polymer matricies has also shown promise in protecting adenoviral vectors from neutralization (Bangari, 2006).

### Clinical Use of Adenoviral Vectors

Exploitation of adenoviruses in medicine started in the late 1950s. Adenovirus serotypes 4 and 7 were first used as an oral vaccine against acute respiratory disease in United States military personnel (Top, 1971). Use of this vaccine for 25 years without significant side effects served as the platform for further development of adenovirus-based vectors for gene transfer. Today, approximately 26% of all gene therapy clinical trials involve recombinant adenoviruses, making them the most widely used vector for gene transfer (Table 4). There are currently 16 trials employing adenovirus-based vectors in the phase II/III stage of clinical testing that focus on treatments for cancer and cardiovascular disease. In 2003, Gencidine (SiBiono, Shenzen, China), a replication deficient adenovirus serotype 5 vector expressing the p53 transgene, was the first gene therapy treatment for cancer to be approved by China's SFDA for worldwide clinical use in head and neck squamous cell carcinoma (Peng, 2005). It and a similar product (INGN 201, Advexin, not yet approved for widespread use (Gabrilovich, 2006)) are currently being tested for treatment of glioma, non-small cell lung cancer, bladder carcinoma and ovarian cancer alone or in combination with chemotherapy and radiation. Because adenoviruses can quickly induce a strong immune response, they can naturally serve as a powerful adjuvant to promote a strong immune response against an encoded antigen for vaccination purposes. Virus encoded with sequences of antigens derived from pathogens such as anthrax, plague, hepatitis C, rabies and SARS successfully induced strong immune responses often correlating with protection of susceptible animals against challenge with the infectious agent (Boyer, 2005; Zhou, 2006). Many of these vectors will soon be tested in clinical vaccination protocols.

### Production and Processing of Recombinant Adenoviruses

Traditionally, recombinant adenoviruses are generated by transfecting E1-complementing human cell lines such as 293, 911, PER.C6 or N52.E6 with: (a) a shuttle plasmid containing the left adenovirus ITR and packaging domain followed by the transgene cassette in the E1 region and (b) a template consisting of most of the adenovirus genome including the right ITR and a stretch of DNA reiterated in the shuttle plasmid. Homologous recombination through the sequences shared by the two DNA molecules creates the full E1-deleted adenovirus genome. Alternative systems for recombination of the plasmids in yeast and bacteria instead of mammalian cells have simplified and accelerated this process. After assembly of the recombinant genome, replication and packaging, adenovirus vectors can easily be produced in large amounts in E1-complementing cells. A significant problem often encountered in 293 cells is the production of replication competent adenoviruses (RCAs) when E1 DNA is acquired by homologous recombination between overlapping sequences contained in the adenoviral DNA inserted in chromosomal DNA of the 293 cells and those present in the vector backbone. Producer cells, like PERC.6 and N52.6, contain minimal E1 sequences to avoid overlap with vector DNA to prevent RCA production (Lusky, 2005).

Production of helper-dependent virus that only contains viral ITRs and packaging signal requires a system that expresses the entire adenovirus genome *in trans*. Due to the complexity of the viral genome, such a system has not yet been constructed. The most effective production system for helper-dependent adenoviruses requires the use of a first generation E1-deleted adenovirus to supply all the necessary genes to support vector DNA amplification and packaging into viral capsids. Infection of 293 cells expressing the *Cre* recombinase (293Cre) with a helper virus with packaging elements framed by *loxP* sites leads to efficient removal of their packaging elements after *Cre*-mediated recombination at the *loxP* recognition sequences (Fig. 10). This and cesium chloride (CsCl) density gradient ultracentrifugation has reduced helper virus contamination levels to 0.1% to 0.01%. Use of the *Cre/loxP* or FLP/frt recombinase systems in cells other than 293 have further reduced RCA and helper contamination to 0.004% to 0.1% (Goncalves, 2006).

Recombinant adenoviral vectors were often purified by CsCl density gradient ultracentrifugation. This is still used for research-scale preparations, but is neither scalable nor efficient for large quantities of clinical grade virus. The most recent scalable purification methods use anion exchange chromatography

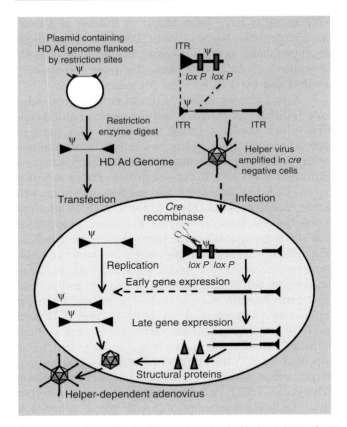

**Figure 10** ■ The *Cre/lox* P-based method of helper-dependent adenovirus (HD-Ad) production. The HD-Ad genome is released from a plasmid by restriction enzyme digestion. The linear virus genome is introduced to cells expressing both the *Cre* recombinase and adenovirus E1 gene products by transfection. Replication of the HD-Ad construct also requires concurrent infection of the cells with a "helper" adenovirus. The packaging signal of this virus is flanked by loxP sites. When added to *Cre* positive cells, packaging sequences are excised by *Cre* recombinase and intact helper particles cannot form. Capsid proteins are made, however, from helper virus sequences and are used to form intact HD-Ad particles. Additional stocks of the helper virus can only be produced in cells that express adenovirus E1 for replication functions but do not express *Cre*, allowing the virus genome to be packaged.

due to the strong affinity of intact virus particles for the resin with respect to that of cellular and individual capsid proteins. Published loading estimates for anion exchange resins range from 0.5 to $5 \times 10^{12}$ virus particles/mL of resin or 0.14 to 1.4 mg of virus/mL resin (Burova, 2005). Gel filtration and immobilized metal affinity chromatography are often used in polishing steps following anion exchange purification of recombinant adenovirus-based products.

The most significant effort to develop formulations to stabilize viruses at ambient temperatures for gene transfer has focused on the adenovirus. Until recently, it was assumed that lyophilization of adenovirus preparations would be the only way to

achieve long-term stability. During the period between 1979 and 1988, numerous reports described liquid formulations that could confer long-term stability of the virus at –20°C and –80°C but very few described stability at 4°C or room temperature (Altaras, 2005). Within the last 6 years, however, an extensive amount of information has been generated in the context of adenovirus stability. Evans et al. and others found that surface adsorption, freeze-thaw damage and free-radical oxidation were the primary inactivation pathways for recombinant adenoviruses (Croyle, 1998; Quick, 2002; Evans, 2004). Use of nonionic surfactants such as polysorbate-80 to prevent adsorption to glass surfaces, cryoprotectants such as sucrose to prevent damage associated with changes in solution pH and virus confirmation during freeze-thaw cycles and free-radical oxidation inhibitors such as histidine, ethanol and ethylenediaminetetraacetic acid (EDTA) can confer a shelf life of 2 years for certain virus preparations at 4°C. The role of other formulation variables, such as virus concentration, purity, divalent cations and solution pH on adeno-virus stability profiles has also been described (Altaras, 2005; Rexroad, 2006).

One of the most significant challenges for adenovirus-based products is the lack of sophisticated techniques for final characterization. Some progress has been made in this area with the recent finding that the penton base and protein IIIa are significantly more labile than other virus capsid proteins (Rexroad, 2003), suggesting that structural transitions in these regions should be monitored during the screening and selection of candidate formulations for long-term stability. It was also originally thought that the virus was much too complex for stability data to follow an Arrhenius relationship. However, using highly sensitive biological and physicochemical methods, it is now clear that adenovirus degradation is a first-order process (Evans, 2004). This provides a platform for rational selection of formulation candidates and suggests that data from short-term accelerated stability studies is useful for predicting the rate of degradation during long-term storage. It is also clear that formulations for recombinant adenoviruses will most likely have to be vector and process specific and tailored to specific nuances associated with a process that makes the virus susceptible to shearing stressors, aggregation and surface adsorption. They will also need to be serotype specific based on the fact that there are significant differences in the amino acid sequences of capsid proteins between the adenovirus groups. These tasks will most likely require significant collaborative efforts between the process engineer and the pharmaceutical scientist.

## Adeno-Associated Virus Vectors

### Biology

The first human AAV was discovered in 1965 as a contaminant of adenovirus preparations (Atchison, 1965). AAV is a non-enveloped parvovirus that requires co-infection with a helper virus in order to replicate. The AAV genome is a 4.7 kb linear, single stranded DNA molecule composed of two large open reading frames (ORFs), *rep* and *cap*, that contain sequences for four replication proteins and three capsid proteins respectively (Fig. 11A). The ORFs are flanked on either side by ITRs, required for genome replication, packaging and integration. The left ORF encodes four replication proteins. Rep 68 and 78 play a role in every aspect of the AAV life cycle such as transcription, viral DNA replication and site-specific integration. Rep 40 and 52 are important for DNA packaging in viral capsids within the nucleus. The right ORF contains sequences for structural capsid proteins.

The icosahedral AAV capsid is 25 nm in diameter (Fig. 11B). It is relatively simple, made up of only 60 copies of three structural capsid proteins, VP1, VP2, and VP3 in a ratio of 1:1:8 respectively. VP3 interacts with cellular receptors and dictates tissue specificity of the virus. A phospholipase domain, essential for virus infectivity, is located in the N-terminus of VP1. The specific role of VP2 is currently unclear. Recently it was found that viable recombinant AAV vectors could be produced without this protein (Warrington, 2004). To date, 9 distinct AAV serotypes have been identified and over 100

AAV variants have been found in human and non-human primate tissues (Wu, 2006). None of these serotypes cause human disease. The biology of AAV serotype 2 (AAV2) has been the most extensively studied and used as a vector for gene transfer.

AAV2 virions utilize heparan sulfate proteoglycans (HSPGs) as primary cellular attachment receptors, which confer a broad tropism to this virus in skeletal muscle, liver, brain, and retina. (Summerford, 1998). Virus internalization is aided by $\alpha v \beta 5$ integrins (Summerford, 1999), fibroblast growth factor receptor type 1 (FGF-1) (Qing, 1999) and the hepatocyte growth factor receptor, c-Met (Kashiwakura, 2005). The virus enters the cell through receptor-mediated endocytosis and is subsequently transported to the nucleus (Fig. 12). In the nucleus, the single-stranded genome must be converted to a double-stranded form for gene expression. Self-complimentary sequences in the viral ITRs form hairpin structures that serve as origins of replication. Rep 68 and 78 bind to the ITRs and mediate replication. The virus relies upon host cellular machinery as well as helper functions supplied by a coinfecting virus such as adenovirus, herpes simplex virus, or vaccinia, in order to replicate (Muzyczka, 2001). Proteins expressed from the helper virus facilitate transcription, AAV gene expression and DNA replication. Release of virus particles from the host is facilitated by the lysogenic properties of the helper virus. In the absence of helper virus, AAV establishes a latent infection within the cell either by site-specific integration into a unique locus on human chromosome 19, AAVS1, or persisting as a stable

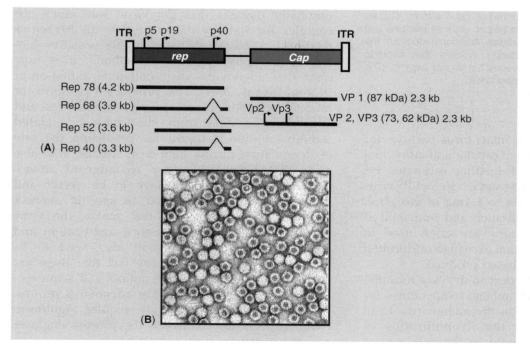

**Figure 11** ■ Adeno-associated virus. (**A**) Genome structure. The *rep* and *cap* sequences are flanked by ITRs. The p5 promoter initiates transcription of Rep78 and Rep68 proteins. The p19 promoter initiates transcription of Rep52 and Rep40 proteins. The p40 promoter initiates transcription of virus capsid proteins. VP2 and VP3 are produced from the same mRNA. Solid dark lines represent mRNA for each gene product. Kinks in the lines represent spliced sequences. (**B**) Electron micrograph of purified adeno-associated virus.

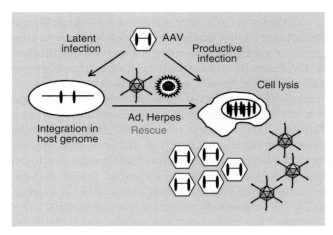

**Figure 12** ■ The AAV infection cycle. AAV can enter cells through receptor-mediated endocytosis. Once in the nucleus, the virus can follow one of two distinct and interchangeable pathways. In the absence of helper virus (adenovirus or herpes simplex), it enters a latent phase. During this phase, the AAV genome integrates into host genomic DNA though sequences located in the viral ITRs. When the cell is infected with a helper virus, AAV gene expression is activated and the virus genome is excised from the host DNA. Once the genome is rescued in this manner, it replicates and is packaged into AAV particles. These particles along with newly formed helper-viruses are released from the cell by helper-induced lysis. The rescue process can also occur after treatment with DNA damaging agents in the absence of helper virus.

episomal complex (Vasileva, 2005). When the cell is re-infected with helper virus, AAV replication occurs. Chemical carcinogens and ultraviolet radiation can also induce AAV to exit its latent state and replicate. In the context of transgene expression, there is initially a slow rise in transgene levels several weeks after administration of recombinant AAV until a stable plateau is reached. The exact reason for the delay in transgene expression is not clear, although it may reflect requirements for cytoplasmic trafficking, vector uncoating and conversion of the single-stranded genome to the double-stranded form necessary for cellular gene expression.

### Suitability of AAVs for Gene Transfer
Recombinant AAV vectors have rapidly gained popularity for gene therapy applications within the last decade, due to their lack of pathogenicity and ability to establish long-term gene expression (Table 5). The viral genome is also simple, making it easy to manipulate. The virus is resistant to many physical and chemical factors, giving AAV a robust stability profile during purification and long-term storage (Croyle, 2001; Wright, 2003). The ability of the virus to integrate in the human chromosome was an initial concern, but it has been found that recombinant AAV vectors that do not express *rep* proteins integrate

at frequencies of approximately $1/3 \times 10^7$ AAV genomes/gene, much lower than the rate of spontaneous mutations in human genes ($1/1 \times 10^5$ mutations/gene)(Cole, 1994; Carter, 2005).

Because recombinant AAV vectors do not contain any viral ORFs, they do not provoke the innate immune response. The primary host response that affects clinical use of AAV vectors, is production of neutralizing antibodies to capsid proteins, which prevent transgene expression upon readministration (Zaiss, 2005). In addition, approximately 80% of the population is seropositive for antibodies to AAV serotype 2 (Erles, 1999). Cellular and humoral immune responses have also been detected against the transgene product encoded in AAV vectors (Zaiss, 2005; Manno, 2006). These responses depend on the nature of the transgene, the promoter used, the route and site of vector administration, the vector dose and genetic predisposition of the host. Induction of tolerance by adoptive transfer of $CD4^+CD25^+$ regulatory T-cells and administration of anti-CD4 and anti-CD40 ligand antibodies, soluble CTLA-4 immunoglobulin fusion proteins or cyclophosphamide with the first dose of vector have been used to dampen this response. Others have changed the AAV serotype with each dose or created vectors pseudotyped with capsids from different AAV strains (Wu, 2006). In contrast to other vectors, AAV has a limited capacity for transgene cassettes. Because they can join via recombination within ITR regions, the transgene cassette can be split over two vectors given simultaneously although transduction efficiency is reduced by the recombination requirement.

### Clinical Use of AAV Vectors
To date, 46 phase I and phase II clinical trials employing recombinant AAV vectors have been initiated (Table 4). Early clinical development of AAV vectors was limited to indications for mono-genetic diseases such as CF, and hemophilia B, but a recent upsurge of trials for other indications was ignited by the impressive safety profile of the virus. The first clinical use of recombinant AAV was to transfer the cystic fibrosis transmembrane-conductance regulator (CFTR) cDNA to the respiratory epithelium for the treatment of CF (Flotte, 1996). These trials were the first to suggest that gene transfer could affect pulmonary function in a positive manner for this disease. Several phase I trials for the treatment of Canavan's, Parkinson's and Alzheimer's disease have shown that AAV-mediated gene transfer to the brain is safe and effective (Carter, 2005; McPhee, 2006). There are currently 4 trials using AAV2 vectors in phase III testing for metastatic hormone-resistant prostate cancer (Simons, 2006).

*Production and Processing of Recombinant AAVs*

Recombinant AAV vectors are constructed by replacing *rep* and *cap* genes with a promoter and transgene flanked by viral ITRs. The recombinant virus genome is cloned in a plasmid that is co-transfected in 293 cells with a separate plasmid containing *rep* and *cap* without ITRs to prevent packaging of these elements in AAV capsids. Because virus replication requires helper sequences, transfected cells were often infected with a low concentration of adenovirus (Fig. 13A). Early purification protocols capitalized on differences in thermostability and density to effectively separate the two viruses. Adenovirus could be inactivated by placing a preparation at 56°C for 30 minutes and removed by density gradient ultracentrifugation. Identification of adenoviral sequences that provide helper functions (E1a, E1b, E2a, E4, and VA1) and cloning them into a third plasmid improved the purity of vector stocks (Fig. 13B). Due to the relative inefficiency of triple transfection during large-scale production, cell lines containing integrated *rep* and *cap* sequences, the AAV genome or both were developed (Fig. 13C). Toxicity of the *rep* and *cap* genes and the need for infection with helper virus continues to complicate AAV production.

Toxicity of CsCl, aggregation of AAV particles and the fact that adenovirus is not completely removed after extensive centrifugation complicates AAV purification by CsCl density gradient ultracentrifugation (Grieger, 2005). Another density separation medium, iodixanol, that is less toxic than CsCl and prevents AAV aggregation has been employed in a single centrifugation step (Burova, 2005). Passage of the AAV fraction over an affinity column consisting of either a heparinized support matrix or a monoclonal antibodies produced against AAV2 significantly increased purity and infectivity of final preparations (Grimm, 1998; Auricchio, 2002). These methods, however, are for specific AAV serotypes. Ion exchange chromatography is the most powerful and versatile method for AAV purification although buffer pH, detergent concentration and column medium must be tailored for each AAV serotype. Infectivity and purity of preparations obtained from these purification strategies are comparable to those obtained from affinity chromatographic methods and are complete within 3 hours.

Few studies have been published that describe systematic efforts to optimize AAV vector formulation and stability. Initial studies demonstrated that AAV is significantly more stable than other recombinant

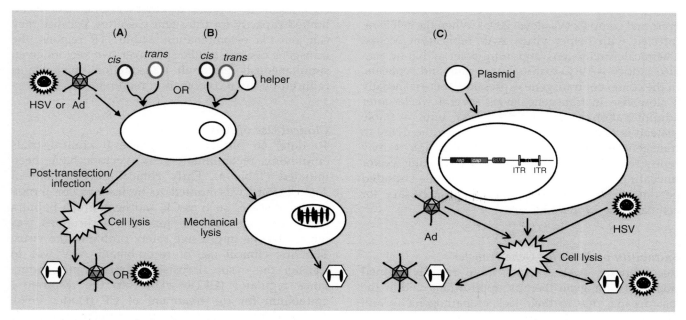

**Figure 13** ■ General overview of methods for production of recombinant AAV by transient transfection. **(A)** Two plasmid method. Cells are transfected with one plasmid, containing AAV ITRs flanking the transgene cassette (*cis*) and another containing AAV *rep* and *cap* sequences without viral ITRs (*trans*). Replication-defective helper virus is also added to the cells to support AAV replication and packaging. When cells show signs of lysis, they are harvested. Extensive purification methods must be in place for efficient separation of AAV from the helper virus. **(B)** Three plasmid method. *Cis* and *trans* plasmids in Scheme A are co-transfected with a third plasmid bearing adenovirus helper sequences. Cells are harvested 48–72 hours after transfection. Only recombinant AAV particles are produced by this method. **(C)** One plasmid method. A single plasmid containing *rep*, *cap* a selectable marker and the transgene cassette flanked by AAV ITRs is introduced into cells by transfection. Cells that contain the integrated plasmid are further propagated by culture in selective media. Helper functions must be provided by infection with a helper virus in this system. As in (A), extensive purification methods must be in place for efficient separation of AAV from the helper virus.

viruses under development for gene transfer. Some have reported that the virus is stable at 4°C in phosphate buffered saline alone for over 4 months before a significant drop in infectious titer was observed (Croyle, 2001). Similar results have been reported at 25°C. Addition of cryoprotectants such as sorbitol and polysorbate 80 have extended the stability of the virus at 4°C for 1 year (Wright, 2003). Lyophilization has also stabilized AAV for over one year at 25°C after a subtle drop in titer due to processing (Croyle, 2001). Like the adenovirus, AAV is susceptible to loss of infectivity after freezing at −80 and −20°C. Use of potassium-based buffers that avoid drastic changes in pH during freezing and the addition of cryoprotectants moderately extended the stability of AAV at sub-zero temperatures (Croyle, 2001; Wright, 2003). Aggregation of virus particles and subsequent loss of infectious titer is a significant issue in preparations purified by column chromatography (Wright, 2005). Unlike density gradient ultracentrifugation, chromatographic techniques cannot distinguish between virus capsids that contain the AAV genome and those that are empty, which promote virus aggregation. Increasing the ionic strength of buffers used during purification and processing and in the final formulation significantly reduces this phenomenon and improves long-term stability.

## ■ Non-Viral Vectors for Gene Transfer

Non-viral vectors were not the agents of choice for gene transfer protocols but problems in clinical trials with recombinant viruses renewed interest in this method of gene transfer. Non-viral vectors generally consist of double-stranded recombinant DNA plasmids alone or encapsulated in cationic polymer or lipid-based formulations. Non-viral vectors offer several important advantages over virus-based methods for gene transfer (Table 5). Their unlimited cloning capacity significantly expands the types of therapeutic transgenes and expression cassettes that can be used for gene transfer. Plasmids, unlike their viral counterparts, are generally non-immunogenic and can easily be readministered multiple times without induction of a prohibitive immune response. Non-viral vectors have a reduced capacity for insertional mutagenesis and a limited ability to produce unwanted by-products in vivo due to homologous recombination. Recombinant DNA plasmids for gene transfer are also relatively easy to manipulate using standard techniques and do not require specialized skills or equipment for large-scale production. They are also inexpensive to produce, especially on a large scale in contrast to viral vectors. Despite all the advantages that non-viral vectors have to offer, their clinical utility is significantly hindered by low transduction efficiency, which stems from non-specific uptake of the vector and poor delivery to the therapeutic target. They also have a limited capacity to override cellular gene silencing mechanisms and, as a result, cannot achieve sustained gene expression. Refinement of delivery methods for non-viral gene transfer and reconstruction of vectors at the molecular level have addressed these issues.

### Construction of Non-Viral Vectors

Identification of cellular and molecular processes associated with gene expression and concurrent advancement of recombinant DNA technology has led to production of highly sophisticated recombinant DNA molecules. Several issues that must be considered when designing a plasmid-based vector are briefly outlined below.

### *Manufacturing Considerations*

*Origin of Replication (ori).* Identification of the *rop* gene as the primary gatekeeper that limits the plasmid number to 20 to 40 copies/cell in bacteria led to the development of the pUC series of plasmids. Elimination of *rop* increased the acceptable copy number to more than 500 copies/cell for plasmids that encode proteins of approximately 1,500 base pairs. Most of the plasmids used in the clinic in the last 2 to 3 years have been constructed using pUC plasmids (Manthorpe, 2005).

*Selection Marker.* Selection markers have commonly been those that conferred resistance to penicillin-based drugs since growth of bacteria in antibiotic supplemented media is convenient, inexpensive and efficient. However, the U.S. Food and Drug Administration has stated that (*a*) selection markers for reagents suitable for human use must have the least impact on human health and should not confer antibiotic resistance to symbiotic bacteria, (*b*) selection by using drugs within the penicillin family could induce adverse reactions in those allergic to these drugs in the event that drug residue remained in purified plasmid preparations, and (*c*) the TN903 gene, conferring resistance to kanamycin, an antibiotic sparingly used in humans, is acceptable for use in plasmids for clinical gene transfer protocols (U.S. Dept. of Health and Human Services, 1998). Despite these recommendations, the risk of introduction of antibiotic resistance is still significant in protocols that require high doses of plasmid.

### *Considerations for Gene Expression*

Advances in recombinant DNA technology suggest that properties associated with viral vectors can be mimicked by elements that facilitate nuclear maintenance and replication of plasmid constructs.

*Site-Specific Integration.* Viral integration in the human chromosome is driven by site-specific recombinases (SSR) that recognize unique sites within pathogen and host genomes. SSRs derived from bacteriophage that do not require bacterial cofactors for stable integration have been used for gene transfer (Glover, 2006). The most efficient integrase, φC31, integrates at a number of sites in the human genome and has significant potential for treatment of recessive genetic disorders (Thyagarajan, 2001). Proximity of integration sites to tumor-suppressor genes and genes that regulate cell proliferation is currently unknown and must be investigated prior to clinical testing.

*Extra-Chromosomal Replication and Stability.* SV40 and Epstein–Barr virus (EBV) viruses replicate episomally in mammalian cells via Tag and EBV nuclear antigen 1 (EBNA1) proteins respectively. Inclusion of viral sequences with the corresponding viral protein that promotes segregation of viral episomes during cell division can markedly sustain the expression of a therapeutic transgene. Unfortunately, viral proteins like Tag and EBNA1 can disable retinoblastoma and p53 tumor suppressor pathways, making them unsuitable for human gene transfer. To address this problem, a plasmid in which the scaffold/matrix attachment region (S/MAR) from the human-β-interferon gene cluster was generated (Glover, 2006). Mitotic stability of this plasmid is conferred by interaction of the S/MAR element with components of the nuclear matrix. This plasmid has been maintained for over 100 divisions in CHO and HeLa cells (Piechaczek, 1999). The safety and stability of S/MAR-based episomal-based plasmids in vivo has not been established. Extensive testing must be completed before they can be considered for human use.

*Human Artificial Chromosomes.* Chromosomes replicate and maintain a low, defined copy number within host cells and accommodate many large genes and regulatory elements. Human artificial chromosomes (HACs) are susceptible to recombination and often integrate into and disrupt the host genome in an unpredictable manner. However, use of HACs to provide long-term expression of HPRT and CFTR transgenes has been described (Grimes, 2001; Auriche, 2002). The size of HACs prevents them from being packaged in viral vectors. Non-viral delivery methods for HACs have not been successful in vivo. Thus, even though elegant recombinant DNA molecules for gene transfer have been constructed, therapeutic efficacy relies on efficient methods of gene delivery.

## Delivery Methods for Non-Viral Gene Transfer

Naked DNA is susceptible to nuclease degradation in the systemic circulation and is taken up in an inefficient, non-specific manner in many tissues. Physical methods used for gene transfer involve disruption of cell membranes. Chemical methods facilitate interaction with tissue targets and transport across cell membranes.

### Physical Methods for Gene Transfer

The earliest techniques to deliver recombinant DNA to cellular targets: microinjection, particle bombardment and electroporation, were rudimentary and severe (Table 6). Microinjection, direct injection of DNA or RNA into the cytoplasm or nucleus of a single cell is the simplest and most effective method for physical delivery of genetic material to cells. This transduces 100% of the recipient cells and minimizes waste of plasmid DNA, but requires highly specialized equipment and skills. It is harsh to the cell since it involves mechanical puncture of plasma and nuclear membranes and is generally restricted to ex vivo gene transfer of cultured cells or embryonic stem cells for production of transgenic animals.

*Particle Bombardment.* Particle bombardment, using a "gene gun," was first used to transfect plant cells and was later adapted for gene transfer in mammalian cells and tissues. Gold particles are coated with recombinant DNA and propelled by an electric spark or helium discharge into the target cell or tissue. Two principal devices available for gene transfer are the Accell (Agracetus, Inc.) and the Helios (BioRad Laboratories) gene guns. Transduction efficiency and distribution of gene expression relies upon particle size, timing of delivery and particle acceleration. This technology has been primarily used for genetic immunization. The benefit of particle bombardment is high levels of transgene expression with very low doses of DNA. DNA-loading capacity of the particles and the limited depth of penetration have limited the utility of this method. Although gene transfer by particle bombardment has been shown to be safe and well tolerated in the clinic, cells that directly encounter DNA-coated particles can be severely damaged.

*Electroporation.* Electroporation, exposes the cell membrane to high-intensity pulses of electricity that transiently destabilize the cell membrane and make it highly permeable to plasmid DNA. Successful delivery with this method has been reported in muscle, skin, liver and solid tumors. Commercially available electroporation devices consist of a pulse generator and an applicator with several specialized electrodes tailored for delivery to specific tissues and organs. Several physical (pulse duration, electric field strength) and

| | Advantages | Disadvantages |
|---|---|---|
| Naked DNA | No special skills needed<br>Easy to produce | Low transduction efficiency<br>Transient gene expression |
| **Physical methods** | | |
| Microinjection | Up to 100% transduction efficiency (nuclear injection) | Requires highly specialized skills for delivery<br>Limited to ex vivo delivery |
| Gene gun | Easy to perform<br>Effective immunization with low amount of DNA | Poor tissue penetration |
| Electroporation | High transduction efficiency | Transient gene expression<br>Toxicity, tissue damage<br>Highly invasive |
| Sonoporation | Method well tolerated for other applications | Transient gene expression<br>Toxicity not yet established |
| Laser irradiation | Can achieve 100% transduction efficiency | Special skills and expensive equipment necessary |
| Magentofection | Safety of method established in the clinic | Poor efficiency with naked DNA |
| **Chemical methods** | | |
| Liposomes | Easy to produce<br>Fusion liposomes improve transduction efficiency | Transient gene expression<br>Toxicity, mildly immunogenic |
| Cationic polymers | Easy to manipulate for targeting | Transient gene expression<br>Toxicity, mildly immunogenic |

*Source*: From Mehier-Humbert and Guy, 2005; Conwell and Huang, 2005; Miyazaki et al., 2006.

**Table 6** ■ Summary of non-viral methods used for gene transfer.

biological (DNA concentration and confirmation and cell size) factors can influence the efficiency of gene transfer and must be optimized based upon the cell type and size of the DNA molecule (Cemazar, 2006). Toxicity of this procedure is cell-specific, and muscle contraction and pain have been reported. The most significant issue limiting the clinical utility of electroporation is unevenly distributed transgene expression in tissue. Several studies have suggested that electroporation can elicit an immune response (Lefesvre, 2002; Babiuk, 2004; Cemazar, 2006).

*Sonoporation.* Within the last 10 years, newer, less invasive methods for gene transfer have been developed. Sonoporation enhances cell membrane permeability by acoustic cavitation through ultrasound. Ultrasound waves collapse active bubbles, releasing energy that disrupts adjacent cell membranes. This technique was first tested for gene transfer in vitro with an ultrasound contrast agent, Albumex, composed of elastic and compressible gas-filled microbubbles to serve as cavitation nuclei and lower the transfection threshold of cultured cells (Bao, 1997). Recently, in vivo gene transfer has been reported with this technique (Miller 1999; Huber, 2000). Efficiency of gene transfer

depends upon transducer frequency, acoustic pressure, pulse duration, and length of exposure. The bubble shell composition and the type of entrapped gas in the contrast agent can also affect gene transfer. A commercial device is available for in vitro and in vivo use (Sonitron, Protech International). Both diagnostic and therapeutic ultrasound have excellent safety profiles in the clinic (Mehier-Humbert, 2005).

*Laser Irradiation.* Laser irradiation, involves focusing a laser beam on a target cell and modifying permeability by thermal effects. Although the mechanism of gene transfer by this method is not completely understood, transduction efficiency relies upon differences in osmotic pressure between the cytoplasm and the surrounding medium. Laser irradiation induces minimal cell damage because permeabilization is transient and very fast. Although this technique can achieve 100% transduction efficiency without affecting cell growth and division, it is not widely used due to the expense and size of the laser source and specialized skills needed for successful application.

*Magnetofection.* Magnetofection, involves attachment of magnetic polymer-coated iron oxide nanoparticles to DNA, a transfection reagent or viral vector by salt-induced colloidal aggregation (Plank, 2003). Magnetic particles are concentrated in target cells by an external magnetic field that pulls the particles across plasma membranes into the cytoplasm. High transduction efficiencies have been achieved with this method in vivo in the gastrointestinal tract and blood vessels (Scherer, 2003). Vector type (viral vs. non-viral), dose, composition and incubation time influence transduction. The apparatus needed for this technique is simple and inexpensive. This method is safe and has been used clinically for delivery of chemotherapeutic agents (Bertram, 2006). Toxicity has been attributed to specific transfection reagents and not the technique itself. The main advantage of magnetofection is that it increases bioavailability of recombinant DNA and reduces the amount needed for effective gene transfer.

*Hydroporation.* Hydroporation or hydrodynamic gene delivery, involves injection of large volumes of solution into the circulation to overcome the physical barriers of the endothelium and the cell membrane. Utility of hydrodynamic gene delivery was first established when Liu et al. and Zhang et al. reported significant gene transfer in the liver of mice after rapid injection of large volume DNA solutions representing 8% to 10% of the total body weight (Liu, 1999; Zhang, 1999). Hydrodynamic delivery of genes to the muscle and kidney has also been described (Al-Dosari, 2005). This technique requires only a needle and syringe. Saline is often used for hydrodynamic procedures, however, Ringers solution and phosphate buffered saline have also been employed. The dose of DNA delivered by hydrodynamic delivery ranges from 0.1 to 10 mg/kg. Although marked transgene expression has been achieved without tissue damage, an increase blood pressure and decrease heart rate due to the volume introduced into the system has been noted (Zhang, 2004). Transient increases in tissue-specific parameters such as serum transaminases after administration to the liver and creatinine kinase after muscle delivery have also been reported. Hydroporation has been limited to small animals for functional and mechanistic studies. Lack of appropriate catheters for administration to larger animals is a limitation that must be overcome for further assessment of this technique in humans.

### Chemical Methods for Gene Transfer

*Cationic Liposomes.* Liposomal gene delivery was the first non-viral system to reach clinical trials due to the pioneering work of Felgner and colleagues that described the natural interaction of cationic liposomes with the negatively charged phosphate backbone of recombinant DNA to form organized structures that

protect the genetic material from degradation (Felgner, 1987). The positive charge along the surface also promoted interaction with the cell membrane and endocytosis.

Interaction of liposomes with DNA is dependent upon pH, charge, and lipid structure. A cationic lipid generally consists of four different functional domains: (*a*) a positively charged head group, (*b*) a spacer of varying length, (*c*) a linker bond, and (*d*) a hydrophobic anchor (Fig. 14). Efforts to improve transduction efficiency of cationic lipoplexes involve the use of neutral "helper" lipids, such as dioleoyl-phosphatidylethanolamine and cholesterol, to stabilize the complex and promote disruption of cell membranes (Karmali, 2006). Addition of other components to enhance DNA-lipid interactions, membrane-permeabilizing agents to facilitate cellular uptake and natural targeting ligands such as transferrin, folate, asialofetuin, or antibodies against cell surface molecules have further improved tissue selectivity and transduction efficiency (Collins, 2006).

*Fusion Liposomes.* Virosomes, or fusion liposomes have been designed to improve vector stability in the endosome and the cytoplasm and facilitate delivery to the nucleus. The first of these viral/non-viral hybrids, the Hemagglutinating Virus of Japan (HVJ) liposome, was prepared from UV-inactivated HVJ particles and liposomes containing DNA complexed with the High Mobility Group-1 (HMG-1) protein (Fig. 15) (Kaneda, 1999). Successful gene transfer is largely due to the hemagglutinin-neuramidase ($H_N$) and fusion glycoproteins (FGP) in the lipid bilayer that facilitate interaction with sialic residues on the cell surface and fuse with the cell membrane, bypassing endocytosis. The HMG-1 protein also promotes gene stabilization within the nucleus. Although, anti-HVJ antibodies have been reported in

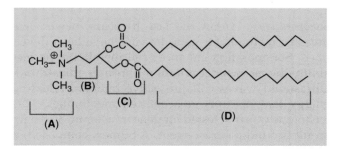

**Figure 14** ■ General structure of a cationic lipid suitable for gene transfer. Cationic lipids contain (**A**) a polar head group, (**B**) a spacer, (**C**) a linker bond, and (**D**) hydrophobic tail groups. Each of these structures can be modified to improve gene transfer.

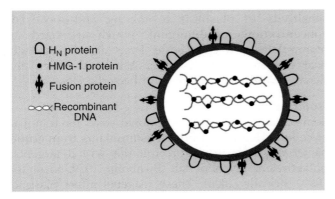

**Figure 15** ■ The hemagglutinating virus of Japan (HVJ) liposome. The HVJ liposome consists of recombinant DNA coated with HMG-1 proteins encased in a liposome prepared from three lipids. Hemagglutinin nuramidase ($H_N$) and fusion glycoproteins isolated from HVJ are interspersed throughout the lipid layer. These novel non-viral vectors have been found to have high transduction efficiency and little toxicity. They have been tested for several applications in vitro and in vivo. Several clinical trials employing this vector are in the planning stages.

several animal models, successful gene transfer has been reported after multiple doses without notable toxicity or inflammatory responses (Hirano, 1998; Hasegawa, 2001). Success of HVJ liposomes led to the development of other virosomes prepared with influenza membrane fusion protein hemagglutinin, cationic-lipid reconstituted influenza virus envelopes and lipoplexes coated with the G glycoprotein of the vesicular stomatitis virus envelope (Shoji, 2004; Cusi, 2006).

*Cationic Polymers.* Cationic polymers condense DNA by neutralizing the charge of the DNA backbone and mediate cellular contact through ionic interactions. Polylysine (PLL) and polyethylenimine (PEI) are the most commonly used cationic polymers. Use of either compound, however, is limited by toxicity. Polymers facilitate tissue-specific gene delivery through covalent attachment of compounds that interact with specific cell surface markers. Attachment of carbohydrates such as lactose and galactose target asialoglycoproteins and aid delivery to hepatocytes. Conjugation of arterial-wall binding peptide aids delivery to endothelial cells. Attachment of antibodies against cell surface molecules induced tissue-specific gene expression and reduced toxicity of DNA-polymer complexes (Lavigne, 2006; Park, 2006). Other biodegradable polymers such as poly($\alpha$-[4-aminobutyl]-L-glycolic acid (PAGA), poly($\beta$-amino ester), poly(2-aminoethyl propylene phosphate, PPE-EA) and poly(D,L-lactide-co-4-hydroxyl-L-proline, PHLP) have reduced toxicity associated with DNA polyplexes and improved gene expression (Park, 2006).

### The Immune Response Against Non-Viral Vectors

The immune response to non-viral DNA complexes is highly dependent upon the dose and route of administration. Low doses have little effect on organ function and tissue histology. Higher doses, especially of cationic liposomes, induce acute inflammation and profound tissue damage (Yew, 2005). Physical properties of the complexes promote aggregation in the circulation, producing large particulates that are readily recognized by the RES (Dash, 1999). The most severe side effects occur after intravenous and intrapulmonary delivery. Strategies to reduce inflammation and toxicity of non-viral vectors involve: removal of CpG motifs in plasmid DNA, minimizing interaction between the complex and the immune system and use of immunosuppressants in the complex.

Elimination of CpG motifs is achieved by: (*a*) amplifying plasmids in bacteria that express Sss I methylase to add a methyl group to cytosine residues, (*b*) use of CpG-free plasmids and/or removal of CpG motifs from plasmids by site-directed mutagenesis, and (*c*) removal of unnecessary prokaryotic sequences by site-specific recombination to create "minimal" plasmids (Yew, 2004; 2005). These actions have reduced the immune response, but have not eliminated it and compromise transduction efficiency. Covalent attachment of poly(ethylene) glycol to the surface of DNA complexes (PEGylation) has improved toxicity and promotes transduction efficiency by preventing aggregation and uptake by the RES (Lee, 2005). PEG molecules are also stabilizing, protective linkers that facilitate attachment of targeting molecules and antibodies (Haag, 2006). Injection of lipids prior to administration of recombinant DNA has reduced cytokine production by 80% in mice by changing the tissue distribution of the plasmid (Zhang, 2006). Creation of "safeplexes", lipo- or polyplexes that contain inflammatory suppressor molecules, has also markedly reduced inflammation and toxicity without compromising gene transfer (Liu, 2004). A combination of each of these approaches will most likely be needed for successful and safe clinical gene transfer.

### Clinical Use of Non-Viral Vectors

Three-fourths of the currently active clinical protocols employing non-viral vectors involve intramuscular injection of plasmids expressing antigenic epitopes of a number of pathogens. Many of these trials involve vaccination against HIV-1 and are in phase I testing (Girard, 2006). One trial employing a three plasmid DNA vaccine for Ebola infection has completed phase I testing and will enter phase II alone and in combination with a recombinant adenovirus vector in a prime-boost dosing regimen (Martin, 2006). Several human trials using non-viral vectors to treat genetic diseases such as hemophilia A, CF, alpha-1-antitrypsin deficiency and Canavan disease illustrate the challenges of permanent correction of a hereditary disorder with a plasmid-based system (O'Connor, 2006). Despite this, some investigators continue to refine and develop additional non-viral systems for treating CF (Lee, 2005).

## Production and Processing of Non-Viral Vectors

One benefit of non-viral vectors for gene transfer is that the production process is rather generic and can be applied to any plasmid preparation regardless of composition or application. Since the current average human dose of plasmid DNA for gene transfer and vaccination is approximately one milligram (Manthorpe, 2005), the primary challenge associated with large-scale production of plasmids is to develop a process that is both scalable and economical. Thus, process development for plasmid-based gene transfer remains an active area of research and development (Schorr, 2006). A standard process for large-scale production of recombinant DNA plasmids consists of five unit operations.

### Fermentation

Fermentation processes must support growth of transformed bacteria and maximize the amount of plasmid produced by each cell. *Escherichia coli* is the most common strain used for plasmid production. Amino acids, nucleosides and the ratio of nitrogen to carbon containing compounds present in a rich media formulation greatly improve plasmid yield (O'Kennedy, 2000).

### Harvest

Bacterial cells are either harvested by centrifugation or microfiltration. Centrifugation under Good Manufacturing Practice (GMP) conditions can be costly, making microfiltration the accepted method of cell harvest (Manthorpe, 2005). This also allows for spent media, metabolic byproducts, extracellular debris and impurities to be washed away prior to purification.

### Lysis

Bacterial cells must be lysed to release the recombinant plasmids. This is one of the most critical steps in the production process since it can significantly affect the amount of usable (covalently closed circular, ccc) and unusable (sheared, partially denatured and open circular) forms of DNA in a preparation. The most widely used method of lysis for clinical-scale manufacturing is treatment with alkaline detergent and precipitation of cellular debris with acetate (Shamlou, 2003). This removes a significant fraction of cellular impurities from the lysate, but increases the sensitivity of plasmids to mixing and localized concentrations of detergent, which are hard to manipulate on a large scale. Lysis of cells through heat exposure addresses this issue and effectively denatures cellular proteins and bacterial DNA.

### Isolation/Purification

Some processes include additional steps for removal of cellular debris and other contaminants from crude bacterial lysates such as precipitation with detergents, polyethylene glycol or salt (Birnboim, 1979; Nicoletti, 1993; Murphy, 2006). These reagents affect plasmid stability and are removed by column chromatography. Size exclusion chromatography can effectively separate plasmid DNA from RNA, proteins and other small molecules present in the cleared lysate. The degree of separation of plasmid DNA from contaminants is highly dependent upon the type and concentration of salt in the running buffer. Resins used in anion exchange chromatography have a high affinity for plasmid DNA and provide maximal sample concentration (Shamlou, 2003; Stadler, 2004; Schorr, 2006). Hydrophobic interaction and thiophilic aromatic chromatography are the methods of choice for selective separation of the different plasmid DNA isoforms and endotoxin reduction.

### Bulk Preparation

After purification, the bulk plasmid is placed in a suitable buffer and formulation by ultrafiltration using a membrane with a pore size of 50 to 100 kDa.

Plasmids for clinical use must be highly characterized. Impurities from production and processing steps are well known. Tests necessary to confirm the identity, purity and potency of a plasmid-based product are well-established and routine. These tests and the current specifications set by the FDA and the World Health Organization are summarized in Table 7.

## THE ROLE OF DRUG METABOLISM IN GENE THERAPY

An important aspect of pre-clinical drug development is evaluation of how a novel compound will influence drug metabolizing enzymes. In vitro, in vivo and clinical observations have documented that infection and inflammation significantly reduces the expression and function of cytochrome P450 (CYP) enzymes (Carcillo, 2003; Aitken, 2006). Understanding the effects of viral and non-viral vectors on CYP and other drug metabolizing enzymes is important since traditional drug regimens are also included in many gene therapy trials. Although this is a new concept in the gene therapy, it has been reported that a single dose of recombinant adenovirus suppresses rat CYP3A2 for 14 days without resolution (Callahan,

| Assay type | Issue | Determined by | Acceptable level in final product |
|---|---|---|---|
| Identity | Cross-contamination with other products | Restriction digest/gel electrophoresis | N/A |
| Purity | Residual bacterial chromosomal DNA | Real-time PCR | <2 µg/mg pDNA |
| | Residual RNA | Analytical HPLC | <0.2 µg/mg pDNA |
| | Residual bacterial protein | BCA protein assay | <3 µg/mg pDNA |
| | Endotoxin | LAL assay | <10 E.U./mg pDNA |
| | Sterility (bacterial and fungal) | Method outlined in CFR 21 610.12 | No growth |
| | Appearance | Visual inspection | Clear solution free of particulates |
| | pH | pH meter | Physiologic (7.0–7.4) but may be product specific |
| | Plasmid confirmation (ccc vs. oc) | HPLC or CGE | >97% ccc |
| Potency | Labeled dose | In vitro ELISA, FACS, RT-PCR Light absorbance ($A_{260}$) | Transgene/plasmid specific |

*Source*: From Manthorpe et al., 2005; USDHHS, 1998; Stadler et al., 2004.

**Table 7** ▪ Quality control assays and "acceptable" levels of impurities in the final plasmid-based product for clinical trials.

2005). CYP3A2 is homologous to human CYP3A4, responsible for the metabolism of approximately 50% of marketed medications. Further study of other gene transfer vectors would be useful to identify potential drug interactions, adverse reactions and clinical failures that may occur during gene therapy clinical trials. This is also of importance since some gene transfer applications rely on metabolism of a medicinal substance to regulate expression of the transgene (see below) while others focus on over-expression of drug metabolizing enzymes to improve the effect of some medicinal compounds.

### ▪ Gene-Directed Enzyme Prodrug Therapy (GDEPT)

One of the primary goals of cancer therapy is to deliver highly potent, cytotoxic compounds to tumors and mestastases and limiting the exposure of normal tissue to these agents. GDEPT is one approach toward this goal where a gene encoding a compound-specific enzyme is delivered directly to tumor cells. The corresponding prodrug is given and is only converted to a cytotoxic agent by the recombinant enzyme in the tumor. Localization of the effects of chemotherapy and the protection of normal cells from cytotoxic effects is further enhanced by the inclusion of tumor-specific promoters that bind transcription factors like hypoxia-inducible factor (HIF)-1 within the tumor microenvironment (Riddick, 2005). Some GDEPT strategies rely on a "bystander effect," where cytotoxic agents produced by transfected cells spread to surrounding cells for arrest and regression of tumor growth, reducing the need for the vector to reach all cells in order for the therapy to be successful (Fig. 16). There are currently 54 active clinical trials employing

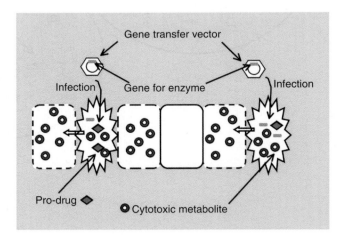

**Figure 16** ▪ The "bystander effect" observed with gene directed-enzyme-prodrug therapy. A recombinant vector expressing an enzyme is given to a patient. The vector induces expression of the enzyme in some but not all of the cells of a particular target. When a pro-drug (diamonds) recognized by the enzyme is given to the patient, cells expressing the enzyme (small bars) metabolize the compound to a highly toxic molecule (double circles). As metabolites accumulate in the cells expressing the enzyme, they eventually kill it to release the toxic compound to surrounding cells. This approach extends the therapeutic effect beyond cells that were transduced by the vector.

the GDEPT approach. Three have achieved phase III status (Wiley, 2006).

Over-expression of the herpes simplex virus thymidine kinase (HSV-tk) gene with gancyclovir represents the clinical standard of GDEPT. This system is selective because gancyclovir, a poor substrate for human monophosphatase kinase, is rapidly converted to the triphosphate form after phosphorylation in a cell expressing HSV-tk (Fig. 17A). The triphosphate competes deoxyguanosine triphosphate during DNA elongation and, once incorporated in a strand, blocks DNA polymerase and induces single strand breaks. To date, the HSV-tk/gancyclovir combination is the only GDEPT approach to reach phase III clinical testing.

Clinical use of 5-Fluorouracil (5-FU) is limited by side effects associated with high doses needed for therapeutic efficacy. Over-expression of bacterial cytosine deaminase and use of the prodrug 5-fluorocytosine (5-FC) has shown promise in treating cancer and minimizing effects in normal cells and tissues. Bacterial cytosine deaminase coverts 5-FC to 5-FU that is then converted to 5-fluorouridine-5-triphosphate (5-FUTP). 5-FUTP prevents nuclear processing of ribosomal and mRNA once it is incorporated into a DNA strand (Fig. 17B). Two phase I trials have demonstrated the safety of the cytosine deaminase/5-FC system in colon carcinoma (Crystal, 1997) and prostate cancer (Freytag, 2002).

The compound 5-aziridinyl-2,4-dinitrobenzamide (CB1954) can be converted to the potent DNA cross-linking mustard metabolite, 5-aziridynyl-4-hydroxylamino-2-nitrobenzaminde by the nitroreductase of *E. coli* (Fig. 17C). The NTR/CB1954 combination is currently being tested in the clinic in the United Kingdom (Wiley, 2006), however, poor-bioavailability

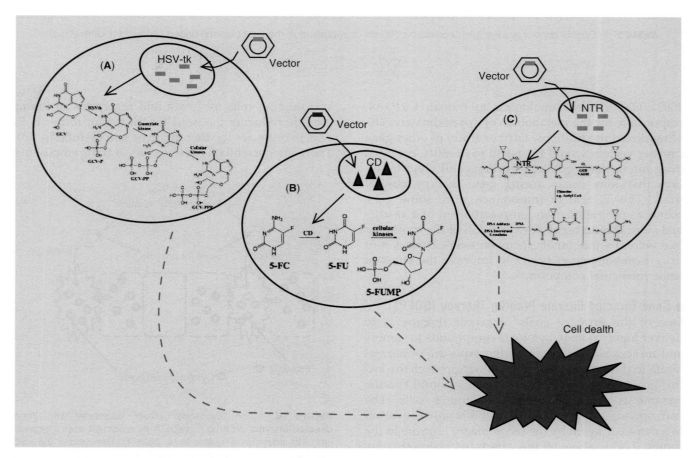

**Figure 17** ■ Models of gene-directed enzyme-prodrug therapy. (**A**) The HSV-tk system. A vector expressing the gene for HSV-tk enters a cellular target. This enzyme is expressed and phosphorylates the drug gancyclovir (GCV). This is subsequently converted to the di- and tri-phosphate forms by guanylate kinase and other cellular kinases. The triphosphate is incorporated into cellular DNA during cell division causing single strand breaks. (**B**) The cytososine deaminase/5-fluorocytosine system. A vector expressing cytosine deaminase (CD) enters a cellular target. Overexpression of CD activates 5-fluorocytosine (5-FC) to 5-fluorouridine (5-FU). 5-FU is converted to mono-, di- and tri-phosphate forms by cellular kinases. Each of these compounds are cytotoxic. (**C**). The nitroreductase/CB1954 system. A vector expressing *E. coli* nitroreductase (NTR) enters a cellular target. Expression of NTR allows the cell to convert the compound CB1954 to a potent DNA cross-linking agent.

of CB1954 limits the efficacy of this combination (Palmer, 2004). The design of highly potent prodrugs for nitroreductase with improved bioavailability is necessary for further work with this system.

## ■ Systems for Pharmacological Regulation of Gene Expression

Strict regulation of gene expression in a consistent manner when and where the transgene is needed is a requirement for successful clinical implementation of gene therapy. Several systems consisting of a chimeric promoter containing a specific tandem operator (Op) placed adjacent to a minimal promoter ($P_{min}$) that drives expression of the therapeutic transgene are under development (Fig. 18). The chimeric promoter is activated by binding of a transactivator (TA) complex to the Op. The TA complex consists of a DNA binding domain (DB) and a ligand binding (LB) domain, capable of interacting with an orally active compound. The compound facilitates formation of the TA complex and dictates gene expression or repression. Regulated gene expression systems currently under development are responsive to small-molecule drugs such as antibiotics, steroids, immunosuppressants and their derivatives (Goverdhana, 2005). In an optimized regulated gene expression system, each component must be non-immunogenic, safe and well tolerated. Transgene expression must be undetectable when repressed and highest when induced. The inducer is reversible and compact in size for efficient

incorporation in gene delivery systems. The regulating compound should be non-toxic, able to distribute to the target tissue and have a half-life of a few hours so that gene expression can be altered quickly. These issues are common to the development of traditional pharmaceutical compounds and are areas in which the pharmacist and the pharmaceutical scientist can make significant contributions.

The most widely tested regulated gene expression systems are the TET-ON/TET-OFF and Rapamycin/Rapalog dimerizer systems (Fig. 19) (Goverdhana, 2005; Vilaboa, 2006). They have been engineered primarily in recombinant adenovirus, AAV and retrovirus vectors (Goverdhana, 2005; Weber, 2006). Although all of the systems currently under investigation are in pre-clinical testing, they are on the brink of entering clinical trials. While these systems involve dosing and control of a single therapeutic transgene, development of elaborate semi-synthetic gene networks, capable of interacting seamlessly with cellular processes to produce self-sustained, feedback-controlled and physiologically triggered transgene expression is underway. This approach, if successful in the clinic, will most likely become the premiere technology of molecular medicine.

The majority of pharmacologically regulated gene expression systems have been tested in animal models of cancer and hormone-related diseases. One approach for the treatment of certain malignancies is the adoptive transfer of T-cells. A problem with this method, however, is that the cells may recognize both normal and malignant tissue and cause fatal graft-

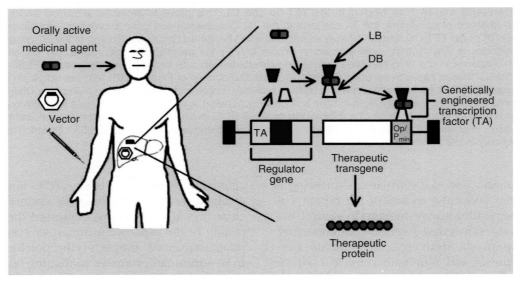

**Figure 18** ■ General concept of pharmacological regulation of gene expression. The patient is given a single dose of a recombinant vector containing sequences for regulatory elements and the transgene cassette. The regulator gene contains sequences for a ligand binding (LB) molecule and a DNA binding (DB) molecule. Both molecules are capable of interacting with an orally active compound that facilitates the formation of the transactivation (TA) complex that cannot form in the absence of this compound. Once formed, the TA complex binds to an Op or minimal promoter (Op/$P_{min}$) placed in front of the therapeutic transgene. Transgene expression will occur only when the TA complex not the DNA binding protein alone binds to the Op/$P_{min}$ sequence.

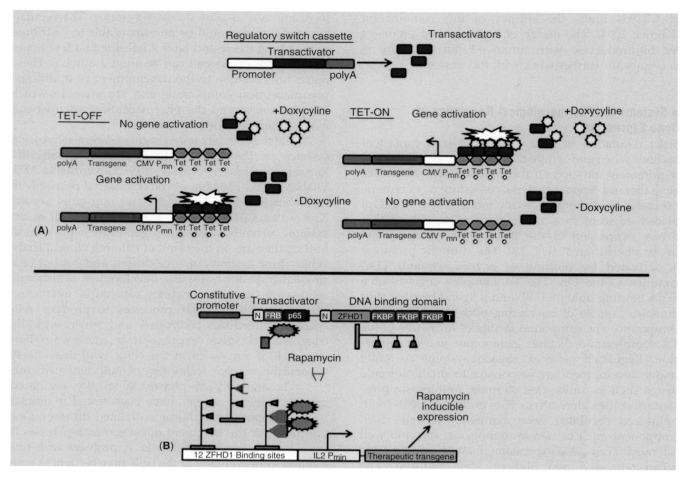

**Figure 19** ■ Examples of pharmacologically regulated gene expression systems. (**A**) Tetracycline dependent regulatory systems. This expression system consists of two distinct constructs. The first construct contains sequences for the transactivator protein (TA). In the TET-OFF system, interaction of a tetracycline molecule or derivative (such as doxycycline) with the TA causes a change in confirmation that prevents the TA from binding to the TET-Op (Tet O). This prevents promoter activation and subsequent gene expression. In the absence of doxycyline, the TA can bind to the Tet O sequence and gene expression commences. Interaction of doxycyline with the TA of the TET-ON system initiates a confirmational change that promotes binding of the TA complex to Tet O that drives gene expression. In this system, gene expression occurs only in the presence of doxycycline. (**B**) Rapamycin dependent regulatory system. Rapamycin is a drug capable of interacting simultaneously with two cellular polypeptides: FKBP12 and FRAP. In this system, the transactivation cassette encodes the rapamycin-binding domain of FRAP (FRB) with the activation domain from the p65 subunit of human NFKB. A second transactivating domain encodes 3 copies of FKBP fused to the unique DNA binding domain, ZFHD-1. Both transactivating protein sequences contain a nuclear localization signal (N). The transgene cassette contains 12 copies of the recognition site for ZFHD-1 upstream of a minimal interleukin-2 (IL-2) promoter that initiates expression and production of the therapeutic transgene only after 12 copies of the complete transactivation complex bind to the ZFHD-1 region. The transactivation complex can form only in the presence of rapamycin.

versus-host-disease. Use of a retrovirus expressing a Fas suicide gene under the control of the rapamycin dimerizer system, allows investigators to control the fate of adoptively transferred T-cells by administering AP1903, a rapamycin derivative, to activate Fas-mediated apoptosis and eliminate cells that attack normal tissue (Berger, 2004). Pharmacologically regulated gene expression systems have also been applied in models of arthritis, hemophilia B, chronic hepatitis B infection, and tuberculosis (Weber, 2006). One of the most promising studies demonstrated the ability of a regulatable system to respond to pharmacological activation over time (Rivera, 2005). Sixteen primates received two recombinant AAV vectors by intramuscular injection. One virus expressed the transcription factors of the rapamycin dimerizer system while the other expressed rhesus erythropoietin downstream from a minimal promoter containing binding sites for the regulated transcription factors. All animals expressed rhesus erythropoietin in a dose-dependent, reversible manner in response to rapamycin or its analogs. One animal was studied for a period of 6 years. The response of this primate is illustrated in Figure 20.

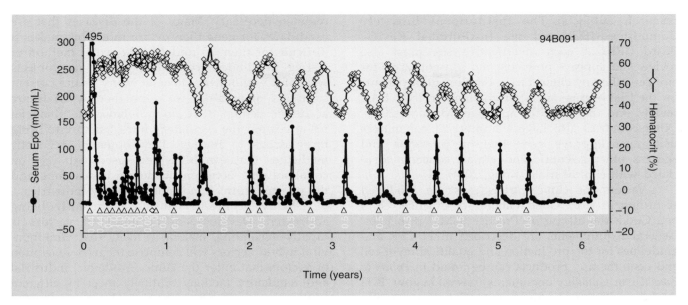

**Figure 20** ■ Long-term regulated gene expression of rhesus erythropoietin in non-human primates using recombinant AAV. A non-human primate was given a single intramuscular dose of a recombinant AAV ($3.9 \times 10^{12}$ genome copies/kg) containing sequences necessary for production of a rapamycin-mediated transactivation complex and a separate virus ($11.5 \times 10^{12}$ genome copies/kg) containing inducible rhesus erythropoietin. The primate was given intravenous rapamycin over the course of 6 years. Times of rapamycin administration are highlighted at the bottom of the traces by open triangles and the dose of drug indicated (mg/kg). Erythropoietin levels (●, left vertical axis) peaked at 495 U/ml after the first induction cycle but were responsive to the drug each time it was given. Hematocrit levels responded in a similar manner (◇, right vertical axis). (Additional information can be obtained from Rivera et al., 2005.) *Source*: With permission from *Blood* and the American Society of Hematology.

## REGULATION AND OVERSIGHT OF GENE THERAPY PRODUCTS

Experimental use of gene medicines is initiated only after careful review of the approach and trials monitored to protect the patient. The process to obtain approval for clinical testing from regulatory agencies in the United States is summarized in Figure 20. The Center for Biologics Evaluation and Research (CBER) of the FDA reviews gene therapy Investigational New Drug (IND) applications submitted by an investigator or sponsor. The National Institutes of Health (NIH) establishes guidelines for genetic research and implements policies through the Office of Biotechnology Activities (OBA). The OBA manages the Recombinant DNA Advisory Committee (RAC), a multidisciplinary group at the NIH established in response to public and scientific concern about the ethical, scientific and safety aspects of genetic research. Scientific and ethical review by the RAC is mandatory for clinical trials occurring at or sponsored by institutions receiving NIH funding for recombinant DNA research. Other protocols not meeting these criteria may also be submitted voluntarily for RAC review. The Office for Human Research Protections (OHRP) is responsible for monitoring and implementing compliance and supplying educational materials protecting human

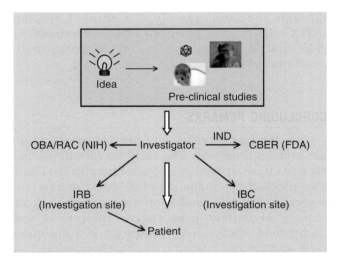

**Figure 21** ■ The approval process for clinical testing of a novel gene medicine. The process starts with an initial concept created by a scientific investigator. The idea is tested in vitro and in vivo in many pre-clinical studies. If the results are promising, the investigator summarizes the approach and pre-clinical data in an IND application that is submitted to the Center for Biologics Evaluation and Research (CBER) at the FDA. The investigator also submits a proposal outlining the details of the clinical trial for review by the RAC under the control of the OBA at the NIH. The same protocol (with any revisions suggested by the RAC) is submitted to the IRB at each location where patients are treated during the trial for review. The IBC at each site must also review the protocol. Only when approval is obtained from each of these groups, can the first patient be enrolled in the trial.

research subjects. The Institutional Biosafety Committee (IBC) and the Institutional Review Board (IRB) at each investigative site must also review and approve protocols and consent forms for any gene therapy clinical trial. Enrollment of patients for the trial begins only after attaining an IND, RAC review, and IBC and IRB approval (Mendell, 2004). Other countries also have a number of committees that must approve gene therapy protocols and address other scientific and ethical concerns associated with clinical trials (Kong, 2004).

Vectors for clinical trials must be produced according to strict Good Laboratory Practice (GLP) and Good Manufacturing Practice (GMP) principles. General requirements are described in 21 CFR and guidelines for the production and qualification of cell and gene therapy products can be found in *Points to Consider* or *Guidance* documents (www.fda.gov). ICH guidance documents for quality-related issues also have application to gene therapy products. Some of these documents are reproduced as chapters in the United States Pharmacopeia (USP) (Seaver, 2000). Reference standards for gene therapy vectors to assist manufacturers in characterizing raw materials, process components and process impurities and for comparative analysis among agents used in different clinical trials are needed. To date, an adenovirus reference standard has been produced and is available through the American Type Culture Collection (ATCC) (Hutchins, 2002). Reference standards for AAV and lentivirus vectors are currently under development (Kiermer, 2005; Flotte, 2006).

## CONCLUDING REMARKS

Within the last 10 years, the field of gene therapy has come a long way. The early vectors developed for gene transfer have now been tested in the clinic. One product has made it to the world market and several are in late phases of testing. Although the biology of current gene transfer vectors is well understood, they can be produced in large quantities and are considered to be highly characterized molecules; several hurdles must be overcome for the field of gene therapy to progress. The immune response against the vector and the therapeutic transgene is the most significant drawback to the use of many vectors for gene transfer. Gene expression systems targeted to tissues that need the transgene is paramount to the success of many gene therapy applications. Thresholds of transgene expression in target tissues vary based on severity of disease and may change over time to accommodate the disease process making continual patient monitoring and adjustment of a given

regimen necessary. Many of the diseases that are candidates for gene therapy are rare. This makes it difficult for them to undergo the usual method of testing in blinded, controlled studies in subjects with and without the disease. Many of the current suppliers of material for gene therapy trials are academic centers that do not have the financial resources nor the regulatory infrastructure to bring these drugs to market. Development of genetic medicines that can be widely used will rely on collaborations between academic institutions and the pharmaceutical and biotechnology industries.

Many of these issues are currently being addressed. Development of non-viral vectors is rapidly expanding, making it likely that viral/non-viral hybrid vectors will comprise the next generation of vectors that enter the clinic. Academic, industrial and regulatory factions routinely meet in different arenas to ensure that clinical trials are conducted properly and in a timely manner. These groups also meet with the public to discuss gene therapy and the current status of the field. Today the question is not: "Will gene therapy be possible?", but instead "When will gene therapy be available?". The paths for the development of therapies that are commonplace today such as bone marrow transplants, monoclonal antibodies, in vitro fertilization and organ transplantation were plagued by many disappointments. Like gene therapy, significant intellectual and economic resources were invested in those therapies and, as tireless efforts persist in this field, doctors of genetic medicine will be at the front line of treating human disease within the next decade.

## REFERENCES

Anonymous (1990). The ADA human gene therapy clinical protocol. Hum Gene Ther 1 (3):327–62.

Anonymous. The Journal of Gene Medicine Clinical Trials Worldwide Database (website) 2007 January 2007 (dated February 14); http://www.wiley.co.uk/genetheraphy.clinical Retrieved November 9, 2006, from http://www.wiley.co.uk/genetherapy/clinical/.

Aghi M, Martuza RL (2005). Oncolytic viral therapies — the clinical experience. Oncogene 24 (52):7802–16.

Aitken AE, Richardson TA, Morgan ET (2006). Regulation of drug-metabolizing enzymes and transporters in inflammation. Annu Rev Pharmacol Toxicol 46:123–49.

Al-Dosari MS, Knapp JE, Liu D (2005). Hydrodynamic delivery. Adv Genet 54:65–82.

Alexander C (2006). Temperature- and pH-responsive smart polymers for gene delivery. Expert Opin Drug Deliv 3 (5):573–81.

Alexander JH, Hafley G, Harrington RA, et al. PREVENT IV Investigators. (2005). Efficacy and safety of edifoligide, an E2F transcription factor decoy, for prevention of vein graft failure following coronary artery bypass graft surgery: PREVENT IV: a randomized controlled trial. JAMA. 294 (19):2446–2454.

Altaras NE, Aunins JG, Evans RK, Kamen A, Konz JO, Wolf JJ (2005). Production and formulation of adenovirus vectors. Adv Biochem Eng Biotechnol 99:193–260.

Argnani R, Lufino M, Manservigi M, Manservigi R (2005). Replication-competent herpes simplex vectors: design and applications. Gene Ther 12 (Suppl 1):S170–7.

Atchison RW, Casto BC, Hammon WM (1965). Adenovirus-Associated Defective Virus Particles. Science 149:754–6.

Auricchio A, Gao GP, Yu QC, et al. (2002). Constitutive and regulated expression of processed insulin following in vivo hepatic gene transfer. Gene Ther 9 (14):963–71.

Auriche C, Carpani D, Conese M, et al. (2002). Functional human CFTR produced by a stable minichromosome. EMBO Rep 3 (9):862–8.

Babiuk S, Baca-Estrada ME, Foldvari M, et al. (2004). Increased gene expression and inflammatory cell infiltration caused by electroporation are both important for improving the efficacy of DNA vaccines. J Biotechnol 110 (1):1–10.

Bangari D S, Mittal SK (2006). Current strategies and future directions for eluding adenoviral vector immunity. Curr Gene Ther 6 (2):215–26.

Bangari DS, Mittal SK (2006). Development of nonhuman adenoviruses as vaccine vectors. Vaccine 24 (7):849–62.

Bao S, Thrall BD, Miller DL (1997). Transfection of a reporter plasmid into cultured cells by sonoporation in vitro. Ultrasound Med Biol 23 (6):953–9.

Beer C, Meyer A, Muller K, Wirth M (2003). The temperature stability of mouse retroviruses depends on the cholesterol levels of viral lipid shell and cellular plasma membrane. Virology 308 (1):137–46.

Bergelson JM, Cunningham JA, Droguett G, et al. (1997). Isolation of a common receptor for Coxsackie B viruses and adenoviruses 2 and 5. Science 275 (5304):1320–3.

Berger C, Blau CA, Huang ML, et al. (2004). Pharmacologically regulated Fas-mediated death of adoptively transferred T cells in a nonhuman primate model. Blood 103 (4):1261–9.

Berk AJ (2005). Recent lessons in gene expression, cell cycle control, and cell biology from adenovirus. Oncogene 24 (52):7673–85.

Bertram J (2006). MATra — Magnet Assisted Transfection: combining nanotechnology and magnetic forces to improve intracellular delivery of nucleic acids. Curr Pharm Biotechnol 7 (4):277–85.

Birnboim HC, Doly J (1979). A rapid alkaline extraction procedure for screening recombinant plasmid DNA. Nucleic Acids Res 7 (6):1513–23.

Blackburn MR, and Kellems RE (2005). Adenosine deaminase deficiency: Metabolic basis of immune deficiency and pulmonary inflammation. Adv Immunol 86:1–41.

Bouchet BP, de Fromentel CC, Puisieux A, Galmarini CM (2006). p53 as a target for anti-cancer drug development. Crit Rev Oncol Hematol 58 (3):190–207.

Boyer JL, Kobinger G, Wilson JM, Crystal RG (2005). Adenovirus-based genetic vaccines for biodefense. Hum Gene Ther 16 (2):157–68.

Burova E, Ioffe E (2005). Chromatographic purification of recombinant adenoviral and adeno-associated viral vectors: Methods and implications. Gene Ther 12 (Suppl. 1):S5–17.

Callahan SM, Ming X, Lu SK, Brunner LJ, Croyle MA (2005). Considerations for use of recombinant adenoviral vectors: dose effect on hepatic cytochromes P450. J Pharmacol Exp Ther 312 (2):492–501.

Carcillo JA, Doughty L, Kofos et al. (2003). Cytochrome P450 mediated-drug metabolism is reduced in children with sepsis-induced multiple organ failure. Intensive Care Med 29 (6):980–4.

Carter BJ (2005). Adeno-Associated Virus Vectors in Clinical Trials. Hum Gene Ther 16 (5):541–50.

Cavazzana-Calvo M, Hacein-Bey S, de Saint Basile G, et al. (2000). Gene therapy of human severe combined immunodeficiency (SCID)-X1 disease. Science 288 (5466):669–72.

Cemazar M, Golzio M, Sersa G, Rols MP, Teissie J (2006). Electrically-assisted nucleic acids delivery to tissues in vivo: where do we stand? Curr Pharm Des 12 (29):3817–25.

Cole J, Skopek TR (1994). International Commission for Protection Against Environmental Mutagens and Carcinogens. Working paper no. 3. Somatic mutant frequency, mutation rates and mutational spectra in the human population in vivo. Mutat Res 304 (1):33–105.

Collins L (2006). Nonviral vectors. Methods Mol Biol 333 (201–26).

Conte MS, Bandyk DF, Clowes AW, et al. PREVENT III Investigators. (2006). Results of PREVENT III: A multicenter, randomized trial of edifoligide for the prevention of vein graft failure in lower extremity bypass surgery. J Vasc Surg 43 (4):742–51.

Cronin J, Zhang XY, Reiser J (2005). Altering the tropism of lentiviral vectors through pseudotyping. Curr Gene Ther 5 (4):387–98.

Croyle MA, Cheng X, Wilson JM (2001). Development of formulations that enhance the physical stability of viral vectors for human gene therapy. Gene Ther 8 (17):1281–91.

Croyle MA, Roessler BJ, Davidson BL, Hilfinger JM, Amidon GL (1998). Factors that influence stability of recombinant adenoviral preparations for human gene therapy. Pharm Dev Technol 3 (3):373–83.

Cruz PE, Silva AC, Roldao A, Carmo M, Carrondo MJ, Alves PM (2006). Screening of novel excipients for improving the stability of retroviral and adenoviral vectors. Biotechnol Prog 22 (2):568–76.

Crystal RG, Hirschowitz E, Lieberman M, et al. (1997). Phase I study of direct administration of a replication deficient adenovirus vector containing the E. coli cytosine deaminase gene to metastatic colon carcinoma of the liver in association with the oral administration of the pro-drug 5-fluorocytosine. Hum Gene Ther 8 (8):985–1001.

Cusi M G (2006). Applications of influenza virosomes as a delivery system. Hum Vaccin 2 (1):1–7.

Dash PR, Read ML, Barrett LB, Wolfert MA, Seymour LW (1999). Factors affecting blood clearance and in vivo distribution of polyelectrolyte complexes for gene delivery. Gene Ther 6 (4):643–50.

de Jong RN, van der Vliet PC, Brenkman AB (2003). Adenovirus DNA replication: Protein priming, jumping back and the role of the DNA binding protein DBP. Curr Top Microbiol Immunol 272:187–211.

Dechecchi MC, Melotti P, Bonizzato A, Santacatterina M, Chilosi M, Cabrini G (2001). Heparan sulfate glycosaminoglycans are receptors sufficient to mediate the initial binding of adenovirus types 2 and 5. J Virol 75 (18):8772–80.

Demeneix B, Hassani Z, Behr JP (2004). Towards multifunctional synthetic vectors. Curr Gene Ther 4 (4): 445–55.

Dropulic B, June CH (2006). Gene-based immunotherapy for human immunodeficiency virus infection and acquired immunodeficiency syndrome. Hum Gene Ther 17 (6):577–88.

Edelstein ML, Abedi MR, Wixon J, Edelstein R.M. (2004). Gene therapy clinical trials worldwide 1989–2004 — an overview. J Gene Med 6 (6):597–602.

Erles K, Sebokova P Schlehofer, JR (1999). Update on the prevalence of serum antibodies (IgG and IgM) to adeno-associated virus (AAV). J Med Virol 59 (3):406–11.

ErtlHC (2005). Challenges of immune responses in gene replacement therapy. IDrugs 8 (9):736–8.

Evans RK, Nawrocki DK, Isopi, LA, et al. (2004). Development of stable liquid formulations for adenovirus-based vaccines. J Pharm Sci 93 (10):2458–75.

Felgner PL, Gadek TR., Holm M, et al. (1987). Lipofection: A highly efficient, lipid-mediated DNA-transfection procedure. Proc Natl Acad Sci USA 84 (21):7413–7.

Flotte T, Carter B, Conrad C, et al. (1996). A phase I study of an adeno-associated virus-CFTR gene vector in adult CF patients with mild lung disease. Hum Gene Ther 7 (9):1145–9.

Flotte TR, Burd P, Snyder RO (2006). Utility of a recombinant adeno-associated viral vector reference standard. November 10: Article can be found on website of the Williamsburg Bioprocessing Foundation www.wilbio.com.

Fortuin FD, Vale P, Losordo DW, et al. (2003). One-year follow-up of direct myocardial gene transfer of vascular endothelial growth factor-2 using naked plasmid deoxyribonucleic acid by way of thoracotomy in no-option patients. Am J Cardiol 924:436–9.

Freytag S Khil O, M, Stricker M, et al. (2002). Phase I study of replication-competent adenovirus-mediated double suicide gene therapy for the treatment of locally recurrent prostate cancer. Cancer Res 62 (17):4968–76.

Gabrilovich DI (2006). INGN 201 (Advexin): Adenoviral p53 gene therapy for cancer. Exp Opin Biol Ther 6 (8):823–32.

Girard MP, Osmanov SK, Kieny MP (2006). A review of vaccine research and development: The human immunodeficiency virus (HIV). Vaccine 24 (19):4062–81.

Glover DJ, Lipps HJ, Jans DA (2006). Towards safe, non-viral therapeutic gene expression in humans. Nat Rev Genet 6 (4):299–310.

Goncalves MA, de Vries AA (2006). Adenovirus: From foe to friend. Rev Med Virol 16 (3):167–86.

Goverdhana S, Puntel M, Xiong W, et al. (2005). Regulatable gene expression systems for gene therapy applications: progress and future challenges. Mol Ther 12 (2):189–211.

Grieger JC, Samulski RJ (2005). Adeno-associated virus as a gene therapy vector: Vector development, production and clinical applications. Adv Biochem Eng Biotechnol 99:119–45.

Grimes BR, Schindelhauer D, McGill NI, Ross A, Ebersole TA, Cooke HJ (2001). Stable gene expression from a mammalian artificial chromosome. EMBO Rep 2 (10):910–4.

Grimm D, Kern A, Rittner K, (1998). Novel tools for production and purification of recombinant adenoassociated virus vectors. Hum Gene Ther 9 (18):2745–60.

Grossman M, Rader DJ, Muller DW, et al. (1995). A pilot study of ex vivo gene therapy for homozygous familial hypercholesterolaemia. Nat Med 1 (11):1148–54.

Haag R, Kratz F (2006). Polymer therapeutics: Concepts and applications. Angew Chem Int Ed Engl 45 (8):1198–215.

Hacein-Bey-Abina S, Le Deist F, Carlier F, et al. (2002). Sustained correction of X-linked severe combined immunodeficiency by ex vivo gene therapy. New Engl J Med 346 (16):1185–93.

Hacein-Bey-Abina S, von Kalle C, SchmidtM, et al. (2003). A serious adverse event after successful gene therapy for X-linked severe combined immunodeficiency. New Engl J Med 348 (3):255–6.

Hacein-Bey-Abina S, Von Kalle C, Schmidt M, et al. (2003). LMO2-associated clonal T cell proliferation in two patients after gene therapy for SCID-X1. Science 302 (5644):415–9.

Hasegawa H, Shimada M, Yonemitsu Y, Sugimachi K (2001). Preclinical and therapeutic utility of HVJ liposomes as a gene transfer vector for hepatocellular carcinoma using herpes simplex virus thymidine kinase. Cancer Gene Ther 8 (4):252–8.

High KA (2003). Gene transfer as an approach to treating hemophilia. Semin Thromb Hemost 29 (1):107–20.

Hirano T, Fujimoto J, Ueki T, et al. (1998). Persistent gene expression in rat liver in vivo by repetitive transfections using HVJ-liposome. Gene Ther 5 (4):459–64.

Hong SS, Karayan L, Tournier J, Curiel DT, Boulanger PA (1997). Adenovirus type 5 fiber knob binds to MHC class I alpha2 domain at the surface of human epithelial and B lymphoblastoid cells. EMBO J 16 (9):2294–306.

Huber PE, Pfisterer P (2000). In vitro and in vivo transfection of plasmid DNA in the Dunning prostate tumor R3327-AT1 is enhanced by focused ultrasound. Gene Ther 7 (17):1516–25.

Hutchins B (2002). Development of a reference material for characterizing adenovirus vectors. Bioprocess J 1(1):25–8.

Kaiser J (2005). Gene therapy. Panel urges limits on X-SCID trials. Science 307 (5715):1544–5.

Kaneda Y (1999). Development of a novel fusogenic viral liposome system (HVJ-liposomes) and its applications to the treatment of acquired diseases. Mol Membr Biol 16 (1):119–22.

Karmali PP, Chaudhuri A (2007). Cationic liposomes as non-viral carriers of gene medicines: Resolved issues, open questions, and future promises. Med Res Rev 27(5):696–722.

Kashiwakura Y, Tamayose K, Iwabuchi K, et al. (2005). Hepatocyte growth factor receptor is a coreceptor for adeno-associated virus type 2 infection. J Virol 79 (1):609–14.

Kiermer V, Borellini F, Lu X, et al. (2005). Report from the Lentivirus Vector Working Group: Issues for developing assays and reference materials for detection replication-competent lentivirus in production lots of lentivirus vectors. Bioprocess J 4 (2):39–42.

Kommareddy S, Tiwari SB, Amiji MM (2005). Long-circulating polymeric nanovectors for tumor-selective gene delivery. Technol Cancer Res Treat 4 (6):615–25.

Kong WM (2004). The regulation of gene therapy research in competent adult patients, today and tomorrow: Implications of EU Directive 2001/20/EC. Med Law Rev 12 (2):164–80.

Kresge KJ (2005). Clinical trials yield promising results from two adenovirus-based vaccines. IAVI Rep 9 (4):24.

Lavigne MD, Gorecki DC (2006). Emerging vectors and targeting methods for nonviral gene therapy. Expert Opin Emerg Drugs 11 (3):541–57.

Le Doux JM, Morgan JR, Yarmush ML (1998). Removal of proteoglycans increases efficiency of retroviral gene transfer. Biotechnol Bioeng 58 (1):23–34.

Lee M, Kim SW (2005). Polyethylene glycol-conjugated copolymers for plasmid DNA delivery. Pharm Res 22 (1):1–10.

Lee TW, Matthews DA, Blair GE (2005). Novel molecular approaches to cystic fibrosis gene therapy. Biochem J 387 (Pt. 1):1–15.

Lefesvre P, Attema J, van Bekkum D (2002). A comparison of efficacy and toxicity between electroporation and adenoviral gene transfer. BMC Mol Biol 3 (12):1–13.

Levine BL, Humeau LM, Boyer J, et al. (2006). Gene transfer in humans using a conditionally replicating lentiviral vector. Proc Natl Acad Sci USA 103 (46):17372–7.

Lichtenstein DL, Toth K, Doronin K, Tollefson AE, Wold WS (2004). Functions and mechanisms of action of the adenovirus E3 proteins. Int Rev Immunol 23 (1–2):75–111.

Liu F, Shollenberger LM, Huang L (2004). Non-immunostimulatory nonviral vectors. FASEB J18 (14):1779–81.

Liu F, Song Y, Liu D (1999). Hydrodynamics-based transfection in animals by systemic administration of plasmid DNA. Gene Ther 6 (7):1258–66.

Losordo DW, Vale PR, Symes JF, et al. (1998). Gene therapy for myocardial angiogenesis: initial clinical results with direct myocardial injection of phVEGF165 as sole therapy for myocardial ischemia. Circulation 98 (25):2800–4.

Lundstrom K (2004). Gene therapy applications of viral vectors. Technol Cancer Res Treat 3 (5):467–77.

Lusky M (2005). Good manufacturing practice production of adenoviral vectors for clinical trials. Hum Gene Ther 16 (3):281–91.

Macpherson JL, Boyd MP, Arndt AJ, et al. (2005). Long-term survival and concomitant gene expression of ribozyme-transduced CD4+ T-lymphocytes in HIV-infected patients. J Gene Med 7 (5):552–64.

Majhen D, Ambriovic-Ristov A (2006). Adenoviral vectors—how to use them in cancer gene therapy? Virus Res 119 (2):121–33.

Manilla P, Rebello T, Afable C, et al. (2005). Regulatory considerations for novel gene therapy products: A review of the process leading to the first clinical lentiviral vector. Hum Gene Ther 16 (1):17–25.

Mangeat B, Trono D (2005). Lentiviral vectors and anti-retroviral vector intrinsic immunity. Hum Gene Ther 16 (8):913–20.

Mann MJ, Whittemore AD, Donaldson MC, et al. (1999). Ex-vivo gene therapy of human vascular bypass grafts with E2F decoy: The PREVENT single-centre, randomised, controlled trial. Lancet 354 (9189):1493–8.

Manno CS, Pierce GF, Arruda VR, et al. (2006). Successful transduction of liver in hemophilia by AAV-Factor IX and limitations imposed by the host immune response. Nat Med 12 (3):342–7.

Manthorpe M, Hobart P, Hermanson G, et al. (2005). Plasmid vaccines and therapeutics: From design to applications. Adv Biochem Eng Biotechnol 99:41–92.

Markert JM, Medlock MD, Rabkin SD, et al. (2000). Conditionally replicating herpes simplex virus mutant, G207 for the treatment of malignant glioma: results of a phase I trial. Gene Ther 7 (10):867–74.

Martin JE, Sullivan NJ, Enama ME, et al. (2006). A DNA vaccine for Ebola virus is safe and immunogenic in a phase I clinical trial. Clin Vacc Immunol 2006 13 (11):1267–77.

McConnell MJ, Imperiale MJ (2004). Biology of adenovirus and its use as a vector for gene therapy. Hum Gene Ther 15 (11):1022–33.

McPhee SW, Janson CG, Li C, et al. (2006). Immune responses to AAV in a phase I study for Canavan disease. J Gene Med 8 (5):577–88.

Medina-Kauwe LK (2003). Endocytosis of adenovirus and adenovirus capsid proteins. Adv Drug Deliv Rev 55 (11):1485–96.

Mehier-Humbert S, Guy RH (2005). Physical methods for gene transfer: Improving the kinetics of gene delivery into cells. Adv Drug Deliv Rev 57 (5):733–53.

Melo LG, Pachori AS, Gnecchi M, Dzau VJ (2006). Genetic therapies for cardiovascular diseases. Trend Mol Med 11 (5):240–50.

Mendell JR, Miller A (2004). Gene transfer for neurologic disease: Agencies, policies, and process. Neurology 63 (12):2225–32.

Merten OW (2004). State-of-the-art of the production of retroviral vectors. J Gene Med 6 (Suppl. 1):S105–24.

Miller DL, Bao S, Gies RA, Thrall BD (1999). Ultrasonic enhancement of gene transfection in murine melanoma tumors. Ultrasound Med Biol 25 (9):1425–30.

Mizuguchi H, Hayakawa T (2004). Targeted adenovirus vectors. Hum Gene Ther 15 (11):1034–44.

Morgan RA, Walker R, Carter CS, et al. (2005). Preferential survival of CD4+ T lymphocytes engineered with anti-human immunodeficiency virus (HIV) genes in HIV-infected individuals. Hum Gene Ther 16 (9):1065–74.

Murphy JC, Winters MA, Sagar SL (2006). Large-scale, nonchromatographic purification of plasmid DNA. Meth Mol Med 127:351–62.

Muruve DA (2004). The innate immune response to adenovirus vectors. Hum Gene Ther 15 (12):1157-66.

Muul LM, Tuschong LM, Soenen SL, et al. (2003). Persistence and expression of the adenosine deaminase gene for 12 years and immune reaction to gene transfer components: long-term results of the first clinical gene therapy trial. Blood 101 (7):2563–9.

Muzyczka N, Berns K (2001). *Parvoviridae:* The viruses and their replication. In: Knipe D, Howley P, Griffen D, Lamb R, Martin M, Roizman B, Straus S, eds. Fields Virology, Vol. 2. Philadelphia, PA: Lippincott Williams & Wilkins, 2001, 2327–47.

Nam CH, Rabbitts TH (2006). The role of LMO2 in development and in T cell leukemia after chromosomal translocation or retroviral insertion. Mol Ther 13 (1):15–25.

Nazir SA, Metcalf JP (2005). Innate immune response to adenovirus. J Investig Med 53 (6):292–304.

Nemerow GR, Stewart PL (1999). Role of $a_v$ integrins in adenovirus cell entry and gene delivery. Microbiol. Mol Biol Rev 63 (3):725–34.

Nevins JR (1987). Regulation of early adenovirus gene expression. Microbiol Rev 51 (4):419–30.

Nicoletti VG, Condorelli DF (1993). Optimized PEG method for rapid plasmid DNA purification: high yield from "midi-prep". Biotechniques 14:532–6.

Nwanegbo E, Vardas E, Gao W, et al. (2004). Prevalence of neutralizing antibodies to adenoviral serotypes 5 and 35 in the adult populations of The Gambia, South Africa, and the United States. Clin Diagn Lab Immunol 11 (2):351–7.

O'Connor TP, Crystal RG (2006). Genetic medicines: treatment strategies for hereditary disorders. Nat Rev Genet 7 (4):261–76.

O'Kennedy RD, Baldwin C, Keshavarz-Moore E (2000). Effects of growth medium selection on plasmid DNA production and initial processing steps. J Biotechnol 76 (2–3):175–83.

Oupicky D, Ogris M, Howard KA, Dash PR, Ulbrich K, Seymour LW (2002). Importance of lateral and steric stabilization of polyelectrolyte gene delivery vectors for extended systemic circulation. Mol Ther 5 (4):463–72.

Palmer DH, Mautner V, Mirza D, et al. (2004). Virus-directed enzyme prodrug therapy: intratumoral administration of a replication-deficient adenovirus encoding nitroreductase to patients with resectable liver cancer. J Clin Oncol 22 (9):1546–52.

Park TG, Jeong JH, Kim SW (2006). Current status of polymeric gene delivery systems. Adv Drug Deliv Rev 58 (4):467–86.

Peng Z (2005). Current status of Gencidine in China: Recombinant human Ad-p53 for treatment of cancers. Hum Gene Ther 16:1016–27.

Phillips JE, Gersbach CA, Garcia AJ (2007). Virus-based gene therapy strategies for bone regeneration. Biomaterials 28 (2):211–29.

Piechaczek C, Fetzer C, Baiker A, Bode J, Lipps HJ (1999). A vector based on the SV40 origin of replication and chromosomal S/MARs replicates episomally in CHO cells. Nucleic Acids Res 27 (2):426–8.

Plank C, Anton M, Rudolph C, Rosenecker J, Krotz F (2003). Enhancing and targeting nucleic acid delivery by magnetic force. Expert Opin Biol Ther 3 (5):745–58.

Qing K, Mah C, Hansen J, Zhou S, Dwarki V, Srivastava A (1999). Human fibroblast growth factor receptor 1 is a co-receptor for infection by adeno-associated virus 2. Nat Med 5 (1):71–7.

Quick KS, Miao C, Gerding K, Croyle MA (2002). Dynamic light scattering as a useful tool for the physical characterization of recombinant viral vectors during production and development. Mol Ther 5 (5):S56–7.

Ranga U, Woffendin C, Verma S, et al. (1998). Enhanced T cell engraftment after retroviral delivery of an antiviral gene in HIV-infected individuals. Proc Natl Acad Sci USA 95 (3):1201–6.

Raper SE, Chirmule N, Lee FS, et al. (2003). Fatal systemic inflammatory response syndrome in a ornithine transcarbamylase deficient patient following adenoviral gene transfer. Mol Genet Metab 80 (1–2):148–58.

Raper SE, Yudkoff M, Chirmule N, et al. (2002). A pilot study of in vivo liver-directed gene transfer with an adenoviral vector in partial ornithine transcarbamylase deficiency. Hum Gene Ther 13 (1):163–75.

Read ML, Logan A, Seymour LW (2005). Barriers to gene delivery using synthetic vectors. Adv Genet 53:19–46.

Rexroad J, Evans RK, Middaugh CR (2006). Effect of pH and ionic strength on the physical stability of adenovirus type 5. J Pharm Sci 95 (2):237–47.

Rexroad J, Wiethoff CM, Green AP, Kierstead TD, Scott MO, Middaugh CR (2003). Structural stability of adenovirus type 5. J Pharm Sci 92 (3):665–78.

Riddick DS, Lee C, Ramji S, et al. (2005). Cancer chemotherapy and drug metabolism. Drug Metab Dispos 33 (8):1083–96.

Rivera VM, Gao GP, Grant RL, et al. (2005). Long-term pharmacologically regulated expression of erythropoietin in primates following AAV-mediated gene transfer. Blood 105 (4):1424–30.

Roberts DM, Nanda A, Havenga MJ, et al. (2006). Hexon-chimaeric adenovirus serotype 5 vectors circumvent pre-existing anti-vector immunity. Nature 441 (7090):239–43.

Rodrigues T, Carrondo MJ, Alves PM, Cruz PE (2007). Purification of retroviral vectors for clinical application: Biological implications and technological challenges. J Biotechnol 127 (3):520–41.

Rodrigues T, Carvalho A, Roldao A, Carrondo MJ, Alves PM, Cruz PE (2006). Screening anion-exchange chromatographic matrices for isolation of onco-retroviral vectors. J Chromatogr B Analyt Technol Biomed Life Sci 837 (1–2):59–68.

Rowe WP, Huebner RJ, Gilmore LK, Parrott RH, Ward TG (1953). Isolation of a cytopathogenic agent from human adenoids undergoing spontaneous degeneration in tissue culture. Proc Soc Exp Biol Med 84 (3):570–3.

Scherer F, Anton M, Schillinger U, et al. (2003). Magnetofection: Enhancing and targeting gene delivery by magnetic force in vitro and in vivo. Gene Ther 9 (2):102–9.

Schorr J, Moritz P, Breul A, Scheef M (2006). Production of plasmid DNA in industrial quantities according to cGMP guidelines. Meth Mol Med 127:339–50.

Seaver S (2000). A new United States Pharmacopeia (USP) Chapter 1046: Cell and Gene Therapy Products. Cytotherapy 2 (1):45–9.

Secretariat G (2005). Recommendations of the Gene Therapy Advisory Committee/Committee on Safety of Medicines Working Party on Retroviruses. Hum Gene Ther 16 (10):1237–9.

Segura MM, Kamen A, Garnier A (2006). Downstream processing of oncoretroviral and lentiviral gene therapy vectors. Biotechnol Adv 24 (3):321–37.

Shamlou PA (2003). Scaleable processes for the manufacture of therapeutic quantities of plasmid DNA. Biotechnol Appl Biochem 37 (Pt. 3): 207–18.

Shoji J, Tanihara Y, Uchiyama T, Kawai A. (2004). Preparation of virosomes coated with the vesicular stomatitis virus glycoprotein as efficient gene transfer vehicles for animal cells. Microbiol Immunol 48 (3):163–74.

Simons JW, Sacks N. (2006). Granulocyte–macrophage colony-stimulating factor-transduced allogeneic cancer cellular immunotherapy: The GVAX vaccine for prostate cancer. Urol Oncol 24 (5):419–24.

Springer ML (2006). A balancing act: Therapeutic approaches for the modulation of angiogenesis. Curr Opin Investig Drugs 7 (3):243–50.

Stadler J, Lemmens R, Nyhammar T (2004). Plasmid DNA purification. J Gene Med 6 (Suppl. 1):S54–66.

Sumida SM, Truitt DM, Lemckert AA, et al. (2005). Neutralizing antibodies to adenovirus serotype 5 vaccine vectors are directed primarily against the adenovirus hexon protein. J Immunol 174 (11):7179–85.

Summerford C, Samulski RJ (1998). Membrane-associated heparan sulfate proteoglycan is a receptor for adeno-associated virus type 2 virions. J Virol 72 (2):1438–45.

Summerford C, Bartlett JS, Samulski RJ (1999). AlphaVbeta5 integrin: A co-receptor for adeno-associated virus type 2 infection. Nat Med 5 (1):78–82.

Thyagarajan B, Olivares EC, Hollis RP, Ginsburg DS, Calos MP (2001). Site-specific genomic integration in mammalian cells mediated by phage phiC31 integrase. Mol Cell Biol 21 (12): 3926–34.

Tiera MJ, Winnik FO, Fernandes JC (2006). Synthetic and natural polycations for gene therapy: state of the art and new perspectives. Curr Gene Ther 6 (1):59–71.

Top FHJ, Buescher EL, Bancroft WH, Russell PK (1971). Immunization with live types 7 and 4 adenovirus vaccines. II. Antibody response and protective effect against acute respiratory disease due to adenovirus type 7. J Infect Dis 124 (2):155–60.

Top FHJ, Grossman RA, Bartelloni PJ, et al. (1971). Immunization with live types 7 and 4 adenovirus vaccines. I. Safety, infectivity, antigenicity, and potency of adenovirus type 7 vaccine in humans. J Infect Dis 124 (2):148–54.

US Dept. of Health and Human Services (1998). Guidance for Industry: Guidance for Human Somatic Cell Therapy and Gene Therapy. Rockville, MD, Center for Biologics Evaluation and Research, United States Food and Drug Administration, 18.

Vahakangas E, Yla-Herttuala S (2005). Gene therapy of atherosclerosis. Handb Exp Pharmacol 170:785–807.

Varghese S, Rabkin SD (2002). Oncolytic herpes simplex virus vectors for cancer virotherapy. Cancer Gene Ther 9 (12):967–78.

Vasileva A, Jessberger R (2005). Precise hit: Adeno-associated virus in gene targeting. Nat Rev Microbiol 3 (11):837–47.

Vilaboa N, Voellmy R (2006). Regulatable gene expression systems for gene therapy. Curr Gene Ther 6 (4):421–38.

Wagner E, Culmsee C, Boeckle S (2005). Targeting of polyplexes: Toward synthetic virus vector systems. Adv Genet 53:333–54.

Wang Y, Yuan F (2006). Delivery of viral vectors to tumor cells: extracellular transport, systemic distribution, and strategies for improvement. Ann Biomed Eng 34(1):114–27.

Warrington Jr KH, Gorbatyuk OS, Harrison JK, Opie SR, Zolotukhin S, Muzyczka N (2004). Adeno-associated virus type 2 VP2 capsid protein is nonessential and can tolerate large peptide insertions at its N terminus. J Virol 78 (12):6595–609.

Weber W, Fussenegger M. (2006). Pharmacologic transgene control systems for gene therapy. J Gene Med 8 (5):535–56.

Weiss DJ (2002). Delivery of gene transfer vectors to lung: Obstacles and the role of adjunct techniques for airway administration. Mol Ther 6 (2):148–52.

Weitzman MD (2005). Functions of the adenovirus E4 proteins and their impact on viral vectors. Front Biosci 10:1106–17.

Wright JF, Le T, Prado J, et al. (2005). Identification of factors that contribute to recombinant AAV2 particle aggregation and methods to prevent its occurrence during vector purification and formulation. Mol Ther 12 (1):171–8.

Wright JF, Qu G, Tang C, Sommer JM (2003). Recombinant adeno-associated virus: Formulation challenges and strategies for a gene therapy vector. Curr Opin Drug Discov Dev 6 (2):174–8.

Wu Z, Asokan A, Samulski RJ (2006). Adeno-associated virus serotypes: Vector toolkit for human gene therapy. Mol Ther 14 (3):316–27.

Xu ZL, Mizuguchi H, Sakurai F, et al. (2005). Approaches to improving the kinetics of adenovirus-delivered genes and gene products. Adv Drug Deliv Rev 57 (5):781–802.

Yew NS, Cheng SH (2004). Reducing the immunostimulatory activity of CpG-containing plasmid DNA vectors for non-viral gene therapy. Expert Opin Drug Deliv 1 (1):115–25.

Yew NS, Scheule RK (2005). Toxicity of cationic lipid-DNA complexes. Adv Genet 53:189–214.

Zaiss AK, Muruve DA (2005). Immune responses to adeno-associated virus vectors. Curr Gene Ther 5 (3):323–31.

Zhang G, Budker V, Wolff JA (1999). High levels of foreign gene expression in hepatocytes after tail vein injections of naked plasmid DNA. Hum Gene Ther 10 (10):1735–7.

Zhang G, Gao X, Song YK, et al. (2004). Hydroporation as the mechanism of hydrodynamic delivery. Gene Ther 11 (8):675–82.

Zhang JS, Liu F, Conwell CC, Tan Y, Huang L (2006). Mechanistic studies of sequential injection of cationic liposome and plasmid DNA. Mol Ther 13 (2):429–37.

Zhang X, Godbey WT (2006). Viral vectors for gene delivery in tissue engineering. Adv Drug Deliv Rev 58 (4):515–34.

Zhou D, Ertl HC (2006). Therapeutic potential of adenovirus as a vaccine vector for chronic virus infections. Expert Opin Biol Ther 6 (1):63–72.

## FURTHER READING

Curiel DT, Douglas JT, eds. (2005). Cancer Gene Therapy. Totowa: Humana Press.

Neff CF, ed. (2005). Exploring Science and Medical Discoveries — Gene Therapy. Farmington Hills: Greenhaven Press, 2005.

Schleef M (2005). DNA Pharmaceuticals: Formulation and Delivery in Gene Therapy DNA Vaccination and Immunotherapy. Hoboken: John Wiley & Sons, 2005.

# 9

# Oligonucleotides

*Raymond M. Schiffelers and Enrico Mastrobattista*
*Department of Pharmaceutical Sciences, Utrecht University, Utrecht, The Netherlands*

## INTRODUCTION

Oligonucleotides (ONs) are (short) chains of (chemically modified) ribo- or deoxyribonucleotides. Their ability to bind to chromosomal DNA or mRNA through Watson–Crick and Hoogsteen base-pairing offers possibilities for highly specific intervention in gene transcription, translation, repair, and recombination for therapeutic applications. In theory, a sequence of 15 to 17 bases occurs only once in the human genome, which would allow specific manipulation of single genes for ONs beyond this size range. In addition, therapeutic effects of ONs can be obtained through sequence-specific binding of transcription factors and intramolecular folding into complex three-dimensional structures that can bind to and interfere with the function of biomolecules. Finally, cells display specific receptors for ONs with associated immunological responses that can be of therapeutic value.

Due to this multitude of possible effects of nucleic acids, ONs can be very potent molecules, yet interpretation of the mechanism of therapeutic action of a specific oligonucleotide sequence is not straightforward (Stein et al., 2005). Apart from the desired activity, ONs are inclined to display (sequence-specific) unintended effects. Partial sequence homology may affect expression of genes other than the targeted gene (known as off-target effects), immune responses may be induced, and binding to proteins and peptides can alter their activity.

sOther characteristics of ONs also impede clear-cut application as therapeutics. Their physicochemical characteristics induce rapid uptake by macrophages and excretion by the kidneys hindering target tissue accumulation. In addition, spontaneous passage over cell membranes for intracellular applications is difficult. Finally, ONs are sensitive to the action of nucleases leading to their degradation. Over the years a number of different modifications have been developed that overcome (part of) these problems (Fig. 1) (Kurreck, 2003). Many of the clinically studied ONs contain one or more of these modified nucleotides.

## INTERFERING WITH GENE EXPRESSION

Triple helix-forming oligonucleotides, antisense, small interfering RNA (siRNA), microRNA (miRNA), transcription factor decoys, ribozymes, DNAzymes, and external guide sequences (EGS) are all members of the class of ONs that can knock down gene expression, albeit that they function at different stages of the gene expression process.

In eukaryotes, transcription takes place in the nucleus, and translation is located in the cytoplasm. To initiate transcription of a gene, promoters and transcription factors are required, whose action is further complemented by the action of enhancers, binding of specific proteins to regulatory DNA sequences, and methylation of CpG islands in the promoter region. RNA polymerase produces pre-mRNA molecules that are capped at their 5′-ends and receive a poly(A) tail at their 3′-ends. Nearly all mRNA precursors are spliced. Introns are excised and exons are joined to form the final mRNA sequence. Different splicing can form alternative sequences. Subsequently, mRNA binds to the ribosomes. Ribosomes are composed of rRNA and proteins and "read" the mRNA sequence. With the help of tRNA carrying the appropriate amino acids, the protein is formed. The process of transcription and translation is shown in Figure 2.

### ■ Triple Helix-Forming Oligonucleotides

Triple helix-forming oligonucleotides, also known as TFO, act at the level of transcription of mRNA. Triple helix formation occurs when a polypurine or polypyrimidine DNA or RNA oligonucleotide binds to a polypurine/polypyrimidine region of genomic DNA. Triple helix-forming ONs can bind specifically in the major groove of such stretches of DNA to the polypurine strand, forming (reverse) Hoogsteen hydrogen bonds (Fig. 3) (Rogers et al., 2005).

As a result of this binding, triplex-forming ONs can prevent transcription initiation or elongation by binding promoter, gene or regulatory DNA regions (Fig. 4). The concept has been validated in vivo,

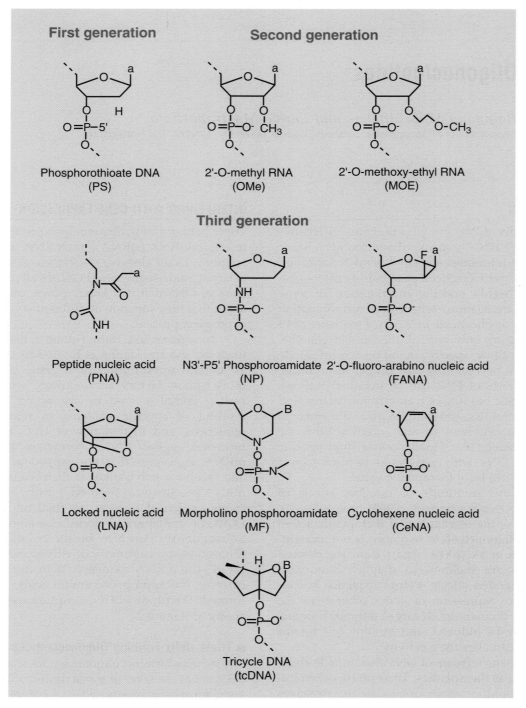

**Figure 1** Popular chemical modifications to improve nuclease resistance and distribution profile of oligonucleotides.

but suffers some drawbacks for straightforward application. Because insertion of the third strand in the duplex requires the negatively charged backbones of the nucleic acid strands to come close, it is often difficult to find sufficiently long uninterrupted polypurine sequences in the genome that overcome the electrostatic repulsion and provide stable triplex binding. The use of chemically modified nucleic acids, like peptide nucleic acid (PNA) that bear no charge in their backbone, strongly facilitates triplex formation and seems especially important for this application.

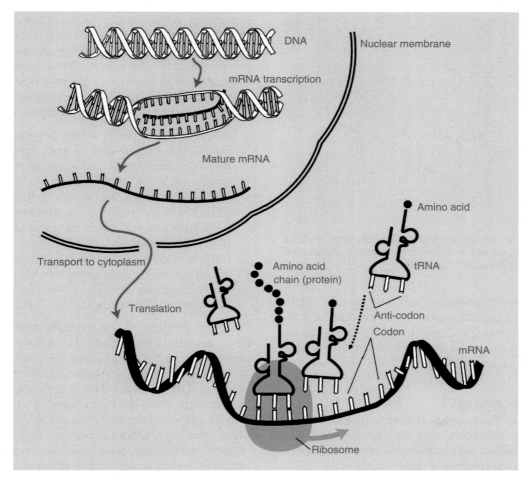

**Figure 2** ▪ Transcription and translation. The synthesis of proteins starts with transcription. DNA is transcribed to RNA to produce mRNA. This happens in the nucleus by RNA polymerase. During transcription the chromosomes are locally decondensed, so that the genes present at this site can be read. Only certain genes are actively transcribed at a certain time depending on the cell's needs. The activity of the genes is determined by transcription factors/enhancers and promoters as well as other internal cellular signals. After splicing of the mRNA, capping and tailing, the mature mRNA is transported to the cytoplasm, where it becomes active in the translation. The translation starts when ribosomes bind mRNA. The ribosomes mediate mRNA-codon to tRNA-anti-codon binding and couple the amino acids to form a polypeptide. *Source*: Courtesy of National Human Genome Research Institute, NIH, Bethesda, MD, USA.

Triplex-forming ONs have also been used for site-directed mutagenesis with or without the use of coupled mutagens, as well as homologous-site-specific recombination using triple-forming ONs alone or in combination with a donor fragment to correct genetic disorders. This application will be discussed in the section on gene repair.

■ **Transcription Factor Decoys**

Transcription factors are nuclear proteins that usually stimulate and occasionally downregulate gene expression by binding to specific DNA sequences, approximately 6 to 10 base-pairs in length, in promoter or enhancer regions of the genes that they influence. The corresponding decoys are ONs that match the attachment site for the transcription factor, known as consensus sequence, thus luring the transcription

factor away from its natural target and thereby altering gene expression (Fig. 5) (Tomita et al., 2004).

The facts that many transcription factors are involved in regulation of a certain gene and that many genes are controlled by a single transcription factor represent important limitations to the decoy approach, especially when decoy action is only desired in the pathological tissue.

Clinically, this strategy has been evaluated in patients at risk of post-operative neo-intimal hyperplasia after bypass vein grafting. The ONs, edifoligide, was delivered to grafts intraoperatively by ex vivo pressure-mediated transfection, and was designed to target E2F, a transcription factor that regulates a family of genes involved in smooth muscle cell proliferation. While pre-clinical studies demonstrated beneficial effects, a series of clinical trials yielded mixed results from reduced graft failure to no

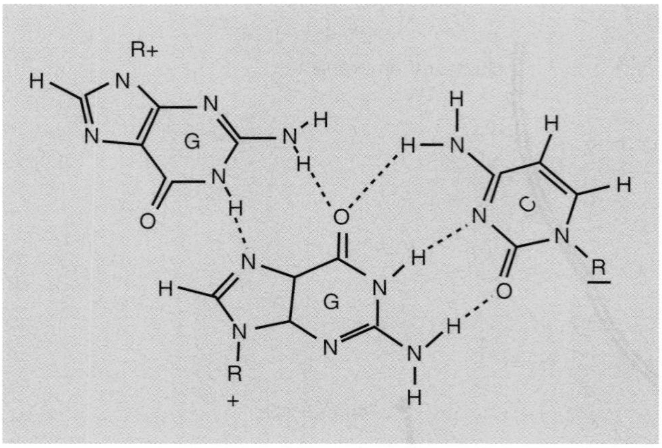

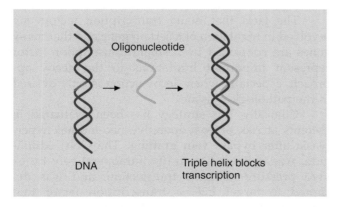

**Figure 3** ▦ Triple helices are formed through Watson–Crick basepairing combined with Hoogsteen basepairing, shown here for guanosine = guanosine ≡ cytosine.

benefit compared to placebo (Conti and Hunter, 2005). The studies did indicate good safety of this local ex vivo treatment strategy. Current clinical studies focus on topical administration of NFκB decoys for atopic dermatitis (Dajee et al., 2006).

### ▪ Antisense/Ribozymes/EGS

The function of ONs to act as antisense molecules was discovered by Zamecnik and Stephenson in 1978, making it the oldest oligonucleotide-based therapeutic approach (Stephenson and Zamecnik, 1978; Zamecnik and Stephenson, 1978). Many of the difficulties associated with the use of ONs for medical applications have consequently been encountered for antisense first, explaining why clinical progress has been difficult. Improvements in synthetic chemistry, knowledge of genome, transcriptome, and proteome, and delivery issues have revived interest in the

**Figure 4** ▦ Mechanism of action of triple helix-forming oligonucleotides. The oligonucleotide interacts with DNA via Hoogsteen basepairing and thereby prevents mRNA transcription.

technology (Chan et al., 2006). "Classical" antisense ONs are single-stranded DNA or RNA molecules that generally consist of 13 to 25 nucleotides. They are complementary to a sense mRNA sequence and can hybridize to it through Watson–Crick base-pairing. Three classes of translation-inhibiting ONs can be distinguished based on their mechanism of action:

- mRNA-blocking ONs, which physically prevent or inhibit the progression of splicing or translation through binding of complementary mRNA sequences (Fig. 6).
- mRNA cleaving ONs, which induce degradation of mRNA by binding complementary mRNA sequences and recruiting the cytoplasmic nuclease RNase H (Aboul-Fadl, 2005).
- mRNA cleaving ONs, which induce degradation of mRNA by recruiting nuclear RNase P via EGS, or by nuclease activity of the nucleic acid itself (ribozymes/DNAzymes) (Fig. 7) (Lilley, 2005).

The majority of the clinically studied antisense ONs act through RNase H. RNase H-mediated knockdown generally reaches >80% downregulation of protein and mRNA expression. In contrast to blocking ONs, RNase H-recruiting antisense ONs can inhibit protein expression without a priori restrictions to the region of the mRNA that is targeted. Most blocking ONs, however, require targeting regions within the 5'-untranslated region or AUG initiation codon region as the ribosome is apparently able to remove bound antisense molecules in the coding region.

One antisense drug has so far been introduced to the market: Fomivirsen (Vitravene®), for the treatment of cytomegalovirus-induced retinitis in AIDS patients (Jabs and Griffiths, 2002). Vitravene® is injected into the vitreous at a dose of 165 μg or 330 μg/eye in 25 μl, once weekly for 3 weeks, followed by 2 weekly administrations. Reported side effects are related to irritation and inflammation of the eye likely caused by the injection procedure. The ON has a thioate backbone which limits nuclease degradation. Local injection at the pathological site improves target cell accumulation.

This successful introduction is overshadowed by failures in phase III clinical trials of a number of products in recent years. Alicaforsen did not induce clinical remissions compared to placebo in patients with Crohn's disease, and Affinitak™ (targeting protein kinase C-alpha) and oblimersen (Genasense®; Bcl-2 antisense oligonucleotide) failed to substantially prolong survival in cancer patients. Nevertheless, the experiences from these trials have provided new insights into the use of alicaforsen and Genasense®, and consequently, these compounds are still in clinical trials for one or more specific indications. Table 1

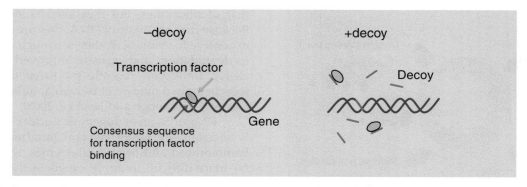

**Figure 5** ■ Mechanism of action of transcription factor decoys. Transcription factor decoys match the consensus attachment site of the factor and thereby prevent it from binding to the DNA, inhibiting the factor's modulating activity on gene expression level.

shows a list of antisense molecules that are currently in clinical trials.

Although sequence specificity is one of the most attractive features for antisense application, there are reports that show that knockdown of related genes with only limited sequence homology can occur. In addition, the effects of oblimersen appear only partly due to Bcl-2 downregulation but can also be attributed to immune stimulation and mitochondrial apoptosis activation independent of Bcl-2 (Gekeler et al., 2006; Lai et al., 2006).

Ribozymes and DNAzymes are molecules that combine a mRNA binding sequence with a catalytic domain and are capable of cleaving mRNA molecules. They are potentially capable of multiple turnovers. Several different types of ribozymes are found in nature: the hammerhead, hairpin, hepatitis delta virus (HDV), Varkud satellite RNA, group I and II introns and the RNA subunit of RNase P. Smaller ribozymes, like hammerhead and hairpin, consist of 40 to 150 nucleotides. But other ribozymes can be hundreds of nucleotides long and fold into protein-like structures

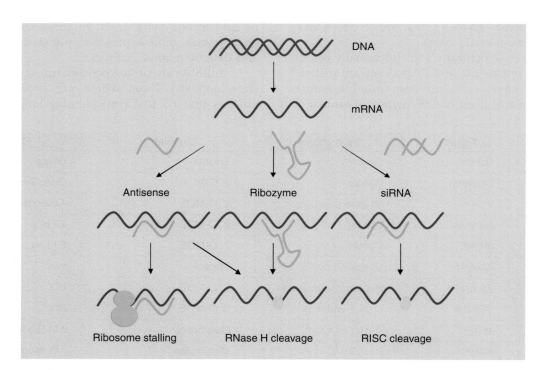

**Figure 6** ■ Mechanism of action of oligonucleotides that act at the level of mRNA. Antisense oligonucleotides can inhibit mRNA translation by sterically blocking translation or inducing RNaseH-mediated mRNA cleavage. In the ribzyme/DNAzyme approach, the oligonucleotide posseses mRNA degradative properties or functions as a recruiting factor (known as EGS) for endogenous ribozymes (RNaseP). Finally, siRNA- and miRNA-based strategies make use of short dsRNAmolecules which unwind and bind complementary mRNA in the RISC, which subsequently cleaves the mRNA.

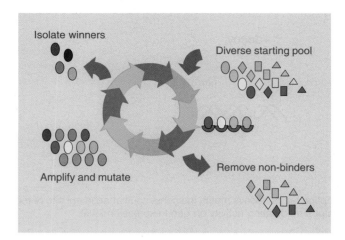

**Figure 7** ▥ General scheme for SELEX-based selection of aptamers. A pool of randomized oligonucleotides is subjected to selection steps whereby the oligonucleotides with higher activity become enriched in the population. By increasing stringency of the selection steps and competition between oligonucleotides in a Darwinian manner, molecular evolution toward oligonucleotides with higher binding affinity takes place.

containing single- and double-stranded regions, base-triplets, loops, bulges, and junctions (like RNaseP).

Ribozymes have been applied clinically. In a study in HIV patients, hematopoietic progenitor cells, were transduced ex vivo using a retroviral vector carrying an anti-HIV-1 ribozyme. Sustained output of ribozyme expressing mature myeloid and T-lymphoid cells was detected, showing that the concept may work (Macpherson et al., 2005).

DNAzymes structurally and functionally resemble ribozymes, but are made of DNA. They are artificial molecules and have, so far, not been found in nature. The working mechanism of DNAzymes is similar to that of ribozymes, but they offer some advantages. Because they are made of DNA, they are easier and less expensive to synthesize, they are much more resistant to degradation, and possess improved catalytic efficiency. DNAzyme recently produced therapeutic effects in animal models of ischemia, inflammation and cancer (Fiammengo and Jaschke, 2005).

RNaseP is an endogenous nuclear ribozyme that is substantially larger (several hundred bases) than hammerhead and hairpin ribozymes, which makes it far more difficult to apply exogenously (Trang et al., 2004). However, by making use of ONs that function as so-called small EGS, they can together with the mRNA form a structure that resembles the endogenous target of RNaseP and thereby recruits the enzyme to digest the mRNA-oligonucleotide sequence combination (Tafech et al., 2006). This concept has not yet been validated in vivo.

## ▪ siRNA/miRNA

miRNA and siRNA are double-stranded RNA (dsRNA) ONs of 21 to 26 base-pairs that can cause gene silencing, a process known as RNA interference (RNAi) (Fig. 8) (Sen and Blau, 2006). In 1998, RNAi was first described in the nematode *Caenorhabditis elegans*. This silencing phenomenon also occurs in plants, protozoa, fungi, and animals and appears to be conserved in all eukaryotes and may even play a role in prokaryotic cells. It is an important process in endogenous gene expression/translation regulation and defense against pathogens.

miRNAs are produced from transcripts that form stem-loop structures. These are processed in the nucleus into 65 to 75 nucleotides long pre-miRNA

| Antisense | Target | Indications | Chemistry | Company |
|---|---|---|---|---|
| Genasense | Bcl-2 | Cancer | Thioate | Genta |
| OGX-011 | Clusterin | Cancer | 2′ O-MOE[a] | OncoGenex |
| ATL1102 | VLA-4 | Multiple sclerosis | 2′ O-MOE | Antisense Therapeutics |
| LY2181308 | Survivin | Cancer | 2′ O-MOE | Eli Lilly |
| LY2275796 | eIF-4E | Cancer | 2′ O-MOE | Eli Lilly |
| Alicaforsen | ICAM-1 | Ulcerative colitis | Thioate | Isis |
| ISIS 301012 | ApoB100 | Hypercholesterolemia | 2′ O-MOE | Isis |
| ISIS 113715 | PTP-1B | Type 2 diabetes | 2′ O-MOE | Isis |
| Resten | MYC | Restenosis | Morpholino | AVI Biopharma |
| AVI-4065 | RdRP | Hepatitis C virus | Morpholino | AVI Biopharma |
| AVI-4557 | CYP450 3A4 | Drug metabolism | Morpholino | AVI Biopharma |
| LErafAON | c-raf | Cancer irradiation | Liposome-encapsulated | NeoPharm |

[a] 2′O-MOE = 2′-O-methoxy ethyl.

**Table 1** ▥ Antisense molecules currently in clinical trials.

followed by transport to the cytoplasm. Pre-miRNA is further cleaved by an enzyme complex known as Dicer-complex to form miRNA, which is loaded into the RNA-induced silencing complex (RISC) that can bind and cleave homologous mRNA. siRNA are produced from endogenous or exogenous long dsRNA precursors that are also cleaved by Dicer and loaded into RISC. The presence of long dsRNA in mammalian cells induces an interferon response, which results in non-specific inhibition of translation, and cell death. Therefore, in mammalian systems, the shorter siRNA is used which largely circumvents this response. Next to the direct endonucleolytic cleavage of mRNAs via RISC, miRNA and siRNA appear also to act at other levels. They have been shown to affect methylation of promoters, increase degradation of mRNA (not

mediated by RISC), block protein translation, and enhance protein degradation.

Since the discovery of the process, a remarkably rapid progress has been made, and several compounds are currently clinically investigated. This rapid progress is partly due to the strong potency of the RNAi technique which seems to silence gene expression far more efficiently than antisense approaches; partly, also because much has been learned from previous nucleic acid-based clinical trials. Acuity Pharmaceuticals and Sirna Therapeutics Inc. focus on macular degeneration as therapeutic target with VEGF-inhibiting siRNAs named Cand5 and siRNA-027, respectively. Alnylam Pharmaceuticals has started a clinical trial on RSV-infection with ALN-RSV-01 inhibiting a viral gene.

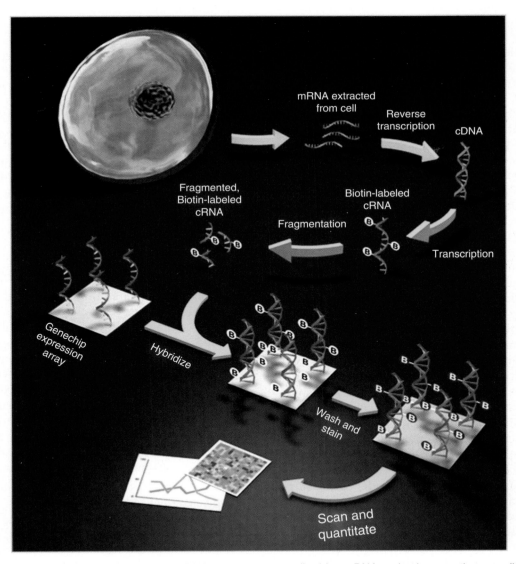

**Figure 8** ■ Application of microarrays. Isolated mRNA is reverse transcribed into cDNA and subsequently transcribed into labeled cRNA. Fragments of the cRNA can hybridize to complementary oligonucleotides from genes of interest, which are spotted at known locations. Quantification of bound cRNA yields a gene expression profile. *Source*: Courtesy of Jiang Jong, Bioteach, Canada.

## DIRECT BINDING TO NON-NUCLEIC ACIDS

The ability of nucleic acids to fold into complex three-dimensional structures through regions of (partial) complementarity allows them to bind to virtually any molecule with nano- to picomolar affinity (Proske et al., 2005). This high affinity is supported by data on their extreme specificity. A nucleic acid sequence specifically binding theophylline has a million times higher affinity for theophylline than caffeine, molecules which differ by only one methyl group.

### ■ Aptamers/Riboswitches

Aptamers and riboswitches are single-stranded ONs of either DNA or RNA, generally about 60 nucleotides long, which fold into well-defined three-dimensional structures. They bind to their target molecule by complementary shape interactions accompanied by charge and hydrophobic interactions and hydrogen bridges. The target can be small molecules or macromolecules. Aptamers are isolated artificially, whereas riboswitches occur naturally (Tucker and Breaker, 2005). Several viruses have been shown to encode small, structured RNAs that bind to viral or cellular proteins with high affinity and specificity. It was demonstrated that these RNAs could modulate the activity of proteins essential for viral replication or inhibit the activity of proteins involved in cellular antiviral responses. Also the genomes of prokaryotes have been shown to contain nutrient responsive riboswitches to regulate gene expression.

Synthetically, such compounds can be identified by subjecting large libraries of nucleic acid molecules to a panning procedure (Fig. 9). This selection process has been named systematic evolution of ligands by exponential enrichment (SELEX). The resulting ligands are called aptamers. The SELEX process starts by generating a large library of randomized RNA sequences. This library contains up to 1015 different nucleic acid molecules that fold into different structures depending on their sequence. The library is incubated with the structure of interest, and those RNAs present in the library that bind the protein are separated from those that do not. The obtained RNAs are then amplified by reverse transcriptase-PCR and in vitro transcribed to generate a pool of RNAs that have been enriched for those that bind the target of interest. This selection and amplification process is repeated (usually 8–12 rounds) under increasingly stringent binding conditions to promote Darwinian selection until the RNA ligands with the highest affinity for the target protein are isolated. This molecular evolution process can also be performed with DNA, circumventing the need for reverse transcription before PCR and in vitro transcription. Automation has reduced aptamer in vitro selection

times from months to days, making aptamers suitable for application in high throughput target validation. Aptamers can bind to proteins for therapeutic use, like antibodies do. However, antibody selection requires a biological system. The selection of aptamers is a chemical process, therefore it can target almost any protein. In contrast to antibodies, aptamers are prone to bind to functional domains of the target protein (for reasons unknown), such as substrate binding pockets or allosteric sites, thereby modulating the biological function of the molecule. A common problem upon the therapeutic development of aptamers is that they can be so specific for the human version of a target protein that they have poor cross-reactivity with orthologs of the target from other animal species, making their pre-clinical evaluation difficult. Toggle SELEX is a possible solution in which selection occurs alternating between pre-clinical and clinical target (White et al., 2001).

One aptamer targeting VEGF, pegaptanib (Macugen®), is marketed for wet age-related macular degeneration (Ng et al., 2006). The PEGylated aptamer (for PEGylation see Chapters 5 and 11) is injected in the vitreous at a dose of 1.65 mg (0.3 mg of which is aptamer)/eye in 90 µl every 6 weeks. Adverse effects included endophtalmitis and bleeding events in the eye, likely related to the injection procedure. The compound also appeared to exhibit effects in diabetic retinopathy. To increase stability several nucleotides are 2′-O-methyl and 2′-O-fluoro modified and the aptamer is conjugated to polyethylene glycol, which stabilizes siRNA in solution and facilitates clinical delivery.

## GENE REPAIR

### ■ Triplex Helix-Forming Oligonucleotides

The triplex-forming ONs have been used for site-directed mutagenesis with or without the use of coupled mutagens, as well as homologous-site-specific recombination using triplex-forming ONs alone, or in combination with a donor fragment to correct genetic disorders (Kalish and Glazer, 2005). Although the site-specificity is an important benefit for this technique, a complete understanding of the molecular mechanisms involved is still lacking, and rates of mutagenesis or gene correction are still too poor ($\leq 0.1\%$) to warrant clinical development.

### ■ Antisense-Induced Exon Skipping

The exon skipping technique tries to restore the reading frame by artificially removing one or more exons before or after the deletion or point mutation in the mRNA. The most popular disease target to work on is Duchenne's muscular dystrophy which, using this technique could be changed into the

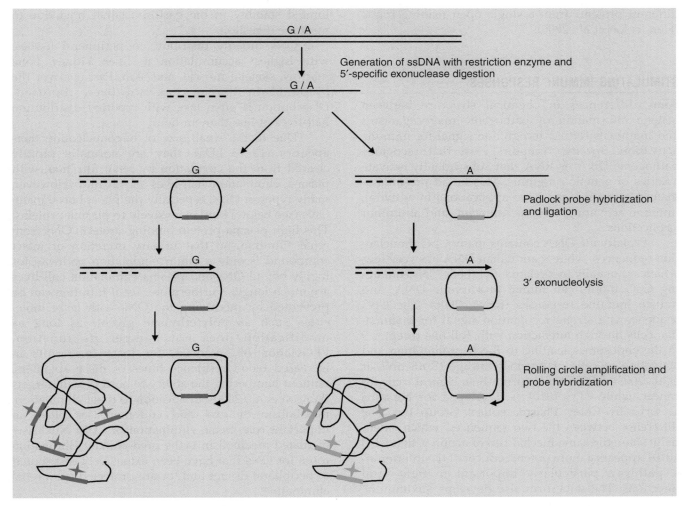

**Figure 9** ▪ In situ genotyping using allele-specific padlock probes and rolling circle amplification (RCA). After fixation of the cells, genomic DNA is cut and made single stranded at the allele position using restriction enzymes and a 5′-specific exonuclease, respectively. Padlock probes are allowed to anneal and ends are closed by ligation to form a circle. RCA is initiated using the target strand as primers, after the protruding 3′-ends of the target strand were removed by the 3′-exonucleolytic activity of the DNA polymerase. In this way multiple copies of the padlock probe are appended onto the 3′-end of the genomic DNA. By using fluorescently labeled oligonucleotides the 3′ tag can be visualized in cells, allowing in situ detection of single DNA molecules.

much milder Becker's dystrophy (Wilton and Fletcher, 2005).

Exons can be skipped from the mRNA with antisense oligoribonucleotides. They attach inside the exon to be removed, or at its borders. The ONs interfere with the splicing machinery so that the targeted exons are no longer included in the mRNA. In Duchenne's disease, if the missing amino acids are part of the central region of the dystrophin, they are often not essential, and the resulting shorter protein can still perform its stabilizing role of the muscle cell membrane. The technique is currently in clinical trials for Duchenne's dystrophy, sponsored by the Imperial College London, UK, after demonstrating pre-clinical efficacy in mice and dogs (Fall et al., 2006; McClorey et al., 2006).

■ **Antisense-Induced Ribonucleoprotein Inhibition**

Antisense ONs can be used to inhibit or alter the functions of ribonucleoproteins by specifically binding to the RNA part of the ribonucleoprotein. For example, telomerase, the enzyme involved in preventing the shortening of telomere ends after each cell division, can be inhibited by using ONs directed against the hTERT domain (i.e., RNA binding domain) (Folini et al., 2002). Antisense-induced telomerase inhibition resulted in progressive shortening of telomere ends and in some cases induction of apoptosis. As telomerase activity is found in many types of cancer, antisense inhibition of telomerase may be an effective approach for cancer treatment. Furthermore, antisense ONs have been used for programmed ribosomal frame-shifting to produce different proteins from a single open reading frame (Henderson et al., 2006).

## STIMULATING IMMUNE RESPONSES

Some differences in chemical structure between genetic information of pathogenic microorganisms and mammals form a recognition signal for immune activation. Specific receptors exist that recognize pathogenic DNA or RNA that subsequently activate a series of genetic programs. This broad pro-inflammatory activation can have applications in antiviral, immune activating, vaccine adjuvant, and antitumor applications.

Prokaryotic DNA contains many CpG dinucleotide sequences, while mammalian DNA has very few, which are usually methylated. Synthetic ONs containing CpG motifs can mimic prokaryotic DNA, and induce immune responses (Krieg, 2006). The CpG sequence is a strong recognition signal for mammalian cells through interaction with Toll-like receptor 9 in the endosomes leading to B-cell proliferation and activation of cells of myeloid lineage (Rothenfusser et al., 2003). CPG 7909 is currently in clinical trials for cancer, while CPG 10101 is developed for hepatitis C virus by Coley Pharmaceutical Group Inc. The difference between the two sequences, which essentially share the same mechanism of action is that CPG 10101 appears a more potent inducer of the interferon-α pathway, particularly important to fight viral infections. The same firm also develops VaxImmune as a support for vaccination protocols, which is based on the same immunostimulatory principle.

In a similar manner, dsRNA can be a predictor of viral infection and Toll-like receptor 3 recognizes dsRNA in the endosomes. In particular, synthetic dsRNA composed of poly-inosinic and poly-cytidylic acids are strong activators (poly-IC). It is clinically tested as poly-ICLC (Hiltonol™) by Oncovir Inc., a poly-lysine complexed formulation of poly-IC, to protect the dsRNA from nuclease action. The system is being developed for the treatment of glioma patients with or without supportive chemotherapy.

## PHARMACOKINETICS OF OLIGONUCLEOTIDE-BASED THERAPEUTICS

Pharmacokinetic studies with different types of ONs (in particular phosphorothioate-ONs) have demonstrated that ONs are rapidly absorbed from parenteral sites. Bioavailability of ONs can be as high as 90% after intradermal injections. Oral bioavailability, however, is generally very low due to their large molecular weight, multiple charges at physiological pH, and limited stability in the gastrointestinal tract due to nuclease digestion.

ONs broadly distribute to peripheral tissues, with highest accumulation in liver, kidney, bone marrow, skeletal muscle, and skin. Passage over the blood–brain barrier has not been reported. Distribution is often fast, with reported distribution half-lives of less than an hour.

Due to the small size of oligonucleotide therapeutics (10–13 kDa), they are normally rapidly cleared from the circulation by renal filtration, with plasma elimination half-lives of <10 min. However, many types of ONs, especially the phosphorothioate-ONs (see below) bind extensively to plasma proteins. This high plasma protein binding protects ONs from renal filtration, so that urinary excretion of intact compound is only a minor elimination pathway for highly bound ONs and plasma elimination half-lives are much longer. Furthermore, renal filtration can be prevented by modifying the ONs with large molecules such as poly(ethylene glycol) as long as modification does not hamper its function. PEGylation of aptamers, for instance, results in increased blood residence times of these aptamers, without hampering the ability to bind protein targets (Watson et al., 2000). In addition to renal elimination, metabolism by exo- and endonucleases plays an important role in the elimination of ONs. Nuclease-mediated metabolism is the predominant elimination route for ONs that have been extensively distributed to peripheral tissues and/or are protected from renal elimination.

## IMPROVING OLIGONUCLEOTIDE STABILITY

Nuclease resistance of AS-ONs can be improved by modifying the backbone of the ONs. Since the early 60s of the last century, several chemical modifications have been introduced to prevent such enzymatic degradation. The first generation DNA analogs consisted of the phosphorothioate (PS) ONs, in which one of the non-bridging oxygen atoms in the phosphodiester bond is replaced by sulfur (Fig. 1). These PS-ONs are more stable in serum, but also show higher binding to proteins that than unmodified ONs, which can cause toxicity problems. However, protein binding also contributes to the increased circulation half-life seen for PS-ON (40–60 hours), presumably due to reduced renal excretion. The second generation ONs are those containing alkyl modifications at the 2' position of the ribose unit (Fig. 1). Although less toxic than the PS-ONs, they have the disadvantage to be a poor substrate for RNase H and thus can only inhibit translation by forming a steric block. However, ONs consisting of 2'-O-(2-methoxyethyl) ONs have greatly improved plasma and tissue half-lives (up to 30 days), presumably due to reduced clearance by nuclease attack. Third generation ONs consist of a variety of different chemical modifications all with the aim to improve stability, pharmacokinetics, and interaction with RNA (Fig. 1). Examples are protein nucleic acids (PNAs) that have a polyamide backbone rather than a deoxyribose phosphate backbone, locked nucleic acids (LNAs) that have a methylene bridge between the $2'$-oxygen of the ribose and the $4'$-carbon, and morpholino nucleic acids containing a non-ionic morpholino subunit instead of a ribose, interlinked by a phosphoroamidate bond (Fig. 1). These third generation ONs all have in common the superior stability and RNA binding properties, but all lack RNase H activation. Therefore, chimeras of third generation ONs with DNA have been made that combine good stability and effective RNase H activation.

Modification of ribozymes or aptamers to obtain better stability and resistance against nucleolytic degradation is even more challenging, as such alterations most likely results in loss of respectively enzymatic or binding activity. The effect of each nucleotide modification on the stability and activity of the ribozyme or aptamer often have to be established empirically. The serum half-life of a DNA ribozyme could be 10-fold increased by protecting the $3'$-end with inverted nucleotides (Sun et al., 1999).

Stability of siRNA in cell culture and serum is generally not a limiting factor due to thermal instability of RNase A. However, for protection against intracellular nucleases further enhancement of stability might be required. This can be achieved by inserting modified nucleotides on either ends of the siRNA. However, one needs to be aware that the amount and chemical nature of modified nucleotides may influence the gene silencing efficacy of siRNA (Amarzguioui et al., 2003). siRNA is generally rapidly cleared.

## IMPROVING CELLULAR UPTAKE

Beside metabolic elimination by nucleases, the poor cellular uptake of ONs poses a problem for therapeutic application of ONs. Compared to conventional drugs, ONs are relatively large and polyanionic, making passage over cellular membranes virtually impossible. Cellular uptake of ONs can be improved in vitro and in vivo by physical methods, chemically modifying the ONs or by making use of specialized delivery systems.

Electroporation of tissue after local injection of ONs results in improved cellular uptake. Due to high voltage pulses, transient perforations in the cell membrane occur that allow passage of ONs into the cytosol. This technique can of course only be applied for delivery of ONs in vitro and in vivo to tissues readily available for electroporation (e.g., skin, skeletal muscle, or superficial tumor tissue).

Grafting ONs with cationic groups in order to reduce the ionic repulsion between ON and cell membrane represents an alternative strategy to enhance cellular uptake. Synthetic guanidinium-containing ONs (GONs) showed improved duplex and triplex stability in addition to enhanced cellular uptake (Deglane et al., 2006). The uptake pattern suggests that these cationic ONs are internalized by endocytosis, although cytosolic localization could also be observed.

Alternatively, cell-penetrating peptides (CPPs) can be conjugated to ONs with the purpose to enhance membrane translocation. CPPs are small basic peptides derived from protein transduction domains present in a variety of proteins which have strong membrane translocating properties. Conjugation of such a CPP called transportan to PNAs resulted in enhanced cellular uptake in a dose-dependent manner with preservation of antisense activity of the PNA.

Lipid modification of siRNA has also been proven to be beneficial for cellular uptake and subsequent gene silencing. siRNA against apoB mRNA, which was modified by attaching a cholesterol group to the $3'$ terminus of the sense strand, showed increased silencing of the gene encoding for apolipoprotein B compared to the unmodified siRNA after intravenous injection into mice (Soutschek et al., 2004).

Another strategy involves the use of sophisticated delivery systems to enhance cellular uptake and to target ONs to specific tissues or cells. Most of the delivery systems for ONs are based on complexation of ONs with cationic molecules, of which cationic lipids (e.g., Lipofectamine™) are the most common. The complexation has a dual function: it protects the ONs from nuclease attack and enhances cellular internalization. By shielding the cationic complexes with large polyethylene glycol polymers displaying targeting ligands, such complexes can be targeted to specific cell types. This has been demonstrated for the delivery of siRNA to angiogenic vascular endothelial cells (Schiffelers et al., 2004). Targeting can also be accomplished by covalently coupling the ONs to antibodies. In this way, PNAs conjugated to an anti-transferrin receptor monoclonal antibody could be transported over the blood–brain barrier (Shi et al., 2000).

## DIAGNOSTIC APPLICATIONS

Apart from the direct application of ONs in medicine as therapeutics, they also fulfill an increasingly important role as diagnostic agents. The highly specific binding of complementary oligonucleotide sequences can be used to detect gene expression profiles and mutations, whereas aptamers can be used to detect presence of specific compounds. PCR amplification of specific nucleic sequences can provide information on the presence and abundance of this particular sequence. For example, the Amplicor HIV-1 Monitor v1.5 assays manufactured by Roche Diagnostics are currently approved for in vitro diagnostic use to determine viral load in blood samples.

Other applications, like microarrays, do not focus on single genes but provide an overview of the "transcriptome" (Fig. 8). A DNA microarray consists of ONs of approximately 25 bases that are spotted on a chip in an orderly arrangement, representing the genes of interest of an organism. Each ON is spotted at a specific location on the array so that the location of each ON with corresponding gene is known. Robotic spotters can currently place tens of thousands of ONs accurately on one slide of a few square centimeters. Each spot contains identical single-stranded ONs that are strongly attached to the slide surface, allowing cellular DNA or RNA to be labeled and hybridized to the complementary sequence on the array. By quantifying the binding of the labeled DNA or RNA to the specific spots, the abundance of each species can be determined and related to the corresponding gene.

In 2004, the FDA approved the first microarray AmpliChip CYP450 for clinical use. The AmpliChip CYP450 provides complete coverage of the gene variations, including duplications and deletion, of the cytochrome P450 enzymes 2D6 and 2C19. These genes are involved in the metabolism of approximately 25% of all prescription drugs. It could be regarded as an important step towards personalized medicine.

The inherent specificity and selectivity of aptamers makes these ONs very useful to detect disease-associated molecules, in a similar manner as antibody-based immunoassays. However, they are not in clinical use yet.

Padlock probes can also be used for diagnostic applications (Nilsson et al., 1994). They consist of long ONs, whose ends are complementary to adjacent target sequences. Upon hybridization, the ends of the ONs are brought together, allowing ligation of the ON ends into a closed and intertwined circle that cannot be replaced by the complementary DNA strand. This closed circle can then be amplified by rolling circle amplification, a powerful and robust DNA amplification method based on the mesophilic Phi29 DNA polymerase, allowing amplification of the padlock signal to detectable levels (Fig. 9). Padlock probes are more specific than conventional antisense ONs, as misannealing of either one of the ends does not result in proper ligation of the ends, and thus prevents circularization of the padlock probe. It has been used for multiplex detection of pathogens in biological samples (Szemes et al., 2005), single nucleotide polymorphisms (Bakht and Qi, 2005) and miRNA (Jonstrup et al., 2006), but also for in situ genotyping of individual DNA molecules (Larsson et al., 2004).

## PERSPECTIVES

At present, two ON-based drugs are marketed, Vitravene® and Macugen®. Both contain chemically modified nucleotides and both are injected in the vitreous, i.e., at the site of the disease process. These choices reflect two of the main difficulties in applying ONs as therapeutics: (1) ONs are sensitive towards nucleases, (2) ONs have difficulties in reaching the target site. As one of the marketed drugs is an aptamer, this target site accumulation is apparently even complicated for ONs that act extracellularly, let alone for oligonucleotide classes that need to interact with intracellular machinery for their action. Current chemical modifications are increasingly able to circumvent these problems by introducing functional groups that offer nuclease resistance and enhanced cellular uptake. Nevertheless, specificity of delivery to the target cell population remains problematic, interaction with the normal cellular machinery may be distorted, and it continues to be unclear what the consequences are of incorporation of these modified nucleotides into normal metabolism.

One of the most promising strategies to circumvent heavy chemical modifications and improve target cell delivery appears the use of nanotechnology. Complexing nucleic acids within nanoparticles, increases their apparent molecular weight preventing renal excretion, protecting against nuclease digestion, and improving target cell recognition and uptake. Targeted delivery seems especially important in view of the plethora of activities nucleic acids can display. It seems hardly possible to find nucleic acid sequences that will act through a single pathway and not interact with any of the other pathways. Limiting the number of cell types where the nucleic acids distribute to will likely contribute to reduce side effects.

## REFERENCES

Aboul-Fadl T (2005). Antisense oligonucleotides: The state of the art. Curr Med Chem 12(19):2193–214.

Amarzguioui M, Holen T, Babaie E, Prydz H (2003). Tolerance for mutations and chemical modifications in siRNA. Nucleic Acids Res 31(2):589–95.

Bakht S, Qi X (2005). Ligation-mediated rolling-circle amplification-based approaches to single nucleotide polymorphism detection. Expert Rev Mol Diagnos 5(1):111–6.

Chan JH, Lim S, Wong WS (2006). Antisense oligonucleotides: From design to therapeutic application. Clin Exp Pharmacol Physiol 33(5–6):533–40.

Conti VR, Hunter GC (2005). Gene therapy and vein graft patency in coronary artery bypass graft surgery. JAMA 294(19):2495–7.

Dajee M, et al. (2006). Blockade of experimental atopic dermatitis via topical NF-kappaB decoy oligonucleotide. J Invest Dermatol 126(8):1792–803.

Deglane G, Abes S, Michel T, et al. (2006). Impact of the guanidinium group on hybridization and cellular uptake of cationic oligonucleotides. Chem Bio Chem 7(4):684–92.

Fall AM, Johnsen R, Honeyman K, Iversen P, Fletcher S, Wilton SD (2006). Induction of revertant fibres in the mdx mouse using antisense oligonucleotides. Genet Vaccines Ther 4:3.

Fiammengo R, Jaschke A (2005). Nucleic acid enzymes. Curr Opin Biotechnol 16(6):614–21.

Folini M, Pennati M, Zaffaroni N (2002). Targeting human telomerase by antisense oligonucleotides and ribozymes. Curr Med Chem Anticanc Agent 2(5):605–12.

Gekeler V, et al. (2006). G3139 and other CpG-containing immunostimulatory phosphorothioate oligodeoxynucleotides are potent suppressors of the growth of human tumor xenografts in nude mice. Oligonucleotides 16(1):83–93.

Henderson CM, Anderson CB, Howard MT (2006). Antisense-induced ribosomal frameshifting. Nucleic Acid Res 34(15):4302–10.

Jabs DA, Griffiths PD (2002). Fomivirsen for the treatment of cytomegalovirus retinitis. Am J Ophthalmol 133(4):552–6.

Jonstrup SP, Koch J, Kjems J (2006). A microRNA detection system based on padlock probes and rolling circle amplification. RNA 12(9):1747–52.

Kalish JM, Glazer PM (2005). Targeted genome modification via triple helix formation. Ann N Y Acad Sci 1058:151–61.

Krieg AM (2006). Therapeutic potential of Toll-like receptor 9 activation. Nat Rev Drug Discov 5(6):471–84.

Kurreck J (2003). Antisense technologies. Improvement through novel chemical modifications. Eur J Biochem 270(8):1628–44.

Lai JC, Tan W, Benimetskaya L, Miller P, Colombini M, Stein CA (2006). A pharmacologic target of G3139 in melanoma cells may be the mitochondrial VDAC. Proc Natl Acad Sci USA 103(19):7494–9.

Larsson C, Koch J, Nygren A, et al. (2004). In situ genotyping individual DNA molecules by target-primed rolling-circle amplification of padlock probes. Nat Method 1(3):227–32.

Lilley DM (2005). Structure, folding, and mechanisms of ribozymes. Curr Opin Struct Biol 15(3):313–23.

Macpherson JL, et al. (2005). Long-term survival and concomitant gene expression of ribozyme-transduced CD4+ T-lymphocytes in HIV-infected patients. J Gene Med 7(5):552–64.

McClorey G, Moulton HM, Iversen PL, Fletcher S, Wilton SD (2006). Antisense oligonucleotide-induced exon skipping restores dystrophin expression in vitro in a canine model of DMD. Gene Ther 13 (19):1373–81.

Ng EW, Shima DT, Calias P, Cunningham Jr ET, Guyer DR, Adamis AP (2006). Pegaptanib, a targeted anti-VEGF aptamer for ocular vascular disease 5(2):123–32.

Nilsson M, Malmgren H, Samiotaki M, Kwiatkowski M, Chowdhary BP, Landegren U (1994). Padlock probes: Circularizing oligonucleotides for localized DNA detection. Science 265(5181):2085–8.

Proske D, Blank M, Buhmann R, Resch A (2005). Aptamers — basic research, drug development, and clinical applications. Appl Microbiol Biotechnol 69(4):367–74.

Rogers FA, Lloyd JA, Glazer PM (2005). Triplex-forming oligonucleotides as potential tools for modulation of gene expression. Curr Med Chem Anticanc Agent 5(4):319–26.

Rothenfusser S, Tuma E, Wagner M, Endres S, Hartmann G (2003). Recent advances in immunostimulatory CpG oligonucleotides. Curr Opin Mol Ther 5 (2):98–106.

Schiffelers RM, Woodle MC, Scaria P (2004). Pharmaceutical prospects for RNA interference. Pharm Res 21(1):1–7.

Sen GL, Blau HM (2006). A brief history of RNAi: The silence of the genes. Faseb J 20(9):1293–9.

Shi N, Boado RJ, Pardridge WM (2000). Antisense imaging of gene expression in the brain in vivo. Proc Natl Acad Sci USA 97(26):14709–14.

Soutschek J, et al. (2004). Therapeutic silencing of an endogenous gene by systemic administration of modified siRNAs. Nature 432(7014):173–8.

Stein CA, Benimetskaya L, Mani S (2005). Antisense strategies for oncogene inactivation. Semin Oncol 32(6):563–72.

Stephenson ML, Zamecnik PC (1978). Inhibition of Rous sarcoma viral RNA translation by a specific oligodeoxyribonucleotide. Proc Natl Acad Sci USA 75 (1):285–8.

Sun LQ, Cairns MJ, Gerlach WL, Witherington C, Wang L, King A (1999). Suppression of smooth muscle cell proliferation by a c-myc RNA-cleaving deoxyribozyme. J Biol Chem 274(24):17236–41.

Szemes M, Bonants P, de Weerdt M, Baner J, Landegren U, Schoen CD (2005). Diagnostic application of padlock probes — Multiplex detection of plant pathogens using universal microarrays. Nucleic Acids Res 33(8):1–13.

Tafech A, Bassett T, Sparanese D, Lee CH (2006). Destroying RNA as a therapeutic approach. Curr Med Chem 13(8):863–81.

Tomita N, Azuma H, Kaneda Y, Ogihara T, Morishita R (2004). Application of decoy oligodeoxynucleotides-based approach to renal diseases. Curr Drug Target 5(8):717–33.

Trang P, Kim K, Liu F (2004). Developing RNase P ribozymes for gene-targeting and antiviral therapy. Cell Microbiol 6(6):499–508.

Tucker BJ, Breaker RR (2005). Riboswitches as versatile gene control elements. Curr Opin Struct Biol 15(3):342–8.

Watson SR, Chang YF, O'Connell D, Weigand L, Ringquist S Parma DH (2000). Anti-L-selectin aptamers: Binding characteristics, pharmacokinetic parameters, and activity against an intravascular target in vivo. Antisense Nucleic Acid Drug Dev 10(2):63–75.

White R, Rusconi C, Scardino E, et al. (2001). Generation of species cross-reactive aptamers using "toggle" SELEX. Mol Ther 4(6):567–73.

Wilton SD, Fletcher S (2005). Antisense oligonucleotides, exon skipping and the dystrophin gene transcript. Acta Myol 24(3):222–9.

Zamecnik PC, Stephenson ML (1978). Inhibition of Rous sarcoma virus replication and cell transformation by a specific oligodeoxynucleotide. Proc Natl Acad Sci USA 75(1):280–4.

## FURTHER READING

Cho-Chung YS, Gewirtz AM, Stein CA (2005). Therapeutic oligonucleotides: Transcriptional and translational strategies for silencing gene expression. Ann NY Acad Sci USA.Kalota A, Dondeti VR, Gewirtz AM (2006). Progress in the development of nucleic acid therapeutics. Handb Exp Pharmacol 173:173–96.

Klussmann S (2006). The aptamer handbook: Functional oligonucleotides and their applications. Weinheim, Germany: Wiley–VCH Verlag.Phillips MI (2004). Antisense therapeutics. Methods in Molecular Medicine. Totowa, NJ: Humana Press.

Raz E (2000). Immunostimulatory DNA Sequences. Berlin, Germany: Springer.Xie FY, Woodle MC, Lu PY (2006). Harnessing in vivo siRNA delivery for drug discovery and therapeutic development. Drug Discov Today 11 (1–2):67–73.

# 10

# Hematopoietic Growth Factors

*MaryAnn Foote*
*MaryAnne Foote Associates, Westlake Village, California, U.S.A.*

### PHARMACOTHERAPY INFORMATION

Further information on the applied pharmacotherapy with hematopoietic growth factors can be found in the following frequently used textbooks:

- **Applied Therapeutics: The Clinical Use of Drugs** (*Koda-Kimble, MA, et al., Eds.*), 8th edition, Lippincott Williams & Wilkins, Baltimore 2005: Chapters 32, 86, 87, 89, 90, 91, 92.
- **Pharmacotherapy: A Pathophysiologic Approach** (*DiPiro, JT, et al., Eds.*), 6th edition, McGraw-Hill, New York 2005: Chapters 44, 102, 120, 123, 124, 125, 131, 134.
- **Textbook of Therapeutics: Drug and Disease Management** (*Helms, RA, et al., Eds.*), 8th edition, Lippincott Williams & Wilkins, Baltimore 2006: Chapters 32, 43, 65, 92.

## INTRODUCTION

Blood cells are vital to life: they transport oxygen and carbon dioxide, contribute to host immunity, and facilitate blood clotting. An intricate, multistep process allows immature precursor cells in the bone marrow to differentiate, mature, and become functional blood cells. Ordinarily, this well-regulated process allows for replacement of cells lost through daily physiologic activities. The process is also capable of producing adequate and appropriate cells for fighting infection and for replacing cell losses due to hemorrhaging or destruction. The process of production and maturation of blood cells is called hematopoiesis.

In the early 1900s, scientists recognized the presence of circulating factors that regulate hematopoiesis. It took approximately 50 years, until cell culture systems were developed that could sustain cell colonies in vitro, to definitively prove the activity of these proteins. The growth and survival of early blood cells required the presence of specific factors, called colony-stimulating factors (CSF). However, hematopoietic growth factor (HGF) is the preferred term because it is more precise than the term based on laboratory observations of the effects of these factors.

Efforts to purify HGFs progressed throughout the 1970s and early 1980s. Blood and other materials (e.g., bone marrow and urine) contain extremely small amounts of growth factors. The presence of many growth factors confounded the search for a single growth factor with a specific activity. Scientific progress was slow until it became possible to purify sufficient quantities to fully evaluate the characteristics and biologic potential of the isolated materials. The introduction of recombinant DNA technology triggered a flurry of studies and an information explosion. Many HGFs have been isolated; some have been studied extensively, and a few have been made for clinical or commercial use.

## HEMATOPOIESIS

Hematopoiesis is mediated by a series of growth factors that act individually and in various combinations involving complex feedback mechanisms to stimulate the proliferation, differentiation, and function of hematopoietic cells.

Ten types of mature blood cells have been identified, each derived from primitive hematopoietic stem cells in the bone marrow. The most primitive pool of pluripotent stem cells comprises approximately 0.1% of the nucleated cells of the bone marrow, and 5% of these cells may be actively cycling at a given time. The stem cell pool maintains itself, seemingly without extensive depletion, by asymmetrical cell division. When a stem cell divides, one daughter cell remains in the stem cell pool and the other becomes a committed colony-forming unit (CFU). CFUs proliferate at a greater rate than the other stem cells and are more limited in self-renewal than pluripotent hematopoietic stem cells. The proliferation and differentiation are regulated by a number of things, including HGFs. These HGFs eventually convert the dividing cells into a population of terminally differentiated functional cells.

Cells committed to the myeloid pathway can develop into:

- red blood cells (erythrocytes)
- platelets (thrombocytes)
- monocytes and macrophages
- granulocytes (neutrophils, eosinophils, and basophils)
- tissue mast cells

Cells committed to the lymphoid pathway give rise to:

- B- or T-lymphocytes
- plasma cells

This chapter focuses on growth factors that are produced by recombinant DNA technology (identified by the prefix "rh" which identifies a recombinant human form of the endogenous protein) and marketed in at least one country.

## CHEMICAL DESCRIPTION OF HEMATOPOIETIC GROWTH FACTORS

Hematopoietic growth factors are generally glycoproteins, which can be distinguished by their amino acid sequence and glycosylation pattern (carbohydrate linkages). The recombinant HGFs, however, are not always glycoproteins. In spite of the lack of the carbohydrate moieties, they may still assume the structure necessary to exert the same biologic activity of the glycosylated form. In some cases, however, additional carbohydrates have been engineered and added to the native CSF to increase circulating half-life. Most HGFs are single-chain polypeptides. The carbohydrate content varies by growth factor and production method, which in turn affects the molecular weight but not necessarily the biologic activity.

Each HGF is encoded by a specific gene. Production of the recombinant proteins is accomplished by first identifying the gene in question, isolating it by various techniques, inserting the gene of interest into a plasmid, and then expressing the protein of interest in a biologic system (e.g., bacteria, yeast, or mammalian cells) to produce recombinant growth factors.

The HGFs that will be discussed in detail include:

- the white cell factors factors, granulocyte colony-stimulating factor (G-CSF) and granulocyte-macrophage colony-stimulating factor (GM-CSF);
- the red cell factors, the erythropoietins (EPO) and darbepoetin alfa;
- the platelet factors, thrombopoietin (TPO), megakaryocyte growth and development factor (MGDF), and interleukin-11 (IL-11) (see Chapter 11); and
- an early acting HGF, stem cell factor (SCF).

A summary of the HGFs and their activities is provided in Table 1.

### ■ Chemical Properties and Marketing Information for the Myeloid Factors, G-CSF and GM-CSF

The chemical properties of the myeloid HGFs, G-CSF and GM-CSF, have been characterized (Table 2). The gene that encodes for G-CSF is located on chromosome 17 and the mature G-CSF polypeptide has 174 amino acids. The gene that encodes for GM-CSF is located on chromosome 4 and the mature polypeptide has 127 or 128 amino acids. Filgrastim, a rhG-CSF, is marketed by several companies under several trade names throughout the world. Lenograstim, another rhG-CSF, is not marketed in the United States but is marketed in other countries under several trade

| Factor | Abbreviation | Molecular weight (kDa) | Target cells | Actions |
|---|---|---|---|---|
| Granulocyte colony-stimulating factor | G-CSF | 18 | Granulocyte progenitors, mature neutrophils | Increase neutrophil counts |
| Granulocyte-macrophage colony-stimulating factor | GM-CSF | 14–35 | Granulocyte, macrophage progenitors, eosinophil progenitors | Increase neutrophil, eosinophil, and monocyte counts |
| Erythropoietin | EPO | 34–39 | Erythroid progenitors | Increase red blood cell counts |
| Stem cell factor | SCF | | Granulocyte-erythroid progenitors, lymphoid progenitors, natural killer cells | Increase pluripotent stem cells and progenitor cells for all other cell types |
| Thrombopoietin | TPO | 35 | Stem cells, megakaryocytes, erythroid progenitors | Increase platelet counts |
| Interleukin-11 | IL-11 | 23 | Early hematopoietic progenitors, megakaryocytes | Increase platelet counts |

**Table 1** ■ Hematopoietic growth factors and their activities.

| | G-CSF | GM-CSF |
|---|---|---|
| Nonproprietary name | Filgrastim, lenograstim, pegfilgrastim | Molgramostim, sargramostim |
| Chromosome location | 17 | 4 |
| Amino acids | 174[a] | 127 or 128[b] |
| Glycosylation | O-linked (lenograstim) | N-linked (sargramostim) |
| Pegylation | Pegfilgrastim | None |
| Source of gene | Bladder carcinoma cell line (filgrastim, pegfilgrastim), squamous carcinoma cell line (lenograstim) | Human monocyte cell line (molgramostim), Mouse T-lymphoma cell line (sargramostim) |
| Expression system | Escherichia coli (bacteria): filgrastim, pegfilgrastim Chinese hamster ovary cell line (mammalian): lenograstim | Escherichia coli (bacteria): molgramostim Saccharomyces cerevisiae (yeast): sargramostim |

[a] Native G-CSF has two forms, one with 177, which is less active than the other form with 174 amino acids; filgrastim has an N-terminal methionine.
[b] Molgramostim has 128 amino acids; sargramostim has 127.
Source: From Nagata et al., 1986; Souza et al., 1986; Gronski et al., 1988.

**Table 2** ■ Characteristics of the marketed myeloid growth factors, rhG-CSF and rhGM-CSF.

names. Molgramostim and sargramostim are two versions of rhGM-CSF; the former is marketed in Europe and the latter, in the United States, under several trade names. For a review of rhG-CSF, see Welte et al. (1996); for a review of rhGM-CSF, see Armitage (1998).

Pegfilgrastim, a long-acting form of filgrastim, is marketed as Neulasta® in Australia, Canada, the European Union, Switzerland, and the United States. For a review of pegfilgratim, see Molineux (2004).

## ■ Chemical Properties and Marketing Information for EPO

The gene that encodes EPO is located on chromosome 7. The mature polypeptide has 165 amino acids, two disulfide bonds, and three N- and one O-linked carbohydrate chains. Unlike G-CSF and GM-CSF, EPO requires glycosylation for its in vivo biologic activity. EPO is heavily glycosylated, which increases the molecular weight from 18.4 kDa for the unglycosylated molecule to approximately 34 kDa. Two rhEPO products are marketed and both are expressed in Chinese hamster ovary cells. Epoetin alfa is available in the United States, Japan, and China, under different trade names. The second recombinant erythropoietin is epoetin beta, which is available in Europe and Japan, again under different trade names. Both recombinant products have the same primary amino acid sequence and almost identical glycosylation (Veys et al., 1992). For a review of EPO and the role of the kidney in erythropoiesis, see Jacobson et al. (2000).

Darbepoetin alfa is a glycoengineered erythropoietin with more carbohydrate than rhEPO, increased molecular weight, and increased number of sialic acids (Elliott et al., 2004). It is marketed in many countries as Aranesp®. For a review of erythropoiesis and the different recombinant EPO, see Molineux (2004).

## ■ Chemical Properties and Marketing Information for SCF

The gene for SCF is located on chromosome 12. A longer form ($SCF^{248}$) and a shorter form ($SCF^{220}$) can be expressed, both of which are membrane bound. Soluble $SCF^{165}$ is proteolytically released from $SCF^{248}$. $SCF^{220}$ lacks the proteolytic cleavage site and tends to remain membrane bound. The approved rhSCF (ancestim), marketed as Stemgen® in Canada, Australia, and New Zealand, corresponds to $SCF^{165}$ plus an N-terminal methionine residue. It is recombinantly produced in Escherichia coli and is, therefore, non-glycosylated. Galli et al. (1994), Broudy (1997, Lacerna et al. (2000), and Langley (2004) offer comprehensive reviews of rhSCF.

## ■ Chemical Properties and Marketing Information for TPOs

Factors responsible for megakaryocyte development and platelet production, the TPOs, include the Mpl ligands (TPO and MGDF) and (IL)-11. TPO and MGDF are Mpl ligands; IL-11s not. For convenience, all three molecules will be referred to as TPOs, although it must be remembered that IL-11's receptor is different from those of TPO/MGDF and that IL-11 has also other biologic functions (see Chapter 11).

The existence of a TPO was suggested in 1958 and activity was demonstrated in the early 1960s. In 1990, studies investigating murine leukemia and oncogenes led to the recognition of a new hematopoietin receptor superfamily, Mpl, which was found to be the receptor of an important regulator of thrombopoiesis (Souyri et al., 1990; Vigon et al., 1992). Two forms of Mpl ligand were produced through recombinant DNA technology. The book edited by Kuter et al. (1994a) is a compilation of the biology, molecular, and cellular information about TPO, MGDF, and IL-11; Kaushansky (2005) reviews the molecular mechanisms that control thrombopoiesis.

The gene for TPO is located on chromosome 3. Depending on the source, the mature polypeptide has between 305 and 355 amino acids, which may undergo cleavage to a smaller polypeptide that retains biologic activity. A wide range of molecular weights (18–70 kDa) has been reported for active molecules (Kaushansky, 1995). At this time, no recombinant Mpl ligands are commercially available.

The gene for IL-11 is located on chromosome 19. IL-11 has multilineage effects. The precursor protein consists of 199 amino acids. IL-11 is rich in proline residues, and it lacks cysteine residues and disulfide bonds common to other HGFs (Du and Williams, 1997).

Oprelvekin (rhIL-11) is a non-glycosylated polypeptide, 177 amino acids in length and approximately 19 kDa in molecular weight (see Chapter 11). Oprelvekin differs from endogenous IL-11 by a single amino acid—the amino terminal proline—but this difference does not affect bioactivity. Oprelvekin is marketed as Neumega® in the United States.

## PHARMACOLOGY

Hematopoietic growth factors act by binding to specific cell surface receptors. Activation of these receptors results in a cascade of intracellular second messengers and altered gene expression, which in turn induce cellular proliferation, differentiation, or activation. A HGF also may act indirectly by inducing the expression of a gene producing a different HGF or cytokine, which in turn stimulates another target cell. This indirect activity has made it difficult to delineate the pharmacologic activity of individual HGFs and accounts for some of the differences between in vitro and in vivo results. Cell culture studies can be designed to exclude indirect effects, but animal and clinical studies generally reflect the full scope of direct and indirect biologic effects.

### ■ In Vitro Activity

As discussed earlier in this chapter, the hierarchy for hematopoiesis involves many steps and pathways. By definition, the pluripotent stem cell is the progenitor or precursor for all hematopoietic cells.

The complex interactions among progenitor cells and their mature progeny were determined by evaluating the effects of adding HGFs to cell cultures containing immature progenitor cells from the bone marrow.

In addition to their effects on progenitor cells, HGFs bind to and regulate the functional activity of mature cells. Whereas lineage-specific growth factors (e.g., G-CSF and EPO) predominantly affect one cell lineage, multilineage growth factors (e.g., GM-CSF and IL-3) affect more than one cell lineage. This phenomenon is concentration dependent. The GM-CSF concentrations that regulate monocytes and granulocytes (5–20 pg/mL)

are lower than those for eosinophils and platelets (20–2000 pg/mL) (Metcalf, 1990).

### ■ In Vivo Activity

The in vivo activity of HGFs can be assessed by measuring endogenous concentrations under different conditions or by administering growth factors to animals or humans. Although the in vivo results are often consistent with those predicted by in vitro studies, differences can be observed and may be the result of interspecies variability. Other reasons for in vivo and in vitro variability include differences in clearance, pharmacokinetics, and glycosylation. Table 3 summarizes cellular sources, endogenous serum levels, and stimuli for release of growth factors.

### ■ Cellular Sources and Stimuli for Release

T-lymphocytes, monocytes/macrophages, fibroblasts, and endothelial cells are the major cellular sources of

| Hematopoietic growth factor (normal range in serum) | Cellular source | Stimuli for release |
|---|---|---|
| G-CSF (9–51 pg/mL) | Monocytes | Lipopolysaccharide induction |
| | Fibroblasts | TNF-α, IL-1 |
| | Endothelial cells | TNF-α, IL-1 |
| | Bone marrow stromal cells | Cytokine activation |
| GM-CSF (0.4–2 pg/mL) | T-cells | Antigens, lectins, IL-1 |
| | Monocytes | Lipopolysaccharide induction |
| | Fibroblasts | TNF-α, IL-1 |
| | Endothelial cells | TNF-α, IL-1 |
| EPO (3–7 mU/mL) | Kidney | Hypoxia |
| | Liver | Hypoxia |
| TPO (20–300 pg/mL) | Kidney | Constitutively expressed |
| | Liver | Constitutively expressed |
| SCF (1200–1900 pg/mL) | Fibroblasts | Constitutively expressed |
| | Bone marrow stroma | Constitutively expressed |

*Source*: From Groopman et al., 1989; Kuter et al., 1994b; Lok et al, 1994; Nichol et al., 1995.

**Table 3**  Cellular sources, endogenous levels and stimuli for release of hematopoietic growth factors in humans.

most HGFs, excluding EPO, TPO, and darbepoetin alfa. EPO is produced primarily (>90%) in the adult kidney (Jacobson et al., 2000). The liver also produces some EPO (<10%), but the amount is insufficient to maintain normal red blood cell formation. TPO is produced in the liver and the kidney (Kuter, 1997).

Many inflammatory stimuli are capable of promoting the cellular release of HGFs (Table 3). Antigens, lectins, and IL-1 can signal T-lymphocytes to produce GM-CSF and IL-3. Endotoxins such as lipopolysaccharides can induce monocytes/macrophages to release G-CSF and GM-CSF. IL-1 and tumor necrosis factor alpha (TNF-α), produced by activated monocytes, can trigger the release of G-CSF and GM-CSF by fibroblasts and endothelial cells. In addition, these findings suggest that HGFs play a major role in host response to infection or antigen challenge and may also play a limited role in maintaining normal hematopoiesis (Groopman et al., 1989; Hartung et al., 1999).

## ■ Physiologic Role of G-CSF and GM-CSF

G-CSF, but not GM-CSF, is usually detectable in the blood and increases during infection (Cebon et al., 1994). Mice that lack endogenous G-CSF (i.e., "knockout mice") have chronic neutropenia and impaired neutrophil mobilization (Lieschke et al., 1994). The collective results of these in vivo studies, together with in vitro observations, suggest that the two myeloid growth factors have complementary roles. G-CSF may help maintain neutrophil production during steady-state conditions and increase production during acute situations such as infection. GM-CSF may be a locally active growth factor that remains at the site of infection to localize and activate neutrophils (Rapoport et al., 1992).

In vivo definition of the physiologic role of GM-CSF in steady-state hematopoiesis has been further elucidated by a knockout mouse model (Stanley et al., 1994). Both survival and fertility of GM−/− mice were found to be normal. The peripheral blood of 6- to 7-week old GM−/− mice showed no significant difference from wild-type (normal) mice in terms of hemoglobin, platelets, total white blood cells, neutrophils, lymphocytes, monocytes, or eosinophils. No other differences were noted in bone marrow cellularity, myeloid:erythroid ratios of marrow, or assayed progenitor cells from different lineages. These data suggest that steady-state hematopoietic pathways that might be affected by loss of GM-CSF are redundantly regulated. The most striking finding in the GM-CSF−/− mice was the development of pulmonary disease. At birth, knockout and wild-type mice have similar lung morphology, but by 3 weeks, knockout mice consistently showed focal peribronchovascular

lymphoid aggregate. Older animals had alveoli with large foamy macrophages. The changes were histologically similar to those produced by pulmonary alveolar proteinosis. These changes were not seen in the wild-type animals.

rhG-CSF reduces neutrophil maturation time from 5 days to 1 day, leading to a rapid release of mature neutrophils from the bone marrow into circulation (Lord et al., 1989; 1992). rhGM-CSF does not reduce the mean maturation time. Neutrophils treated with rhG-CSF show normal intravascular half-life (Lord et al., 1989); neutrophils treated with rhGM-CSF have an increased serum half-life of 48 hours (Lord et al., 1989), which may be due to impaired maturation. rhG-CSF enhances chemotaxis by increasing the binding of fMLP (formyl-methionyl-leucyl-phenylalanine) (Colgan et al., 1992). A short incubation (<30 minutes) with rhGM-CSF enhances neutrophil chemotaxis, but incubation >30 minutes results in the inhibition of neutrophil motility (Weisbart and Golde, 1989). Neutrophils treated with rhG-CSF have enhanced superoxide production in response to chemoattractants (Weisbart and Golde, 1989). rhGM-CSF also enhances superoxide production, but optimal priming requires a long incubation period. Clinical studies in patients receiving rhGM-CSF using the skin-window technique showed significantly reduced neutrophil migration compared with healthy volunteers (Dale et al., 1998).

CD34[+] hematopoietic cells harvested from bone marrow, umbilical cord blood, or peripheral blood can be co-cultured with TNF-α and GM-CSF to induce conversion of CD34[+] cells to dendritic cells. Dendritic cells are antigen-presenting cells capable of long-term activation of antibody/antigen complexes (Hart, 1997; Siena et al., 1997). Peripheral blood monocytes co-cultured with IL-4 and GM-CSF can produce dendritic cells. The functional activity of dendritic cells generated using different culture methods can vary considerably (Hart, 1997).

## ■ Physiologic Role of EPO

EPO increases red blood cell count by causing committed erythroid progenitor cells to proliferate and differentiate into normoblasts (a nucleated precursor cell in the erythropoietic lineage). EPO also shifts reticulocytes (mature red blood cells) from the bone marrow into the peripheral circulation. EPO is ordinarily present in plasma in low, but detectable, quantities. Unlike some other HGFs, EPO release is not mediated by inflammatory stimuli. Tissue hypoxia resulting from anemia induces the kidney to increase its production of EPO by a magnitude of a hundredfold or more. Patients with chronic renal failure are unable to produce adequate EPO levels because of the loss of renal function (Erslev, 1991).

rhEPO accelerates erythropoiesis in patients with chronic renal failure and has been used to enhance red cell production after chemotherapy and allogeneic bone marrow transplantation, and to increase red blood cell numbers for presurgical autodonation. Although rhEPO is a late-acting factor, it may synergize with TPO s to stimulate the production of megakaryocyte colony-forming cells (Broudy et al., 1997).

### ■ Physiologic Role of SCF

SCF is an early acting HGF that stimulates the proliferation of primitive hematopoietic and non-hematopoietic cells. In vitro, SCF alone has minimal colony-stimulating activity on hematopoietic progenitor cells; however, it synergistically increases colony-forming or stimulatory activity of other HGFs, including G-CSF, GM-CSF, EPO, MGDF, and IL-2. SCF is produced by bone marrow stroma and has an important role in steady-state hematopoiesis. Unlike most HGFs, SCF circulates in relatively high concentrations in normal human plasma (Langley et al., 1993). The generation of dendritic cells from CD34$^+$ cells is enhanced 2.5-fold by the addition of SCF to the culture cocktail, and is enhanced fivefold if SCF and fit-3 ligand are added (Siena et al., 1997).

### ■ Physiologic Role of TPOs

TPO/MGDF are HGFs that stimulate the production of megakaryocyte precursors, megakaryocytes, and platelets. Endogenous TPO is produced by the liver and enters the peripheral circulation. It eventually reaches the bone marrow and stimulates bone marrow megakaryocytes to produce platelets (Kuter, 1997). Platelet production is subject to a homeostatic regulation, similar to that observed for EPO.

IL-11 has pleiotropic effects on multiple tissues. In terms of thrombopoiesis, IL-11 works synergistically with IL-3, TPO, MGDF, or SCF to stimulate various stages of megakaryocytopoiesis and thrombopoiesis (Du and Williams, 1997). It is possible that IL-11's effects on platelet formation are mediated in part by TPO.

## PHARMACEUTICAL ISSUES

Pharmaceutical issues include the status and source, storage and stability, pharmacokinetics, and pharmacodynamics of HGFs. Unless otherwise indicated, the information in this section is taken from the product package inserts.

### ■ Commercially Available Hematopoietic Growth Factors for Clinical Use

Five types of HGFs are commercially available (Table 4):

- rhG-CSF (filgrastim, lenograstim, and pegfilgrastim)
- rhGM-CSF (molgramostim and sargramostim)
- rhEPO (epoetin alfa, epoetin beta, and darbepoetin alfa)
- rhSCF (ancestim)
- rhIL-11 (oprelvekin) (see Chapter 11)

Recombinant EPO, launched in 1989, was the first recombinant human HGF to be approved for marketing. Filgrastim, lenograstim, and sargramostim followed in 1991. Molgramostim was introduced in 1992. Oprelvekin was approved in 1997, ancestim in 1999, and darbepoetin alfa and pegfilgrastim in 2001. Hematopoietic growth factors may be developed by one company, manufactured by another, and distributed by a third. These arrangements are dynamic, complex, and differ from country to country. Appropriate resources should be checked to determine the licensing and distribution agreements in a particular country. The pharmacist, physician, or other healthcare providers are responsible for reading the current package insert for each product before prescribing, preparing, or administering any recombinant HGF discussed in this chapter. All recombinant human growth factor preparations should be kept from freezing and should not be shaken as shaking can denature the proteins. All preparations should be visually inspected for particulate matter before administration.

### ■ Storage and Stability

#### Filgrastim, Lenograstim, and Pegfilgrasim

Filgrastim is available as single-use prefilled syringes and as single-use vials for subcutaneous or intravenous administration. Filgrastim is stable in liquid form when kept at a suitable temperature. It should be stored in the refrigerator at 2° to 8°C and should not be frozen, but accidental exposure to freezing temperatures does not adversely affect the stability. It can be left at room temperature (25°C) for up to 24 hours. Filgrastim may be diluted in 5% dextrose solution, but it should never be diluted with saline, because saline may cause the product to precipitate.

Lenograstim is available as a lyophilized powder for reconstitution with Sterile Water for Injection, USP. If lenograstim will be administered as an intravenous injection, it must be reconstituted in 0.9% saline or 5% dextrose solution. Reconstituted lenograstim remains stable at room temperature (25°C) for 24 hours. The lenograstim formulation contains human serum albumin.

Pegfilgrastim is supplied as prefilled syringes for subcutaneous administration. Pegfilgrastim should be stored in the refrigerator at 2° to 8°C and

|  | Proper name | Trade name(s) | Countries | Company |
|---|---|---|---|---|
| rhG-CSF | Filgrastim | Neupogen, Granulokine, Gran | EU, USA, Canada, Australia, Japan, Taiwan, Korea, China, Cyprus, Greece | Amgen, Dompe, Genesis Pharma, Esteve-Pensa, Kirin, Sankyo |
|  | Lenograstim | Granocyte, Euprotin, Euprotin, Neutrogin | EU, Australia, Spain, Japan, China | Rhone-Poulenc, Amrad, Almirall, Chugai |
|  | Pegfilgrastim | Neulasta, Neupopeg | EU, Canada, Australia, Switzerland, Cyprus, Greece | Amgen, Dompe, Genesis Pharma |
| rhGM-CSF | Molgramostim | Leucomax, Mielogen | EU, Canada Italy | Schering, Sandoz Schering-Plough |
|  | Sargramostim | Leukine | USA, Canada | Berlex, Wyeth-Ayerst |
| rhEPO | Epoetin alfa | Epogen, Procrit, Eso, Eprex | USA, Japan, China, EU, Australia, Canada | Amgen, Ortho Kirin, Sankyo |
|  | Epoetin beta | Epogin, NeoRecormon | Japan, EU | Chugai, Boehringer Mannheim |
|  | Darbepoetin alfa | Aranesp | EU, Canada, Australia, New Zealand, and other Scandinavian and Middle Eastern countries, Greece, Cyprus | Amgen, Genesis Pharma |
| rhSCF | Ancestim | Stemgen | Canada, Australia | Amgen |
| rhIL-11 | Oprelvekin | Neumega | USA | Wyeth |

*Note*: Not all products are approved for all indications in all countries listed, and marketing agreements are fluid. Refer to current package insert for further information. *Abbreviations*: EU, European Union; UAE, United Arab Emirates; USA, United States of America.

**Table 4** ▪ Status of commercially available hematopoietic growth factors.

should not be frozen. It can be left at room temperature (25°C) for up to 48 hours. Pegfilgrastim should be protected from light.

### Sargramostim and Molgramostim

Sargramostim is supplied in vials as a liquid or as a lyophilized powder to be reconstituted with Sterile Water for Injection, USP or Bacteriostatic Water for Injection, USP. Sargramostim for subcutaneous injection should not be diluted, but if it is to be administered as an intravenous infusion, sargramostim should be diluted in 0.9% saline and in-line filters should not be used. Sargramostim can be stored at 2° to 8°C for 20 days once the vial has been entered; it should be discarded after 20 days.

Molgramostim is supplied as a lyophilized powder to be reconstituted with normal saline, 5% dextrose solution, or Bacteriostatic Water for Injection. Some infusion systems may be incompatible with molgramostim because of significant absorption. Molgramostim should be kept from exposure to light.

### Epoetin Alfa, Epoetin Beta, and Darbepoetin Alfa

Epoetin alfa is supplied as a sterile solution for intravenous or subcutaneous administration. Single-use vials have no preservative, whereas multiple-use vials contain 1% benzyl alcohol as a preservative.

Prefilled syringes are available in some countries. Epoetin alfa should be stored at 2° to 8°C.

Epoetin beta is supplied as a powder for reconstitution with Sterile Water for Injection, USP, containing benzyl alcohol and benzalkonium chloride. Unreconstituted epoetin beta should be stored at 2° to 8°C, but it can be stored for 5 days at room temperature (25°C). The reconstituted solution should be used immediately and lack of refrigeration should be limited to the time needed to prepare the injection.

Darbepoetin alfa is available in single-dose vials, prefilled syringes, and autoinjectors in two solutions: an albumin solution and a polysorbate solution. Darbepoetin alfa should be stored at 2° to 8°C and should be protected from exposure to light.

### Ancestim

Ancestim is supplied as a lyophilized powder for reconsituation. Ancestim is reconstituted with Sterile Water for Injection, USP, and is always administered as a subcutaneous injection. Ancestim should not be administered as an intravenous injection under any circumstance. Ancestim can be reconstituted in advance and stored at 2° to 8°C.

### Oprelvekin

Oprelvekin is supplied as a lyophilized powder for reconstitution with Sterile Water for Injection, USP.

The reconstituted material must be used within three hours of reconstitution whether refrigerated (2–8°C) or kept at room temperature (25°C).

## PHARMACOKINETICS

The pharmacokinetic profiles of HGFs obtained in different studies should not be compared directly due to the clinically relevant differences in doses, administration routes, and study populations. For example, patients with advanced cancer typically receive chemotherapeutic agents, antibiotics, and other therapeutic interventions that may directly alter the disposition of HGFs or affect the organs that metabolize and eliminate these growth factors. Patients undergoing bone marrow transplantation typically are exposed to an even wider variety of therapeutic interventions.

### Filgrastim, Lenograstim, and Pegfilgrastim

Filgrastim exhibits first-order kinetics and increasing plasma concentrations with increasing doses (Roskos et al., 1998). Filgrastim is rapidly absorbed after subcutaneous administration, achieving peak concentrations in 2–8 hours. The elimination half-life of filgrastim is approximately 3.5 hours in both healthy volunteers and patients with cancer, and after intravenous as well as subcutaneous administration.

The pharmacokinetics of lenograstim are dose and time dependent. Peak serum concentration after either subcutaneous or intravenous administration is dose dependent. The serum half-life is 3 to 4 hours for subcutaneous administration and 1 to 1.5 hours for intravenous administration.

Pegfilgrastim has nonlinear pharmacokinetics in patients with cancer and decreased clearance with increased dose; the half-life of pegfilgrastim is 15 to 80 hours after subcutaneous administration. The prolonged half-life is thought to be due to the "self-regulation" of pegfilgrastim and neutrophil binding (Johnston et al., 2000) (see Chapter 5).

### Sargramostim and Molgramostim

Pharmacokinetic parameters of sargramostim are similar between healthy individuals and patients (Armitage, 1998). In patients with advanced cancer, sargramostim is rapidly absorbed after subcutaneous administration, achieving peak concentrations in 2 hours. After intravenous infusion over 2 hours, serum concentrations initially decline rapidly ($t_{1/2 \text{ alpha}}$=12–17 minutes) and then more slowly ($t_{1/2 \text{ beta}}$ = 2 hours). Elimination is primarily by non-renal pathways.

In pharmacokinetic studies with molgramostim, maximum serum concentration and area-under-the-concentration-versus-time curve increased with both subcutaneous and intravenous administration but serum concentration was higher for a longer period of time after intravenous dosing (Armitage, 1998). Immunoreactive molgramostim can be detected in the urine of patients, supporting a renal route of elimination. The reported half-life after intravenous administration is 0.24 to 1.18 hours; mean half-life after subcutaneous administration is 3.6 hours.

### Epoetin Alfa, Epoetin Beta, and Darbepoetin Alfa

Epoetin alfa and epoetin beta follow first-order kinetics (Elliott et al., 2004). Serum concentrations peak 5 to 24 hours after subcutaneous administration and are lower than after intravenous administration. The elimination half-life of intravenously administered rhEPO is 4 to 13 hours in patients with chronic renal failure and approximately 20% shorter in healthy volunteers. The reported elimination half-life is longer after subcutaneous administration and results in more-sustained plasma concentrations (Erslev, 1991; Markham and Bryson, 1995).

Because of its increased carbohydrate content and sialic acid changes, darbepoetin alfa has a threefold longer serum half-life in animal models compared with rhEPO, which was substantiated in a double-blind, randomized, crossover trial in humans (Macdougall et al., 1999). The area-under-the-serum-concentration-time curve was significantly greater for darbepoetin alfa compared with rhEPO, and volume of distribution was similar for both products. The peak concentration of darbepoetin alfa administered subcutaneously was about 10% of that after intravenous administration, and bioavailability was approximately 37% by the subcutaneous route. The longer half-life of darbepoetin alfa may confer a clinical advantage over rhEPO by allowing less frequent dosing when treating patients for anemia of chronic renal failure or anemia associated with cancer or chemotherapy or both.

### Ancestim

Ancestim follows first-order kinetics after a single subcutaneous injection to normal healthy volunteers and to patients with cancer. After subcutaneous administration (dose range 5–15 µg/kg) to healthy men, ancestim was absorbed slowly, reaching peak concentrations between 8 and 72 hours. The mean absorption half-life was 41 hours, with an initial lag time of approximately 2 hours. Elimination is also first order, with a half-life of 5 hours; hence, absorption is rate limiting. In patients with cancer, a single dose of 5 to 50 µg/kg produced a mean peak serum concentration approximately 15 hours after administration. Both absorption and elimination followed first-order kinetics with a $t_{1/2}$ of 36 and

2.6 hours, respectively. The pharmacokinetics of ancestim are very similar between healthy volunteers and patients with cancer.

## Oprelvekin

Oprelvekin administered as a single, 50 μg/kg dose to men showed a terminal half-life of 6.9±1.7 hours. Clearance of oprelvekin decreases with patient age and clearance in infants and children is 1.2- to 1.6-fold greater than in adults and adolescents.

## PHARMACODYNAMICS

### Filgrastim, Lenograstim, and Pegfilgrastim

All three white cell factors increase neutrophil counts rapidly. Filgrastim and lenograstim have been shown to mobilize hematopoietic progenitor cells into the peripheral circulation. When filgrastim is discontinued, neutrophil counts return to baseline within approximately 4 days in most patients. A single dose of pegfilgrastim increases neutrophil count and $CD34^+$ cell mobilization in a comparable or greater fashion than what is seen with filgrastim (Johnston et al., 2000).

### Sargramostim and Molgramostim

Both sargramostim and molgramostim are multilineage HGFs and as such increase the number of granulocytes, monocytes, macrophages, and T-lymphocytes.

### Epoetin Alfa, Epoetin Beta, and Darbepoetin Alfa

In patients with anemia due to chronic renal failure, administration of rhEPO (three times weekly) increases reticulocyte counts within 10 days. This reticulocyte increase is followed by increases in the red blood cell count, hemoglobin, and hematocrit within 2 to 6 weeks (Eschbach et al., 1989). Several studies with darbepoetin alfa in patients with renal failure or cancer show that red blood cell count is rapidly increased with the use of darbepoetin alfa (Macdougall et al., 1999; Glaspy et al., 2002; Vansteenkiste et al., 2002).

### Ancestim

In phase I/II studies in patients with cancer, ancestim administered over a range of 5 to 25 μg/kg/day, in combination with fixed doses of filgrastim, produced a dose-dependent increase in circulating peripheral blood progenitor cells (PBPCs), including $CD34^+$ cells, compared with the administration of ancestim alone (Glaspy et al., 1995). Patients receiving the cytokine combination had increases in circulating PBPCs that resulted in apheresis yields that were two- to threefold greater than those of patients receiving filgrastim alone.

## Oprelvekin

Oprelvekin administered daily for 14 days to patients who did not have myelosuppression from their chemotherapy caused platelet counts to increase in a dose-dependent manner (Orazi et al., 1995). Platelet counts began to increase between 5 and 9 days after the commencement of dosing; after the cessation of treatment, platelet counts continued to increase for another 7 days. No change in platelet aggregation or activation was noted. Healthy volunteers treated with oprelvekin had mean increases in plasma volume of >20%.

## ESTABLISHED USES

It is impossible to review all literature that explores the investigational use of HGFs. Thus, only the pivotal studies for each established use have been selected to illustrate the benefit of HGFs in patients with hematologic disorders.

Not all uses discussed here have received regulatory approval in all countries (Table 5). Refer to the current product package insert for licensed indications in the country of interest.

### ■ Chemotherapy-Induced Neutropenia

Neutropenia and infection are common dose-limiting effects of cancer chemotherapy. The risk of infection is directly related to the depth and duration of neutropenia. The severity of neutropenia depends on the intensity of the cancer chemotherapy regimen, as well as host- and disease-related factors. Fever may be the only manifestation of infection because underlying immunosuppression often obscures the classic signs and symptoms. Therefore, it is standard practice to administer broad-spectrum antibiotic therapy and even to hospitalize patients who have febrile neutropenia. Furthermore, oncologists may delay the start of subsequent cycles of chemotherapy until neutrophil recovery, decrease the dose of cancer chemotherapy, or both. Although this practice may be deemed necessary to prevent infectious complications, it may also compromise otherwise effective cancer chemotherapy.

### Filgrastim

The phase III pivotal trials for filgrastim demonstrated beneficial effects of the HGF on febrile neutropenia after standard-dose chemotherapy (Crawford et al., 1991; Trillet-Lenoir et al., 1993). In these two randomized, double-blind, placebo-controlled trials involving >300 patients with small-cell lung cancer, filgrastim significantly decreased the incidence, severity, and duration of neutropenia, days of hospitalization and duration of intravenous antibiotic use.

| Molecule | Proper name | Approved uses |
|---|---|---|
| G-CSF | Filgrastim, lenograstim, pegfilgrastim | Treatment of chemotherapy-induced febrile neutropenia, severe chronic neutropenia, aplastic anemia; support of hematopoiesis after bone marrow transplantation; support of induction/consolidation chemotherapy for AML; mobilization of stem cells for transplantation; prevention of infections in HIV/AIDS patients |
| GM-CSF | Molgramostim, sargramostim | Support of hematopoiesis after induction chemotherapy for AML; mobilization of stem cells for transplantation; support of hematopoiesis after bone marrow transplantation; use in bone marrow transplantation failure or engraftment delay |
| EPO | Epoetin alfa, epoetin beta, darbepoietin alfa | Treatment of anemia associated with chronic renal failure; treatment of symptomatic anemia in predialysis patients; increasing yield of autologous blood in presurgery donation programs; treatment of anemia due to zidovudine in HIV/AIDS patients; treatment of chemotherapy-induced anemia |
| SCF | Ancestim | Used in conjunction with filgrastim to increase mobilization of stem cells for autologous transplantation |
| IL-11 | Oprelvekin | Prevention of severe thrombocytopenia and reduction of platelet transfusions after chemotherapy |

*Note*: Not all indications are approved for marketing in all countries.

**Table 5** ■ Summary of approved and investigational uses for selected hematopoietic growth factors as of July 2006.

## Lenograstim

In phase III studies, prophylactic administration of lenograstim shortened the duration of chemotherapy-induced neutropenia in patients with non-myelogenous cancers who received standard-dose chemotherapy or myeloablative chemotherapy followed by bone marrow transplantation (Gisselbrecht et al., 1994; Chevallier et al., 1995). The median neutrophil nadir was significantly higher in patients treated with lenograstim compared with placebo recipients. Incidences of culture-confirmed infections across all cycles were significantly reduced in the lenograstim group during the period of neutropenia. The incidence of all infections in lenograstim-treated patients was lower than in the placebo group, but the difference was not statistically significant.

## Pegfilgrastim

Two double-blind, active-controlled, phase III studies established the utility of pegfilgrastim in patients with cancer who were treated with doxorubicin and docetaxel (Holmes et al., 2002; Green et al., 2003). In the Holmes et al. study, 310 patients were randomly assigned to receive on day 2 of chemotherapy either a single dose of pegfilgrastim or daily injections of filgrastim. The results of the study showed that one dose of pegfilgrastim per chemotherapy cycle was comparable to daily injections of filgrastim in terms of neutrophil nadir and recovery. The Green et al. study used a fixed dose of pegfilgrastim, again compared with daily doses of filgrastim. In this study with 157 patients, one dose of pegfilgrastim per chemotherapy cycle was comparable to daily injections of filgrastim.

## Sargramostim

Sargramostim is not indicated for the reduction of chemotherapy-induced neutropenia, but it is indicated for use after induction chemotherapy in adults aged >55 years with acute myeloid leukemia to shorten time to neutrophil recovery and to reduce the incidence of severe and life-threatening infections. In a phase III multicenter, randomized, double-blind, placebo-controlled study, sargramostim significantly shortened the median duration of neutropenia after induction chemotherapy compared with controls (Rowe et al., 1995). During consolidation chemotherapy, however, the use of sargramostim did not shorten the median time to recovery of neutrophils compared with placebo. The incidence of severe infections and deaths associated with infections was significantly reduced in patients who received sargramostim compared with those who received placebo.

## Molgramostim

In a phase III trial, patients with high-grade non-Hodgkin's lymphoma were administered molgramostim as a subcutaneous injection for 7 days after chemotherapy (Gerhartz et al., 1993). The frequency of infections, periods of neutropenia, days with fever, and days of hospitalization for infection were reduced significantly, and white blood cell counts increased.

## ■ Bone Marrow or Stem Cell Transplantation

Bone marrow transplantation allows for the use of very high doses of chemotherapy, with or without radiotherapy, to eliminate malignant cells from patients with refractory tumors. The procedure involves administering ablative cancer chemotherapy and then infusing bone marrow progenitor cells that were harvested from the patient (autologous transplantation) or a donor (allogeneic transplantation). Before the patient's bone marrow recovers full function, the neutrophil count usually drops to zero and most patients experience profound pancytopenia and require multiple transfusions of blood and blood products. Allogeneic transplantation is more complicated than autologous transplantation because donor white blood cells may recognize host antigens as foreign and attack host tissues. Graft-versus-host disease can be life-threatening and is manifested by epithelial damage in the skin, liver, and gastrointestinal tract. Consequently, recipients of allogeneic transplantation receive immunosuppressive therapy, which further increases the risk of infection. Regardless of the source of the bone marrow, the procedure may necessitate prolonged hospitalization, which increases the cost of treatment.

## Filgrastim

Two randomized, controlled trials have shown the utility of filgrastim in the autologous bone marrow transplantation setting. In one study, filgrastim reduced the median number of days of severe neutropenia compared with placebo (Schmitz et al., 1995). The other showed a statistically significant reduction in the median number of days of severe neutropenia in filgrastim-treated patients and the number of days of febrile neutropenia was reduced significantly, as well (Stahel et al., 1994).

## Lenograstim

A phase III trial of 315 patients demonstrated the beneficial effects of lenograstim on neutrophil recovery in patients receiving either autologous or allogeneic bone marrow transplantation (Gisselbrecht et al., 1994). The data suggest that lenograstim was beneficial for patients <15 years of age, as well as for the general population. No difference was seen between the lenograstim and placebo groups in the frequency of infections, culture-confirmed infections, or neutropenic fever, but the durations of infections and fever were shorter in lenograstim-treated patients. Use of lenograstim also shortened days of hospitalization, antibacterial use, and parenteral nutrition compared with placebo.

## Sargramostim

Sargramostim is indicated to accelerate myeloid recovery after autologous bone marrow transplantation in patients with non-Hodgkin's lymphoma, acute lymphoblastic leukemia, or Hodgkin's disease. It is also indicated in patients undergoing allogeneic transplantation from human leukocyte antigen (HLA)-matched related donors. In a double-blind, randomized, placebo-controlled study, 128 patients underwent autologous bone marrow transplantation for lymphoid cancer. Sargramostim administered by intravenous infusion over 2 hours was started within

4 hours after bone marrow infusion and continued for 21 days. Sargramostim shortened the duration of neutropenia, antibiotic therapy, and hospitalization (Nemunaitis et al., 1991).

## Molgramostim

Molgramostim is indicated to reduce the duration of neutropenia and its sequelae after bone marrow transplantation for non-myeloid malignancies. Molgramostim accelerated neutrophil recovery in a randomized phase III study in patients with delayed engraftment. Although molgramostim allowed recovery of neutrophil counts, some patients did not respond, and a few responded to treatment but subsequently died (Klingemann et al., 1990; Brandwein et al., 1991).

## ■ Peripheral Blood Progenitor Cell Mobilization for Harvesting and Transplantation

Stem (progenitor) cells found in the blood can be collected and concentrated for infusion after myelosuppressive cancer chemotherapy. PBPC harvesting (or collection) is attractive because it is less invasive than bone marrow harvesting. PBPC harvesting can be performed in the outpatient setting without anesthetizing the donor; it causes less morbidity and mortality, costs less, circumvents donor problems, and is suitable for a larger number of patients.

Hematopoietic growth factors expand the population of circulating hematopoietic progenitor cells and may be used to facilitate peripheral collection, which in turn can be used to supplement and/or replace autologous bone marrow collection. Hematopoietic growth factors can either be combined with chemotherapy to enhance the mobilizing effect of the latter or used alone to induce de novo mobilization.

## Filgrastim

In the United States, filgrastim is indicated to mobilize PBPCs for collection by leukapheresis in patients undergoing myelosuppressive or myeloablative therapy followed by transplantation. In Europe, filgrastim is indicated to mobilize PBPCs in patients undergoing myelosuppressive or myeloablative therapy followed by autologous PBPC transplantation with or without bone marrow transplantation.

Seventeen patients with non-myeloid malignancies who received filgrastim by continuous subcutaneous infusion had a 58-fold increase in the numbers of granulocyte-macrophage progenitor cells (CFU-GM) in peripheral blood (Sheridan et al., 1992). Progenitor cells were collected by three leukapheresis procedures and infused after high-dose chemotherapy to augment autologous bone marrow rescue and post-transplant filgrastim therapy. The time to platelet recovery was shorter in patients who received filgrastim-mobilized PBPCs compared with controls. A prospective randomized trial in lymphoma patients compared the effects of filgrastim-mobilized PBPCs or autologous bone marrow infused after high-dose chemotherapy. In this study, filgrastim-mobilized PBPCs significantly reduced the number of platelet transfusions and the time to platelet and neutrophil recovery. It also led to an earlier hospital discharge compared with patients receiving autologous marrow (Schmitz et al., 1996).

### Sargramostim

Sargramostim is indicated to mobilize PBPCs in patients undergoing myelosuppressive or myeloablative therapy followed by autologous PBPC transplantation. It is also indicated to further accelerate myeloid recovery after PBPC transplantation. A trial of sargramostim alone, filgrastim alone, or the combination in normal donors showed a greater median CD34$^+$ cell yield with the combination or with filgrastim alone compared with sargramostim alone (Lane et al., 1995).

A prospective, randomized, open-label trial directly compared the effects of filgrastim and sargramostim used prophylactically in hematologic recovery and resource utilization after myelosuppressive chemotherapy (Weaver et al., 2000). One hundred and fifty-eight patients with breast cancer, malignant lymphoma, or multiple myeloma were enrolled and received myelosuppressive chemotherapy. Starting the day after the completion of chemotherapy, patients received filgrastim or sargramostim or the combination of sargramostim followed by filgrastim. Patients treated with filgrastim alone had significantly faster neutrophil recovery, lower incidence of fever, less intravenous antibiotic use, and fewer hospital admissions compared with patients treated with sargramostim alone. Patients treated with sargramostim followed by filgrastim had significantly faster neutrophil recovery, lower incidence of fever, less intravenous antibiotic use, and fewer hospital admissions compared with patients treated with sargramostim alone. Patients treated with filgrastim alone did not have significant differences in clinical endpoints compared with patients treated with the growth factor combination, but did have a more rapid neutrophil recovery.

### Molgramostim

Molgramostim has been studied in combination and in sequence with rhG-CSF for mobilization of PBPCs (Winter et al., 1996). The combination of the two growth factors resulted in dramatic and sustained increases in peripheral blood GM-CFUs. In patients receiving rhG-CSF with molgramostim, PBPC cell content increased nearly 80-fold.

### Ancestim

A number of randomized, controlled studies, including a pivotal phase III trial, were done to evaluate the efficacy of ancestim plus filgrastim compared with filgrastim alone to mobilize PBPCs in patients who were chemotherapy naive or who had received moderate to extensive prior chemotherapy or radiation therapy. Patients in these studies had tumors that are often treated with high-dose chemotherapy and PBPC support (i.e., breast cancer, non-Hodgkin's lymphoma, Hodgkin's disease, myeloma, and ovarian cancer). The phase III trial evaluated ancestim plus filgrastim in a cytokine-only mobilization regimen (Shpall et al., 1999). The primary endpoint of this study was reduction in the number of leukaphereses. The combination of ancestim and filgrastim resulted in a statistically significant reduction in the number of leukaphereses needed to reach the CD34$^+$ cell target compared with mobilization with filgrastim alone. A median of four leukaphereses was needed in the ancestim plus filgrastim group compared with six or more in the filgrastim-alone group.

## ■ Severe Chronic Neutropenia

Severe chronic neutropenia may be present from birth (congenital), be periodic (cyclic), or have an unknown etiology (idiopathic). The condition is manifested by decreased neutrophil counts, recurrent fever, chronic oropharyngeal inflammation, and severe infection.

### Filgrastim

Filgrastim is indicated to reduce the incidence and duration of these sequelae. In a phase III study, 123 patients were randomized to receive filgrastim immediately or after a 4-months observation period (Dale et al., 1993). Filgrastim was given by subcutaneous injection at doses of 3.45 µg/kg/day for idiopathic neutropenia, 5.75 µg/kg/day for cyclic neutropenia, and 11.50 µg/kg twice daily for congenital neutropenia. The dose was adjusted to maintain the median monthly absolute neutrophil count between 1.5 and $10 \times 10^9$/L. Hematologic responses were evident within a few days. Ninety percent of patients achieved complete responses: improved bone marrow morphology and a lower incidence and duration of infection-related events.

## ■ AIDS

Patients infected with HIV often have neutropenia, anemia, and/or thrombocytopenia. These hematologic abnormalities may occur as a direct result of HIV infection, as secondary effects of comorbid conditions, or because of chronic myelosuppressive therapy. Antiviral therapy must be interrupted in up to half of the patients because of drug-induced neutropenia (Foote and Welch, 1999; Welch and Foote, 1999).

## Filgrastim

Filgrastim has been approved in Australia, Canada, the European Union, and Japan for use in patients with HIV infection for the reversal of clinically significant neutropenia and for the subsequent maintenance of adequate neutrophil counts during treatment with antiviral and/or other myelosuppressive medications when other options to manage neutropenia are inappropriate. A phase III study reported the effect of filgrastim on the incidence of severe neutropenia in patients with advanced HIV infection and its effect on the prevention of infectious morbidity (Kuritzkes et al., 1998). Two hundred and fifty-eight patients enrolled in the 24-week study, and 201 completed it. Filgrastim was administered daily at $1\,\mu/kg$ and adjusted up to $10\,\mu g/kg/day$ or intermittently at $300\,\mu g$ daily 1 to 3 days per week. Patients in a control group received filgrastim only if severe neutropenia (defined as a neutrophil count $<0.5 \times 10^9/L$) developed. Both daily and intermittent administration of filgrastim lowered the incidence of bacterial infection rates compared with patients in the control group. Overall, filgrastim-treated patients developed 31% fewer bacterial infections than did control patients. Use of filgrastim produced significant reductions in the risk of severe bacterial infections and the number of days of hospitalization.

## rhEPO

A randomized, double-blind, placebo-controlled study in 63 patients with AIDS treated with zidovudine showed that the addition of rhEPO three times a week reduced the number of transfusions of packed red blood cells and the number of units of packed red blood cells (Fischl et al., 1990). A significantly higher rate of increase in hematocrit was observed in patients treated with rhEPO when their native EPO concentrations were less than $500\,IU/L$.

Various additional dosing regimens of filgrastim have been used alone or in combination with rhEPO to reverse the dose-limiting hematologic toxicity of ganciclovir or zidovudine (Miles et al., 1991).

### ■ Anemia

Anemia, a low number of red blood cells, a decreased volume of red blood cells, or a reduced hemoglobin concentration, has many causes. The symptoms of anemia may include fatigue, dizziness, headache, chest pain, shortness of breath, and depression. Anemia is associated with increases in illness and death in patients with chronic renal failure, cancer, or HIV infection. Use of an erythropoietic factor has many advantages for patients with anemia associated with cancer, chemotherapy, or renal failure.

## rhEPO

In a phase III study of 333 patients with anemia and end-stage renal disease, epoetin alfa increased the hematocrit and eliminated the need for red blood cell transfusions in nearly all patients (Eschbach et al., 1989). The response was dose dependent, evident within 2 weeks, and maximal at 6 to 10 weeks of dosing.

In patients with cancer receiving chemotherapy, rhEPO increases hemoglobin values and decreases the need for blood transfusions (Abels et al., 1991). In patients with HIV/AIDS, rhEPO increased hemoglobin levels even when administered concomitantly with zidovudine therapy (Henry et al., 1992).

## Darbepoetin Alfa

Darbepoetin alfa was designed by introducing five amino acid changes into the primary sequence of EPO to create two extra consensus N-linked carbohydrate sites (Egrie et al., 2003; Elliott et al., 2004). Because of its increased carbohydrate content and sialic acid changes, darbepoetin alfa has a threefold longer serum half-life in animal models compared with rhEPO, which was substantiated in a double-blind, randomized, crossover trial in humans (Macdougall et al., 1999). The area-under-the-serum-concentration-time curve was significantly greater for darbepoetin alfa compared with rhEPO, and volume of distribution was similar for both products. The peak concentration of darbepoetin alfa administered subcutaneously was about 10% of that after intravenous administration, and bioavailability was approximately 37% by the subcutaneous route. The longer half-life of darbepoetin alfa may confer a clinical advantage over rhEPO by allowing less frequent dosing when treating patients for anemia of chronic renal failure or anemia associated with cancer or chemotherapy or both.

### ■ Thrombocytopenia

Oprelvekin is licensed for use for the prevention of severe thrombocytopenia and the reduction of platelet transfusions after chemotherapy. In a placebo-controlled trial of women receiving chemotherapy for breast cancer, oprelvekin 25 or $50\,\mu g/kg$ produced dose-related increases in mean platelet counts and a reduction in chemotherapy-induced thrombocytopenia (Tepler et al., 1996).

## TOXICITIES

Many HGFs, especially multipotential factors that act on early progenitor cells, are associated with constitutional symptoms, such as fever, chills, rash, myalgia, injection-site reaction, and edema. The safety of individual HGFs depends on their receptor sites and the effects of secondary cytokine release.

| Product | Contraindications, adverse effects, and warnings |
|---|---|
| Filgrastim | Contraindicated in patients with known hypersensitivity to *E. coli*-derived proteins, filgrastim, or any component. Allergic reactions and adult respiratory syndrome have been reported. Rare splenic rupture and severe sickle cell crises, in some cases causing death, have been reported. Product should not be administered with chemotherapy or radiotherapy but only 24 hours before or 24 hours after their delivery. The most common adverse effects are bone pain and flu-like symptoms |
| Lenograstim | Contraindicated in patients with known hypersensitivity to the product or its components. Not to be used to increase dose intensity of cytotoxic chemotherapy beyond established doses and should not be administered to patients with myeloid malignancies (other than de novo acute myeloid leukemia) or concurrently with cytotoxic chemotherapy. Rare pulmonary adverse effects and splenic rupture reported in patients using G-CSF. The most common adverse effects are flu-like symptoms, nausea, vomiting, bone pain, and headache |
| Pegfilgrastim | Contraindicated in patients with known hypersensitivity to *E. coli*-derived proteins, pegfilgrastim, filgrastim, or any component of finished product. Rare cases of splenic rupture, some resulting in death, have been reported. Allergic reactions, including anaphylaxis, have been reported as have episodes of severe sickle cell crisis in patients with sickle cell disease. Should not be delivered 14 days before or 24 hours after chemotherapy or radiotherapy. Most common adverse effects are bone pain, flu-like symptoms, nausea, vomiting, and diarrhea |
| Sargramostim | Contraindicated in patients with excessive leukemic myeloid blasts in blood or bone marrow; in patients with known hypersensitivity to GM-CSF or any component of finished product; and with chemotherapy and radiotherapy. Edema, capillary leak syndrome, plural effusions, pericardial effusions, respiratory symptoms caused by granulocyte sequestration in lungs; occasional supraventricular arrhythmias, and occasional renal and hepatic dysfunction. Most common adverse effects are flu-like symptoms, and nausea and vomiting |
| Molgramostim | First dose must be administered under close medical supervision. Close supervision required in patients with preexisting pulmonary disease. Acute severe and life-threatening hypersensitivity reactions have occurred. Infrequent pleuritis, pleural effusion, pericarditis, and pericardial effusion. Most common adverse events are flu-like symptoms, dyspnea, nausea, vomiting, non-specific chest pain, and hypotension |
| Epoetin alfa | Contraindicated in patients with uncontrolled hypertension, known sensitivity to mammalian cell-derived products, and known hypersensitivity to albumin. Increased thrombotic events, seizures, and pure red cell aplasia have been reported. May increase risk of cardiovascular events, including death. The most common adverse effects reported are hypertension, headache, arthralgia, nausea, pyrexia, fatigue, diarrhea, vomiting, and edema |
| Epoetin beta | Contraindicated in patients with known hypersensitivity to epoetin beta or any component of the finished product, uncontrolled blood pressure, heart disease (in patients donating their own blood). Caution advised for patients with phenylketonuria. May increase risk of cardiovascular events, including death. The most common adverse effects are decreased iron load, injection site reactions (rash or hives), severe allergic reactions, and flu-like symptoms. In patients with chronic kidney disease, increased blood pressure, headache, convulsions, low blood pressure, and pure red cell aplasia have been reported |
| Darbepoetin alfa | Contraindicated in patients with uncontrolled hypertension or known hypersensitivity to darbepoetin alfa or any component of the finished product. May increase risk of cardiovascular events, including death. Hypertension, seizures, thrombotic events, and pure red cell aplasia have been reported. The most common adverse effects are edema, hypertension, hypotension, headache, diarrhea, myalgia, infection, and fatigue |
| Ancestim | Intravenous administration is contraindicated and all doses should be administered under supervision of medical staff with medication and equipment for resuscitation nearby. Prophylaxis with antihistamines is required. Ancestim should be administered with filgrastim, and not as a single agent. The most common adverse effects are injection site reactions, nausea, tachycardia, respiratory symptoms, and distant skin reactions |
| Oprelvekin | Contraindicated in patients with history of hypersensitivity to oprelvekin or any components of the finished product. Allergic or hypersensitivity reactions, including anaphylaxis, have been reported. Not indicated for use after myeloablative chemotherapy. Known serious effects include fluid retention, anemia, and cardiovascular events. The most common adverse effects were edema, tachycardia, atrial fibrillation/flutter, oral moniliasis, dyspnea, pleural effusions, and conjunctival infection |

*Note*: Refer to current package insert for updated information.

**Table 6** ■ Contraindications, adverse effects, and warnings per July 2006 package inserts.

Determination of the relative toxicity of HGFs is difficult because of the lack of comparative studies and confounding effects of different reporting methods and different cancer chemotherapy regimens. For example, patients who undergo bone marrow transplantation experience toxicity that may obscure HGF-related adverse effects. Formulations with different levels of glycosylation may also play a role.

Because these products are recombinant proteins, a small risk of developing antibodies is possible. Development of neutralizing antibodies required the cessation of clinical development of MGDF and, more recently, a form of rhEPO caused a sudden spike in the number of patients who developed pure red cell aplasia (Casadevall et al., 2002; Gershon et al., 2002).

All drugs that are effective have inherent adverse effects, but compliance with guidelines and dosage regimens approved by regulatory authorities can lessen untoward effects. Use of rhEPO in treatment regimens outside the currently approved labeling and guidelines increased mortality in patients with head-and-neck cancer (Henke et al, 2003; Leyland-Jones and Mahmud, 2004. Unfortunately, abuse of rhEPO by athletes is another problem (Catlin et al., 2003).

Again, the healthcare provider is responsible for consulting the current product package insert of all medicines for precautions, warnings, and possible drug interactions. A summary of the most common adverse events is presented (Table 6), as listed in the current package inserts, but it should not be considered to be comprehensive or inclusive.

## CONCLUDING REMARKS

Hematopoietic growth factors have had a significant impact on the ancillary treatment of cancer: prevention of infections associated with chemotherapy-induced neutropenia, chemotherapy-induced thrombocytopenia, and chemotherapy-induced anemia. Patients with other diseases, such as severe chronic neutropenia and HIV/AIDS, have been helped by the administration of recombinant HGFs. Some factors have been more commercially successful than others, i.e., the white cell factors, while the interleukins that once held such great promise, have only one representative. The pharmacist has an important role in assisting with studies of new and improved HGFs, alone or in combination, as well as the day-to-day care of patients who are treated with these products.

Basic understanding of HGFs and their clinical potential continues to grow, and the discovery of new factors and how all factors interact will undoubtedly be an area of research for some time.

## REFERENCES

Abels RL, Larholt KM, Krantz KDA, Bryant EC (1991). Recombinant human erythropoietin (r-HuEPO) for the treatment of the anemia of cancer. In: Murphy MJ, ed. Blood Cell Growth Factors. Dayton, OH: Alpha Med Press, 121–41.

Armitage JO (1998). Emerging applications of recombinant human granulocyte colony-stimulating factor. Blood 92:4491–508.

Brandwein JM, Nayar R, Baker MA, et al. (1991). GM-CSF therapy for delayed engraftment after autologous bone marrow transplantation. Exp Hematol 19:191–5.

Broudy VC (1997). Stem cell factor and hematopoiesis. Blood 90:1345–64.

Broudy VC, Lin NL, Sabath DF, Papayannopoulou T, Kaushansky K (1997). Human platelets display high-affinity receptors for thrombopoietins. Blood 89:1896–904.

Casadevall N, Nataf J, Viron B, et al. (2002). Pure red-cell aplasia and anti-erythropoietin antibodies in patients treated with recombinant erythropoietin. New Eng J Med 346:469–75.

Catlin DH, Hatton CK, Lasne F (2003). Abuse of recombinant erythropoietins by athletes. In: Molineux G, Foote MA, Elliott SG, eds. Erythropoitins and Erythropoiesis. Molecular, Cellular, Preclinicall, and Clinical Biology. Basel, Switzerland: Birkhauser, 205–27.

Cebon I, Layton JE, Maher D, Morstyn G (1994). Endogenous haemopoietic growth factors in neutropenia and infection. Br J Haematol 86:265–74.

Chevallier B, Chollet P, Merrouche Y, et al. (1995). Lenograstim prevents morbidity from intensive induction chemotherapy in the treatment of inflammatory breast cancer. J Clin Onc 13:1564–71.

Colgan SP, Gasper PW, Thrall MA, Boone TC, Blancquaert AMB, Bruyninckx WJ (1992). Neutrophil function in normal and Chediak–Higashi syndrome cats following administration of recombinant canine granulocyte colony-stimulating factor. Exp Hematol 20:1229–34.

Crawford J, Ozer H, Stoller R, et al. (1991). Reduction by granulocyte colony-stimulating factor of fever and neutropenia induced by chemotherapy in patients with small-cell lung cancer. New Eng J Med 325:164–70.

Dale DC, Bonilla MA, Davis MW, Nakanishi AM, Hammond WP, Kurtzberg J, et al. (1993). A randomized controlled phase III trial of recombinant human granulocyte colony-stimulating factor (filgrastim) for treatment of severe chronic neutropenia. Blood 81:2496–502.

Dale DC, Liles WC, Llewellyn C, Price TH (1998). Effects of granulocyte-macrophage colony-stimulating factor (GM-CSF) on neutrophil kinetics and function in normal human volunteers. Am J Hematol 57:7–15.

Du XX, Williams DA (1997). lnterleukin-11: Review of molecular, cell biology, and clinical use. Blood 89:3897–908.

Egrie JC, Dwyer E, Browne JK, Hitz A, Lykos M (2003). Darbepoetin alfa has a longer circulating half-life and greater in vivo potency than recombinant human erythropoietin. Exp Hematol 31:290–9.

Elliott S, Egrie J, Browne J, et al. (2004). Control of rHuEPO biological activity: The role of carbohydrate. Exp Hematol 32:1146–55.

Elliott S, Heatherington AC, Foote MA (2004). Erythropoietic factors. In: Morstyn G, Foote MA, Lieschke GJ, eds. Hematopoietic Growth Factors in Oncology: Basic Science and Clinical Therapeutics. Totowa, NJ: Humana Press, 97–123.

Erslev AJ (1991). Erythropoietin. New Eng J Med 324:1339–44.

Eschbach JW, Abdulhadi MH, Browne JK, et al. (1989). Recombinant human erythropoietin in anemic patients with end-stage renal disease. Results of a phase III multicenter trial. Ann Int Med 111:992–1000.

Fischl M, Galpin JE, Levine JD, et al. (1990). Recombinant human erythropoietin for patients with AIDS treated with zidovudine. New Eng J Med 322:1488–93.

Galli SJ, Zsebo KM, Geissler EM (1994). The kit ligand, SCF. Adv Immunol 55:1–96.

Gerhartz HH, Englehard M, Meusers P, et al. (1993). Randomized, double-blind, placebo-controlled, phase III study of recombinant human granulocyte-macrophage colony-stimulating factor as adjunct to induction treatment of high-grade malignant non-Hodgkin's lymphomas. Blood 82:2329–39.

Gerson SK, Luksenburg H, Cote TR, Braun MM (2002). Pure red-cell aplasia and recombinant erythropoietin. New Eng J Med 346:1584–6.

Gisselbrecht C, Prentice HG, Bacligalupo A, et al. (1994). Placebo-controlled phase III trial of lenograstim in bone marrow transplantation. Lancet 343:696–700.

Glaspy JA, Shpall EJ, LeMaistre CF, et al. (1995). Peripheral blood progenitor cell mobilization utilizing stem cell factor in combination with filgrastim in breast cancer patients. Blood 90:2939–51.

Glaspy JA, Jadeja JS, Justice G, et al. (2002). Darbepoetin alfa given every 1 or 2 weeks alleviates anaemia associated with cancer chemotherapy. Br J Cancer 87:268–76.

Green MD, Koelbl H, Baselga J, et al. (2003). A randomized double-blind multicenter phase II study of fixed-dose single-administration pegfilgrastim versus daily filgrastim in patients receiving myelosuppressive chemotherapy. Ann Oncol 14:29–35.

Grichnik JM, Crawford J, Jiminez F, et al. (1995). Human recombinant stem-cell factor induces melanocytic hyperplasia in susceptible patients. J Am Acad Dermatol 33:577–83.

Gronski P, Badziong W, Habermann P, et al. (1988). Escherichia coli derived human granulocyte-macrophage colony-stimulating factor (rh GM-CSF) available for clinical trials. Behring Inst Mitteilungen 83:246–9.

Groopman JE, Molina JM, Scadden DT (1989). Hematopoietic growth factors. Biology and clinical applications. New Eng J Med 321:1449–59.

Hart D (1997). Dendritic cells: Unique leukocyte populations which control the primary immune response. Blood 90:3245–87.

Hartung T, Doecke WD, Bundschuh D, et al. (1999). Effect of filgrastim treatment on inflammatory cytokines and lymphocyte functions. Clin Pharmacol Ther 66:415–24.

Henke M, Laszig R, Rube C, et al. (2003). Erythropoietin used to treat head and neck cancer patients with anemia undergoing radiotherapy: Randomised, double-blind, placebo-controlled trial. Lancet 362:1255–60.

Holmes FA, O'Shaughnessy JA, Vukelja S, et al. (2002). Blinded, randomized, multicenter study to evaluate single administration pegfilgrastim once per cycle versus daily filgrastim as an adjunct to chemotherapy in patients with high-risk stage II or stage III/IV breast cancer. J Clin Oncol 20:727–31.

Jacobson JO, Goldwasser E, Fried W, Plzak L (2000). Role of the kidney in erythropoiesis. J Am Soc Nephrol 11:589–92.

Johnston E, Crawford J, Blackwell S, et al. (2000). Randomized, dose-escalation study of SD/01 compared with daily filgrastim in patients receiving chemotherapy. J Clin Oncol 18:2522–28.

Kaushansky K (1995). Thrombopoietin: Basic biology, clinical promise. Int J Hematol 62:7–15.

Kauchansky K (2005). The molecular mechanisms that control thrombopoiesis. J Clin Inv 115:3339–47.

Klingemann HG, Eaves AC, Barnett MJ, et al. (1990). Recombinant GM-CSF in patients with poor graft function after bone marrow transplantation. Clin Inv Med 13:77–81.

Kuritzkes DR, Parenti D, Ward D, et al. (1998). Filgrastim prevents severe neutropenia and reduces infective morbidity in patients with advanced HIV infection: results of a randomized, multicenter, controlled trial. AIDS 12:65–74.

Kuter DJ, Hunt P, Sheridan W, Zucker-Franklin D, eds. (1994a). Thromobopoiesis and Thrombopoeitin. Totowa, NJ: Humana Press, 412.

Kuter DJ, Beeler DL, Rosenberg RD (1994b). The purification of megapoietin: A physiological regulator of megakaryocyte growth and platelet production. Proc Natl Acad Sci USA 91:11104–8.

Kuter DJ (1997). The regulation of platelet production in vivo. In: Kuter DJ, Hunt P, Sheridan W, Zucker-Franklin D, eds. Thrombopoiesis and Thrombopoietins. Totowa, NJ: Humana Press, 377–97.

Lacerna L, Sheridan WP, Basser R, et al. (2000). Stem cell factor. In: Ho AD, Haas R, Champlin RE, eds. Hematopoietic Stem Cell Transplantation. New York: Marcel Dekker, 31–46:

Lane TA, Law P, Maruyama M, et al. (1995). Harvesting and enrichment of hematopoietic progenitor cells mobilized into the peripheral blood of normal donors by granulocyte-macrophage colony-stimulating factor (GM-CSF) or G-CSF: potential role in allogeneic marrow transplantation. Blood 25:275–82.

Langley KE (2004). Stem cell factor and its receptor, c-Kit. In: Morstyn G, Foote MA, Lieschke GJ, eds. Hematopoietic Growth Factors in Oncology. Totowa, NJ: Humana Press 153–84.

Langley KE, Bennett LG, Wypych J, et al. (1993). Soluble stem cell factor in human serum. Blood 81:656–60.

Leyland-Jones B, Mahmud S (2004). Erythropoietin to treat anaemia in patients with head and neck cancer. Lancet 363:80.

Lieschke GJ, Grail D, Hodgson G, et al. (1994). Mice lacking granulocyte colony-stimulating factor have chronic neutropenia, granulocyte and macrophage progenitor cell deficiency, and impaired neutrophil mobilization. Blood 84:1737–46.

Lok S, Kaushansky K, Holly RD, et al. (1994). Cloning and expression of murine thrombopoietin cDNA and stimulation of platelet production in vivo. Nature 369:565–8.

Lord BI, Bronchud MH, Owens S, et al. (1989). The kinetics of human granulopoiesis following treatment with granulocyte colony-stimulating factor in vivo. Proc Natl Acad Sci USA 86:9499–503.

Lord BI, Gurney H, Chang J, Thatcher N, Crowther D, Dexter TM (1992). Haemopoietic cell kinetics in humans treated with rGM-CSF. Int J Cancer 50:26–31.

Macdougall IC, Gray SJ, Elston O, et al. (1999). Pharmacokinetics of novel erythropoiesis stimulating protein compared with epoetin alfa in dialysis patients. J Am Soc Nephrol 10:2392–5.

Markham A, Bryson HM (1995). Epoetin alpha. A review of its pharmacodynamic and pharmacokinetic properties and therapeutic use in nonrenal applications. Drugs 49:232–54.

Metcalf D (1990). The colony stimulating factors. Discovery, development, and clinical applications. Cancer 65:2185–95.

Miles SA, Mitsuyasu RT, Moreno J, et al. (1991). Combined therapy with recombinant granulocyte colony-stimulating factor and erythropoietin decreases hematologic toxicity from zidovudine. Blood 77:2109–17.

Molineux G (2004). The design and development of pegfilgrastim (PEG-rmetHuG-CSF, Neulasta). Curr Pharmaceut Design, 10:1235–44.

Molineux G, Foote MA, Elliott SG (2003). Erythropoietins and Erythropoiesis: Molecular, Cellular, Preclinical, and Clinical Biology. Basel, Switzerland: Birkhasuer, 269.

Nagata S, Tsuchiya M, Asano S, et al. (1986). Molecular cloning and expression of cDNA for human granulocyte-colony stimulating factor. Nature 319:415–8.

Nemunaitis J, Rabinowe SN, Singer JW, et al. (1991). Recombinant granulocyte-macrophage colony-stimulating factor after autologous bone marrow transplantation for lymphoid cancer. New Eng J Med 324:1773–78.

Nichol JL, Hokom MM, Hornkohl A, et al. (1995). Megakaryocyte growth and development factor. Analyses of in vitro effects on human megakaryopoiesis and endogenous serum levels during chemotherapy-induced thrombocytopenia. J Clin Invest 95:2973–8.

Orazi A, Cooper RJ, Tong J, et al. (1996). Effects of recombinant IL-11 (Neumega rhIL-11 growth factor) on megakaryocytopoiesis in human bone marrow. Exp Hematol 24:1289–97.

Rapoport AP, Abboud CN, DiPersio JF (1992). Granulocyte macrophage colony-stimulating factor (GM-CSF) and granulocyte colony-stimulating factor (G-CSF): Receptor biology, signal transduction, and neutrophil activation. Blood Rev 6:43–57.

Roskos LK, Cheung EN, Vincent M, Foote MA, Morstyn G (1998). Pharmacology of filgrastim (r-metHuG-CSF). In: Morstyn G, Dexter TM, Foote MA, eds. Filgrastim (r-metHuG-CSF) in Clinical Practice. New York: Marcel Dekker, 51–71.

Rowe JM, Andersen JW, Mazza JJ, et al. (1995). A randomized placebo-controlled phase III study of granulocyte-macrophage colony-stimulating factor in adult patients (>55 to 70 years of age) with acute myelogenous leukemia: A study of the Eastern Cooperative Oncology Group (E1490). Blood 86:457–62.

Schmitz N, Dreger P, Zander AR, et al. (1995). Results of a randomised, controlled, multicentre study of recombinant human granulocyte colony-stimulating factor (filgrastim) in patients with Hodgkin's disease and non-Hodgkin's lymphoma undergoing autologous bone marrow transplantation. Bone Marrow Transpl 15:261–6.

Schmitz N, Linch DC, Dreger P, et al. (1996). Randomised trial of filgrastim-mobilised peripheral blood progenitor cell transplantation versus autologous bone-marrow transplantation in lymphoma patients. Lancet 10:353–7.

Shpall EJ, Wheeler CA, Turner SA, et al. (1999). A randomized phase 3 study of peripheral blood progenitor cell mobilization with stem cell factor and filgrastim in high-risk breast cancer patients. Blood 93:2491–501.

Sheridan WP, Begley CG, Juttner CA, et al. (1992). Effect of peripheral-blood progenitor cells mobilised by filgrastim (G-CSF) on platelet recovery after high-dose chemotherapy. Lancet 339:640–4.

Siena S, Nicola M, Mortorini R, Anichini A, Bregni M, Parmiani G, Gianni AM (1997). Expansion of immunostimulatory dendritic cells from peripheral blood of patients with cancer. Oncologist 2:65–9.

Souyri M, Vigon I, Penciolelli J-F, Tambourin P, Wendling F (1990). A putative truncated cytokine receptor gene transduced by the myeloproliferative leukemia virus immortalizes hematopoietic progenitors. Cell 63:1137–47.

Souza LM, Boone TC, Gabrilove J, et al. (1986). Recombinant human granulocyte colony-stimulating factor: Effects on normal and leukemic myeloid cells. Science 232:61–5.

Stahel RA, Jost LM, Cerny T, et al. (1994). Randomized study of recombinant human granulocyte colony-stimulating factor after high-dose chemotherapy and autologous bone marrow transplantation for high-risk lymphoid malignancies. J Clin Oncol 12:1931–8.

Stanley E, Lieschke GJ, Grail D, et al. (1994). Granulocyte/macrophage colony-stimulating factor-deficient mice show no perturbation of hematopoiesis but develop a characteristic pulmonary pathology. Proc Natl Acad Sci USA 91:5592–6.

Tepler I, Elias L, Smith JW, et al. (1996). A randomized placebo-controlled trial of recombinant human interleukin-11 in cancer patients with severe thrombocytopenia due to chemotherapy. Blood 87:3607–14.

Trillet-Lenoir V, Green J, Manegold C, et al. (1993). Recombinant granulocyte colony stimulating factor reduces infectious complications of cytotoxic chemotherapy. Eur J Cancer 29A:319–24.

Vansteenkiste J, Pirker R, Massuti B, et al. (2002). Double-blind, placebo-controlled, randomized phase III trial of darbepoetin alfa in lung cancer patients receiving chemotherapy. J Nat Cancer Inst 94:1211–20.

Veys N, Vanholder, R, Lameire N (1992). Pain at the injection site of subcutaneously administered erythropoietin in maintenance hemodialysis patients: A comparison of two brands of erythropoietin. Am J Nephrol 12:68–72.

Vigon I, Mornon JP, Cocault L, et al. (1992). Molecular cloning and characterization of MPL, the human homolog of the v-mpl oncogene: Identification of a member of the HGF receptor superfamily. Proc Natl Acad Sci USA 89:5640–4.

Weaver C, Schulman K, Wilson-Relyea B, Birch R, West W, Buchner CD (2000). Randomized trial of filgrastim, sargramostim, or sequential sargramostim and filgrastim after myelosuppressive chemotherapy for the harvesting of peripheral-blood stem cells. J Clin Oncol 18:43–53.

Weisbart RH, Golde DW (1989). Physiology of granulocyte and macrophage colony-stimulating factors in host defense. Hematol Oncol Clin North Am 3:401–9.

Welte K, Gabrilove J, Bronchud MJ, Platzer E, Morstyn G (1996). Filgrastim (r-metHuG-CSF): The first 10 years. Blood 88:1907–29.

Winter JN, Lazarus HM, Rademaker A, et al. (1996). Phase I/II study of combined granulocyte colony-stimulating factor and granulocyte-macrophage colony-stimulating factor administration for the mobilization of hematopoietic progenitor cells. J Clin Oncol 14:277–86.

# Interferons and Interleukins

*Jean-Charles Ryff*
*Biotech Research and Innovation Network, Basel, Switzerland*

*Ronald W. Bordens*
*Schering-Plough Corporation, Kenilworth, New Jersey, U.S.A.*

*Sidney Pestka*
*Department of Molecular Genetics, Microbiology, and Immunology, University of Medicine and Dentistry of New Jersey–Robert Wood Johnson Medical School, Piscataway, New Jersey, U.S.A.*

## PHARMACOTHERAPY INFORMATION

Further information on the applied pharmacotherapy with interferons and interleukin can be found in the following frequently used textbooks:

- **Applied Therapeutics: The Clinical Use of Drugs** (Koda-Kimble, MA, et al., Eds.), 8th edition,Lippincott Williams & Wilkins, Baltimore 2005: Chapters 35, 43, 70, 73, 88, 90, 91, 92.
- **Pharmacotherapy: A Pathophysiologic Approach** (DiPiro, JT, et al., Eds.), 6th edition, McGraw-Hill, New York 2005: Chapters 40, 53, 89, 97, 124, 127,129, 131, 132, 133.
- **Textbook of Therapeutics: Drug and Disease Management** (Helms, RA, et al., Eds.), 8th edition, Lippincott Williams & Wilkins, Baltimore 2006: Chapters 9, 33, 46, 49, 65, 93, 103.

## INTRODUCTION

In 1957 a substance was described (Isaacs and Lindenmann, 1957) that was produced by virus-infected cell cultures and "interfered" with infection by other viruses; it was called interferon (IFN). Over the following decades it was realized that "IFN" comprises a family of related proteins with several additional properties. Starting in the 1960s various "factors" produced primarily by white blood cells (WBC) as well as other cell supernatants were described which acted in various ways on other WBCs or somatic cells. They were usually given a descriptive name either associated with their cell of origin or their activity on other cells resulting in a myriad of names. The application of molecular technology allowed us to determine that some cytokines had multiple activities and that different cytokines had similar overlapping activities. A systematic classification based on genetic structure and protein characterization has been effective. The interactive networks and cascades of cytokines, IFN, interleukins (IL), growth factors (GF), chemokines (CK), their receptors (r or R) and signaling pathways are highly complex and will be further explored in this chapter.

*Cytokine* is a term coined in 1974 by Stanley Cohen in an attempt at a more systematic approach to the numerous regulatory proteins secreted by hemopoietic and nonhemopoietic cells. Cytokines play a critical role in modulating the innate and adaptive immune systems. They are multifunctional peptides that are now known to be produced by normal and neoplastic cells, apart from those of the immune system. These local messengers and signaling molecules are involved in the development of the immune system, cell growth and differentiation, repair mechanisms and the inflammatory cascade. Functionally, immunological cytokines can be classified as T-helper cells type 1 (Th1; proinflammatory), e.g., IL-2, IL-12, IL-18, IFN$\gamma$, or type 2 (Th2; anti-inflammatory) stimulating, e.g., IL-4, IL-10, IL-13, TGF-$\beta$. Cytokines include:

*a) IFNs*: Proteins produced by eukaryotic cells in response to viral infections, tumors and other biological inducers. They promote an antiviral state in other, neighboring cells and also help to regulate the immune response. They exhibit a variety of other activities and represent a wide family of proteins.

*b) ILs*: A group of cytokines mainly secreted by leukocytes and primarily affecting growth and differentiation of hematopoietic and immune cells. They are also produced by other normal and malignant cells and are of central importance in the regulation of hematopoiesis, immunity, inflammation, tissue remodeling, and embryonic development.

*c) GFs*: Proteins that activate cellular proliferation and/or differentiation. Many GFs stimulate cellular division in numerous different cell types,

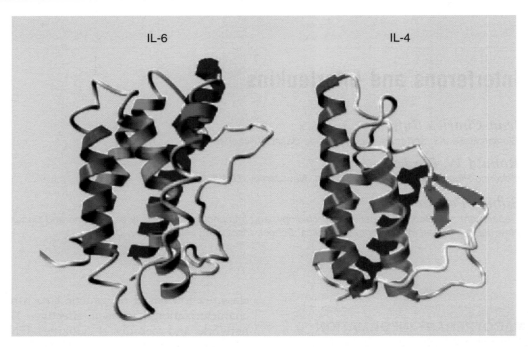

**Figure 1** ■ Class-1 helical cytokines. Class-1 helical cytokines fold into a bundle of four tightly packed α-helices. On the basis of their helix length, class-I helical cytokines are characterized as long chain, such as IL-6, or short chain, such as IL-4. *Source*: From Huising et al., 2006.

others are specific to a particular cell type. They promote proliferation of connective tissue, glial and smooth muscle cells, enhance normal wound healing and promote proliferation and differentiation of erythrocytes (erythropoietin). Hematopoietic GFs are reviewed in Chapter 10. Some ILs have a function overlap to GF, e.g., IL-2, IL-3, IL-11 (Table 2).

*d) CKs (chemotactic cytokines)*: A large family of structurally related low-molecular-weight proteins with potent leukocyte activation and/or chemotactic activity. "CXC" (or α) and "C–C" (or β) CK subsets are based on presence or absence of an amino acid between the first two of four conserved cysteines. A third subset, "C," has only two cysteines and to date only one member, IL-16, has been identified. The fourth subgroup, the C–X3–C CK has three amino acid residues between the first two cysteines.

*e) Others*: Such as tumor necrosis factors (TNF)-α and -β and transforming GF (TGF)-α, -β and -γ.

All cytokines act by binding to specific transmembrane receptors. In general these receptors have two main components: a low affinity ligand-binding domain that ensures ligand specificity and a high affinity effector domain activating target gene promoters via an intracellular signaling pathway (see also Chapters 10 and 13).

Their action is described as:

■ *Autocrine*, if the cytokine acts on the cell that secretes it,

■ *Paracrine*, if the action is restricted to the immediate vicinity of a cytokine's secretion, or

■ *Endocrine*, if the cytokine diffuses to distant regions of the body to affect different tissues.

## INTERFERONS: NOMENCLATURE AND FUNCTIONS

IFNs are a family of naturally occurring proteins and glycoproteins with molecular weights of 16,776 to 22,093 Da produced and secreted by cells in response to viral infections and to synthetic or biological inducers. By interacting with their specific heterodimeric receptors on the surface of cells, the IFNs initiate a broad and varied array of signals that induce cellular antiviral states, modulate inflammatory responses, inhibit or stimulate cell growth, produce or inhibit apoptosis, and modulate many components of the immune system. Structurally, they are part of the helical cytokine family (Fig. 1). During the past 25 years, major research efforts have been undertaken to understand the signaling mechanisms through which these cytokines induce their effects. Figure 2, as an example, illustrates the Janus-activated kinase–signal transducer and activator of transcription (JAK-STAT), the best characterized IFN signaling pathway. However, coordination and cooperation of multiple distinct signaling cascades, including the mitogen-activated protein kinase p38 cascade and the phosphatidylinositol 3-kinase cascade, are required

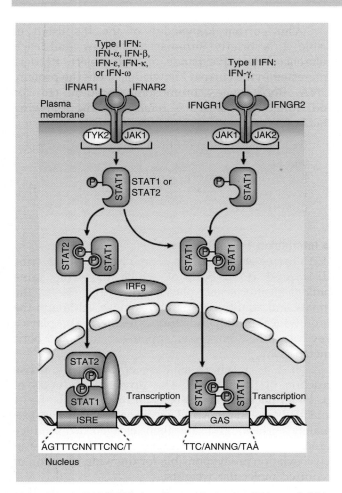

**Figure 2** ■ JAK-STAT signaling pathway for IFNα and IFNγ. *Note*: Recent data suggest that Stat1 is a dimer even before phosphorylation (Braunstein et al. 2003; Ota et al., 2004). *Abbreviations*: GAS, IFNγ-activated site; IFNAR, IFNα receptor; IFNGR, IFNγ receptor; IRF9, IFN regulated factor 9; ISRE, IFN stimulated response element; JAK, Janus-activated kinase; STAT, signal transducer and activator of transcription; TyK2, tyrosine kinase. *Source*: From Platanias, 2005.

for the generation of responses to IFNs (Platanias, 2005). (For a review of the IFN signaling pathways see Special Issue: The Neoclassical Pathways of Interferon Signaling. Journal of Interferon and Cytokine Research 2005; 25:731–811.) Many of the symptoms of acute viral infections are the consequence of the high systemic IFNα response induced by the infecting viruses particularly during the viremic phase.

Human type I IFNs comprise 13 different IFNα isoforms or subtypes with varying specificities, e.g. affinities to different cell types, and downstream activities. Although there are 13 human IFNα proteins, two of them (IFNα1 and IFNα13) are identical proteins so that the total number of type I IFNs are often listed as 12 (Pestka, 1981a,b, 1986). There is also one subtype each for IFNβ (beta), IFNε (epsilon), IFNκ (kappa) and IFNω (omega). Their ability to establish

an "antiviral state" is the distinctive fundamental property of type I IFNs (Sen, 2001). They are produced by most cells, however, certain types seem to be more selectively expressed, e.g., IFNκ by keratinocytes (LaFleur et al., 2001).

Type II IFN consists of a single representative: IFNγ (gamma) (Pestka, 1981a,b, 1986). IFNγ or immune IFN plays an essential role in cell-mediated immune responses. It is produced by NK cells, dendritic cells, cytotoxic T cells, progenitor Th0 cells and Th1 cells.

IFNα2, -β and -γ are the most extensively studied to date. All IFNs and IFN-like cytokines have been recently reviewed in Pestka et al. (2004a).

The names for the human IFNs presently approved by the Human Genome Nomenclature Committee (HGNC) are listed in Table 1. (For an exhaustive review see Meager, 2006).

## INTERLEUKINS: NOMENCLATURE AND FUNCTIONS

ILs are primarily a collection of immune cell growth, differentiation and maturation factors. Collectively they orchestrate a precise and efficient immune response to toxins and pathogens, including cancer cells, recognized as foreign. As is the case for IFNs, ILs bind to related specific cell surface receptors which activate similar intracellular signaling cascades (Lutfalla et al., 2003; Pestka et al., 2004b; Huising et al., 2006). Many ILs, primarily those with proinflammatory function, are intrinsically toxic either directly or indirectly, i.e., through induction of toxic gene products. Therefore the human body has an elaborate system of checks and balances that, under (patho)-physiological conditions, regulates the magnitude and duration of an immune response. Under biological conditions, ILs usually have a short circulation time, and their production is regulated by positive and negative feedback loops. Furthermore their effect is mostly localized, and in some cases soluble receptors (sR) or neutralizing antibodies limit their dissemination. Specific receptor antagonists can also control their activity.

Table 2 lists the ILs for which the protein and gene structure have been characterized. Their names and symbols have been approved by the HGNC.

Under physiological conditions, the relative concentrations of agonistic and antagonistic ILs establish a delicate balance in driving pro- and anti-inflammatory processes. This balance can be disturbed by various pathogenic agents or mechanisms:

- Infectious agents or toxins
- Allergens
- Malignant tumors
- Genetic variants

| Symbol | Name |
|---|---|
| IFNα1 | Interferon, alpha 1 |
| IFNα2 | Interferon, alpha 2 |
| IFNα4 | Interferon, alpha 4 |
| IFNα5 | Interferon, alpha 5 |
| IFNα6 | Interferon, alpha 6 |
| IFNα7 | Interferon, alpha 7 |
| IFNα8 | Interferon, alpha 8 |
| IFNα10 | Interferon, alpha 10 |
| IFNα13 | Interferon, alpha 13[a] |
| IFNα14 | Interferon, alpha 14 |
| IFNα16 | Interferon, alpha 16 |
| IFNα17 | Interferon, alpha 17 |
| IFNα21 | Interferon, alpha 21 |
| IFNβ1 | Interferon, beta-1, fibroblast |
| IFNε1 | Interferon, epsilon-1 |
| IFNκ | Interferon, kappa |
| IFNω1 | Interferon, omega-1 |
| IFNγ | Interferon, gamma |

*Note*: There are, in addition, a number of interferon pseudogenes (nonfunctional and related to interferon genes) mentioned for completion's sake: IFNα22, IFNv (nu) 1, IFNPs 11, 12, 20, 23 and 24, IFNω P2, 4, 5, 9, 15, 18 and 19.
[a]IFN 13 sequence identical to IFN 1; P, pseudogene.
*Source*: Adapted from the ExPASy and HGNC database.

**Table 1** ■ Human genome nomenclature committee approved human interferon names.

These pathogenic agents or mechanisms result in a self-limited or protracted disequilibrium. Symptoms of disease can be the consequence of an adequate immune response at the end of which the steady-state is reestablished. A brisk inflammatory response is the sign of a healthy immune reaction. In some instances an inadequate response can manifest itself as relapsing remitting progressive disease, e.g. rheumatoid arthritis, asthma, chronic inflammatory bowel disease, multiple sclerosis, chronic hepatitis, or chronic insulitis leading to diabetes mellitus. All have in common that they need a genetic predisposition and an environmental trigger factor to become active, and are at best only partially understood. In many cases these diseases are caused by either insufficient production or overproduction of key ILs. Thus, in principle, once the diagnosis is made these ILs can be therapeutically supplemented or suppressed to restore proper balance (Ryff, 1996).

Our current knowledge of the ILs listed in Table 2 is briefly summarized below and each reference selected expands on the subject. Readers interested in the current knowledge about the protein, DNA, RNA, gene, chromosome location, etc. for individual IFNs or ILs is referred to the following databases:

1. www.genatlas.org (with a links to other databases), or
2. http://au.expasy.org/sprot/, or
3. www.rcsb.org/pdb/ for the 3D models of individual IFNs or ILs.

### ■ Interleukin-1 Family

IL-1 (Towne et al., 2004) is generally used to describe IL-1α and IL-1β both of which have the same biological effects and play a primordial role in the innate and adaptive immune response. Although the prototypical proinflammatory cytokine, it also plays a key role in hematopoiesis, appetite control, and bone metabolism.

IL-1 is released as part of the acute phase reaction of hepatocytes. The primary producers of IL-1 are macrophages, B-cells and neutrophils. IL-1α and IL-1β are synthesized as propeptides of approximately 30 kDa, and are then cleaved to produce products of 159 and 153 amino acids. Differences in glycosylation are responsible for the wide variation of reported molecular weights.

There are several other members of the IL-1 family. One is a naturally occurring inhibitor of IL-1. This IL-1 receptor antagonist (IL-1Ra) has limited sequence similarity to either IL-1α or IL-1β, but does have the ability to bind to the IL-1 receptors. Lacking IL-1 activity, it acts as a useful blocker of the receptor. A recombinant IL-1Ra has been investigated for its potential use in sepsis; however, the clinical trials were inconclusive. Recombinant IL-1Ra has however been used successfully in treatment of rheumatoid arthritis and is marketed under the name of Kineret® (see section "Therapeutic Use of Recombinant Interleukins").

### ■ Interleukin 2

IL-2 (Nelson, 2004) is a typical four α helix cytokine originally described as T-cell GF (TCGF). Synthesized and secreted primarily by T-cells, IL-2 can stimulate the growth, differentiation and activation of T-cells, B-cells, and NK-cells. The new understanding of IL-2 biology is that its major physiological effect is to promote self-tolerance by suppressing T-cell response in vivo. Three chains comprise the cellular high affinity IL-2 receptor—the α, β and γ chains. IL-15 is closely related to IL-2 with which it shares

| Symbol | Protein name | Previous symbol | Aliases |
|---|---|---|---|
| IL-1A | Interleukin-1, alpha | IL1 | IL-1 alpha, hematopoietin-1 |
| IL-1B | Interleukin-1, beta | | IL-1 beta, catabolin |
| IL-1F5 | Interleukin-1 family, member 5 | | Interleukin-1 delta, interleukin-1 receptor antagonist homolog 1, IL-1-related protein 3 |
| IL-1F6 | Interleukin-1 family, member 6 | | Interleukin-1 epsilon |
| IL-1F7 | Interleukin-1 family, member 7 | | Interleukin-1 zeta, interleukin-1 homolog 4, interleukin-1-related protein 1 |
| IL-1F8 | Interleukin-1 family, member 8 | | Interleukin-1 eta, interleukin-1 homolog 2 |
| IL-1F9 | Interleukin-1 family, member 9 | | Interleukin-1 epsilon, interleukin-1 homolog, 1IL-1-related protein 2 |
| IL-1F10 | Interleukin-1 family, member 10 | | Interleukin-1 receptor antagonist-like FIL1 theta, interleukin-1 theta, interleukin-1 HY2 |
| IL-2 | Interleukin-2 | | T-cell growth factor (TCGF) aldesleukin |
| IL-3 | Interleukin-3 | | Multi-CSF |
| IL-4 | Interleukin-4 | | BSF1 |
| IL-5 | Interleukin-5 | | T-cell replacing factor, TRF eosinophil differentiation factor (EDF) B cell differentiation factor I |
| IL-6 | Interleukin-6 | IFNB2 | Interferon beta-2, B-cell stimulatory factor 2, hepatocyte stimulatory factor, hybridoma growth factor, CTL differentiation factor |
| IL-7 | Interleukin-7 | | |
| IL-8 | Interleukin-8 | | CXCL8 (chemokine) monocyte-derived neutrophil chemotactic factor, T-cell chemotactic factor, neutrophil-activating protein 1, granulocyte chemotactic protein 1, monocyte-derived neutrophil-activating peptide (MONAP), emoctakin |
| IL-9 | Interleukin-9 | | TCGF P40, P40 cytokine |
| IL-10 | Interleukin-10 | | Cytokine synthesis inhibitory factor CSIF, tumor growth inhibitory factor TGIF, IL-10A |
| IL-11 | Interleukin-11 | | Adipogenesis inhibitory factor, AGIF oprelvekin (see Chapter 10) |
| IL-12A | Interleukin-12A | NKSF1 | Cytotoxic lymphocyte maturation factor 35 kDa subunit, CLMF p35 NK cell stimulatory factor chain 1, NKSF1, IL:12 p35 |
| IL-12B | Interleukin-12B | NKSF2 | Cytotoxic lymphocyte maturation factor 40 kDa subunit, CLMF p40 NK cell stimulatory factor chain 2 NKSF2, IL-12 p40 |
| IL-13 | Interleukin-13 | | P600 |
| IL-15 | Interleukin-15 | | |
| IL-16 | Interleukin-16 | | Lympho chemoattractant factor, LCF "C" chemokine |
| IL-17A | Interleukin-17A | IL-17 | Cytotoxic T-lymphocyte-associated antigen 8, CTLA-8 |
| IL-17B | Interleukin-17B | | Cytokine-like protein Zcyto7 neuronal interleukin-17-related factor interleukin-20 |
| IL-17C | Interleukin-17C | | Cytokine CX2 |
| IL-17D | Interleukin-17D | | Interleukin-27 |
| IL-17F | Interleukin-17F | | Interleukin-24, cytokine ML-1 |
| IL-18 | Interleukin-18 | | Interferon-gamma-inducing factor, interleukin-1 gamma, interleukin-1 family, member 4, iboctadekin |

**Table 2** ■ Human genome nomenclature committee approved interleukin names. (*Continued on next page*)

| Symbol | Protein name | Previous symbol | Aliases |
|--------|-------------|-----------------|---------|
| IL-19 | Interleukin-19 | | Melanoma differentiation-associated protein-like protein, IL-10C |
| IL-20 | Interleukin-20 | | Four alpha helix cytokine, ZCYTO10 |
| IL-21 | Interleukin-21 | | Za11 |
| IL-22 | Interleukin-22 | | IL-10-related T-cell-derived-inducible factor, Zcyto18, IL-TIF, IL-D110, TIFa, TIFIL-23 |
| IL23A | Interleukin 23A | | IL-23, IL-23A, SGRF, IL23P19 |
| IL-24 | Interleukin-24 | ST16 | Suppression of tumorigenicity 16 protein, melanoma differentiation-associated gene 7 protein |
| IL-25 | Interleukin-25 | IL-17E | Interleukin-17E |
| IL-26 | Interleukin-26 | | AK155 protein |
| IL-27B | Interleukin-27 beta chain | IL-30 | EBV-induced gene 3 protein |
| IL-28A | Interleukin-28 | | IFN lambda-2, ZCYTO20 |
| IL-28B | Interleukin-28B | | IFN lambda-3, IFN lambda-4 ZCYTO22 |
| IL-29 | Interleukin-29 | | IFN lambda-1, ZCYTO21 |
| IL-31 | Interleukin-31 | | |
| IL-32 | Interleukin-32 | | NK cell protein 4, TAIF, TAIFb, TAIFd |
| IL-33[a] | Interleukin-33 | | Interleukin-1 family, member 11 |

[a] As of August 1st 2006 (last update), IL-33 was not approved by the HGNC; the symbols IL-14 and IL-30 are no longer used as approved nomenclature (Schmitz et al., 2005).
*Abbreviations*: TCGF, T-cell growth factor; EDF, eosinophil differentiation factor.
*Source*: Adapted from ExPASy and HGNC.

**Table 2** ■ (*Continued*) Human genome nomenclature committee approved interleukin names.

the β and γ signaling receptor subunits. A soluble form of the IL-2R capable of binding IL-2, a truncated version of the α chain without cytoplasmic tail, has been found in human serum (sR). High levels of IL-2sR have been found in patients with a wide variety of disorders, including chronic hepatitis C, HIV infection, cancer, solid organ transplant rejection, and arthritis. Soluble IL-2R can bind released IL-2 prior to its binding to cells to prevent overflow or over-stimulation. Several other cytokine and adhesion molecule receptors also have circulating forms. This is one manner in which the immunological cascade maintains its checks and balances.

■ **Interleukin 3**

IL-3 (Konishi et al., 1999) is a multicolony stimulating, hematopoietic GF which stimulates the generation of hematopoietic progenitors of every lineage. Administration of IL-3 produces an increase in erythrocytes, neutrophils, eosinophils, monocytes and platelets. IL-3, however, is not involved in constitutive hematopoiesis but rather in inductive hematopoiesis upon exposure to immunological stress. IL-3 can act synergistically or additively with other hematopoietic GFs.

■ **Interleukin 4**

IL-4 (Steinke and Borish, 2001) is produced by Th2 cells and by mast cells, basophils, and eosinophils. It stimulates B-cell proliferation and activation, induces class switch to IgE and IgG$_1$ expression from B-cells, as well as class II Major Histocompatibility Complex (MHC) expression. In addition it induces the differentiation of eosinophils and activity of cytotoxic T-cells. IL-4 regulates the differentiation of helper T-cells to the Th2 type. These T-cells produce the cytokines IL-4, IL-5, IL-9, and IL-13, which can all participate in the allergic response. IL-4 regulates the production of IgE by B-lymphocytes. It also has the ability to stimulate CK production and mucus hypersecretion by epithelial cells. IL-4 can elicit many responses, some of which are associated with allergy and asthma.

## ■ Interleukin 5

IL-5 (Greenfeder et al., 2001) acts as a homodimer originally known as T-cell replacement factor (TRF), eosinophil differentiation factor (EDF) and B-cell GF (BCGFII). It is produced by a number of cell types. It acts on the eosinophilic lineage, stimulating eosinophil expansion and chemotaxis and also has activity on basophils. In humans IL-5 is a very selective cytokine as only eosinophils and basophils express IL-5 receptors.

## ■ Interleukin 6

IL-6 (Heinrich et al., 1990) is produced by lymphoid and nonlymphoid cells. By stimulating hepatocytes to produce "acute phase proteins" it plays a central role in the "acute phase reaction." It is also responsible for the reactive thrombocytosis seen in acute inflammatory processes by stimulating thrombopoietin (TPO) (Kaushansky, 2005). IL-6 was formerly known as IFN$\beta_2$ for its weak antiviral activity. IL-6 is also associated with insulin resistance in obese individuals (Esposito et al., 2003).

## ■ Interleukin 7

IL-7 (Fry and Mackall, 2002) is a glycosylated essentially tissue-derived cytokine. Its primary sources are stromal and epithelial cells in various locations including intestinal epithelium, liver and to a lesser degree dendritic cells. IL-7 acts primarily on pre-B-cells to stimulate their differentiation. It can also stimulate the development of human T-cells. IL-7 is classified as a type I short chain cytokine of the hematopoietin family which also includes IL-2, IL-3, IL-4, IL-5, GM-CSF, IL-9, IL-13, IL-15, M-CSF and stem cell factor (SCF).

## ■ Interleukin 8

IL-8 (Remick, 2005) is a 6 to 8 kDa CXC CK, a potent chemoattractant for neutrophils. It affects the proinflammatory effector side, including the stimulation of neutrophil degranulation and the enhancement of neutrophil adherence to endothelial cells. It is produced by monocytes, macrophages, fibroblasts, keratinocytes and endothelial cells. Elevated levels of IL-8 have been found in psoriatic arthritis, synovial fluid and synovium. IL-8 has been implicated in angiogenesis.

## ■ Interleukin 9

IL-9 (Zhou et al., 2001) is a Th2 cytokine originally characterized as a factor produced by activated T-cells and able to support the long-term growth of some T-helper clones. IL-9 activities extend to various cell types including mast cells, B-lymphocytes, hemopoietic progenitors, eosinophils, lung epithelial cells, neuronal precursors and T-lymphocytes. Increased IL-9 production has been implicated in major pathologies such as asthma supported by its effects on IgE production, mucus production, mast cell differentiation, eosinophil activation and bronchial hyperresponsiveness. IL-9 stimulates the growth of murine thymic lymphomas and an autocrine loop has been suggested in Hodgkin lymphoma. Finally, IL-9 is required for an efficient immune response against intestinal parasites. IL-9 exerts its effects through a receptor that belongs to the hemopoietic receptor superfamily and consists of two chains, also involved in IL-2, IL-4, IL-7, and IL-15 signaling.

## ■ Interleukin 10

Macrophages are the major source of IL-10 (Asadullah, 2004), which Th2 cell subsets, monocytes and several other cells can also synthesize. It is a homodimer, whereby each monomer consists of 160 amino acids with a MW of 18.5 kDa. IL-10 is a major endogenous anti-inflammatory mediator which acts by profoundly inhibiting the synthesis of proinflammatory molecules. A number of molecules produced under stress conditions including reactive oxygen species stimulate IL-10 synthesis. Recombinant human IL-10 has been tested in clinical trials in rheumatoid arthritis, inflammatory bowel disease, psoriasis, organ transplantation, and chronic hepatitis C. The results are mixed, however they give new insight into the immunobiology of IL-10 and suggest that the IL-10/IL-10R system may become a new therapeutic target. Several novel IL-10 related class 2 cytokines have recently been discovered (Pestka et al., 2004b). These include IL-19, -20, -22, -24, -26, -28A, -28B and -29. The receptor complexes for IL-22, IL-26, IL-28A, IL-28B and IL-29 are distinct from that used by IL-10; however, all of these cytokines use a common second chain, IL-10 receptor-2 (IL-10R2; CRF2-4), to assemble their active receptor complexes (Donnelly et al. 2004; Pestka et al., 2004b).

## ■ Interleukin 11

IL-11 (Du and Williams, 1997) initially described as hematopoietic factor with thrombopoietic activity has subsequently been shown to be expressed and active in many other tissues including brain, spinal cord neurons, gut, and testes. IL-11 acts synergistically with other cytokines such as IL-3, -4, -7, -12, -13, SCF and GM-CSF to stimulate various stages and lineages of hematopoiesis and in particular with IL-3 and TPO, also termed megakaryocyte growth and development factor (MGDF), to stimulate various stages of megakaryocytopoiesis and thrombopoiesis. Treatment with IL-11 results in production, differentiation, and maturation of megakaryocytes. IL-11 also has a direct effect on erythroid progenitors and also modulates the differentiation and maturation of myeloid progenitor cells. Alveolar and bronchial epithelial cells produce IL-11, which is upregulated by inflammatory cytokines and respiratory syncitial virus (RSV) suggesting that it plays a role in pulmonary inflammation. IL-11 also is an important regulator of bone metabolism.

## ■ Interleukin 12

IL-12 (Adorini, 1999) is a 75-kDa heterodimeric proinflammatory cytokine composed of two covalently linked glycosylated chains: p35 and p40. It is produced predominantly by activated monocytes and dendritic cells, enhances proliferation and cytolytic activity of NK- and T-cells, and stimulates their IFNγ production, guiding them toward a Th1 response while it inhibits Th2 cells. Because of these properties, the regulation of IL-12 production and its alteration in certain disease states have major relevance for the modulation of immune and allergic responses, and recombinant IL-12 has several potential therapeutic uses in infectious diseases, allergy, and cancer.

## ■ Interleukin 13

Human IL-13 (Wills-Karp, 2004) is a 17 kDa glycoprotein cloned from activated T-cells. IL-13 was first recognized for its effects on B cells and monocytes, where it upregulated class II expression, promoted IgE class switching and inhibited inflammatory cytokine production. IL-13 possesses several unique effector functions that distinguish it from IL-4. Resistance to most gastrointestinal nematodes is mediated by type-2 cytokine responses, in which IL-13 plays a dominant role. By regulating cell-mediated immunity, IL-13 modulates resistance to intracellular organisms. In the lung, IL-13 is the central mediator of allergic asthma, where it regulates eosinophilic inflammation, mucus secretion, and airway hyperresponsiveness. IL-13 can also inhibit tumor immunosurveillance. Thus, inhibitors of IL-13 might be effective as cancer immunotherapeutics by boosting type-1-associated antitumor defenses. Investigations into the mechanisms that regulate IL-13 production and/or function have shown that IL-4, IL-9, IL-10, IL-12, IL-18, IL-25, IFNγ, TGF-β, TNF-α, and the IL-4/IL-13 receptor complex play important roles in this process.

## ■ Interleukin 15

IL-15 (Fehniger and Caligiuri, 2001) shares the IL-2βγ receptor complex components IL-2Rβ (CD122) and IL-2Rγ (CD132), however specificity is conferred by a unique α-chain (IL-15Rα) completing the IL-15Rαβγ heterotrimeric high affinity receptor complex. IL-15 exhibits characteristics of IL-2 such as stimulation of T-cells, but the third receptor chain (IL-15Rα) distinguishes its activities and specificities. In addition, IL-15 and its receptor have a much wider tissue distribution than IL-2 and its receptor.

## ■ Interleukin 16

IL-16 (Cruikshank et al., 1998) is a proinflammatory cytokine, which induces chemotaxis of CD4+ T-cells, monocytes and eosinophils. It has been shown to play a role in asthma (El Bassam et al., 2005), Crohn's Disease (CD) (Middel et al., 2001) and systemic lupus erythematosus (SLE) (Lee et al., 1998). IL-16 also inhibits human (HIV) and simian (SIV) immunodeficiency virus. A neuronal form of IL-16 detected in neurons of the cerebellum and hippocampus has been described (Kurschner and Yuzaki, 1999).

## ■ Interleukin 17 Family

IL-17 (Kolls and Lindén, 2004) a homodimeric glycoprotein more recently renamed IL-17A is the prototypic IL-17 family member. It is produced by activated T-cells, but its receptor is expressed in every tissue examined. Subsequently, five additional family members IL-17B to IL-17F have been discovered. The importance of this family of cytokines and their receptors expressed in disparate tissues goes beyond the modulation of T-cell-mediated inflammatory response and importance in effective host defense against gram-negative bacteria. IL-17 cytokines have also a role in the homeostasis of tissues and the progression of diseases such as arthritis (Gaffen, 2004; Lubberts et al., 2005), and cancer, e.g. prostate cancer (Moseley et al., 2003).

## ■ Interleukin 18

IL-18 (Liu et al., 2000) shares unique structural features with the IL-1 family, but it does not have the usual four-helix structure rather an all β-pleated sheet structure. It is produced by activated macrophages such as Kupffer cells of the liver and other resident macrophages from which the mature protein is released. IL-18 is an early inducer of the Th1 response, costimulating, with IL-12, the production of IFNγ, TNF-α, GM-CSF and IL-2. IL-18 is associated with the Metabolic Syndrome and coronary vascular disease (Hung et al., 2005).

## ■ Interleukin 19

IL-19 (Gallagher et al., 2000; Chang et al., 2003) is a newly discovered member of the IL-10 family whose function is presently undefined. The induction of IL-19 in human monocytes is downregulated by IFNγ and upregulated by IL-4. IL-19 plays a role in the Th1/Th2 system. IL-19 is able to influence the maturation of human T-cells. CD4+ T-cells resulting from staphylococcal enterotoxin B (SEB) stimulation in the presence of IL-19 contained a higher proportion of IL-4 producing cells than those developing in the absence of IL-19. This observation was complemented by the observation that fewer IFNγ cells accrued in the presence of IL-19, thereby suggesting that IL-19 altered the balance of Th1/Th2 cells in favor of Th2 cells. Furthermore, in cultures of whole peripheral blood mononuclear cells (PBMC) IL-19 upregulated IL-4 and downregulated IFNγ in a dose-dependent manner.

## ■ Interleukin 20

IL-20 (Blumberg et al., 2001) was originally identified from a keratinocyte library, mRNA isolated from skin and trachea. Analysis of the entire coding sequence yielded a 176 amino acid sequence classified as a helical cytokine member of the IL-10 family. IL-1β, TGF-α and epidermal GF (EGF), factors known to be involved with proliferative and proinflammatory signals in the skin, enhance the response to IL-20. Two orphan class 2 cytokine receptors, both expressed in skin, have been discovered and labeled IL-20Rα and IL-20Rβ; both are required for IL-20 binding and mRNA for both are markedly upregulated in psoriatic compared to normal skin.

## ■ Interleukin 21

IL-21 (Sivakumar et al., 2004), a four-helix cytokine, is a new member of the IL-2 family of cytokines that utilize the common γ-chain receptor subunit for signal transduction. The heterodimeric IL-21R has a IL-21-specific subunit besides the γ-chain. IL-21 expression is restricted primarily to activated CD4+ T-cells. IL-21 expression seems transient and stage specific during T-cell differentiation. It is required for normal humoral immunity and regulates antibody production in cooperation with IL-4. IL-21 also regulates cell-mediated immunity by inducing IFNγ, TNF-α, synthesis of perforin and granzyme B leading to cytolytic activity. It can cooperate with other cytokines to generate potent killer T-cells and thus has antitumor activity. Lastly it also has inhibitory activity by inducing IL-10. Thus, altogether, it is responsible for the coordination of the initiation and cessation of an immune response.

## ■ Interleukin 22

IL-22 (Kotenko et al., 2001a,b; Boniface et al., 2005) belongs to a family of cytokines structurally related to IL-10, including IL-19, IL-20, IL-24, and IL-26. In contrast to IL-10, it has proinflammatory activities: it upregulates the production of acute phase proteins and pancreatitis-associated protein 1. The IL-22 receptor is composed of an IL-22-binding chain, IL-22R1 and the IL-10R2 subunit, which is shared with the IL-10R. IL-22 is produced by activated human Th cells and mast cells. A soluble IL-22-binding protein, IL22RBP, encoded by a distinct gene, has been identified. This sR, which has 34% amino acid identity to the extracellular domain of the IL-22R1, binds IL-22 and antagonizes its functional activities. The skin is also a target for IL-22; high IL-22 expression has been detected in the skin of patients with T-cell-mediated dermatoses. Normal human epidermal keratinocytes express a functional receptor for IL-22 but not for IL-10. IL-22 plays a role in skin inflammatory processes and wound healing.

## ■ Interleukin 23

IL-23 (Aggarwal et al., 2003) is a heterodimeric cytokine comprising the IL-12 p40 subunit and an IL-23-specific p19 subunit. It is produced by activated dendritic cells and acts on memory CD4+ T-cells. IL-23 induces IL-17 and thus plays an early role in defense against gram-negative infection. It is also pivotal for establishing and maintaining organ-specific inflammatory autoimmune disease. IL-23 and IL-27 both have potent antitumor activity even against poorly immunogenic tumors using different effector mechanisms.

## ■ Interleukin 24

IL-24 (Jiang et al., 1996; Wang and Liang, 2005) is a novel member of the IL-10 family secreted by activated PBMC and the ligand for two heterodimeric receptors, IL-22R1/IL-20R2 and IL-20R1/IL-20R2. The latter is also a receptor chain for IL-20. Under physiological conditions, the major sources of IL-24 are activated monocytes and Th2 cells, whereas the major IL-24 target tissues, based on the receptor expression pattern, are nonhematopoietic in origin, and include skin, lung and reproductive tissues. Structurally and functionally, IL-24 is highly conserved across species. It has shown antiangiogenic activity and its gene is a tumor suppressor gene (Ishikawa et al., 2005).

## ■ Interleukin 25

IL-25 (Fort et al., 2001), although structurally related to IL-17, is a protein of approximately 17 kDa. It is produced by Th2-polarized T-cells, and its biological effects differ markedly from those of the previously described IL-17 family members. IL-25 induces IL-4, -5 and -13 and causes histological changes in the lungs and GI tract, including eosinophilic and mononuclear infiltrates, increased mucus production, and epithelial cell hyperplasia and hypertrophy. IL-12 appears to be a key cytokine for the development of Th2-associated pathologies such as asthma and other allergic reactions, as well as antiparasitic response.

## ■ Interleukin 26

IL-26 (Fickenscher and Pirzer, 2004; Hör, 2004) is a polypeptide of 177 amino acids and is part of the IL-10 family. IL-26 is produced in activated Th1 memory cells, to some extent in NK cells, but neither in Th2 or regulatory T-cells, nor in monocytes or B-cells. IL-26 is normally expressed by various sorts of T-cells at low levels, and specifically overexpressed by T-cells after *Herpesvirus saimiri* (HVS) transformation. It binds to a heterodimeric receptor postulated to be comprised of the IL-20R1 and IL-10R2 chains. Targeting epithelial cells, the T-cell lymphokine IL-26 is likely to play a role in local mechanisms of mucosal and cutaneous immunity.

## ■ Interleukin 27

IL-27 (Villarino and Hunter, 2004) is a novel heterodimeric cytokine of the IL-12 family that consists of EBI3, an IL-12p40-related protein, and p28, a newly discovered IL-12p35-related polypeptide. It is produced by antigen-presenting cells and specifically acts on naïve T-cells. IL-27 synergizes with IL-12 to produce IFNγ and does not support Th2 cytokine production by activated T-cells. Recent evidence however suggests that this receptor/ligand pair is also required to suppress a variety of immune cell effector processes, including proliferation and cytokine production. There is some evidence for the protective role of IL-27 from inflammatory autoimmune diseases and it has been shown to have antitumor effects in animal models (Hisada et al., 2004).

## ■ Interleukin 28 and Interleukin 29

Recently, the human genomic sequence for a family of three cytokines, designated IL-28A, IL-28B and IL-29 (Sheppard, 2002), that are distantly related to type I IFNs and the IL-10 family has been described (Pestka et al., 2004a,b). Like type I IFNs, IL-28 and IL-29 are induced by viral infection and have antiviral activity. However, IL-28 and IL-29 interact with a heterodimeric class 2 cytokine receptor that consists of the IL-10 receptor 2 (IL-10R2) and an orphan class 2 receptor chain, designated IL-28R1. This newly described cytokine family may serve as an alternative to type I IFNs in providing immunity to viral infection.

## ■ Interleukin 31

IL-31 (Bilsborough et al., 2006) is a newly discovered four-helix bundle cytokine preferentially expressed by activated T-cells with a Th2 bias. Together with IL-4 and IL-13, IL-31 has been implicated in the pathogenesis of atopic dermatitis because they are produced by a subset of T-cells that home to the skin. IL-31 signals through a heterodimeric receptor constitutively expressed by epithelial cells including keratinocytes. IL-31 stimulated keratinocytes induce a whole array of inflammatory CKs which also facilitate the recruitment of lymphocytes, monocytes and polymorphonuclear cells to the epidermis.

## ■ Interleukin 32

IL-32 (Kim et al., 2005) is a recently characterized polypeptide which was described several years ago as natural killer cell transcript 4 (NK4) of activated T-cells and NK-cells and belongs to the proinflammatory cytokines. It induces TNF-α and MIP-2, a CK, in different cells via the signal pathway of proinflammatory cytokines. To date it has been detected in higher concentration in some of the patients with sepsis compared to healthy individuals.

## ■ Interleukin 33

IL-33 (Schmitz et al., 2005), unlike other members of the IL-1 ligand family, which are all proinflammatory, has a major role in the development of a Th2 type immune response by inducing IL-5 and IL-13. Human smooth muscle cells as well as epithelial cells forming bronchus and small airways show constitutive expression of IL-33 mRNA; in lung or dermal fibroblasts and keratinocytes IL-33 mRNA is induced after activation with TNF-α and IL-1β. Activated dendritic cells and macrophages are the only hematopoietic cells showing low quantities of IL-33 mRNA. In addition, IL-33 and IL-18 are the only known IL-1 family member genes not located on chromosome 2.

# THERAPEUTIC USE OF RECOMBINANT INTERFERONS

## ■ IFNα Therapeutics

Together with recombinant human insulin and growth hormone, recombinant IFNα was one of the first rDNA-derived pharmaceuticals. The drive to produce recombinant IFN and other rDNA-derived pharmaceuticals developed from the need to obtain large amounts of a well-defined, purified protein for large-scale therapeutic use (Pestka, 1981a,b, 1986). Availability of the necessary basic technologies (see Chapters 1 through 3) made this possible. The history of IFNα given in the attached case history is well suited to illustrate most of the issues that need to be addressed in developing recombinant proteins. Starting in the early 1980s, a number of cytokines produced by recombinant gene technology were developed to become innovative therapeutic modalities called biologicals or biopharmaceuticals. Table 3 summarizes the recombinant IFNs approved for therapeutic use.

| Recombinant interferons | Company | 1st indication | 1st approval |
|---|---|---|---|
| **Interferon-α** | | | |
| IFNα2a produced in *Escherichia coli*; Roferon A | Hoffmann–La Roche (Basel, Switzerland) | Hairy cell leukemia | 1986 (EU and USA) |
| IFNα2b produced in *E. coli;* Intron A; Viraferon; Alfatronol | Schering-Plough (Kenilworth, NJ, USA) | Hairy cell leukemia | 1986 (USA and EU) |
| IFNαcon1, synthetic type I IFN produced in *E. coli;* Infergen | Amgen (Thousand Oaks, USA); Yamanouchi Europe (Leiderdorp, The Netherlands, EU) | Chronic hepatitis C | 2001 (USA) |
| **Interferon-β** | | | |
| IFNβ1a produced in CHO cells; Rebif | Serono (Geneva, Switzerland) | Relapsing/remitting multiple sclerosis | 1998 (EU), 2002 (USA) |
| IFNβ1a produced in CHO cells; Avonex | Biogen (Cambridge, MA, USA) | Relapsing/remitting multiple sclerosis | 1997 (EU), 1996 (USA) |
| IFNβ1b Cys17 Ser substitution; produced in *E. coli;* Betaferon | Schering AG (Berlin, Germany) | Relapsing/remitting multiple sclerosis | 1995 (EU) |
| IFNβ1b, Cys17 Ser substitution; produced in *E. coli;* Betaseron | Berlex Labs/Chiron (Richmond/Emeryville, CA, USA) | Relapsing/remitting multiple sclerosis | 1993 (USA) |
| **Interferon-γ** | | | |
| Actimmune (IFNγ1b; produced in *E. coli*) | Genentech (San Francisco CA, USA); InterMune (Palo Alto, CA, USA) | Chronic granulomatous disease | 1990 (USA) |

*Source*: Adapted from Walsh, 2006.

**Table 3** Interferons approved as biopharmaceuticals approved in the United States and Europe.

IFNα2 was developed independently by Hoffmann-LaRoche Ltd. (IFNα2a; Roferon A) and Schering Plough Corporation (IFNα2b; Intron A). Both were obtained by recombinant DNA technology in *Escherichia coli*, consist of 165 amino acids with an approximate molecular weight of 19 kDa and differ by one amino acid in position 23: Lys for IFNα2a and Arg for IFNα2b (Pestka, 1986). For all practical purposes there is no difference between these two products in terms of pharmacological properties or clinical application.

The metabolism of IFNα2a is consistent with that of alpha IFNs in general and is therefore used as example. Alpha IFNs are totally filtered through the glomeruli and undergo rapid proteolytic degradation during tubular reabsorption (see Chapter 5). Liver metabolism and subsequent biliary excretion are considered minor pathways of elimination for alpha IFNs. After intramuscular (IM) and subcutaneous (SC) administrations of 36 MIU, peak serum concentrations range from 1500 to 2580 pg/mL (mean 2020 pg/mL) at a mean time to peak of 3.8 hr and from 1250 to 2320 pg/mL (mean 1730 pg/mL) at a mean time to peak of 7.3 hr, respectively. The apparent fraction of the dose absorbed after IM injection is >80%. The pharmacokinetics of IFNα2a after single IM doses to patients with disseminated cancer are similar to those found in healthy volunteers. Dose proportional increases in serum concentrations are observed after single doses up to 198 MIU. There are no changes in the distribution or elimination of IFNα2a during twice daily (0.5 to 36 MIU), once daily (1 to 54 MIU), or three times weekly (1 to 136 MIU) dosing regimens up to 28 days of dosing. Multiple IM doses of IFNα2a result in an accumulation of two to four times the serum concentrations seen after a single dose.

Roferon A and Intron A are approved for the following indications: chronic hepatitis B and C, Kaposi's sarcoma, renal cell carcinoma, malignant melanoma, carcinoid tumor, multiple myeloma, non-Hodgkin lymphoma (NHL), hairy cell leukemia, chronic myelogenous leukemia, thrombocytosis associated with chronic myelogenous leukemia, and other myeloproliferative disorders. The approved indications vary depending on company and regulatory policies; for detailed information as well as for the recommended dosing the reader is referred to the respective product information current in their countries.

The adverse event profile for the three IFNα is the same; it is generally more or less well tolerated depending on the dose regimen used and subjectively consists primarily of the "influenza-like symptoms" named as such because they mimic the symptoms of early influenza. This, of course, should come as no surprise as these symptoms are caused by peaks of endogenous IFN stimulated by the influenza virus infection. For a detailed reporting of all adverse events, the reader is referred to the product information for each product.

Given the principle that the toxicity of a given medication is defined by its peak, i.e. by the time it is above a toxic threshold concentration and the efficacy by the trough concentration, i.e., the time the substance is below the therapeutic level, it would be desirable to obtain a therapeutic regimen which minimizes fluctuations; a constant therapeutic drug concentration would be an ideal goal. The first step toward that goal, as a proof of concept, was to model a long-acting IFN using an insulin pump to inject patients with chronic hepatitis C with IFNα2a at predetermined rates per hour for 28 days. A similar study was performed in patients with renal cell carcinoma. These studies indicated that IFNα2a at a constant dose was indeed better tolerated while showing activity when administered by continuous SC infusion (Ludwig et al., 1990; Carreño et al., 1992). The next step therefore was to develop a new longer acting molecule by attaching several polyethylene glycol (PEG) chains to the native IFN molecule (see section "Pegylated IFNs and Interleukins: The Next Generation").

*Roferon A* is supplied as prefilled syringes containing 3, 4.5, 6 or 9 MIU in 0.5 mL, or as cartridges containing 18 MIU/mL for SC injection only, or as vials each containing 3, 6, 9 or 36 MIU in 1 mL, or multidose injectable solution containing 9 MIU (each 0.3 mL contains 3 MIU) or 18 MIU of IFNα2a (each mL contains 6 MIU) for SC or IM injection. All presentations are human serum albumin (HSA)-free liquid formulations with 7.21 mg sodium chloride, 0.2 mg polysorbate 80, 10 mg benzyl alcohol (as a preservative), 0.77 mg ammonium acetate and sterile water for injections.

*Intron A* is supplied as vials containing 10, 15 or 50 MIU as lyophilisate and a vial with 1 mL of diluent for reconstitution containing 20 mg glycine, 2.3 mg sodium phosphate dibasic, 0.55 mg sodium phosphate monobasic and 1.0 mg HSA, or as solution vials containing 10 MIU as single dose, 18 MIU or 25 MIU as multidose with 7.5 mg sodium chloride, 1.8 mg sodium phosphate dibasic, 3 mg sodium phosphate monobasic, 0.1 mg edetate disodium, 0.1 mg polysorbate 80, and 1.5 mg m-cresol as a preservative per mL for SC, IM or intralesional injection, or solution in multidose pens containing 6 doses of 3, 5 or 10 MIU IFNα2b per 0.2 mL and adjuvants as above for SC injection.

*Infergen* (IFN alphacon-1) is a synthetic "consensus" IFN consisting of 166 amino acids and not occurring in nature. It was genetically engineered in *E. coli* by Amgen. The amino acid sequence of the product is derived by comparison of the sequences of several natural IFNα subtypes and assigning the most frequently observed amino acid in each corresponding position. Infergen is supplied as single-dose, preservative-free vials containing either 9 μg (0.3 mL) or 15 μg (5 mL) of IFN alphacon-1 for SC injection.

## ■ IFNβ Therapeutics

Three IFNβ-products (Table 3) are marketed worldwide for the treatment of multiple sclerosis: the first was Berlex's Betaseron, marketed by Schering AG as Betaferon in Europe. It is IFNβ1b with 165 amino acids and an approximate molecular weight of 18,500 Da, a cysteines-17-serine substitution. It is produced in *E. coli*, which was then the standard method. It is nonglycosylated, as without further engineering glycosylation is not possible in the *E. coli* system (Wacker et al., 2002) (see Chapters 2 and 3). Independently, Biogen and Serono developed a glycosylated IFNβ1a produced in Chinese hamster ovary cells. Thus, not only is the amino acid sequence of these IFNβs identical to that of natural fibroblast-derived human IFN beta, but they are also glycosylated, each containing a single N-linked complex carbohydrate moiety. The two products are marketed as Avonex and Rebif, respectively. All three products are indicated for the treatment of multiple sclerosis.

Glycosylating proteins fundamentally alter their pharmacokinetic and pharmacodynamic properties. The nonglycosylated IFNβ1b (IFNβ$_{ser17}$) has the expected short circulation time: time to peak concentration ($C_{max}$) between 1 and 8 hr with a mean peak serum IFN concentration of 40 IU/mL after a single SC injection of 0.5 mg (16 MIU). Bioavailability is about 50%. Patients receiving single intravenous (IV) doses up to 2.0 mg (64 MIU) show an increase in serum concentrations which is dose proportional. Mean terminal elimination half-life values ranged from 8.0 min to 4.3 hr. Thrice weekly IV dosing for 2 weeks resulted in no accumulation of IFNβ1b in sera of patients. Pharmacokinetic parameters after single and multiple IV doses were comparable. Following every other day SC administration of 0.25 mg (8 MIU) IFNβ1b in healthy volunteers, biologic response marker levels (neopterin, β$_2$-microglobulin, MxA protein, and IL-10) increased significantly above baseline 6 to 12 hr after the first dose. Biologic response marker levels peaked between 40 and 124 hr and remained elevated above baseline throughout the 7-day study (168 hr).

Glycosylated IFNβ1a such as Rebif, on the other hand, is slower to reach $C_{max}$, with a median 16 hr and the serum elimination half-life is $69 \pm 37$ hr (mean ± SD). In healthy volunteers a single SC injection of 60 µg (~18 MIU) of IFNβ1a resulted in a $C_{max}$ of $5.1 \pm 1.7$ IU/mL. Following every other day SC injections in healthy volunteers, an increase in AUC of approximately 240% was observed, suggesting that accumulation of IFNβ1a occurs after repeated administration. Biological response markers [e.g., 2′, 5′-oligoadenylate synthetase (OAS), neopterin and β₂-microglobulin] are induced by IFNβ1a following a single SC administration of 60 µg. Intracellular 2′, 5′-OAS peaked between 12 and 24 hr and β₂-microglobulin and neopterin serum concentrations showed a maximum at approximately 24 to 48 hr. All three markers remained elevated for up to 4 days. Administration of 22 µg (6 MIU) IFNβ1a three times per week inhibited mitogen-induced release of proinflammatory cytokines (IFNγ, IL-1, IL-6, TNF-α and TNF-β) by PBMC that, on average, was near double that observed with IFNβ1a administered once per week at either 22 (6 MIU) or 66 µg (12 MIU).

*Betaseron/Betaferon* is formulated as a sterile powder with a 0.54% sodium chloride solution as diluent. Reconstituted it presents as 0.25 mg (8 MIU of antiviral activity) per mL. The recommended dose is 0.25 mg injected SC every other day.

*Avonex* is formulated as a lyophilized powder for IM injection. After reconstitution with the supplied diluent (sterile water for injection) each vial contains 30 µg of IFNβ1a, 15 mg HSA, 5.8 mg sodium chloride, 5.7 mg dibasic sodium phosphate and 1.2 mg monobasic sodium phosphate in 1.0 mL at a pH of approximately 7.3, or as a prefilled syringe with a sterile solution for IM injection containing 0.5 mL with 30 µg of IFNβ1a, 0.79 mg sodium acetate trihydrate, 0.25 mg glacial acetic acid, 15.8 mg arginine hydrochloride and 0.025 mg polysorbate 20 in water for injection at a pH of approximately 4.8. The recommended dosage is 30 µg injected IM once a week.

*Rebif* is supplied in prefilled 0.5 mL syringes: each 0.5 mL contains either 22 µg (6 MIU) or 44 µg (12 MIU) of IFNβ1a, 2 or 4 mg HSA, 27.3 mg mannitol, 0.4 mg sodium acetate, and water for injection. The recommended dosage is 22 µg (6 MIU) given three times per week by SC injection. This dose is effective in the majority of patients to delay progression of the disease. Patients with a higher degree of disability (EDSS, Expanded Disability Status Scale; Kurtzke, 1983) of 4 or higher) may require a dose of 44 µg (12 MIU) three times per week.

The adverse event profile for the three IFNβ is similar to IFNα; it is generally reasonably well tolerated and subjectively again consists primarily of the "influenza-like symptoms." For a detailed reporting of all adverse events, the reader is referred to the product information for each biopharmaceutical.

## ■ IFNγ Therapeutics

*Actimmune* (recombinant IFNγ1b; immune IFN) is a single-chain polypeptide containing 140 amino acids. It is produced by genetically engineered *E. coli* containing the DNA which encodes for the human protein. It is a highly purified sterile solution consisting of noncovalent dimers of two identical 16,465 Da monomers. Actimmune is slowly absorbed, after IM injection of 100 µg/m², a $C_{max}$ of 1.5 ng/mL is reached in approximately 4 hr, and after SC injection a $C_{max}$ of 0.6 ng/mL is reached in 7 hr. The apparent fraction of dose absorbed is > 89%. The mean half-life after IV administration was 38 min and after IM and SC dosing with 100 µg/m² were 2.9 and 5.9 hr, respectively. Multiple-dose SC pharmacokinetics showed no accumulation of Actimmune after 12 consecutive daily injections of 100 µg/m².

*Actimmune* is a solution filled in a single-dose vial for SC injection. Each 0.5 mL contains: 100 µg (2 MIU) of IFNγ1b, formulated in 20 mg mannitol, 0.36 mg sodium succinate, 0.05 mg polysorbate 20 and sterile water for injection. The dosage for the treatment of patients with chronic granulomatous disease or severe, malignant osteopetrosis is 50 µg/m² (1 MIU/m²) for patients whose body surface area is greater than 0.5 m² and 1.5 µg/kg/dose for patients whose body surface area is equal to or less than 0.5 m².

The adverse event profile of IFNγ is similar to IFNγ; it is generally well tolerated and subjectively consists primarily of the "influenza-like symptoms." For a detailed reporting of all adverse events, the reader is referred to the Actimmune product information.

## THERAPEUTIC USE OF RECOMBINANT INTERLEUKINS

In general, the approach to the development of ILs as a therapeutic modality is even more complex than for IFNs. Most ILs are embedded in a regulatory network and so far the pharmacological use of ILs has been somewhat disappointing. This was largely due to our lack of understanding of the role of these molecules and of the best way to use them; they are less well studied than IFNs. IL-2, for example, was initially developed by oncologists in the days when "go in fast, hit them hard and get out" was the prevalent strategy. Terms like maximal tolerated dose (which we called minimal poisonous dose) actually defined the dose at which a given drug was in most cases no longer tolerated. Thus IL-2 was given an undeserved bad reputation. Similar thinking nearly killed the development of IFNα for the treatment of chronic viral hepatitis and was ultimately the main reason for discontinuing the development of IL-2 in chronic hepatitis B (Pardo et al., 1997; Artillo et al., 1998) and IL-12 in chronic hepatitis B and C (Zeuzem et al., 1999; Carreño et al., 2000; Pockros et al., 2003). In spite of this progress has been made and our understanding of the complexities of such substances and their antagonists is growing.

## ■ Aldesleukin

*Proleukin* (aldesleukin), a nonglycosylated human recombinant IL-2 product, is a highly purified protein with a molecular weight of approximately 15 kDa. The chemical name is des-alanyl-1, serine-125 human IL-2. It is produced by recombinant DNA technology using a genetically engineered *E. coli* containing an analog of the human IL-2 gene. The modified human IL-2 gene encodes a modified human IL-2 differing from the native form: the molecule has no N-terminal alanine; the codon for this amino acid was deleted during the genetic engineering procedure; serine was substituted for cysteine at amino acid position 125. Aldesleukin exists as biologically active, noncovalently bound microaggregates with an average size of 27 recombinant IL-2 molecules. The pharmacokinetic profile of aldesleukin is characterized by high plasma concentrations following a short IV infusion, rapid distribution into the extravascular space and elimination from the body by metabolism in the kidneys with little or no bioactive protein excreted in the urine. Studies of IV aldesleukin indicate that upon completion of infusion, approximately 30% of the administered dose is detectable in plasma. Observed serum levels are dose proportional. The distribution and elimination half-life after a 5-min IV infusion are 13 and 85 min, respectively. In humans and animals, aldesleukin is cleared from the circulation by both glomerular filtration and peritubular extraction in the kidney. The rapid clearance of aldesleukin has led to dosage schedules characterized by frequent, short infusions. The adverse event profile of IL-2 is similar to that seen for IFNs and many ILs; it is generally reasonably well tolerated and subjectively consists primarily of the "influenza-like symptoms." For a detailed reporting of all adverse events, rarely severe, the reader is referred to the product information for Proleukin.

Proleukin is supplied as a sterile, lyophilized cake in single-use vials intended for IV injection. After reconstitution with 1.2 mL sterile water for injection, each mL contains 18 MIU (1.1 mg) aldesleukin, 50 mg mannitol and 0.18 mg sodium dodecyl sulfate, without preservatives, buffered with approximately 0.17 mg monobasic and 0.89 mg dibasic sodium phosphate to a pH of 7.5. It is indicated for the treatment of adults with metastatic renal cell carcinoma or metastatic melanoma. Each treatment course consists of two 5-day treatment cycles: 600,000 IU/kg (0.037 mg/kg) are administered every 8 hr by a 15-min

IV infusion for a maximum of 14 doses. Following 9 days of rest, the schedule is repeated for another 14 doses, or a maximum of 28 doses per course, as tolerated.

## ■ Oprelvekin

*Neumega* (oprelvekin) a nonglycosylated IL-11 is produced in *E. coli* by recombinant DNA technology and has 177 amino acids in length and a molecular mass of approximately 19 kDa. It differs from the 178 amino acid length of native IL-11 in lacking the amino-terminal proline residue. It is used as a thrombopoietic GF that directly stimulates the proliferation of hematopoietic stem cells and megakaryocyte progenitor cells and induces megakaryocyte maturation resulting in increased platelet production. Pharmacokinetics shows a rapid clearance from the serum and distribution to highly perfused organs. The kidneys are the primary route of elimination and little intact product can be found in the urine (see Chapter 5). After injection the $C_{max}$ of $17.4 \pm 5.4$ ng/mL is reached after $3.2 \pm 2.4$ hr ($T_{max}$) with a half-life of $6.9 \pm 1.7$ hr. The absolute bioavailability is >80%. There is no accumulation after multiple doses. Patients with severely impaired renal function show a marked decrease in clearance to 40% of that seen in subjects with normal renal function.

Neumega is supplied as single-use vials containing 5 mg of oprelvekin (specific activity approximately $8 \times 10^6$ U/mg) as a sterile lyophilized powder with 23 mg of glycine, 1.6 mg of dibasic sodium phosphate heptahydrate, and 0.55 mg monobasic sodium phosphate monohydrate. When reconstituted with 1 mL of sterile water for injection, the solution has a pH of 7.0. It is indicated for the prevention of severe thrombocytopenia following myelosuppressive chemotherapy. The recommended dose is 50 μg/kg given once daily by SC injection after a chemotherapy cycle in courses of 10 to 21 days. Platelet counts should be monitored to assess the optimal course of therapy. Treatment beyond 21 days is not recommended. Oprelvekin is generally well tolerated. Reported adverse events, mainly as a consequence of fluid retention, include edema, tachycardia/palpitations, dyspnea, and oral moniliasis. For a detailed reporting of all adverse events, rarely severe, the reader is referred to the product information for Neumega.

## ■ Anakinra

*Kineret* (anakinra) is a recombinant, nonglycosylated form of the human IL-1 receptor antagonist (IL-1Ra) produced using an *E. coli* bacterial expression system. It consists of 153 amino acids, has a molecular weight of 17.3 kDa, and differs from native human IL-1Ra in that it has the addition of a single methionine residue at its amino terminus. The absolute bioavailability of Kineret

| Recombinant interleukins | Company | 1st indication | 1st approval |
|---|---|---|---|
| Proleukin (aldesleukin; IL-2, lacking N-terminal alanine, C125 S substitution, produced in *E. coli*) | Chiron Therapeutics (Emeryville, CA, USA) | RCC (renal-cell carcinoma) | 1992 (EU and USA) |
| Neumega (oprelvekin; IL-11, lacking N-terminal proline produced in *E. coli.*) | Genetics Institute/Wyeth Pharmaceuticals, (Philadelphia, PA, USA) | Prevention of chemotherapy induced thrombocytopenia | 1997 (USA) |
| Kineret (anakinra; IL-1 receptor antagonist (produced in *E. coli*) | Amgen (Thousand Oaks, CA, USA) | RA (rheumatoid arthritis) | 2001 (USA) |

*Source*: Adapted from *Nature Biotechnology* 2006, 24:769–76.

**Table 4** ▪ Interleukins approved as biopharmaceuticals worldwide.

after a 70 mg SC bolus injection is 95%. $C_{max}$ occurs 3 to 7 hr after SC administration at clinically relevant doses (1 to 2 mg/kg) with half-life ranging from 4 to 6 hr. There is no accumulation of Kineret after daily SC doses for up to 24 weeks. The mean plasma clearance with mild and moderate (creatinine clearance 50–80 mL/min and 30–49 mL/min) renal insufficiency was reduced by 16% and 50%, respectively. In severe renal insufficiency and end-stage renal disease (creatinine clearance <30 mL/min), mean plasma clearance declined by 70% and 75%, respectively. Less than 2.5% of the administered dose is removed by hemodialysis or continuous peritoneal dialysis. A dose schedule change should be considered for subjects with severe renal insufficiency or end-stage renal disease.

Kineret is supplied in single-use prefilled glass syringes with 27 gauge needles as a sterile, clear, preservative-free solution for daily SC administration. Each prefilled glass syringe contains: 0.67 mL (100 mg) of anakinra in a solution (pH 6.5) containing 1.29 mg sodium citrate, 5.48 mg sodium chloride, 0.12 mg disodium EDTA, and 0.70 mg polysorbate 80 in water for injection. It is indicated for the reduction in signs and symptoms and slowing the progression of structural damage in moderately to severely active rheumatoid arthritis and can be used alone or in combination with DMARDs other than TNF-blocking agents (see

Chapter 18). The recommended dose for the treatment of patients with rheumatoid arthritis is 100 mg/day. Patients with severe renal insufficiency or end-stage renal disease should receive 100 mg every other day. Anakinra is generally well-tolerated, the most common adverse reaction is injection-site reactions, the most serious adverse reactions neutropenia, particularly when used in combination with TNF-blocking agents, and serious infections. For a detailed reporting of all adverse events, rarely severe, the reader is referred to the product information for Kineret.

## PEGYLATED INTERFERONS AND INTERLEUKINS: THE NEXT GENERATION

Since 1977 it has been known that PEG conjugated proteins are frequently more effective than their native parent molecule. Our understanding of PEG chemistry and how it affects the behavior of a biopharmaceutical has increased with the number of PEGylated proteins developed as therapeutic agents (Table 5 gives some examples). PEG is inert, nontoxic, nonimmunogenic and in its most common form either linear or branched terminated with hydroxyl groups that can be activated to couple to the desired target protein. It has been approved for human administration by mouth, injection, and topical application. Its general structure is:

| PEGylated recombinant interferons | | | |
|---|---|---|---|
| Pegasys (PEGylated IFNα2a produced in *E. coli*) | Hoffman–La Roche (Basel, Switzerland) | Chronic hepatitis B and C | 2002 (EU and USA) |
| ViraferonPeg (PEGylated IFNα2b produced in *E. coli*) | Schering-Plough (Kenilworth, NJ, USA) | Chronic hepatitis C | 2000 (EU) |
| PegIntron (PEGylated IFNα2b produced in *E. coli*) | Schering-Plough (Kenilworth, NJ, USA) | Chronic hepatitis C | 2000 (EU), 2001 (USA) |

*Source*: Adapted from Walsh, 2006.

**Table 5** ▪ PEGylated interferons approved in the United States and Europe.

*Bifunctional linear PEG (diol):*

$$HO-(CH_2CH_2)_n-CH_2CH_2-OH$$

For polypeptide modification one hydroxyl group is usually inactivated by conversion to monomethoxy or mPEG and becomes monofunctional, i.e., only one hydroxyl group is activated during the PEGylation process, thus avoiding the formation of interprotein (oligomerization) or intraprotein bridges:

*Monofunctional linear mPEG:*

$$CH_3O-(CH_2CH_2O)_n-CH_2CH_2-OH$$

To couple PEG to a molecule such as polypeptides, polysaccharides, polynucleotides or small organic molecules it is necessary to chemically activate it. This is done by preparing a PEG derivative with a functional group chosen according to the desired profile for the final product. In addition to the linear PEGs, branched structures have proven useful for peptide and protein modifications:

*Branched PEG:*

$$CH_3O-CH_2CH_2(OCH_2CH_2)_nO-\overset{\overset{O}{\|}}{C}-NH-CH-\overset{\overset{O}{\|}}{C}-X$$
$$\underset{CH_3O-CH_2CH_2(OCH_2CH_2)_nO-\overset{\overset{O}{\|}}{C}-NH}{O\ (CH_2)_4}$$

Branched PEG or PEG2 have a number of advantages over linear structures:

- Attached to proteins they "act" much larger than a linear mPEG of the same MW.
- Two PEG chains are added per attachment site, reducing the chance of protein inactivation.
- More effective in protecting proteins from proteolysis, reducing antigenicity and immunogenicity.

Depending on the desired use for the PEG-modified molecule different PEGylation strategies can be chosen, for example:

- Multiple shorter chain PEGylation if the biological activity should be preserved.
- A weak PEG-protein bond if a slow release effect is desired.
- A branched chain with high MW and a strong bond if prolonged circulation and receptor saturation is the goal.

Table 5 lists some of the PEGylated protein pharmaceuticals on the market or in various phases of development with appropriate references. For a more in-depth review of PEG chemistries and characteristics the interested reader is referred to Roberts et al. (2002) and Bailon et al. (2001).

The development of rhIFNα from the native, unmodified molecule to the PEGylated form with the desired pharmacological profile is an example of how the understanding of PEG chemistry progressed with experience (Zeuzem et al., 2003). Increasing the length of the PEG chain resulted in progressively longer circulating half-life due to protracted resorption and lower clearance, ultimately resulting in a near constant serum concentration over an entire week summarized in Figure 3.

The first PEGylated IFN, IFNα2a, used a linear, 5 kDa mPEG with a weak urethane PEG-IFNα2a link. Clinical trials conducted with this compound were unsuccessful because the blood circulation half-life for the conjugate (Fig. 3B) was only slightly improved relative to that of the native protein (Fig. 3A) (Wills, 1990). Development of the product was therefore halted at Phase II clinical trials (Zeuzem et al., 2003). The second compound was developed by Schering Plough, Kenilworth, New Jersey in collaboration with Enzon Pharmaceutical Inc, Bridgewater, New Jersey. It made use of a longer (12 kDa), linear PEG with an urethane linkage to IFNα2b. The chosen strategy was to combine the advantages of high specific activity with slower serum clearance resulting in PegIntron® (Wang et al., 2002) with markedly improved pharmacological properties allowing once a week administration (Fig. 3C) (Glue et al., 2000). PegIntron, also marketed as Viraferon® in some countries, is approved worldwide for the treatment of chronic hepatitis C.

The development of the third PEGylated IFN, IFNα2a, took a different approach. The strategic goal was to achieve lasting and constant serum concentrations over an entire week. In a collaboration of Roche with Shearwater Polymers in Huntsville, Alabama (now Nektar; San Carlos, California), IFNα2a was linked by a stable amide bond to four different PEG chains of various sizes, structures, and site-attachment numbers. The resulting products were tested for antiviral activity and a variety of pharmacokinetic parameters including half-life, absorption rate, and mean residence time:

- 20-kDa linear mono-PEGIFNα2a,
- 40-kDa linear di-PEGIFNα2a,
- 20-kDa branched mono-PEGIFNα2a
- 40-kDa branched mono-PEGIFNα2a

The 40-kDa, branched PEGylated molecule (later named Pegasys) exhibited sustained absorption, decreased systemic clearance, and an approximate 10-fold increase in serum half-life over regular IFN. The biological activity was similarly prolonged resulting in an optimal pharmacological profile, Figure 3D (Algranati et al., 1999). It was therefore chosen for further clinical development (Reddy et al., 2002) leading to its approval worldwide for the treatment of chronic hepatitis B and C. Pegasys is being tested for the treatment of renal cell carcinoma

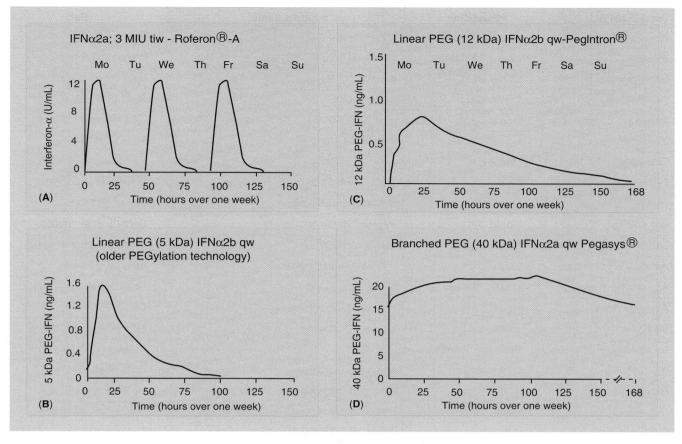

**Figure 3** ■ Pharmacokinetic profiles for IFN and PEG-IFN (repeated dosing).

(Motzer et al., 2002), malignant melanoma, chronic myeloid leukemia (Talpaz et al., 2005) and NHL.

The rapidly growing understanding of the potential of advanced PEGylation chemistry to improve the stability and pharmacological properties of biopharmaceuticals has fostered the development of an increasing number of PEG-biopharmaceuticals. Several of those have proven to offer significant advantages over their native counterparts and found their place in our therapeutic armamentarium. PEG is also used for a variety of other (nonbio) pharmaceutical applications. Table 6 lists several examples of different marketed products and others still in development.

## OUTLOOK AND CONCLUSIONS

There is a very precise and organized order in the intricate function of the immune system to make it work effectively and we are well on our way to map it. For us to fully understand what still appears as complex to some, a lot of hard work still lies ahead. The fundamental approach to cytokine or cytokine antagonist therapy with biopharmaceuticals is to identify diseases caused by insufficient or excessive cytokine production. In the first case, e.g., certain

chronic viral diseases or cancers, appropriate cytokines are used pharmacologically to boost the immune response. Examples include IFNα with antiviral as well as immunomodulatory properties in chronic viral hepatitis, or IL-2 or IL-12 in renal cell cancer and malignant melanoma. For chronic inflammatory or atopic diseases caused by unchecked overproduction of ILs, two options are available: either ILs or receptor antagonists, e.g., humanized monoclonal antibodies (Remicade or Enbrel; see Chapter 18) or IL-1R antagonist (Kineret, see above) in rheumatoid arthritis, or downregulation of the excessively produced IL using its antagonistic cytokine, e.g., PEGylated IL-12 in asthma (Leonard and Sur, 2003) or IL-10 in psoriasis (Asadullah et al., 2004).

Although, in relation to the magnitude of the potential of cytokines and anticytokines, the undeniable success stories to date may appear modest, they do set the scene. In parallel with the exponential boost of basic knowledge initiated by mastering the tools of biotechnology our understanding of the complex systems we are dealing with has progressed. Diagnostic and pharmacological applications are following closely behind, as well as the capability to monitor the effect of our interventions accurately. As a

| Protein name | PEGylation | Product name | Ref. |
|---|---|---|---|
| IFNα2a | Branched, 40 kDa | Pegasys | Reddy (2002) |
| IFNα2b | Linear, 12 kDa | PegIntron | Wang (2002) |
| Interferon β | Linear, 20 kDa | mPEGIFNβ 1b$_{20,000}$ | Baker et al. (2006) |
| Interleukin-2 | Linear, 5 kDa | multiPEGIL-2 | Pettit et al. (1997) |
| Interleukin-6 | Linear, 5 kDa | multiPEGIL-6 | Tsunoda et al. (2001) |
| Interleukin-15 | Linear, 5 kDa | multiPEGIL-15 | Pettit et al. (1997) |
| TNF-αLys(-) | Linear, 5 kDa | monoPEG TNF-α$_{5,000}$ | Yamamoto et al. (2003) |
| Erythropoietin[a] | 60 kDa | Mircera (Ro 50-3821; mPEG epoetin$_{60,000}$) | Schellekens (2006) |
| G-CSF[a] | Linear, 20 kDa | Neulasta (pegfilgrastim) | Lyman (2005) |
| GM-CSF[a] | Linear, 5 kDa | Pegsargramostim | Doherty et al. (2005) |
| MGDF[a] | Linear, 20 kDa | PEG rHuMGDF | Kuter and Begley (2002) |
| Adenosine deaminase | Linear, 5 kDa | Adagen (pegademase) | FDA Drug Label |
| Arginine deiminase | Linear, 20 kDa | ADI-SS PEG$_{20'000}$ | Holtsberg et al. (2002) |
| Asparaginase | Linear, 5 kDa | Oncaspar (pegaspargase) | Cao et al. (1990) |
| Insulin | Linear, 5 kDa | Exubera (rhInsulin) | Adis R&D profile (2004) |
| Leptin | Branched, 42 kDa | PEG-OB | Hukshorn et al. (2000) |
| rhGH analog[c] | Linear, 5 kDa | Somavert (pegvisomant) | Ross et al. (2001) |
| RNA aptamer | 40 kDa | Macugen (pegaptanib) | Ng et al. (2006) |
| Doxorubicin | Linear, 2 kDa | Doxil (doxorubicin HCl liposome injection) | Product information |
| PEG-hydrogel | <20 kDa | SprayGel Adhesion Barrier | Ferland (2001) |
| PEG-hydrogel | Unknown | FocalSeal Tissue Sealant | Henney (2000) |

[a] See Chapter 10: Hematopoietic Growth Factors.
[b] See Chapter 12: Insulin.
[c] See Chapter 13: Growth Hormones.

**Table 6** ■ Examples of PEGylated biopharmaceuticals.

consequence, an interesting paradigm shift in our approach to many diseases has taken place. Atherosclerosis (von der Thüsen et al., 2003), psoriasis (Barry and Kirby, 2004), insulitis (Knip, 1997), insulin resistance (Shoelson et al., 2006), and asthma (Barnes et al., 1998) as examples for chronic inflammatory diseases in which ILs and other cytokines play central roles are becoming therapeutic targets for treatment with biopharmaceuticals. A huge amount of knowledge and experience is available; what is sometimes missing is an integrative view of the many islands of knowledge: "Join the dots to see the greater picture." We must start thinking four-dimensionally: Look at the 3D network of immune and other cells or tissues, cytokines, their receptors and the cascade of events their interaction triggers and, in addition, how this constellation changes over time. For example depending on context and time when IL-12 is given, it may induce Th1 cytokines or boost a Th2 response (Biedermann et al., 2006). We need to understand the dynamic processes of acute self-limited and relapsing-remitting progressive diseases consequent to unbalanced cytokine response in order to optimally intervene and re-establish a state of health. The tools are there: polymerase chain reaction, genomics, sequencing, proteomics, microarrays (see Chapters 1 and 7). Time is an essential factor as we need to learn to recognize potential or established disease early when intervention is often more effective. Time is lastly also a consideration when treating patients, as a beneficial response can require weeks, months, years or a lifetime of therapy.

There are still issues in need of solutions: how to manage toxicities of some, mainly the proinflammatory cytokines, particularly for their therapeutic use in cancer. Better understanding of the interaction with their receptors, where those receptors are expressed, the dynamics of that expression, and the actions of cascade their interaction induces. Can we develop a computer model to visualize and help us understand the intricacies of the immune system better? Can biopharmaceuticals be targeted for better efficacy and less toxicity? How much can cell and animal models tell us? Will gene therapy ultimately displace pharmacological replacement or inhibition of cytokines (Yang et al., 2002; Spitzweg and Morris, 2004, Kawakami, 2005)?

In conclusion, IFNs as well as ILs and their antagonists have shown their usefulness in clinical medicine establishing a proof of concept. Ongoing research is looking for innovative approaches to the treatment of various diseases by developing the full potential of this promising biopharmaceutical approach. In addition to their use for therapeutic interventions, future research will also focus the application of IFNs and ILs towards prevention of diseases. Success in terms of marketable products, however, will require hard work, creativity and persistence.

## REFERENCES

Adis R&D Profile. Insulin Inhalation–Pfizer/Nektar Therapeutics: HMR 4006, Inhaled PEG-Insulin—Nektar, PEGylated Insulin—Nektar. Drugs in R&D 2004; 5:166–70.

Adorini L. Interleukin-12, a key cytokine in Th1-mediated autoimmune diseases. Cell Mol Life Sci 1999; 55:1610–25.

Aggarwal S, Ghilardi N, Xie M-H, et al. Interleukin-23 promotes a distinct CD4 T cell activation state characterised by the production of IL-17. J Biol Chem 2003; 278:1910–14.

Algranati NE, Sy S, Modi M A branched methoxy 40-kDa polyethylene glycol (PEG) moiety optimizes the pharmacokinetics of peginterferon alpha-2a (PEG-IFN) and may explain its enhanced efficacy in chronic hepatitis C. Hepatology 1999; 40(Suppl. ):190A.

Artillo S, Pastore G, Alberti A, et al. Double-blind, randomized controlled trial of interleukin-2 for the treatment of chronic hepatitis B. J Med Virol 1998; 54:167–72.

Asadullah K, Sabat R, Friederich M, et al. Interleukin-10: an important immunoregulatory cytokine with major impact on psoriasis. Cur Drug Targets Inflamm Allergy 2004; 3:185–92.

Bailon P, Palleroni, A, Schaffer CA, et al. Rational design of a potent, long-lasting form of interferon: A 40 kDa branched polyethylene glycol-conjugated interferon α-2a for the treatment of hepatitis C. Bioconjugate Chem 2001; 12:195–202.

Baker DP, Lin EY, Lin K, et al. N-terminally PEGylated human interferon-beta-1a with improved pharmacokinetic properties and in vivo efficacy in a melanoma angiogenesis model. Bioconjug Chem 2006; 17:179–88.

Barnes PJ, Fan Chung K, Page CP. Inflammatory mediators of asthma: an update. Pharmacol Rev 1998; 50:517–96.

Barry J, Kirby B. Novel biologic therapies for psoriasis. Expert Opin Biol Ther 2004; 4:975–987.

Biedermann T, Lametschwandtner G, Tangemann K, et al. IL-12 instructs skin homing of human Th2 cells. J Immunol 2006; 177:3763–70.

Bilsborough J, Leung DYM, Maurer M, et al. IL-31 is associated with cutaneous lymphocyte antigen-positive skin homing T cells in patients with atopic dermatitis. J Allergy Clin Immunol 2006; 117:418–25.

Blumberg H, Conklin D, Xu WF, et al. Interleukin-20: discovery, receptor identification, and role in epidermal function. Cell 2001; 104:9–19.

Boniface K, Bernard F-X, Garcia M, et al. IL-22 Inhibits epidermal differentiation and induces proinflammatory gene expression and migration of human keratinocytes. J Immunol 2005; 174:3695–702.

Braunstein J, Brutsaert S, Olson R, et al. STATs dimerize in the absence of phosphorylation. J Biol Chem 2003; 278:34133–40.

Cao SG, Zhao QY, Ding ZT, et al. Chemical modification of enzyme molecules to improve their characteristics. Ann NY Acad Sci 1990; 613:460–7.

Carreño V, Zeuzem S, Hopf U, et al. A phase I/II study of recombinant human interleukin-12 in patients with chronic hepatitis B. J Hepatol 2000; 32:317–24.

Carreño V, Tapia L, Ryff JC, et al. Treatment of chronic hepatitis C by continuous subcutaneous infusion of interferon-alpha. J Med Virol 1992; 37:215–9.

Chang C, Magracheva E, Kozlov S, et al. Crystal structure of interleukin-19 defines a new subfamily of helical cytokines. J Biol Chem 2003; 278:3308–13.

Cruikshank WW, Kornfeld H, Center DM. Signaling and function of interleukin-16. Int Rev Immunol 1998; 16:523–40.

Doherty DH, Rosendahl MS, Smith DJ, et al. Site-specific pegylation of engineered cysteine analogs of recombinant human granulocyte-macrophage colony-stimulating factor. Bioconjug Chem 2005; 16:1291–8.

Donnelly RP, Sheikh F, Kotenko SV. The expanded family of class II cytokines that share the IL-10 receptor-2 (IL-10R2) chain. J Leukocyte Biol 2004; 76:314–21.

Du X, Williams DA. Interleikin-11: Review of molecular, cell biology, and clinical use. Blood 1997; 89:3897–908.

El Bassam S, Pinsonneault S, Kornfeld H, et al. Interleukin-16 inhibits interleukin-13 production by allergen-stimulated blood mononuclear cells. Immunology 2005; 117:89–96.

Esposito K, Pontillo A, DiPalo C, et al. Effect of weight loss and lifestyle changes on vascular inflammatory markers in obese women. JAMA 2003; 289:1799–804.

ExPASy http://au.expasy.org/uniprot/Q9UBH0—(**Expert Protein Analysis System**) proteomics server of the Swiss Institute of Bioinformatics (SIB).

Fehniger TA, Caligiuri MA. Interleukin 15: biology and relevance to human disease. Blood 2001; 97:14–32.

Fickenscher H, Pirzer H. Interleukin-26. International Immunopharmacology 2004; 4:609–13.

Fort MM, Cheung J, Yen D, et al. IL-25 Induces IL-4, IL-5, and IL-13 and Th2-associated pathologies in vivo. Immunity 2001; 15:985–95.

Fry TJ, Mackall CL. Interleukin-7: from bench to clinic. Blood 2002; 99:3892–904.

Gaffen SL. Biology of recently discovered cytokines: interleukin-17—a unique inflammatory cytokine with roles in bone biology and arthritis. Arthritis Res Ther 2004; 6:240–7.

Gallagher G, Dickensheets H, Eskdale J, et al. Cloning, expression and initial characterization of interleukin-19 (IL-19) a novel homologue of human interleukin-10 (IL-10). Genes Immun 2000; 1:442–50.

Glue P, Fang JWS, Rouzier-Panis R, et al. Pegylated interferon-α2b: pharmacokinetics, pharmacodynamics, safety, and preliminary efficacy data. Clin Pharm Ther 2000; 68:556–67.

Greenfeder S, Umland SP, Cuss FM, et al. Th2 cytokines and asthma: the role of interleukin-5 in allergic eosinophilic disease. Respir Res 2001; 2:71–9.

Heinrich PC, Castell JV, Andus T. Interleukin-6 and the acute phase response. Biochem J 1990; 265:621–35.

Henney JM. Surgical sealant for lung cancer. JAMA 2000; 284:685.

HGNC—www.gene.ucl.ac.uk/nomenclature/—Gene Families and Grouping–Interferons (IFN)–Interleukins and interleukin receptor genes (IL).

Hisada M, Kamiya S, Fujita K, et al. Potent antitumor activity of interleukin-27. Cancer Res 2004; 64:1152–6.

Holtsberg FW, Ensor CM, Steiner MR, et al. Poly(ethylene glycol) (PEG) conjugated arginine deiminase: effects of PEG formulations on its pharmacological properties. J Control Release 2002; 80:259–71.

Hör S, Pirzer H, Dumoutier L, et al. The T-cell lymphokine interleukin-26 targets epithelial cells through the interleukin-20 receptor 1 and interleukin-10 receptor 2 chains. J Biol Chem 2004; 279:33343–51.

Huising MO, Cruiswijck CP, Flik G. Phylogeny and evolution of class-I helical cytokines. J Endocrinology 2006; 189:1–25.

Hukshorn CJ, Saris WHM, Westerterp-Plantenga MS, et al. Weekly subcutaneous pegylated recombinant native human leptin (PEG-OB) administration in obese men. J Clin Endo & Metabol 2000; 85:4003–9.

Hung J, McQuillan BM, Chapman CML, et al. Elevated interleukin-18 levels are associated with the metabolic syndrome independent of obesity and insulin resistance. Arterioscl Thromb Vasc Biol 2005; 25:1268–73.

Isaacs A, Lindenmann J. Virus interference I: the interferon. Proc R Soc Ser B 1957; 147:258–67.

Ishikawa S, Nakagawa T, Miyahara R, et al. Expression of MDA-7/IL-24 and its clinical significance in resected non–small cell lung cancer. Clin Cancer Res 2005; 11:1198–202.

Jiang H, Su ZZ, Lin JJ, et al. The melanoma differentiation associated gene mda-7 suppresses cancer cell growth. Proc Natl Acad Sci (PNAS) USA 1996; 93:9160–5.

Kaushansky K. The molecular mechanisms that control thrombopoiesis. J Clin Invest 2005; 115:3339–45.

Kawakami K. Cancer gene therapy utilizing interleukin-13 receptor alpha2 chain. Cur Gene Ther 2005; 5:213–23.

Kim S-H, Han S-Y, Azam T, et al. Interleukin 32: a cytokine and inducer of TNF. Immunity 2005; 22:131–42.

Knip M. Disease-associated autoimmunity and prevention of insulin-dependent diabetes mellitus. Ann Med 1997; 29:447–51.

Kolls JK, Lindén A. Interleukin-17 family members and inflammation. Immunity 2004; 21:467–76.

Konishi Y, Harano T, Tabira T. Neurotrophic effect of interleukin-3 (IL-13) and its mechanisms of action in the nervous system. CNS Drug Rev 1990; 5:265–80.

Kotenko SV, Izotova LS, Mirochnitchenko OV, et al. Identification of the functional IL-TIF (IL-22) receptor complex: the IL-10R2 chain (IL-10Rβ) is a common chain of both IL-10 and IL-TIF (IL-22) receptor complexes. J Biol Chem 2001a; 276:2725–32.

Kotenko SV, Izotova LS, Mirochnitchenko OV, et al. Identification, cloning and characterization of a novel soluble receptor which binds IL-22, and neutralizes its activity. J. Immunol 2001b; 166:7096–103.

Kurschner C, Yuzaki M. Neuronal interleukin-16 (NIL-16): a dual function PDZ domain protein. J Neurosci 1999; 19:7770–80.

Kuter DJ, Begley CG. Recombinant human thrombopoietin: basic biology and evaluation of clinical studies. Blood 2002; 100:3457–69.

Kurtzke JF. Rating neurologic impairment in multiple sclerosis: an expanded disability status scale (EDSS). Neurology 1983; 33:1444–52.

LaFleur DW, Nardelli B, Tsareva T, et al. Interferon-κ, a novel type I interferon expressed in human keratinocytes. J Biol Chem 2001; 276:39765–71.

Lee S, Kaneko H, Sekigawa I, et al. Circulating interleukin-16 in systemic lupus erythematosus. Brit J Rheumatol 1998; 37:1334–7.

Leonard P, Sur S. Interleukin-12: potential role in asthma therapy. BioDrugs 2003; 17:1–7.

Liu B, Novick D, Kim S-H, et al. Production of biologically active human interleukin 18 requires its prior synthesis as pro-IL-18. Cytokine 2000; 12:1519–25.

Lubberts E, Koenders MI, van den Berg WB. The role of T-cell interleukin-17 in conducting destructive arthritis: lessons learned from animal models. Arthritis Res Ther 2005; 7:29–37.

Ludwig CU, Ludwig-Habemann R, Obrist R, et al. Improved tolerance of interferon alpha-2a by continuous subcutaneous infusion. Onkologie 1990; 13:117–22.

Lutfalla G, Crollius HR, Stange-Thomman N, et al. Comparative genomic analysis reveals independent expansion of a lineage-specific gene family in vertebrates: the class II cytokine receptors and their ligands in mammals and fish. BMC Genomics 2003; 4:29–44.

Lyman GH. Pegfilgrastim: a granulocyte colony-stimulating factor with sustained duration of action. Expert Opin Biol Ther 2005; 5:1635–46.

Meager A, editor. The interferons: characterization and application. WILEY-VCH, Weinheim; ISBN: 3-527-31180-7.

Middel P, Reich K, Polzien F, et al. Interleukin-16 expression and phenotype of interleukin-16 producing cells in Crohn's disease. Gut 2001; 49:795–803.

Moseley TA, Haudenschild TR, Rose L, et al. Interleukin-17 family and IL-17 receptors. Cytokine & Growth Factor Rev 2003; 14:155–74.

Motzer RJ, Ashok R, Thompson J, et al. Phase II trial of branched peginterferon-α 2a (40 kDa) for patients with advanced renal cell carcinoma. Ann Oncol 2002; 13:1799–805.

Nelson BH. IL-2, Regulatory T-cells, and tolerance. J Immunol 2004; 172:3983–8.

Ng EWM, Shima DT, Calias P, et al. Pegaptanib, a targeted anti-VEGF aptamer for ocular vascular disease. Nature Rev Drug Discov 2006; 5:123–32.

Ota N, Brett TJ, Murphy TL, et al. N-domain-dependent nonphosphorylated STAT4 dimers required for cytokine-driven activation. Nat Immunol 2004; 5:208–15.

Pardo M, Castillo I, Oliva H, et al. A pilot study of recombinant interleukin-2 for treatment of chronic hepatitis C. Hepatology 1997; 26:1318–21.

Pestka S. Interferons. In: Sidney Pestka, edited. Methods in enzymology, vol. 78. New York: Academic Press; 1981a. 632 pp.

Pestka S. Interferons. In: Sidney Pestka, editor. Methods in enzymology, vol. 78. New York: Academic Press; 1981b. 677 pp.

Pestka S. Interferons. In: Sidney Pestka, editor. Methods in enzymology, vol. 119. New York: Academic Press; 1986. 845 pp.

Pestka S, Krause CD, Walter MR. Interferons, interferon-like cytokines and their receptors. Immunol Rev 2004a; 202:8–32.

Pestka S, Krause CD, Sarkar C, et al. IL-10 and related cytokines and receptors. Annual Review of Immunology 2004b; 22:929–79.

Pettit DK, Bonnert TP, Eisenman J, et al. Structure-function studies of interleukin 15 using site-specific mutagenesis, polyethylene glycol conjugation, and homology modeling. J Biol Chem 1997; 272:2312–8.

Platanias L. Mechanism of Type I- and Type II-interferon mediated signaling. Nature Reviews Immunol 2005; 5:375–86.

Pockros P, Patel K, O'Brien CB. A multicenter study of recombinant human interleukin-12 for the treatment of chronic hepatitis C infection in patients with non-responsiveness to previous therapy. Hepatology 2003; 37:1368–74.

Reddy KR, Modi WM, Pedder S. Use of peginterferon alfa-2a (40 KD) (Pegasys) for the treatment of hepatitis C. Advanced Drug Deliv Rev 2002; 54:571–86.

Remick DG. Interleukin-8. Crit Care Med 2005; 33(Suppl.): S466–7.

Roberts MJ, Bentley MD, Harris JM. Chemistry for peptide and protein PEGylation. Adv Drug Deliv Rev 2002; 54:459–76.

Ross RJM, Leung KC, Maamra M, et al. Binding and functional studies with the growth hormone receptor antagonist, B2036-PEG (Pegvisomant), reveal effects of pegylation and evidence that it binds to a receptor dimer. J Clin Endocrinol Metab 2001; 86:1716–23.

Ryff JC. Both cytokines and their antagonists have a place in clinical medicine. Eur Cytokine Netw 1996; 7:437 (Abstract 40).

Schellekens H. Erythropiesis-stimulating agents—present and future. Business briefing: european endocrine review 2006: Touch Briefings Publishers December 2005.

Schmitz J, Owyang A, Oldham E, et al. IL-33, an interleukin-1-like cytokine that signals via the IL-1 receptor-related protein ST2 and induces T helper type 2-associated cytokines. Immunity 2005; 23:479–90.

Sen GC. Viruses and interferons. Annu Rev.Microbiol 2001; 55:255–81.

Sheppard P, Kindsvogel W, Xu W, et al. IL-28, IL-29 and their class II cytokine receptor IL-28R. Nature Immunology 2002; 4:63–8.

Shoelson SE, Lee J, Goldfine AB. Inflammation and insulin resistance. J Clin Invest 2006; 116:1793–801.

Sivakumar PV, Foster DC, Clegg CH. Interleukin-21 is a T-helper cytokine that regulates humoral immunity and cell-mediated anti-tumor responses. Immunology 2004; 112:177–82.

Spitzweg C, Morris JC. Gene therapy for thyroid cancer: current status and future prospects. Thyroid 2004; 14:424–34.

Steinke JW, Borish L. Th2 cytokines and asthma: its role in the pathogenesis of asthma, and targeting it for asthma treatment with interleukin-4 receptor antagonists. Respir Res 2001; 2:66–70.

Talpaz M, Rakhit A, Rittweger K, et al. Phase I evaluation of a 40-kDa branched-chain long-acting PEGylated IFN-A-2a with and without cytarabine in patients with chronic myelogenous leukemia. Clin Cancer Res 2005; 11:6247–455.

Towne J, Garka KE, Renshaw BR, et al. Interleukin (IL)-F6m IL-1F8, and IL-1F9 signal through IL-Rrp2 and IL-1RacP to activate the pathway leading to NF-κB and MAPKs. J Biol Chem 2004; 279: 13677–88.

Tsunoda S, Ishikawa T, Watanabe M, et al. Selective enhancement of thrombopoietic activity of PEGylated interleukin 6 by a simple procedure using a reversible amino-protective reagent. Br J Haematol 2001; 112:181–8.

Villarino AV, Hunter CA. Biology of recently discovered cytokines: discerning the pro- and anti-inflammatory properties of interleukin-27. Arthritis Res Ther 2004; 6:225–33.

von der Thüsen J, Kuiper J, van Berkel TJC, et al. Interleukins in atherosclerosis: molecular pathways and therapeutic potential. Pharmacol Rev 2003; 55:133–66.

Wacker A, Linton D, Hitchen P, et al. N-linked glycosylation in *Campylobacter jejuni* and its functional transfer into *E. coli*. Science 2002; 298:1790–3.

Walsh G. Biopharmaceutisol benchmark 2006. Nat Biotechnol 2006; 24:769–76.

Wang M, Liang P. Interleukin-24 and its receptors. Immunology 2005; 114:166–70.

Wang Y-S, Younster S, Grace M, et al. Structural and biological characterization of pegylated recombinant interferon alpha-2b and its therapeutic implications. Adv Drug Deliv Rev 2002; 54:547–70.

Wills RJ. Clinical pharmacokinetics of interferons. Clin Pharmacokinet 1990; 19:390–9.

Wills-Karp M. Interleukin-13 in asthma pathogenesis. Immunol Rev 2004; 202:175–90.

Yamamoto Y, Tsutsumi Y, Yoshioka, et al. Site-specific PEGylation of a lysin-deficient TNF-α with full bioactivity. Nat Biotechnol 2003; 21:546–52.

Yang Z, Chen M, Wu R. et al. Suppression of autoimmune diabetes by viral IL-10 gene transfer. J Immunol 2002; 168:6479–85.

Zeuzem S, Hopf U, Carreno V, et al. A phase I/II study of recombinant human interleukin-12 in patients with chronic hepatitis C. Hepatology 1999; 29:1280–6.

Zeuzem S, Welsch C, Herrmann E. Pharmacokinetics of peginterferons. Semin Liver Dis 2003; 23(Suppl. 1):S23–8.

Zhou Y, McLane M, Levitt RC. Th2 cytokines and asthma: interleukin-9 as a therapeutic target for asthma. Respir Res 2001; 2:80–4.

## FURTHER READING

Reviews which summarize the referenced subject in more detail:

### ■ Interferons

Meager A, editor. The interferons: characterization and application. WILEY-VCH, Weinheim; ISBN: 3-527-31180-7.

Pestka S, Krause CD, Walter M. Interferons, interferon-like cytokines, and their receptors. Immunological Reviews 2004a; **202**:8–32

Pestka S. Interferons. In: Sidney Pestka, editor. Methods in enzymology, vol. 78. New York: Academic Press; 1981. 632 pp.

Pestka S. Interferons. In: Sidney Pestka, editor. Methods in enzymology, vol. 79. New York: Academic Press; 1981. 677 pp.

Pestka S. Interferons. In: Sidney Pestka, editor. Methods in enzymology, vol. 119. New York: Academic Press 1986. 845 pp.

Special Issue: The neoclassical pathways of interferon signaling. J Interferon Cytokine Res 2005; 25:731–811.

### ■ Interleukins

Pestka S, Krause CD, Sarkar C et al. IL-10 and related cytokines and receptors. Annu Rev Immunol 2004a; 22;929–79.

Sigal LH. Interleukins of current clinical relevance (Part I). J Clin Rheumatol 2004; 10:353–9.

Sigal LH. Interleukins of current clinical relevance (Part II). J Clin Rheumatol 2004; 11:34-–9.

### ■ PEGylation

Bailon P, Palleroni A, Schaffer CA et al. Rational design of a potent, long-lasting form of interferon: a 40 kDa branched polyethylene glycol. Conjugated interferon α-2a for the treatment of hepatitis C. Bioconjugate Chem 2001:12:195–202.

Reddy KR, Modi WM, Pedder S. Use of peginterferon alfa-2a (40 KD) (Pegasys®) for the treatment of hepatitis C. Adv Drug Deliv Rev 2002; 54:571–86.

Roberts MJ, Bentley MD, Harris JM. Chemistry for peptide and protein PEGylation. Adv Drug Deliv Rev 2002; 54:459–76.

Wang Y-S, Youngster S, Grace M et al. Structural and biological characterization of pegylated recombinant interferon alpha-2b and its therapeutic implications. Adv Drug Deliv Rev 2002; 54:547–70.

# 12
# Insulin

*John M. Beals, Michael R. DeFelippis, and Paul M. Kovach*
*Eli Lilly & Company, Lilly Research Laboratories, Indianapolis, Indiana, U.S.A.*

## INTRODUCTION

Insulin was discovered by Banting and Best in 1921 (Bliss, 1982). Soon afterward, manufacturing processes were developed to extract the insulin from porcine and bovine pancreata. From 1921 to 1980, efforts were directed at increasing the purity of the insulin and providing different formulations for altering time-action for improved glucose control (Brange, 1987a,b; Galloway, 1988). Purification was improved by optimizing extraction and processing conditions and by implementing chromatographic processes (size exclusion, ion exchange, and reversed-phase) (Kroeff et al., 1989) to reduce the levels of both general protein impurities as well as insulin-related proteins such as proinsulin and insulin polymers. Formulation development focused on improving chemical stability by moving from acidic to neutral formulations and by modifying the time-action profile through the uses of various levels of zinc and protamine. The evolution of recombinant DNA (rDNA) technology led to the unlimited availability of human insulin, which has eliminated issues with sourcing constraints while providing the patient with a natural exogenous source of insulin. Combining the improved purification methodologies and recombinant DNA technology, manufacturers of insulin are now able to provide the purest human insulin ever made available, >98%. Further advances in rDNA technology, coupled with a detailed understanding of the molecular properties of insulin and knowledge of its endogenous secretion profile, enabled the development of insulin analogs with improved pharmacology relative to existing human insulin products.

## CHEMICAL DESCRIPTION

Insulin, a 51-amino acid protein, is a hormone that is synthesized as a proinsulin precursor in the β-cell of the pancreas and is converted to insulin by enzymatic cleavage. The resulting insulin molecule is composed of two polypeptide chains that are connected by two interchain disulfide bonds (Fig. 1) (Baker et al., 1988). The A-chain is composed of 21 amino acids and the B-chain is composed of 30 amino acids. The interchain disulfide linkages occur between $A^7$–$B^7$ and $A^{20}$–$B^{19}$, respectively. A third intrachain disulfide bond is located in the A-chain, between residues $A^6$ and $A^{11}$.

In addition to human insulin and insulin analog products, which are predominately used today as the first-line therapies for the treatment of diabetes, bovine and porcine insulin preparations have also been made commercially available (Table 1; Fig. 1); however, all major manufacturers of insulin have discontinued production of these products marking an end to future supply of animal-sourced insulin products. Difficulties obtaining sufficient supplies of bovine or porcine pancreata and recent concerns over transmissible spongiform encephalopathies associated with the use of animal-derived materials are major reasons for the product deletions.

The net charge on the insulin molecule is produced from the ionization potential of four glutamic acid residues, four tyrosine residues, two histidine residues, a lysine residue, and an arginine residue, in conjunction with two α-carboxyl and two

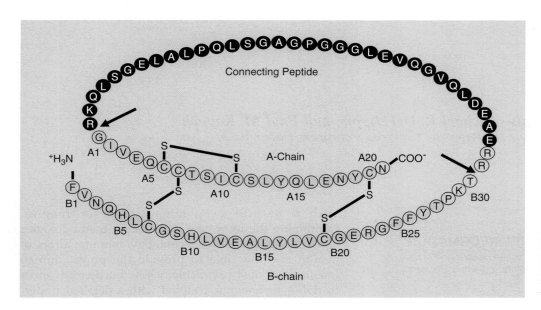

**Figure 1** ▪ Primary sequence of insulin. The colored (yellow) amino acids represent sites of sequence alterations denoted in Table 1.

α-amino groups. Insulin has an isoelectric point (pI) of 5.3 in the denatured state; thus, the insulin molecule is negatively charged at neutral pH (Kaarsholm et al., 1990). This net negative charge-state of insulin has been used in formulation development, as will be discussed later.

In addition to the net charge on insulin, another important intrinsic property of the molecule is its ability to readily associate into dimers and higher order states (Figs. 2 and 3) (Pekar and Frank, 1972). The driving force for dimerization appears to be the formation of favorable hydrophobic interactions at the C-terminus of the B-chain (Ciszak et al., 1995). Insulin can associate into discrete hexameric complexes in the presence of various divalent metal ions, such as zinc at 0.33 g-atom/monomer (Goldman and Carpenter, 1974), where each zinc ion (a total of two) is coordinated by a His$^{B10}$ residue from three monomers. Physiologically, insulin is stored as a zinc-containing hexamer in the β-cells of the pancreas. As will be discussed later, the ability to form discrete hexamers in the presence of zinc has been used to develop therapeutically useful formulations of insulin.

Commercial insulin preparations also contain phenolic excipients (e.g., phenol, m-cresol, or methylparaben) as antimicrobial agents. As represented in Figures 2 and 3D, these phenolic species also bind to specific sites on insulin hexamers, causing a conformational change that increases the chemical stability of insulin in commercial preparations (Brange and Langkjær, 1992). X-ray crystallographic data have identified the location of six phenolic ligand-binding sites on the insulin hexamer and the nature of the conformational change induced by the binding of these ligands (Derewenda et al., 1989). The phenolic ligands are stabilized in a binding pocket between monomers of adjacent dimers by hydrogen bonds

| Species | A$^8$ | A$^{10}$ | A$^{21}$ | B$^3$ | B$^{28}$ | B$^{29}$ | B$^{30}$ | B$^{31}$ | B$^{32}$ |
|---|---|---|---|---|---|---|---|---|---|
| Human (Humulin®, Novolin®) | Thr | Ile | Asn | Asn | Pro | Lys | Thr | — | — |
| Porcine insulin | Thr | Ile | Asn | Asn | Pro | Lys | Ala | — | — |
| Bovine insulin | Ala | Val | Asn | Asn | Pro | Lys | Ala | — | — |
| Insulin lispro (Humalog®) | Thr | Ile | Asn | Asn | Lys | Pro | Thr | — | — |
| Insulin aspart (NovoRapid®, NovoLog®) | Thr | Ile | Asn | Asn | Asp | Lys | Thr | — | — |
| Insulin glulisine (Apidra™) | Thr | Ile | Asn | Lys | Pro | Glu | Thr | | |
| Insulin glargine (Lantus®) | Thr | Ile | Gly | Asn | Pro | Lys | Thr | Arg | Arg |
| Insulin detemir (Levemir®) | Thr | Ile | Asn | Asn | Lys-(*N*-tetra decanoyl) | Pro | | | |

**Table 1** ▪ Amino acid substitutions in animal and insulin analogs.

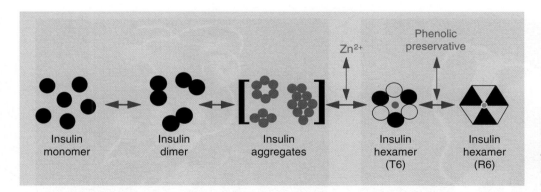

**Figure 2** Schematic representation of insulin association in the presence and absence of zinc and phenolic antimicrobial preservatives.

with the carbonyl oxygen of $Cys^{A6}$ and the amide proton of $Cys^{A11}$ as well as numerous van der Waals contacts. The binding of these ligands stabilizes a conformational change that occurs at the N-terminus of the B-chain in each insulin monomer, shifting the conformational equilibrium of residues B1 to B8 from an extended structure (T-state) to an α-helical structure (R-state). This conformational change is referred to as the T<–> R transition (Brader and Dunn, 1991) and is illustrated in Figure 3D.

In addition to the presence of zinc and phenolic preservatives, modern insulin formulations may contain an isotonicity agent (glycerol or NaCl) and/or a physiologic buffer (sodium phosphate). The former is used to minimize subcutaneous tissue damage and pain on injection. The latter is present to minimize pH drift in some pH-sensitive formulations.

## PHARMACOLOGY AND FORMULATIONS

Normal insulin secretion in the nondiabetic person falls into two categories: (*i*) insulin that is secreted in response to a meal and (*ii*) the background or *basal* insulin that is continually secreted between meals and during the nighttime hours. The pancreatic response to a meal typically results in peak serum insulin levels of 60–80 μU/mL whereas basal serum insulin levels fall within the 5–15 μU/mL range (Galloway and Chance, 1994). Because of these vastly different insulin demands, considerable effort has been expended to develop insulin formulations that meet the pharmacokinetic and pharmacodynamic requirements of each condition. More recently, insulin analogs and insulin analog formulations have been developed to improve pharmacokinetic and pharmacodynamic properties.

### ■ Regular and Rapid-Acting Soluble Formulations
Initial soluble insulin formulations were prepared under acidic conditions and were chemically unstable. In these early formulations, considerable deamidation was identified at $Asn^{A21}$ and significant potency loss

was observed during prolonged storage under acidic conditions. Efforts to improve the chemical stability of these soluble formulations led to the development of neutral, zinc-stabilized solutions.

The insulin in these neutral, regular formulations is chemically stabilized by the addition of zinc (~0.4% relative to the insulin concentration) and phenolic preservatives. As mentioned above, the addition of zinc leads to the formation of discrete hexameric structures (containing 2 Zn atoms per hexamer) that can bind six molecules of phenolic preservatives, e.g., m-cresol (Fig. 2). The binding of these excipients increases the stability of insulin by inducing the formation of a specific hexameric conformation ($R_6$), in which the B1 to B8 region of each monomer is in an α-helical conformation. This in turn decreases the availability of residues involved in deamidation and high-molecular-weight polymer formation (Brange et al., 1992a,b).

The pharmacodynamic profile of this soluble formulation is listed in Table 2. The neutral, regular formulations show peak insulin activity between 2 and 4 hr with a maximum duration of 5 to 8 hr. As with other formulations, the variations in time-action can be attributed to factors such as dose, site of injection, temperature, and the patient's physical activity. Despite the soluble state of insulin in these formulations, a delay in activity is still observed. This delay has been attributed to the time required for the hexamer to dissociate into the dimeric and/or monomeric substituents prior to absorption from the interstitium. This dissociation requires the diffusion of the preservative and insulin from the site of injection, effectively diluting the protein and shifting the equilibrium from hexamers to dimers and monomers (Fig. 4) (Brange et al., 1990). Recent studies exploring the relationship of molecular weight and cumulative dose recovery of various compounds in the popliteal lymph following subcutaneous injection suggest that lymphatic transport may account for approximately 20% of the

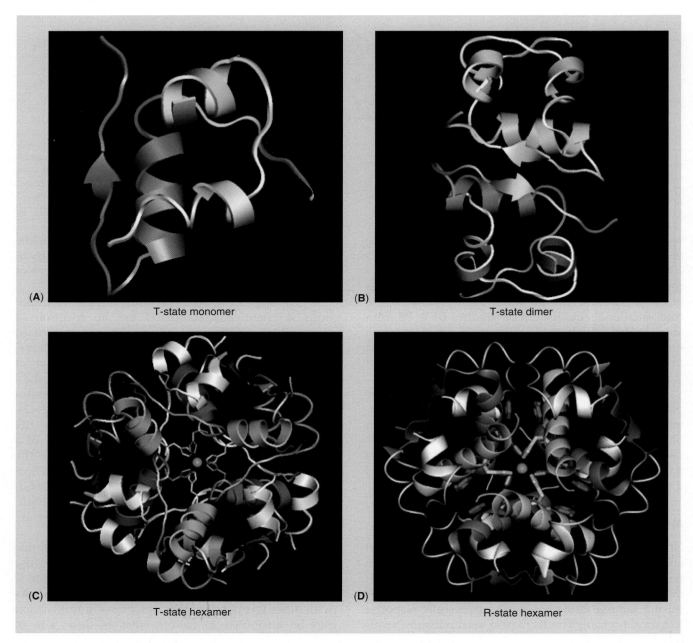

**Figure 3** ■ (**A**) A representation of the secondary and tertiary structures of a T-state monomer of insulin, with the B1–B8 region in an extended conformation. The A-chain is colored white and the B-chain is colored blue. (**B**) A representation of the secondary and tertiary structures of a T-state dimer of insulin. The A-chains are colored white and the B-chains are colored blue and cyan. (**C**) A representation of the secondary and tertiary structures of a T-state hexamer of insulin. The A-chains are colored white, the B-chains are colored blue and cyan, and zinc is colored green. (**D**) A representation of the secondary and tertiary structures of a R-state hexamer of insulin in the presence of preservative. The A-chains are colored white, the B-chains are colored blue and cyan, zinc is colored green, and preservative is colored magenta.

absorption of insulin from the interstitium (Supersaxo et al., 1990; Porter and Charman, 2000). The remaining balance of insulin is predominately absorbed through capillary diffusion.

Monomeric insulin analogs were designed to achieve a more natural response to prandial glucose-level increases while providing convenience to the patient. The pharmacodynamic profiles of these soluble formulations are listed in Table 3. The development of monomeric analogs of insulin for the treatment of insulin-dependent diabetes mellitus has focused on shifting the self-association properties of insulin to favor the monomeric species and consequently minimizing the delay in time-action

| Type[a] | Description | Appearance | Components | Action (hours)[b] | | |
|---|---|---|---|---|---|---|
| | | | | Onset | Peak | Duration |
| R[c] | Regular soluble insulin injection | Clear solution | Metal ion: zinc (10–40 µg/mL)<br>Buffer: none<br>Preservative: m-cresol (2.5 mg/mL)<br>Isotonicity agent: glycerin (16 mg/mL)<br>pH: 7.25–7.6 | 0.5–1 | 2–4 | 5–8 |
| N | NPH insulin isophane suspension | Turbid or cloudy suspension | Metal ion: zinc (21–40 µg/mL)<br>Buffer: dibasic sodium phosphate (3.78 mg/mL)<br>Preservative: m-cresol (1.6 mg/mL) phenol (0.73 mg/mL)<br>Isotonicity agent: glycerin (16 mg/mL)<br>Modifying protein: protamine (~0.35 mg/mL)<br>pH: 7.0–7.5 | 1–2 | 2–8 | 14–24 |
| L | Lente insulin zinc suspension | Turbid or cloudy suspension | Metal ion: zinc (120–250 µg/mL)<br>Buffer: sodium acetate (1.6 mg/mL)<br>Preservative: methylparaben (1.0 mg/mL)<br>Isotonicity agent: sodium chloride (7.0 mg/mL)<br>Modifying protein: none<br>pH: 7.0–7.8 | 1–2 | 3–10 | 20–24 |
| U | Ultralente extended insulin zinc suspension | Turbid or cloudy suspension | Metal ion: zinc (120–250 µg/mL)<br>Buffer: sodium acetate anhydrous (1.6 mg/mL)<br>Preservative: methylparaben (1.0 mg/mL)<br>Isotonicity agent: sodium chloride (7.0 mg/mL)<br>Modifying protein: none<br>pH: 7.0–7.8 | 0.5–3 | 4–20 | 20–36 |
| 70/30[d] | 70% insulin isophane suspension, 30% regular insulin Injection | Turbid or cloudy suspension | Metal ion: zinc (21–35 µg/mL)<br>Buffer: dibasic sodium phosphate (3.78 mg/mL)<br>Preservative: m-cresol (1.6 mg/mL); phenol (0.73 mg/mL)<br>Isotonicity agent: glycerin (16 mg/mL)<br>Modifying protein: protamine (~0.241 mg/mL)<br>pH: 7.0–7.8 | 0.5 | 2–4 | 14–24 |
| 50/50 | 50% insulin isophane suspension, 50% regular insulin injection | Turbid or cloudy suspension | Metal ion: zinc (21–35 µg/mL)<br>Buffer: dibasic sodium phosphate (3.78 mg/mL)<br>Preservative: m-cresol (1.6 mg/mL); phenol (0.73 mg/mL)<br>Isotonicity agent: glycerin (16 mg/mL)<br>Modifying protein: protamine (~0.172 mg/mL)<br>pH: 7.0–7.8 | 0.5 | 2–4 | 14–24 |

[a] U.S. designation.
[b] The time action profiles of Lilly insulins are the average onset, peak action, and duration of action taken from a composite of studies. The onset, peak and duration of insulin action depends on numerous factors, such as dose, injection site, presence of insulin antibodies, and physical activity. The action times listed represent the generally accepted values in the medical community
[c] Another notable designation is S (Britain). Other soluble formulations have been designed for pump use and include Velosulin® and HOE 21PH.
[d] In Europe the ratio designation is inverted on the label, e.g., 30/70. In addition, other ratios are available in Europe and include 10/90, 20/80, and 40/60 (note: designation).

**Table 2** ■ A list of neutral Humulin® U-100 (~3.5 mg/mL) insulin formulations.

(Brange et al., 1988, 1990; Brems et al., 1992). One such monomeric analog, Lys[B28]Pro[B29]-human insulin (Humalog® or Liprolog®; insulin lispro; Eli Lilly & Co., Lilly Corporate Center, Indianapolis, IN) has been developed and does have a more rapid time-action profile, with a peak activity of approximately 1 hr (Howey et al., 1994). The sequence inversion at positions B28 and B29 yields an analog with reduced self-association behavior compared to human insulin (Fig. 1; Table 1); however, insulin lispro can be stabilized in a preservative-dependent hexameric complex that provides the necessary chemical and physical stability required by insulin preparations. Despite the hexameric complexation of this analog, insulin lispro retains its rapid time-action. Based on the crystal structure of the insulin lispro hexameric complex, Ciszak et al. (1995) have hypothesized that the reduced dimerization properties of the analog, coupled with the preservative dependence, yields a hexameric complex that readily dissociates into

| Type[a] | Description | Appearance | Components | Action (hours)[b] | | |
|---|---|---|---|---|---|---|
| | | | | Onset | Peak | Duration |
| Humalog® | Rapid-acting soluble insulin analog for injection | Aqueous, clear, and colorless solution | Metal ion: zinc (19.7 μg/mL)<br>Buffer: dibasic sodium phosphate (1.88 mg/mL)<br>Preservative: m-cresol (3.15 mg/mL); phenol (trace)<br>Isotonicity agent: glycerin (16 mg/mL)<br>pH: 7.0–7.8 | 0.25–0.5 | 0.5–2.5 | <5 |
| Humalog Mix 75/25™ | 75% insulin lispro protamine suspension and 25% insulin lispro for injection | Turbid or cloudy suspension | Metal ion: zinc (25 μg/mL)<br>Buffer: dibasic sodium phosphate (3.78 mg/mL)<br>Preservative: m-cresol (1.76 mg/mL); phenol (0.715 mg/mL)<br>Isotonicity agent: glycerin (16 mg/mL)<br>Modifying protein: protamine (0.28 mg/mL)<br>pH: 7.0–7.8 | 0.25–0.5 | 0.2–2.5 | 14–24 |
| NovoLog® | Rapid-acting soluble insulin analog for injection | Aqueous, clear, and colorless solution | Metal ion: zinc (19.6 μg/mL)<br>Buffer: disodium hydrogen phosphate dihydrate (1.25 mg/mL)<br>Preservative: m-cresol (1.72 mg/mL); phenol (1.50 mg/mL)<br>Isotonicity agent: glycerin (16 mg/mL) sodium chloride (0.58 mg/mL)<br>pH: 7.2–7.6 | 0.25[c] | 0.75–1.5[c] | 3–5[c] |
| Novolog Mix 70/30 | 70% insulin aspart protamine suspension and 30% insulin aspart for injection | Turbid or cloudy suspension | Metal ion: zinc (19.6 μg/mL)<br>Buffer: dibasic sodium phosphate (1.25 mg/mL)<br>Preservative: m-cresol (1.72 mg/mL); phenol (1.50 mg/mL)<br>Isotonicity agent: sodium chloride (0.58 mg/mL) mannitol (36.4 mg/mL)<br>Modifying protein: protamine (0.33 mg/mL)<br>pH: 7.2–7.44 | <0.5[d] | 1–4[d]pppp | <24[d] |
| Apidra™ | Rapid-acting soluble insulin analog for injection | Aqueous, clear, and colorless solution | Metal ion: none<br>Buffer: tromethamine (6 mg/mL)<br>Preservative: m-cresol (3.15 mg/mL)<br>Isotonicity agent: sodium chloride (5 mg/mL)<br>Stabilizing agent: polysorbate 20, (0.01 mg/mL)<br>pH: ~7.3 | ~0.3[c] | 0.5–1.5[c] | ~5.3[c] |
| Lantus® | Long-acting soluble insulin analog for injection | Aqueous, clear, and colorless solution | Metal ion: zinc (30 μg/mL)<br>Buffer: none<br>Preservative: m-cresol (2.7 mg/mL)<br>Isotonicity agent: glycerin (20 mg 85%/mL)<br>Modifying protein: none<br>pH: ~4 | constant release with no pronounced peak[c] | | 10.8 –> 24.0[d] |
| Levemir® | Long-acting soluble insulin analog for injection | Aqueous, clear, and colorless solution | Metal ion: zinc (65.4 μg/mL)<br>Buffer: dibasic sodium phosphate (0.89 mg/mL)<br>Preservative: m-cresol (2.06 mg/mL); phenol (1.8 mg/mL)<br>Isotonicity agent: mannitol (30 mg/mL) sodium chloride (1.17 mg/mL)<br>Modifying protein: none<br>pH: 7.4 | | 3–14[c] | 5.7–23.2[c] |

[a] U.S. designation.

[b] The time action profiles of Lilly insulins are the average onset, peak action, and duration of action taken from a composite of studies. The onset, peak and duration of insulin action depends on numerous factors, such as dose, injection site, presence of insulin antibodies, and physical activity. The action times listed represent the generally accepted values in the medical community.

[c] DRUGDEX® System [Internet database]. Greenwood Village, Co; Thomson Micromedex. Updated periodically.

[d] PDR® Electronic Library™ [Internet database]. Greenwood Village, Co; Thomson Micromedex. Updated periodically.

**Table 3** ▪ A list of human-based U-100 (~3.5 mg/mL) insulin analog formulations.

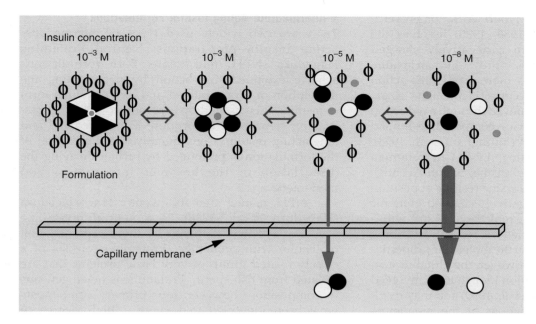

**Figure 4** ■ A schematic representation of insulin dissociation after subcutaneous administration.

monomers after rapid diffusion of the phenolic preservative into the subcutaneous tissue at the site of injection (Fig. 5). Consequently, the substantial dilution ($10^5$) of the human insulin zinc hexamers is not necessary for the analog to dissociate from hexamers to monomers/dimers, which is required for absorption.

It is important to highlight that the properties engineered into Humalog not only provide the patient with a more convenient therapy, but also improve control of postprandial hyperglycemia and reduce the frequency of severe hypoglycemic events (Anderson et al., 1997; Holleman et al., 1997).

Since the introduction of insulin lispro, two additional rapid-acting insulin analogs have been introduced to the market. The amino acid modifications made to the human insulin sequence to produce these analogs are depicted in Table 1. Like insulin lispro, both analogs are supplied as neutral pH solutions containing phenolic preservative. The design strategy for $Asp^{B28}$-human insulin (NovoRapid® or NovoLog®; insulin aspart; Novo Nordisk A/S,

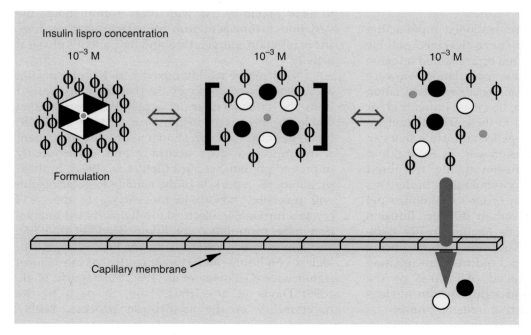

**Figure 5** ■ A schematic representation of insulin lispro dissociation after subcutaneous administration.

Corporate Headquarters, Novo Allé, Bagsvaerd, Denmark) (Brange et al., 1988, 1990) involves the replacement of Pro$^{B28}$ with a negatively charged aspartic acid residue. Like Lys$^{B28}$Pro$^{B29}$-human insulin, Asp$^{B28}$-human insulin has a more rapid time-action following subcutaneous injection (Heinemann et al., 1997). This rapid action is achieved through a reduction in the self-association behavior compared to human insulin (Brange et al., 1990; Whittingham et al., 1998). The other rapid-acting analog, Lys$^{B3}$-Glu$^{B29}$-human insulin (Apidra$^{TM}$, insulin glulisine; Sanofi-Aventis), involves a substitution of the lysine residue at position 29 of the B-chain with a negatively charged glutamic acid. Additionally, this analog replaces the Asn$^{B3}$ with a positively charged lysine. Scientific reports describing the impact of these changes on the molecular properties of this analog are lacking. However, the glutamic acid substitution occurs at a position known to be involved in dimer formation (Brange et al., 1990) and may result in disruption of key interactions at the monomer–monomer interface. The Asn residue at position 3 of the B-chain plays no direct role in insulin self-association (Brange et al., 1990), but it is flanked by two amino acids involved in the assembly of the $Zn^{2+}$ insulin hexamer. Despite the limited physicochemical information on insulin glulisine, studies conducted in persons with either Type 1 or Type 2 diabetes (Dailey et al., 2004; Dreyer et al., 2005) confirm the analog displays similar pharmacological properties as insulin lispro. Interestingly, insulin glulisine is not formulated in the presence of zinc as are the other rapid-acting analogs. Instead, insulin glulisine is formulated in the presence of a stabilizing agent (polysorbate 20) (Table 3). The surfactant in the formulation presumably minimizes higher order association and contributes to more rapid adsorption of the monomeric species.

In addition to the aforementioned rapid-acting formulations, manufacturers have designed soluble formulations for use in external or implanted infusion pumps. In most respects, these formulations are very similar to Regular insulin (i.e., hexameric association state, preservative, and zinc); however, buffer and/or surfactants may be included in these formulations to minimize the physical aggregation of insulin that can lead to clogging of the infusion sets. In early pump systems, gas-permeable infusion tubing was used with the external pumps. Consequently a buffer was added to the formulation in order to minimize pH changes due to dissolved carbon dioxide. Infusion tubing composed of materials having greater resistance to carbon dioxide diffusion is currently being used and the potential for pH-induced precipitation of insulin is greatly reduced. All three of the commercially available rapid-acting insulin analogs are approved for use in external infusion pumps.

## ■ Intermediate-Acting Insulin Formulations

There are two widely used types of intermediate-acting insulin preparations: Neutral Protamine Hagedorn (NPH) and Lente. Both formulations achieve extended time-action by necessitating the dissolution of a precipitated and/or crystalline form of insulin. This dissolution is presumed to be the rate-limiting step in the absorption of intermediate- and long-acting insulin. Consequently, the time-action of the formulation is prolonged by further delaying the dissociation of the hexamer into dimers and monomers.

NPH, named after its inventor H.C. Hagedorn (Hagedorn et al., 1936), is a neutral crystalline suspension that is prepared by the cocrystallization of insulin with protamine. Protamine consists of a closely related group of very basic proteins that are isolated from fish sperm. Protamine is heterogeneous in composition; however, four primary components have been identified and show a high degree of sequence homology (Hoffmann et al., 1990). In general, protamine is ~30 amino acids in length and has an amino acid composition that is primarily composed of arginine, 65–70%. Using crystallization conditions identified by Krayenbühl and Rosenberg (1946), oblong tetragonal NPH insulin crystals with volumes between 1 and $20\,\mu m^3$ can be consistently prepared from protamine and insulin (Deckert, 1980). These formulations, by design, have very minimal levels of soluble insulin or protamine in solution. The condition at which no measurable protamine or insulin exists in solution after crystallization is referred to as the isophane point.

NPH has an onset of action from 1 to 2 hr, peak activity from 2 to 8 hr, and duration of activity from 14 to 24 hr (Table 2). As with other formulations, the variations in time-action are due to factors such as dose, site of injection, temperature, and the patient's physical activity.

NPH can be readily mixed with Regular insulin either extemporaneously by the patient or as obtained from the manufacturer in a premixed formulation (Table 2). Premixed insulin, e.g., 70/30 or 50/50 NPH/Regular, has been shown to provide the patient with improved dose accuracy and consequently improved glycemic control (Bell et al., 1991). In these preparations, a portion of the soluble Regular insulin will reversibly adsorb to the surface of the NPH crystals through an electrostatically mediated interaction under formulation conditions (Dodd et al., 1995); however, this adsorption is reversible under physiological conditions and consequently has no clinical significance (Galloway et al., 1982; Hamaguchi et al., 1990; Davis et al., 1991). Due, in part, to the reversibility of the adsorption process, NPH/

Regular mixtures are uniquely stable and have a two-year shelf life.

The rapid-acting insulin analog, insulin lispro, can be extemporaneously mixed with NPH; however, such mixtures must be injected immediately upon preparation due to the potential for exchange between the soluble and suspension components upon long-term storage. Exchange refers to the release of human insulin from the NPH crystals into the solution phase and concomitant loss of the analog into the crystalline phase. The presence of human insulin in solution could diminish the rapid time-action effect of the analog. One way to overcome the problem of exchange is to prepare mixtures containing the same insulin species in both the suspension and the solution phases, analogous to human insulin Regular/NPH preparations. However, this approach requires an NPH-like preparation of the rapid-acting analog.

An NPH-like suspension of $Lys^{B28}$, $Pro^{B29}$-human insulin has been prepared and its physicochemical properties relative to human insulin NPH have been described (DeFelippis et al., 1998). In order to prepare the appropriate crystalline form of the analog, significant modifications to the NPH crystallization procedure are required. The differences between the crystallization conditions have been proposed to result from the reduced self-association properties of $Lys^{B28}$, $Pro^{B29}$-human insulin.

Pharmacological studies reported for the $Lys^{B28}$, $Pro^{B29}$-human insulin NPH-like suspension, commonly referred to as neutral protamine lispro (NPL) (Janssen et al., 1997; DeFelippis et al., 1998) indicate that the pharmacokinetic and pharmacodynamic properties of this analog suspension are analogous to human insulin NPH. The availability of NPL suspension allows for the preparation of homogeneous, biphasic mixture preparations containing intermediate-acting NPL and rapid-acting solutions of $Lys^{B28}$, $Pro^{B29}$-human insulin that are not impacted by exchange between solution and crystalline forms.

As with $Lys^{B28}$, $Pro^{B29}$-human insulin, premixed formulations of the $Asp^{B28}$-human insulin have been prepared in which rapid-acting soluble insulin aspart has been combined with a protamine-retarded crystalline preparation of insulin aspart (Balschmidt, 1996). Clinical data on $Lys^{B28}$, $Pro^{B29}$-human insulin mixtures and those composed of $Asp^{B28}$-insulin have been reported in the literature (Weyer et al., 1997; Heise et al., 1998). The pharmacological properties of the rapid-acting analogs are preserved in these stable mixtures (Table 3). Premixed formulations of both rapid-acting analogs are now commercially available in many countries.

Immunogenicity issues with protamine have been documented in a small percentage of diabetic patients (Kurtz et al., 1983; Nell and Thomas, 1988). Individuals who show sensitivity to the protamine in NPH formulations are routinely switched to Lente or Ultralente preparations to control their basal glucose levels.

Lente insulin is a zinc insulin suspension that was designed for single daily injection (Hallas-Møller et al., 1952). Lente insulin is a mixture of two insoluble forms of insulin, 70% rhombohedral zinc insulin crystals (Ultralente component) and 30% amorphous insulin particles (Semilente component). The pH of the formulation is neutral and contains acetate and excess zinc. The surplus zinc in the formulation presumably binds to weak-binding metal sites on the insulin hexamer surface, reducing the solubility of the insulin, and thus slowing the time-action of the insulin (Deckert, 1980). The crystal volume of the Ultralente component is routinely between 200 and 1200 $\mu m^3$ (Deckert, 1980).

Lente has an onset of action of 1–2 hr, peak activity from 3 to 10 hr, and duration of action from 20 to 24 hr (Table 2). As with other formulations, the variations in observed time-action are due to factors such as dose, site of injection, temperature, and the patient's physical activity.

The mixability of Lente with Regular insulin is restricted to extemporaneous mixtures that are used immediately upon preparation (Deckert, 1980; Galloway et al., 1982). Prolonged storage of Lente/Regular insulin mixtures leads to a change in the course of effect due to precipitation of the insulin from the Regular section (Deckert, 1980). The precipitation of Regular insulin is presumably due to binding of the surplus zinc found in the Lente formulation to weak-binding sites on the insulin hexamer. Use of Lente insulin among persons with diabetes continues to decline and its continued commercial viability is in doubt.

## ■ Long-Acting Insulin Formulations

The normal human pancreas secretes approximately 1 unit of insulin (0.035 mg) per hour to maintain basal glycemic control. Adequate basal insulin levels are a critical component of diabetes therapy because they regulate hepatic glucose output, which is essential for energy production by the brain. Consequently, long-acting insulin formulation must provide a very different pharmacokinetic profile than "meal-time" insulin formulation.

There are three long-acting insulin preparations currently commercially available: Ultralente, which was developed in the 1950s and two insulin analogs, Lantus® (insulin glargine) and Levemir® (insulin detemir), which have been recently approved (Table 1; Fig. 1). Ultralente and Lantus derive their protracted time-action profiles from the slow and relatively constant dissolution of solid particles in the subcutaneous tissue. This slow dissolution precedes the dissociation of insulin into absorbable units, and thus the *rate of absorption* (units per hour) into the bloodstream is significantly decreased in comparison to that of a solution (mealtime) formulation. Levemir, on the other hand, achieves its protracted effect by a combination of structural interactions and physiological binding events (Havelund et al., 2004).

Ultralente is analogous to NPH insulin in that they are both formulated as crystalline insulin suspensions. However, the preparations differ in several key aspects. For one, under microscopic examination, the larger rhombohedral Ultralente microcrystals are notably different than the much smaller rod-shaped NPH microcrystals. This difference originates from the different crystallization conditions employed to prepare these formulations as well as the excipients used. Ultralente contains no protamine and is crystallized at pH 5.5 in the presence of zinc, NaCl, and acetate buffer. The subsequent formulation process involves adjustment of the pH to a final value of 7.4, with the addition of excess zinc and methylparaben as an antimicrobial agent (preservative). The different formulation excipients used for Ultralente in comparison to NPH are a reflection of the different way in which the insulin molecules are complexed into the respective crystal lattices. NPH crystals are believed to be composed of zinc insulin hexamers stabilized as a complex with protamine and preservative molecules (Balschmidt et al., 1991), whereas, Ultralente crystals incorporate zinc insulin hexamers only (Brange, 1987a; Yip et al., 1998). A consequence of this composition is that methylparaben must be utilized as the preservative for Ultralente formulations because, unlike phenol and m-cresol, it does not interact with and destabilize the Ultralente crystal lattice.

As with all suspension products, Ultralente insulin should be uniformly resuspended prior to withdrawal of the dose from the vial to ensure accurate dosage. Ultralente has an onset of action of 0.5 to 3 hr, peak activity between 4 and 20 hr, and duration of action from 20 to 36 hr (Table 2). Similar to other insulin formulations, the variations in time-action are due to factors such as dose, site of injection, temperature, and the patient's physical activity. Ultralente may be mixed with Regular insulin and Humalog, although its use in mixtures is constrained to extemporaneous mixing with immediate use for the reasons outlined for Lente. Much like the Lente insulin formulation use of Ultralente is declining and its commercial manufacturing may soon cease.

Insulin glargine (Lantus; $Gly^{A21}$, $Arg^{B31}$, $Arg^{B32}$ human insulin; Sanofi-Aventis), is a long-acting insulin analog, whose amino acid sequence modifications are highlighted in Table 1 and Figure 1. This analog differs from human insulin in that the amino acid asparagine is replaced with glycine at position A21 and two arginine residues have been added to the C-terminus of the B-chain. The impact of the additional arginine residues is to shift the pI from a pH of 5.4 to 6.7, thereby producing an insulin analog that is soluble at acidic pH values, but is less soluble at the neutral pH of subcutaneous tissue. Lantus is a solution formulation prepared under acidic conditions, pH 4.0. The introduction of glycine at position A21 yields a protein with acceptable chemical stability under acidic formulation conditions, since the native asparagine is susceptible to acid-mediated degradation and reduced potency. Thus, the changes to the molecular sequence of insulin have been made to improve chemical stability and to modulate absorption from the subcutaneous tissue, resulting in an analog that has approximately the same potency as human insulin. The Lantus formulation is a clear solution that incorporates zinc and m-cresol (preservative) at a pH value of 4. Consequently, Lantus does not need to be resuspended prior to dosing. Immediately following injection into the subcutaneous tissue, the insulin glargine precipitates due to the pH change, forming a slowly dissolving precipitate. This results in a relatively constant rate of absorption over 10.8 to 24 hr with no pronounced peak (Table 3). This profile allows once-daily dosing as a patient's basal insulin. As with all insulin preparations, the time course of Lantus may vary in different individuals or at different times in the same individual and the rate of absorption is dependent on blood supply, temperature, and the patient's physical activity. Lantus should not be diluted or mixed with any other solution or insulin, as will be discussed below.

Insulin detemir (Levemir; $Lys^{B29}$(*N*-tetradecanoyl)des(B30)human insulin; Novo-Nordisk A/S) utilizes acylation of insulin with a fatty acid moiety as a means to achieve a protracted pharmacological effect. As shown in Table 1 and Figure 1, the B30 threonine residue of human insulin is eliminated in insulin detemir and a 14-carbon, myristoyl fatty acid is covalently attached to the ε-amino group of $Lys^{B29}$. The analog forms a zinc hexamer at neutral pH in a preserved solution. Clinical studies have reported that insulin detemir displays lower pharmacokinetic and pharmacodynamic variability than NPH (Hermansen et al., 2001; Vague et al., 2003). An approximate description of the pharmacodynamic profile of Levemir is listed in Table 3. This analog appears to display a slower onset of action than NPH without a pronounced peak (Heinemann et al., 1999). However, whether the duration of the protracted effect can truly be considered sufficient enough to warrant classification of insulin detemir as a long-acting insulin remains a subject of debate since published clinical studies of this insulin analog are typically referenced to intermediate-acting NPH.

Binding of the tetradecanoyl-acylated insulin to albumin was originally proposed as the underlying mechanism behind the observed prolonged effect for the modified insulin analog; however, recent investigations on insulin detemir have determined that the mechanism is more complex (Havelund et al., 2004). It has been proposed that subcutaneous absorption is initially delayed as a result of hexamer stability and dihexamerization. Such interactions between hexamers are a likely consequence of the symmetrical arrangement of fatty acid moieties around the outside of the hexamers (Whittingham et al., 2004), as shown by X-ray crystallographic studies. These associated forms further bind to albumin within the injection site depot. Additional prolongation may result due to albumin binding.

## PHARMACEUTICAL CONCERNS

### ■ Chemical Stability of Insulin Formulations

Insulin has two primary routes of chemical degradation upon storage and use: hydrolytic transformation of amide to acid groups and formation of covalent dimers and higher order polymers. Primarily the pH, the storage temperature, and the components of the specific formulation influence the rate of formation of these degradation products. The purity of insulin formulations is typically assessed by high-performance liquid chromatography using reversed-phase and size exclusion separation modes (USP Monographs: Insulin, 2006). In acidic solution, the main degradation reaction is the transformation of asparagine (Asn) at the terminal 21 position of the A-chain to aspartic acid. This reaction is relatively facile at low pH, but is extremely slow at neutral pH (Brange et al., 1992b). This was the primary degradation route in early soluble (acidic) insulin formulations. However, the development of neutral solutions and suspensions has diminished the importance of this degradation route. Stability studies of neutral solutions indicate that the amount of A21 desamido insulin does not change upon storage. Thus, the relatively small amounts of this bioactive material present in the formulation arise either from the source insulin or from pharmaceutical process operations.

The deamidation of the $Asn^{B3}$ of the B-chain is the primary degradation mechanism at neutral pH. The reaction proceeds through the formation of a cyclic imide that results in two products, aspartic acid (Asp) and iso-aspartic acid (iso-Asp) (Brennan and Clarke, 1994). This reaction occurs relatively slowly in neutral solution (approximately 1/12 the rate of A21 desamido formation in acid solution) (Brange et al., 1992b). The relative amounts of these products are influenced by the flexibility of the B-chain, with approximate ratios of Asp:iso-Asp of 1:2 and 2:1 for solution and crystalline formulations, respectively. As noted earlier, the use of phenolic preservatives provides a stabilizing effect on the insulin hexamer that reduces the formation of the cyclic imide, as evidenced by reduced deamidation. The rate of formation also depends on temperature; typical rates of formation are approximately 2% per year at 5°C. Studies have shown B3 deamidated insulin to be essentially fully potent (Chance, 1995).

High-molecular-weight protein (HMWP) products form at both storage and room temperatures. Covalent dimers that form between two insulin molecules are the primary condensation products in marketed insulin products. There is evidence that insulin-protamine heterodimers also form in NPH suspensions (Brange et al., 1992a). At higher temperatures, the probability of forming higher order insulin oligomers increases. The rate of formation of HMWP is less than that of hydrolytic reactions; typical rates are less than 0.5% per year for soluble neutral Regular insulin formulations at 5°C. The rate of formation can be affected by the strength of the insulin formulation or by the addition of glycerol as an isotonicity agent. The latter increases the rate of HMWP formation presumably by introducing impurities such as glyceraldehyde. HMWP formation is believed to also occur as a result of a reaction between the N-terminal B1 phenylalanine amino group and the C-terminal A21 asparagine of a second insulin molecule (Darrington and Anderson, 1995).

Disulfide exchange leading to polymer formation is also possible at basic pH; however, the rate for these reactions is very slow under neutral pH formulation conditions. The quality of excipients such as glycerol is also critical because small amounts of aldehyde and other glycerol-related chemical impurities can accelerate the formation of HMWP. The biopotency of HMWP is significantly less (1/10 to 1/5 of insulin) than monomeric species (Chance, 1995).

Unfortunately, no chemical stability data has been published with regard to the insulin analog formulations containing insulin lispro, insulin aspart, insulin glulisine, insulin glargine, or insulin detemir; however, it is reasonable to presume that similar chemical degradation pathways are present to varying extents in these compounds. Moreover, since some analogs are formulated under acidic conditions, e.g., Lantus is formulated at pH 4.0, or have been modified with hydrophobic moieties, e.g., Levemir, it is reasonable to presume that alternate chemical degradation pathways may be operable.

## Physical Stability of Insulin Formulations

The physical stability of insulin formulations is mediated by noncovalent aggregation of insulin. Hydrophobic forces typically drive the aggregation although electrostatics plays a subtle but important role. Aggregation typically leads to a loss in potency of the formulation, and therefore should be avoided. Extreme aggregation may lead to the formation of fibrils of insulin. The physical stability of insulin formulations is readily assessed by visual observation for macroscopic characteristics as well as by instrumental methods such as light and differential phase contrast microscopy. Various particle-sizing techniques also may be used to characterize microscopic phenomena.

In general, insulin solutions have good physical stability. Physical changes in soluble formulations may be manifested as color or clarity change or, in extreme situations, the formation of a precipitate. Insulin suspensions, such as NPH or Lente, are the most susceptible to changes in physical stability. These typically occur as a result of both elevated temperature and mechanical stress to the suspension. The increase in temperature favors hydrophobic interactions, while mechanical agitation serves to provide mixing and stress across interfacial boundaries. Nucleation of aggregation in suspensions can lead to conditions described as visible clumping of the suspension or "frosting" of the glass wall of the insulin vial by aggregates. In severe cases, resuspension may be nearly impossible because of caking of the suspension in the vial. Temperatures above normal ambient (>25°C) can accelerate the aggregation process, especially those at or above body temperature (37°C). Normal mechanical mixing of suspensions prior to administration is not deleterious to physical stability. However, vigorous shaking or mixing should be avoided. Consequently, this latter constraint has, in part, led to the observation that patients do not place enough effort into resuspension. Thus, proper emphasis must be placed on training the patient in resuspension of crystalline, amorphous, and premixed formulations of insulin and insulin analogs. The necessity of rigorous resuspension may be the first sign of aggregation and should prompt a careful examination of the formulation to verify its suitability for use.

As with the chemical stability data, information regarding the physical stability of the newer insulin analog formulations containing insulin lispro, insulin aspart, insulin glulisine, insulin glargine, or insulin detemir, have yet to be published. However, it is reasonable to assume that similar constraints regarding extreme agitation and thermal excursions should be avoided to minimize undesirable physical transformations such as precipitation, aggregation, gelation, or fibrillation.

## CLINICAL AND PRACTICE ASPECTS

### Vial Presentations

Insulin is commonly available in 10-mL vials. In the United States, a strength of U-100 (100 U/mL) is the standard, whereas outside the United States both U-100 and U-40 (40 U/mL) are commonly used. It is essential to obtain the proper strength and formulation of insulin in order to maintain glycemic control. In addition, species and brand/method of manufacture are important. Any change in insulin should be made cautiously and only under medical supervision (Galloway, 1988; Brackenridge, 1994). Common formulations, such as Regular, NPH, and Lente, are listed in Table 2 and the newer insulin analog formulations are listed in Table 3. Mixtures of rapid- or fast-acting with intermediate-acting insulin formulation, e.g., NPH/Regular 70/30, NPH/Regular 50/50, Humalog Mix 75/25, and NovoLog Mix 70/30, are a popular choice for glycemic control. The ratio is defined as ratio of protamine-containing fraction/rapid-or fast-acting fraction, e.g., Humalog Mix 75/25 where 75% of a dose is available as insulin lispro protamine suspension and 25% insulin lispro for injection. With regards to NPH:Regular mixtures, caution must be used in the nomenclature because it may vary depending on the country of sale and the governing pharmacopeial body. In the United States, for example, the predominant species is listed first as in N/R 70/30, but in Europe the same formulation is described as R/N 30/70 (Soluble/Isophane) where the base ("normal") ingredient is listed first. Currently an effort is being made to standardize worldwide to the European nomenclature. Mixtures available in the United States include N/R 70/30 and 50/50 while Europe has R/N 10/90, 20/80, 30/70, 40/60, and 50/50.

### Injectors

Insulin syringes should be purchased to match the strength of the insulin that is to be administered (e.g., for U-100 strength use 30- or 100-unit syringes designated for U-100). The gauge of needles available for insulin administration has been reduced to very fine gauges (30–31 gauges) in order to minimize pain during injection. The use of a new needle for each dose maintains the sharp point of the needle and ensures a sterile needle for the injection.

In recent years the availability of insulin pen injectors has made dosing and compliance easier for the patient with diabetes. The first pen injector used a 1.5-mL cartridge of U-100 insulin. A needle was attached to the end of the pen, and the proper dose was selected and then injected by the patient. The cartridge was replaced when the contents were exhausted, typically 3 to 7 days. Currently, 3.0-mL cartridges in U-100 strength for Regular, NPH, and the range of N/R mixtures have become the market standard with regard to size and strength. The advantages of the pen injectors are primarily better compliance for the patient through a variety of factors including more accurate and reproducible dose control, easier transport of the drug, more discrete dose administration, timelier dose administration, and greater convenience.

## ■ Continuous Subcutaneous Insulin Infusion—External Pumps

As previously mentioned, solution formulations of human insulin specifically designed for continuous subcutaneous insulin infusion (CSII) are commercially available. CSII systems were traditionally used by a small population of diabetic patients, but have become more popular with the recent introduction of rapid-acting insulin analogs. Currently, all three rapid-acting insulin analog formulations have received regulatory approval for this mode of delivery; however, specific in vitro data demonstrating the appropriate physicochemical stability for CSII has only been reported for insulin lispro (DeFelippis et al., 2006). Pump devices contain glass or plastic reservoirs that must be hand-filled from vial presentations by the patient. Some pumps have been specifically designed to accept the same glass 3-mL cartridges used in pen injector systems. Due to concerns over the impact of elevated temperature exposure and mechanical stress on the integrity of the insulin molecule along with the increased risk of microbial contamination, reservoirs, infusion sets, catheters and insulin must be replaced and a new infusion site selected every 48 hr or less.

## ■ Noninvasive Delivery

Since the discovery of insulin there has been a strong desire to overcome the need for injection-based therapy. Progress has been made in the form of needle-free injector systems (Robertson et al., 2000), but these devices have not gained widespread acceptance presumably because administration is not entirely pain free, device costs are high and other factors make it less desirable than traditional injection. Extensive research efforts have also focused on noninvasive routes of administration with attempts made to demonstrate the feasibility of transdermal, nasal, buccal, ocular, pulmonary, oral and even rectal delivery of insulin. Unfortunately, most attempts failed to progress beyond the proof of concept stage because low bioavailability, dose response variability

and other adverse factors seriously called into question commercial viability. This situation has changed for pulmonary and buccal delivery of insulin as products for these routes of administration have been recently approved by regulatory authorities.

Several pulmonary delivery systems specifically aimed at insulin administration have advanced sufficiently through development to enable more extensive studies in human clinical trials and comprehensive reviews examining this work in detail are available (Patton et al., 1999, 2004; Cefalu, 2004). While many of these technologies continue to advance through late-stage development, one insulin pulmonary delivery system, referred to as Exubera®, has recently received regulatory approval in both Europe and the United States. Exubera consists of a dry powder insulin formulation composed of small geometric diameter particles produced by spray drying (Patton, 1998). The powder formulation is packaged into individual blisters and combined with an active device that incorporates a mechanical energy source to achieve dispersion and aerosolization of the particles.

Based on the published clinical trial information, some generalizations about pulmonary insulin administration can be made (Heinemann et al., 2001; Patton et al., 2004). The pharmacokinetic profile of inhaled insulin is characterized by a faster onset compared to subcutaneous administration of solution insulin formulations and at least as fast as rapid-acting insulin analogs; thus, the current delivery systems and formulations are targeted at controlling postprandial glucose excursions. Duration of action is intermediate between that of subcutaneously administered rapid-acting insulin analogs and regular insulin. While the pharmacological properties reported for inhaled insulin seems appropriate to meet prandial insulin requirements, it will not address basal insulin needs. In certain treatment regimes, an injection of a long-acting (basal) insulin preparation will still be required to adequately manage blood glucose levels. Intrapatient variability in pharmacokinetic and pharmacodynamic responses for pulmonary-delivered insulin is low and similar to subcutaneously administered insulin. Estimated bioavailabilities are typically in the range of approximately 10–20% relative to insulin administered by subcutaneous injection. In special patient populations such as smokers, absorption of insulin is significantly greater (Himmelmann et al., 2003) when administered by the pulmonary route. Alterations in pharmacological responses have been similarly observed in other studies conducted in elderly subjects, asthmatics, or individuals with acute respiratory tract infections (Patton et al., 2004). Now that a pulmonary insulin product is commercially available, knowledge about this noninvasive route of administration will continue to increase as broader patient experience is obtained.

In addition to pulmonary insulin, a buccal insulin product, referred to as Oralin™, has been developed consisting of a solution formulation of insulin containing various absorption enhancers needed to achieve mucosal absorption (Modi et al., 2002) and a metered dose inhaler is used to administer a fine mist into the oral cavity. Clinical study results evaluating this buccal delivery system in healthy subjects as well as patients with Type 1 and Type 2 diabetes have been reported (Modi et al., 2002; Cernea et al., 2004). While Oralin has only achieved regulatory approval in Ecuador, it is unknown if the product will have similar success with regulatory agencies in the United States or Europe.

## ■ Storage

Insulin formulations should be stored in a cool place that avoids direct sunlight. Vials or cartridges that are not in active use should be stored under refrigerated (2–8°C) conditions. Vials or cartridges in active use may be stored at ambient temperature. High temperatures, such as those found in non-air-conditioned vehicles in the summer, should be avoided. Insulin formulations should not be frozen; if this occurs, the product should be disposed immediately. Insulin formulations should never be purchased or used past the expiration date on the package.

## ■ Usage

### Resuspension

Insulin suspensions (e.g., NPH, Premixtures, Lente, Ultralente) should be resuspended by gentle back-and-forth mixing and rolling of the vial between the palms to obtain a uniform, milky suspension. The patient should be advised of the resuspension technique for specific insoluble insulin and insulin analog formulations, which is detailed in the package insert. The homogeneity of suspensions is critical to obtaining an accurate dose. Any suspension that fails to provide a homogeneous dispersion of particles should not be used. Cartridges in pen injectors may be suspended in the same manner. However, the smaller size of the container and shape of the injector device may require slight modification of the resuspension method. A glass bead is typically added to cartridges to aid in the resuspension of suspension formulations.

### Dosing

Dose withdrawal should immediately follow the resuspension of any insulin suspension, especially Lente and Ultralente formulations because they settle relatively quickly. The patient should be instructed by his or her doctor, pharmacist, or nurse educator in proper procedures for dose administration. Of particular importance are procedures for disinfecting the container top and injection site. The patient is also advised to use a new needle and syringe for each injection. Reuse of these components, even after cleaning, may lead to contamination of the insulin formulation by microorganisms or by other materials, such as cleaning agents.

### Extemporaneous Mixing

As discussed above in the section on "Intermediate- and Long-acting Insulin Preparations," Regular insulin can be mixed in the syringe with NPH, Lente, and Ultralente. However, only the Regular/NPH mixtures are stable enough to be stored for extended periods of time. The Lente/Regular and Ultralente/Regular formulations can be prepared but *must* be used immediately. Otherwise, the time-action of the Regular component can be affected.

With regards to extemporaneously mixing of the newer insulin analogs, caution must be used. Lantus, due to its acidic pH, should not be mixed with other fast- or rapid-acting insulin formulations which are formulated under neutral pH. If Lantus is mixed with other insulin formulations, the solution may become cloudy due to pI precipitation of both the insulin glargine and the fast- or rapid-acting insulin resulting from pH changes. Consequently, the pharmacokinetic/pharmacodynamic profile, e.g., onset of action, time to peak effect, of Lantus and/or the mixed insulin may be altered in an unpredictable manner. With regard to rapid-acting insulin analogs, extemporaneous mixing with human insulin NPH formulations is acceptable if used immediately. Not under any circumstances should these formulations be stored, as human insulin and insulin analog exchange can occur between solution and the crystalline matter thereby potentially altering time-action profiles of the solution insulin analog. With regard to Levemir, mixing restrictions have not been reported.

## REFERENCES

Anderson JH Jr, Brunelle RL, Keohane P, Koivisto VA, Trautmann ME, Vignati L, et al. Mealtime treatment with insulin analog improves postprandial hyperglycemia and hypoglycemia in patients with non-insulin-dependent diabetes mellitus. Multicenter Insulin Lispro Study Group. Arch Intern Med 1997; 157:1249–55.

Baker EN, Blundell TL, Cutfield JF, Cutfield SM, Dodson EJ, Dodson GG, et al. The structure of 2Zn pig insulin crystals at 1.5 Å resolution. Philos Trans R Soc Lond B 1988; 319:369–456.

Balschmidt P, Benned Hansen F, Dodson EJ, Dodson GG, Korber F. Structure of porcine insulin cocrystallized with clupeine-Z. Acta Crystallogr B 1991; B47: 975–86.

Balschmidt P. (1996) AspB28 Insulin Crystals. United States Patent 5;547:930.

Bell DSH, Clements RS, Perentesis G, Roddam R, Wagenknecht L. Dosage accuracy of self-mixed vs premixed insulin. Arch Intern Med 1991; 151:2265–9.

Bliss M. Who discovered insulin. In: The discovery of insulin. Toronto: McClelland and Stewart Limited; 1982. p. 189–211.

Brackenridge B. Diabetes medicines: insulin. In: Brackenridge B, editor. Managing your diabetes. Indianapolis (Indiana, USA): Eli Lilly and Company; 1994. p. 36–50.

Brader ML, Dunn MF. Insulin hexamers: new conformations and applications. TIBS 1991; 16:341–5.

Brange J. Insulin preparations. In: Galenics of insulin. Berlin: Springer-Verlag; 1987a. p. 17–39.

Brange J. Production of bovine and porcine insulin. In: Galenics of Insulin. Berlin: Springer-Verlag; 1987b. p. 1–5.

Brange J, Havelund S, Hougaard P. Chemical stability of insulin. 2. Formation of higher molecular weight transformation products during storage of pharmaceutical preparations. Pharm Res 1992a; 9:727–34.

Brange J, Langkjær L, Havelund S, Vølund A. Chemical stability of insulin. 1. Hydrolytic degradation during storage of pharmaceutical preparations. Pharm Res 1992b; 9:715–26.

Brange J Langkjær L. Chemical stability of insulin. 3. Influence of excipients, formulation, and pH. Acta Pharm Nord 1992; 4:149–58.

Brange J, Owens DR, Kang S, Vølund A. Monomeric insulins and their experimental and clinical applications. Diabetes Care 1990; 13:923–54.

Brange J, Ribel U, Hansen JF, Dodson G, Hansen MT, Havelund S, et al. Monomeric insulins obtained by protein engineering and their medical implications. Nature 1988; 333:679–82.

Brems DN, Alter LA, Beckage MJ, Chance RE, DiMarchi RD, Green LK, et al. Altering the association properties of insulin by amino acid replacement. Prot Eng 1992; 6:527–33.

Brennan TV, Clarke S. Deamidation and isoasparate formation in model synthetic peptides. In Aswad DW, editor. Deamidation and isoaspartate formation in peptides and proteins. Boca Raton (Florida, USA): CRC Press; 1994. p. 65–90.

Cefalu WT. Concept, strategies, and feasibility of noninvasive insulin delivery. Diabetes Care 2004; 27:239–46.

Cernea S, Kidron M, Wohlgelernter J, Modi P, Raz I. Comparison of pharmacokinetic and pharmacodynamic properties of single-dose oral insulin spray and subcutaneous insulin injection in healthy subjects using the euglycemic clamp technique. Clin Ther 2004; 26:2084–91.

Chance RE. Bioactivity data for insulin related substances. Personal Communication. Indianapolis (Indiana, USA): Eli Lilly and Company; 1995.

Ciszak E, Beals JM, Baker JC, Carter ND, Frank BH, Smith GD. The role of the C-terminal B-chain residues in insulin assembly: the structure of hexameric LysB28ProB29-human insulin. Structure 1995; 3:615–22.

Dailey G, Rosenstock J, Moses RG, Ways K. Insulin glulisine provides improved glycemic control in patients with type 2 diabetes. Diabetes Care 2004; 27:2363–8.

Darrington RT, Anderson BD. Effects of insulin concentration and self-association on the partitioning of its A-21 cyclic anhydride intermediate to desamido insulin and covalent dimer. Pharmcol Res 1995; 12:1077–84.

Davis SN, Thompson CJ, Brown MD, Home PD, Alberti KGMM. A comparison of the pharmacokinetics and metabolic effects of Human Regular and NPH mixtures. Diabetes Res Clin Pract 1991; 13:107–18.

Deckert T. Intermediate-acting insulin preparations: NPH and Lente. Diabetes Care 1980; 3:623–6.

DeFelippis MR, Bakaysa DL, Bell MA, Heady MA, Li S, Pye S, et al. Preparation and characterization of a cocrystalline suspension of [LysB28,ProB29]-human insulin analogue. J Pharm Sci 1998; 87:170–6.

DeFelippis MR, Bell MA, Heyob JA, Storms SM. In vitro stability of insulin lispro in continuous subcutaneous insulin infusion. Diabetes Technol Ther 2006 (June); 8(3): 358–68.

Derewenda U, Derewenda Z, Dodson EJ, Dodson GG, Reynolds CD, Smith GD, et al. Phenol stabilizes more helix in a new symmetrical zinc insulin hexamer. Nature 1989; 338:594–6.

Dodd SW, Havel HA, Kovach PM, Lakshminarayan C, Redmon MP, Sargeant CM, et al. Reversible adsorption of soluble hexameric insulin onto the surface of insulin crystals cocrystallized with protamine: an electrostatic interaction. Pharmcol Res 1995; 12:60–8.

Dreyer M, Prager R, Robinson A, Busch K, Ellis G, Souhami E, et al. Efficacy and safety of insulin glulisine in patients with type 1 diabetes. Horm Metab Res 2005; 37:702–7.

Galloway JA. Chemistry and clinical use of insulin. In: Galloway JA, Potvin JH, Shuman CR, editors. Diabetes mellitus. 9th ed. Indianapolis (Indiana, USA): Lilly Research Laboratories; 1988. p. 105–33.

Galloway JA, Chance RE. Improving insulin therapy: achievements and challenges. Horm Metab Res 1994; 26:591–8.

Galloway JA, Spradlin CT, Jackson RL, Otto DC, Bechtel LD. Mixtures of intermediate-acting insulin (NPH and Lente) with regular insulin: an update. In: Skyler JS, editor. Insulin update: 1982. Princeton: Exerpta Medica; 1982. p. 111–9.

Goldman J, Carpenter FH. Zinc binding, circular dichroism, and equilibrium sedimentation studies on insulin (bovine) and several of its derivatives. Biochemistry 1974; 13:4566–74.

Hagedorn HC, Jensen BN, Krarup NB, Wodstrup I. Protamine insulinate. JAMA 1936; 106:177–80.

Hallas–Møller K, Jersild M, Petersen K, Schlichtkrull J. Zinc insulin preparations for single daily injection. JAMA 1952; 150:1667–71.

Hamaguchi T, Hashimoto Y, Miyata T, Kishikawa H, Yano T, Fukushima H, et al. Effect of mixing short and intermediate NPH insulin or Zn insulin suspension acting Human insulin on plasma free insulin levels and action profiles. J Jpn Diabet Soc 1990; 33:223–9.

Havelund S, Plum A, Ribel U, Jonassen I, Vølund A, Markussen J, et al. The mechanism of protraction of insulin detemir, a long-acting, acylated analog of human insulin. Pharmcol Res 2004; 21:1498–504.

Heinemann L, Pfützner A, Heise T. Alternative routes of administration as an approach to improve insulin therapy: update on dermal, oral, nasal and pulmonary insulin delivery. Curr Pharm Des 2001; 7:1327–51.

Heinemann L, Sinha K, Weyer C, Loftager M, Hirschberger S, Heise T. Time-action profile of the soluble, fatty acid acylated, long-acting insulin analogue NN304. Diabet Med 1999; 16:332–8.

Heinemann L, Weyer C, Rave K, Stiefelhagen O, Rauhaus M, Heise T. Comparison of the time-action profiles of U40- and U100-regular human insulin and the rapid-acting insulin analogue B28 Asp. Exp Clin Endocrinol Diabetes 1997; 105:140–4.

Heise T, Weyer C, Serwas A, Heinrichs S, Osinga J, Roach P, et al. Time-action profiles of novel premixed preparations of insulin lispro and NPL insulin. Diabetes Care 1998; 21:800–3.

Hermansen K, Madsbad S, Perrild H, Kristensen A, Axelsen M. Comparison of the soluble basal insulin analog insulin detemir with NPH insulin: a randomized open crossover trial in type 1 diabetic subjects on basal-bolus therapy. Diabetes Care 2001; 24:296–301.

Himmelmann A, Jendle J, Mellén A, Petersen AH, Dahl UL, Wollmer P. The impact of smoking on inhaled insulin. Diabetes Care 2003; 26:677–82.

Hoffmann JA, Chance RE, Johnson MG. Purification and analysis of the major components of chum salmon protamine contained in insulin formulations using high-performance liquid chromatography. Protein Expr Purif 1990; 1:127–33.

Howey DC, Bowsher RR, Brunelle RL, Woodworth JR. [Lys (B28),Pro(B29)]-human insulin: a rapidly-absorbed analogue of human insulin. Diabetes 1994; 43:396–402.

Janssen MMJ, Casteleijn S, Devillé W, Popp-Snijders C, Roach P, Heine RJ. Nighttime insulin kinetics and glycemic control in type 1 diabetic patients following administration of an intermediate-acting lispro preparation. Diabetes Care 1997; 20:1870–3.

Kaarsholm NC, Havelund S, Hougaard P. Ionization behavior of native and mutant insulins: pK Perturbation of B13-Glu in aggregated species. Arch Biochem Biophys 1990; 283:496–502.

Krayenbühl C, Rosenberg T. Crystalline protamine insulin. Rep Steno Hosp (Kbh) 1946; 1:60–73.

Kroeff EP, Owen RA, Campbell EL, Johnson RD, Marks HI. Production scale purification of biosynthetic human insulin by reversed phase high performance liquid chromatography. J Chromatography 1989; 461:45–61.

Kurtz AB, Gray RS, Markanday S, Nabarro JDN. Circulating IgG antibody to protamine in patients treated with protamine-insulins. Diabetologia 1983; 25:322–4.

Modi P, Mihic M, Lewin A. The evolving role of oral insulin in the treatment of diabetes using a novel RapidMist™ System. Diabetes Metab Res Rev 2002; 18(Suppl. 1):S38–42.

Nell LJ, Thomas JW. Frequency and specificity of protamine antibodies in diabetic and control subjects. Diabetes 1988; 37:172–6.

Patton JS, Bukar JG, Eldon MA. Clinical pharmacokinetics and pharmacodynamics of inhaled insulin. Clin Pharmacokinet 2004; 43:781–801.

Patton JS, Bukar J, Nagarajan S. Inhaled insulin. Adv Drug Deliv Rev 1999; 35:235–47.

Patton JS. Deep-lung delivery of proteins. Mod Drug Disc 1998; 1:19–28.

Pekar AH, Frank BH. Conformation of proinsulin. A comparison of insulin and proinsulin self-association at neutral pH. Biochemistry 1972; 11:4013–6.

Porter CJ, Charman SA. Lymphatic transport of proteins after subcutaneous administration. J Pharm Sci 2000; 89:297–310.

Robertson KE, Glazer NB, Campbell RK. The latest developments in insulin injection devices. Diabetes Educ 2000; 26:135–52.

Supersaxo A, Hein WR, Steffen H. Effect of molecular weight on the lymphatic absorption of water-soluble compounds following subcutaneous administration. Pharm Res 1990; 7:167–9.

USP Monographs: insulin. (2006) USP 29-NF 24.

Vague P, Selam J-L, Skeie S, De Leeuw I, Elte JWF, Haahr H, et al. Insulin detemir is associated with more predictable glycemic control and reduced risk of hypoglycemia than NPH insulin in patients with type 1 diabetes on a basal-bolus regimen with premeal insulin aspart. Diabetes Care 2003; 26:590–6.

Weyer C, Heise T, Heinemann L. Insulin aspart in a 30/70 premixed formulation. Diabetes Care 1997; 20:1612–4.

Whittingham JL, Jonassen I, Havelund S, Roberts SM, Dodson EJ, Verma CS, et al. Crystallographic and solution studies of N-lithocholyl insulin: a new generation of prolonged-acting human insulins. Biochemistry 2004; 43:5987–95.

Whittingham JL, Edwards DJ, Antson AA, Clarkson JM, Dodson GG. Interactions of phenol and m-cresol in the insulin hexamer, and their effect on the association properties of B28 pro → Asp insulin analogues. Biochemistry 1998; 37:11516–23.

Yip CM, DeFelippis MR, Frank BH, Brader ML, Ward MD. Structural and morphological characterization of Ultralente insulin crystals by atomic force microscopy: evidence of hydrophobically driven assembly. Biophys J 1998; 75:1172–9.

## FURTHER READING

Bliss M. The discovery of insulin. Toronto: McClelland and Stewart Limited; 1982.

Brange J. Galenics of insulin. Berlin: Springer-Verlag; 1987.

Galloway JA, Potvin JH, Shuman CR. Diabetes mellitus. 9th ed. Indianapolis (Indiana, USA): Lilly Research Laboratories; 1988.

# Growth Hormones

*Melinda Marian*
Schering-Plough Biopharma, Palo Alto, California, U.S.A.
*James Q. Oeswein*
Genentech, Inc. (Retired), South San Francisco, California, U.S.A.

## PHARMACOTHERAPY INFORMATION

Further information on the applied pharmacotherapy with growth hormone can be found in the following frequently used textbooks:

- **Applied Therapeutics: The Clinical Use of Drugs** (*Koda-Kimble, MA, et al., Eds.*), *8th edition, Lippincott Williams & Wilkins, Baltimore 2005*: Chapter 70.
- **Pharmacotherapy: A Pathophysiologic Approach** (*DiPiro, JT, et al., Eds.*), *6th edition, McGraw-Hill, New York 2005*: Chapters 75, 139.
- **Textbook of Therapeutics: Drug and Disease Management** (*Helms, RA, et al., Eds.*), *8th edition, Lippincott Williams & Wilkins, Baltimore 2006*: Chapter 7.

## INTRODUCTION

Human growth hormone (hGH) is a protein hormone essential for normal growth and development in humans. hGH affects many aspects of human metabolism, including lipolysis, the stimulation of protein synthesis and the inhibition of glucose metabolism. hGH was first isolated and identified in the late 1950s from extracts of pituitary glands obtained from cadavers and from patients undergoing hypophysectomy. The first clinical use of these pituitary-extracted hGHs for stimulation of growth in hypopituitary children occurred in 1957 and 1958 (Raben, 1958). From 1958 to 1985 the primary material used for clinical studies was pituitary-derived human growth hormone (pit-hGH). hGH was first cloned in 1979 (Goeddel et al., 1979; Martial et al. 1979). The first use in humans of recombinant human growth hormone (rhGH) was reported in the literature in 1982 (Hintz et al., 1982). The introduction of rhGH coincided with reports of a number of cases of Creutzfeldt–Jakob disease, a fatal degenerative neurological disorder, in patients receiving pit-hGH. Concern over possible contamination of the pit-hGH preparations by the prion responsible for Creutzfeldt–Jakob disease led to the removal of pit-hGH products from the market in the United States in 1985. The initial rhGH preparations were produced in bacteria (*Escherichia coli*) and, unlike endogenous hGH, contained an N-terminal methionine group (met-rhGH). Natural sequence recombinant hGH products have subsequently been produced in bacteria, yeast and mammalian cells.

### hGH Structure and Isohormones

The major, circulating form of hGH is a non-glycosylated, 22 kDa protein composed of 191 amino acid residues linked by disulfide bridges in two peptide loops (Fig. 1). The three-dimensional structure of hGH includes four antiparallel alpha-helical regions (Fig. 2). Helix 4 and Helix 1 have been determined to contain the primary sites for binding to the growth hormone receptor (Wells et al., 1993). Endogenous growth hormone contains a variety of other isoforms including a 20 kDa monomer, disulfide-linked dimers, oligomers, proteolytic fragments, and other modified forms (Lewis et al., 2000; Boguszewski, 2003). The 20 kDa monomer, dimers, oligomers, and other modified forms occur as a result of different gene products, different splicing of hGH mRNA, and post-translational modifications.

There are two hGH genes in humans, the "normal" hGH-N gene and the "variant" hGH-V gene. The hGH-N gene is expressed in the pituitary gland. The hGH-V gene is expressed in the placenta and is responsible for the production of several variant forms of hGH found in pregnant women.

## PHARMACOLOGY

### ■ Growth Hormone Secretion and Regulation

Growth hormone is secreted from somatotrophs in the anterior pituitary. Multiple feedback loops are

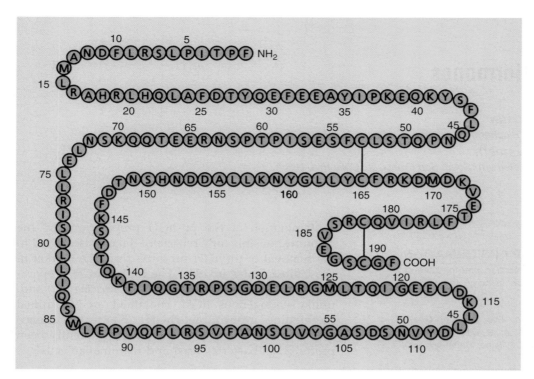

**Figure 1** ▨ Primary structure of recombinant human growth hormone.

present in normal regulation of hGH secretion (Casanueva, 1992; Giustina and Veldhuis 1998) (Fig. 3). Growth hormone release from the pituitary is regulated by a "short loop" of two coupled hypothalamic peptides—a stimulatory peptide, growth hormone releasing hormone (GHRH) and an inhibitory peptide, somatostatin. GHRH and somatostatin are, in turn, regulated by neuronal input to the hypothalamus and the GH secretagogue, ghrelin (Kojima et al., 2001). There is possibly also an "ultrashort loop" in which hGH release is feedback regulated by growth hormone receptors present on the somatotrophs of the pituitary themselves. Growth hormone secretion is also regulated by a "long loop" of peripheral signals including insulin-like growth factor (IGF-1) and other modulators.

Growth hormone secretion changes during human development, with the highest production rates observed during gestation and puberty (Brook and Hindmarsh 1992; Guistina and Veldhuis, 1998). Growth hormone production declines approximately 10 to 15% each decade from age 20 to 70 years. Endogenous hGH secretion also varies with sex, nutritional status, obesity, physical activity, and in a variety of disease states. Endogenous hGH is secreted in periodic bursts over a 24 hour period with great variability in burst frequency, amplitude and duration. There is little detectable hGH released from the pituitary between bursts. The highest endogenous hGH serum concentrations of 10 to 30 ng/mL usually occur at night when the secretory bursts are largest and most frequent.

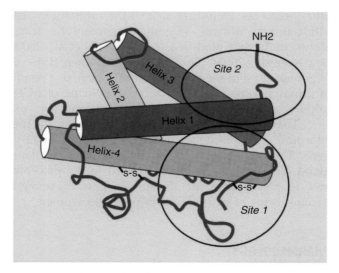

**Figure 2** ▨ Schematic 3-D structure of hGH showing 4 anti-parallel α-helices and receptor binding sites 1 and 2. Approximate positions of the two disulfide bridges (S-S) are also indicated. *Source*: Modified from Wells et al., 1993.

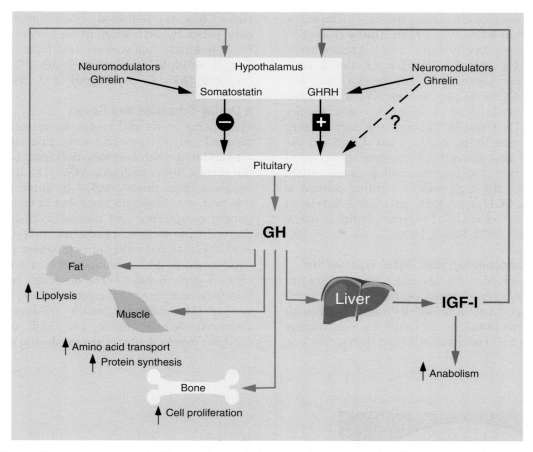

**Figure 3** ▪ Schematic representation of hGH regulation and biologic actions in humans. "Short loop" regulation of hGH secretion occurs between the hypothalamus and pituitary. GHRH stimulates GH release. Somatostatin inhibits GH release. "Long loop" regulation of hGH secretion occurs through peripheral feedback signals, including IGF-1, hGH, and other modulators itself. hGH acts directly on muscle, bone and adipose tissue. Other anabolic actions are generally mediated through IGF-1.

## ▪ Growth Hormone Biologic Actions

hGH has well-defined growth promoting and metabolic actions. hGH stimulates the growth of cartilage and bone directly, through hGH receptors in those tissues, and indirectly, via local increases in IGF-1 (Fig. 3) (Bouillon 1991; Isaksson et al., 2000). Metabolic actions, which may be directly controlled by hGH, include the elevation of circulating glucose levels (diabetogenic effect) and acute increases in circulating concentrations of free fatty acids (lipolytic effect). Other hGH anabolic and metabolic actions believed to be mediated through increases in local or systemic IGF-1 concentrations include: increases in net muscle protein synthesis (anabolic effect); modulation of reproduction in both males and females; maintenance, control and modulation of lymphocyte functions; increases in glomerular filtration rate and renal plasma flow rate (osmoregulation); influences on the release and metabolism of insulin, glucagon, and thyroid hormones (T3, T4); and possible direct effects on pituitary function and neural tissue development

(Le Roith et al. 1991; Casanueva, 1992; Strobl and Thomas, 1994).

## ▪ hGH Receptor and Binding Proteins

The hGH receptor is a member of the hematopoietic cytokine receptor family. It has an extracellular domain consisting of 246 amino acids, a single 24 amino acid transmembrane domain, and a 350 amino acid intracellular domain (Fisker, 2006). The extracellular domain has at least six potential N-glycosylation sites and is usually extensively glycosylated. hGH receptors are found in most tissues in humans. However, the greatest concentration of receptors in humans and other mammals occurs in the liver (Mertani et al., 1995).

As much as 40% to 45% of monomeric hGH circulating in plasma is bound to one of two binding proteins (GHBP) (Fig. 4) (Fisker, 2006). Binding proteins decrease the clearance of hGH from the circulation (Baumann, 1991) and may also serve to dampen the biological effects of hGH by competing with cell receptors for circulating free hGH. The major form of GHBP in humans is a high affinity (Ka = $10^{-9}$ to $10^{-8}$ M), low capacity form which preferentially binds the 22 kDa form of hGH (Herington et al. 1986; Baumann, 1991). Another low affinity (Ka = $10^{-5}$ M), high capacity GHBP is also present which binds the 20 kDa form with equal or slightly greater affinity than the 22 kDa form. In humans, the high affinity GHBP is identical to the extracellular domain of the hGH receptor and arises by proteolytic cleavage of hGH receptors by a process called ecto-domain shedding. Since the high affinity binding protein is derived from hGH receptors, circulating levels of GHBP generally reflect hGH receptor status in many tissues (Hansen, 2002; Fisker, 2006).

### ■ Molecular Endocrinology and Signal Transduction

X-ray crystallographic studies and functional studies of the extracellular domain of the hGH receptor suggest that two receptor molecules form a dimer with a single growth hormone molecule by sequentially binding to Site 1 on Helix 4 of hGH and then to Site 2 on Helix 1 (Fig. 4) (Wells et al., 1993). Signal transduction may occur by activation/phosphorylation of JAK-2 tyrosine kinase followed by activation/phosphorylation of multiple signaling cascades (Herrington and Carter-Su, 2001; Piwien-Pilipuk et al., 2002).

### ■ Dosing Schedules and Routes

The dosing levels and routes for exogenously administered growth hormone were first established for pit-hGH in growth hormone deficient (GHD) patients (Jorgensen, 1991; Laursen, 2004). The initial pit-hGH regimen, three times weekly by intramuscular (IM) injection, was based on a number of factors including patient compliance and limited availability of hGH derived from cadaver pituitaries. Subsequent clinical evaluations found a very strong patient preference for subcutaneous (SC) administration. Furthermore, increased growth rates were observed with daily SC injections compared to the previous two to three times weekly IM injection schedule (Hansen, 2002). The abdomen, deltoid muscle, and thigh are commonly used SC injection sites. Current dosing schedules are

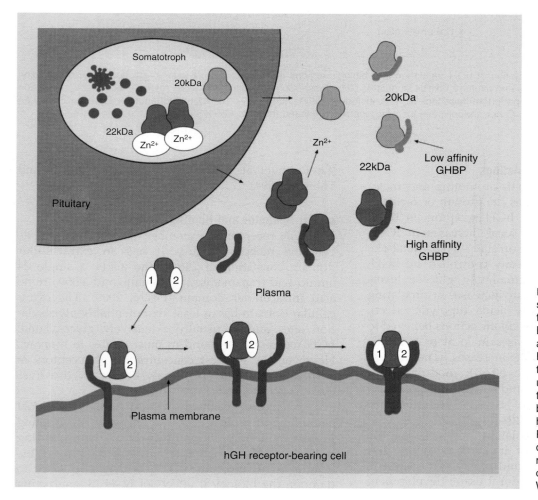

**Figure 4** ■ Growth hormone secreted isoforms, binding proteins and receptor interactions. Both 22 kDa and 20 kDa forms are secreted by the pituitary. Pituitary hGH is stored bound to zinc ($Zn^{2+}$) which is released upon secretion from the pituitary. Secreted hGH is free or bound to either the low or high affinity GHBP in plasma. Receptor activation involves dimerization of two receptor molecules with one molecule of hGH. *Source*: Modified from Wells et al., 1993.

usually daily SC injections, often self-administered with a variety of injection devices.

## ■ Pharmacokinetics and Metabolism

The earliest pharmacokinetic studies were conducted with pit-hGH. The pharmacokinetic profiles of pit-hGH, met-rhGH and rhGH have been compared (Hansen, 2002; Laursen, 2004) and shown to be very similar. The pharmacokinetics of hGH have been studied in normal, healthy children and adults, and a variety of patient populations (Jorgensen, 1991; Hansen, 2002; Laursen, 2004).

Exogenously administered pit-hGH, met-rhGH and rhGH are rapidly cleared following intravenous (IV) injection with terminal half-lives of approximately 15 to 20 minutes (Hansen, 2002; Laursen, 2004). Distribution volumes usually approximate the plasma volume. hGH clearance in normal subjects ranges from 2.2 to 3.0 mL/kg/min. hGH clearance decreases with increasing serum GH concentrations, most likely due to saturation of hGH receptors at concentrations >10 to 15 µg/L (Hansen, 2002). Comparative analyses of total hGH clearance have not shown consistent population differences based on age, sex or body composition. However, hGH clearance is controlled by a complex interaction between free hGH, GHBP-bound hGH and GH receptor status (Hansen, 2002). Individual subject variations in GHBP or GH receptor levels may result in substantial differences in hGH clearance.

hGH is slowly, but relatively completely, absorbed after either IM or SC injection. Time to peak concentration ranges from 2 to 4 hours following IM bolus administration and 4 to 6 hours following SC bolus administration (Jorgensen, 1991; Laursen, 2004). SC administered rhGH is approximately 50% to 80% bioavailable (Laursen, 2004). The rate of absorption of hGH is slightly faster after injection in the abdomen compared with the thigh (Laursen, 2004), but the extent of absorption is comparable. Elimination half-lives following extravascular administration (2–5 hours) are usually longer than the IV terminal half-lives indicating absorption rate-limited kinetics.

hGH pharmacokinetics in the presence of growth hormone deficiency, diabetes, obesity, critical illness or diseases of the thyroid, liver and kidney have been evaluated. Results suggest disposition is not significantly altered compared with normal subjects except in severe liver or kidney dysfunction (Hansen, 2002; Haffner et al., 1994; Owens et al., 1973; Cameron et al., 1972). The reduction in clearance observed in severe liver (30%) or kidney dysfunction (40–75%) is consistent with the role of the liver and kidney as major organs of hGH elimination.

Both the kidney and the liver have been shown to be important in the clearance of hGH in humans (Hansen, 2002). The relative contribution of each organ has not been rigorously quantitated in humans, but the preponderance of studies in laboratory animals and in isolated perfused organ systems suggest a dominant role for the kidney at pharmacologic levels of hGH. Receptor-mediated uptake of hGH by the liver is the major extra-renal clearance mechanism (Harvey, 1995).

## PROTEIN MANUFACTURE, FORMULATION AND STABILITY

Commercially available hGH preparations are summarized in Table 1. All recombinant growth hormones except Serostim®/ Saizen®/ Zorbtive® are produced in bacteria or yeast (*E. coli, S. cerevisiae*). Serostim®/ Saizen®/ Zorbtive® are produced in mammalian cells (C127 mouse cells). Growth hormone produced in *E. coli* may contain an N-terminal methionine residue. Natural sequence rhGH is produced either by enzymatic cleavage of the methionine during the purification procedure or by periplasmic secretion of rhGH into refractile bodies. The rhGH is then released from the refractile bodies by osmotic shock and the protein recovered and purified. rhGH synthesized in mammalian cells is transported across the endoplasmic reticulum and secreted directly into the culture medium from which it is recovered and purified.

Historically, the potency of hGH products was expressed in international units per mg (IU/mg). The initial standard, established in 1982 for pit-hGH preparations, was 2 IU/mg. The standard for rhGH products was 2.6 IU/mg until September 1994. The current WHO standard, established in September 1994, is 3.0 IU/mg. Dosages are usually expressed as IU/kg or $IU/m^2$ in Europe and Japan and as mg/kg in the United States. However, the use of IU dosages is no longer necessary due to the high level of purity and consistent potency of recombinant hGH products.

All current rhGH products are available as lyophilized or liquid preparations. Lyophilized formulations usually include 5 or 10 mg of protein in a glycine and mannitol or sucrose-containing phosphate buffer excipient. The materials are usually reconstituted with sterile water for injection for single use or with bacteriostatic water or bacteriostatic saline for multiple injection use. Liquid formulations of rhGH (Nutropin AQ®, Norditropin®, SimpleXx®) contain mannitol or sodium chloride, histidine or citrate buffer, poloxamer 188 or polysorbate 20 and phenol. Product stability has been very good with shelf lives of approximately 2 years at 2°C to 8°C. A long-acting dosage form of rhGH (Nutropin Depot®) was available from 1999 until 2004.

| Source | Brand names | Product form | Container | Injection device | Manufacturer |
|---|---|---|---|---|---|
| Recombinant protein produced in bacteria (*E. coli*) | Genotropin® Genotonorm | Lyophilized powder | Two-chamber cartridge | Genotropin Pen® Genotropin Miniquick® | Pfizer Inc. (previously KabiVitrum, Pharmacia and Upjohn) |
| | Norditropin® | No longer marketed | NA | NA | Novo Nordisk A/S |
| | Norditropin® SimpleXx® | Liquid | Cartridge | NordiPen® Norditropin NordiFlex® | Novo Nordisk A/S |
| | Nutropin® | Lyophilized powder | Vial | Single use syringe | Genentech, Inc. |
| | Nutropin AQ® | Liquid | Vial Cartridges | Single use syringe Nutropin AQ® Pen | Genentech, Inc. |
| | Nutropin Depot® | No longer marketed | NA | NA | Genentech, Inc. |
| | Humatrope® Umatrope | Lyophilized powder | Vial Cartridges | Single use syringe HumatroPen™ | Eli Lilly & Co. |
| | Bio-Tropin® Scitropin® Zomacton® Growject® | Lyophilized powder | Vial | Single use syringe Zomajet 2 Vision | Ferring Pharmaceuticals Ltd. (formerly Savient/ Bio-Technolgy General Corporation) |
| | Tev-Tropin™ | Lyophilized powder | Vial | Single use syringe | Teva Pharmaceutical Industries Inc. |
| | Omnitrope® Omnitrop | Lyophilized powder | Vial | Single use syringe | Sandoz, GmbH |
| Recombinant protein produced in yeast cells (*S. cerevisiae*) | Valtropin® | Lyophilized powder | Vial | Single use syringe | BioPartners GmbH |
| Recombinant protein produced in mammalian cells (C127 mouse cell line derived) | Serostim® (AIDS wasting) | Lyophilized powder | Vial with click.easy® reconstitution device | SeroJet™ one.click® | Merck Serono SA |
| | Saizen® (growth inadequacy) | Lyophilized powder | Vial with click.easy® reconstitution device | Single use syringe cool.click™ one click® | Merck Serono SA |
| | Zorbtive® (short bowel syndrome) | Lyophilized powder | Vial | Single use syringe | Merck Serono SA |

**Table 1** ▪ Recombinant hGH products.

Nutropin Depot® contained micronized particles of rhGH embedded in biocompatible, biodegradable polylactide-coglycolide (PLGA) microspheres. Omnitrope®/Omnitrop® (US/EU) and Valtropin® (EU only), lyophilized rhGH preparations, were approved for marketing as the first "biosimilar" rhGH products in 2006.

## CLINICAL USAGE

Clinical usage of rhGH has been reviewed for pediatric indications (Harris et al. 2004) and adult indications (Iglesias and Diez 1999; Simpson et al., 2002; Keating and Wellington, 2004).

Investigations of clinical usage of hGH have focused, generally, on two major areas of hGH biologic action: (1) linear growth promotion and (2) modulation of metabolism. Growth promoting indications which have been approved for market include growth hormone deficiency (GHD) and idiopathic short stature (ISS) in children, growth failure associated with chronic renal insufficiency (CRI) in children, growth failure in children born small for gestational age (SGA), short stature in Prader–Willi syndrome (PWS) and Turner syndrome (TS). Modulation of metabolism is the primary biologic action in long-term replacement therapy in adults with GH deficiency of either childhood- or adult-onset, AIDS wasting or cachexia, and in short bowel syndrome (SBS). Additional indications for which hGH has been investigated as a possible therapeutic are summarized in Table 2.

## ■ GHD and ISS in Children

The major indication for therapeutic use of hGH is the long-term replacement treatment for children with classic growth hormone deficiency in whom growth failure is due to a lack of adequate endogenous hGH secretion. Diagnosis of hGH deficiency is usually defined based on an inadequate response to two hGH provocation tests implying a functional deficiency in the production or secretion of hGH from the pituitary gland.

Usual doses range from 0.08–0.35 mg/kg/week administered as daily SC injections in prepubertal children. Doses up to 0.7 mg/kg/week have been used for adolescent subjects to improve final height (Mauras et al., 2000). hGH treatment results in increased growth velocity and, at least in some populations, enhancement in final adult height. The growth response correlates positively with hGH dose and frequency of injections, and negatively with chronological age at onset of treatment. hGH therapy in children is usually continued until growth has been completed, as evidenced by epiphyseal fusion. Partial GHD and ISS comprise a heterogeneous group of growth failure states due to impaired spontaneous hGH secretion, hGH resistance due to low levels of hGH receptors or possible other defects in either secreted hGH or hGH receptors. hGH treatment in these groups results in acceleration of growth and improvement of final height.

## ■ Turner Syndrome

TS is a disease of females caused by partial or total loss of one sex chromosome and is characterized by decreased intrauterine and postnatal growth, short final adult height, incomplete development of the ovaries and secondary sexual characteristics, and other physical abnormalities. Although serum levels

| Growth hormone biologic actions | Clinical indications |
| --- | --- |
| Promotion of linear growth | Classic GHD, partial GHD/idiopathic short stature, Turner syndrome, Down's syndrome, Prader-Willi syndrome, chronic renal insufficiency, cystic fibrosis, Noonan's syndrome, intrauterine growth retardation, Silver-Russel syndrome, thalassemia, hypochondroplasia, spina bifida, myelomeningocele, growth impairment in chronic steroid therapy |
| Modulation of metabolism<br>Stimulation of lipolysis and protein synthesis | Adult GHD, aging, obesity, weight training in athletes, Prader–Willi syndrome, cardiovascular dysfunction |
| Anabolism<br>Stimulation of protein synthesis<br>Improved nitrogen retention<br>Prevention of starvation-induced hypoglycemia | Catabolic states due to chronic disease, infections, surgery, trauma, burns; chronic obstructive pulmonary disease; short bowel syndrome; AIDS |
| Stimulation of collagen formation | Burns, wound healing |
| Stimulation of bone formation | Osteoporosis, fractures |
| Stimulation of conversion of thyroxin (T4) to triiodothyronine (T3) | Hypothyroidism |
| Osmoregulation<br>Increased GFR | Chronic renal disease<br>Increased renal plasma flow |
| Maintenance of immune function | Immune dysfunction |
| Enhancement of gonadotropin action | Female and male infertility |
| Stimulation of lactation | Lactational failure in women |

**Table 2** ■ Growth hormone biologic actions and related clinical investigations.

of hGH and IGF-1 are not consistently low in this population, hGH treatment (0.33–0.45 mg/kg/week), alone or in combination with oxandrolone, significantly improves growth rate and final adult height in this patient group (Pasquino, 2004).

### ■ Prader–Willi Syndrome

PWS is a pediatric disease caused by the functional deletion of the paternal allele of chromosome 15. Clinical manifestations include obesity, hypotonia, short stature, hypogonadism and behavior abnormalities. PWS children have especially high rates of morbidity due to obesity-related illnesses. Growth hormone treatment (0.24–0.48 mg/kg/week) has been shown to improve height and, perhaps more importantly, improve body composition, physical strength and agility in PWS children (Allen and Carrel, 2004).

### ■ Small for Gestational Age

Growth hormone is approved for use in long term treatment of growth failure in children born SGA who fail to manifest catch-up growth. Children born at birth weights and birth lengths more than two standard deviations below the mean are considered SGA. Children who fail to catch up by age two to three are at risk for growing into adults with substantial height deficits (Rappaport, 2004). Growth hormone treatment at doses of 0.24 to 0.48 mg/kg/week can safely induce catch-up growth, normalize height at an earlier age, and improve potential adult height.

### ■ Chronic Renal Insufficiency

Children with renal disease grow slowly, possibly related to defects in metabolism and/or defects in the IGF-1/hGH axis. Basal serum hGH concentrations and IGF-1 responses to hGH stimulation are usually normal. However, there are reported abnormalities in the IGF-binding protein levels in renal disease patients suggesting possible problems with GH/IGF-1 action. Growth hormone therapy (0.35 mg/kg/week) in children with CRI results in significant increases in height velocity (Greenbaum et al., 2004). Increases are best during the first year of treatment for younger children with stable renal disease. Responses are less for children on dialysis or children post-transplant receiving corticosteroids.

### ■ GHD in Adults and the Elderly

Early limitations in hGH supply severely limited treatment of adults with GHD. With the increased supply of recombinant rhGH products, replacement therapy for adults was evaluated and, ultimately, approved as a clinical indication (Simpson et al., 2002). Growth hormone has been used in three GHD adult populations: (1) adults with childhood onset GHD; (2) adults with adult onset GHD usually due to pituitary tumors and subsequent hypophysectomy; and (3) elderly normal adults, 60 years of age or older. Growth hormone treatment (0.04–0.175 mg/kg/week) reduces body fat, increases lean body mass, increases exercise capacity and muscle strength in the elderly and adult GHD patients. Increases in bone density have been observed in some bone types although treatment duration greater than 6 months may be necessary to see significant effects. hGH treatment consistently elevates both serum IGF-1 and insulin levels. Women have also been shown to require higher doses to normalize IGF-1 levels than men, especially women taking oral estrogens.

### ■ Clinical Malnutrition and Wasting Syndromes

Growth hormone is approved for treatment of SBS, a congenital or acquired condition in which less than ~200 cm of small intestine is present. SBS patients have severe fluid and nutrient malabsorption and are often dependent upon intravenous parenteral nutrition (IPN). Administration of growth hormone, 0.1 mg/kg/day for 4 weeks, alone or in combination with glutamine, reduces the volume and frequency of required IPN (Keating and Wellington, 2004). Growth hormone is indicated for use in patients who are also receiving specialized nutritional support. Usage for periods > 4 weeks, or in children, has not been investigated. Usage of growth hormone for SBS remains controversial due to potential risks associated with IGF-1-related fibrosis and cancer (Theiss et al., 2004). Growth hormone is also approved for use in wasting associated with AIDS (Iglesias and Diez, 1999). Growth hormone treatment (~ 0.1 mg/kg daily, max. 6 mg/day), when used with controlled diets, increases body weight and nitrogen retention. rhGH treatment is also under investigation for HIV-associated lipodistrophy, a syndrome of fat re-distribution and metabolic complications resulting from the highly active antiretroviral therapy commonly used in HIV infection (Burgess and Wanke, 2005).

### ■ Other Indications

The use of hGH therapy to ameliorate the negative nitrogen balance seen in patients following surgery, injury or infections have been investigated in a number of studies (Ponting et al., 1988; Jeevanandam et al., 1995; Voerman et al. 1995; Takala et al., 1999). Treatment with hGH alone improved nitrogen and phosphorous retention and increased body weight. Several studies have demonstrated improved bone mineral density (BMD) with hGH administration in GH-deficient adults (Hansen, 2002). Positive effects are best demonstrated with long-term administration (>1 year), as

short-term (<3 months) therapy can produce apparent decreases in BMD due to increased bone re-modeling. Studies of hGH effects in burns have shown significant effectiveness in acceleration of healing in skin graft sites and improvements in growth in burned children (Herndon and Tompkins, 2004). Growth hormone has been shown to significantly reduce multiple disease symptoms and improve well-being in Crohn's disease, a chronic inflammatory disorder of the bowel (Slonim et al., 2000; Theiss et al., 2004). Growth hormone has also shown benefit in cardiovascular recovery and function in congestive heart failure (Colao et al., 2004). Several studies have indicated growth hormone treatment improves growth, pulmonary function and clinical status in children with cystic fibrosis (Hardin, 2004).

### ■ Safety Concerns

hGH has been widely used for many years and has been proven to be remarkably safe in pediatric indications (Growth Hormone Research Society, 2001). Adverse events have been reported in a small number of children and include benign intracranial hypertension, glucose intolerance, and the development of anti-hGH antibodies. The antibodies have not been positively correlated with a loss in efficacy. Growth hormone therapy is also not associated with increased risk of malignancies or tumor recurrence (Growth Hormone Research Society, 2001; Sklar et al., 2002). However, growth hormone treatment should generally not be initiated in children until one year or more after completion of anti-neoplastic therapy.

Growth hormone has caused significant, dose limiting, fluid retention in adult populations resulting in increased body weight, swollen joints and arthralgias and carpal tunnel syndrome (Carroll et al., 2001). Symptoms were usually transient and resolved upon reduction of hGH dosage or upon discontinuation of hGH treatment. Growth hormone administration has been associated with increased mortality in clinical trials in critically ill, intensive-care patients with acute catabolism (Takala et al., 1999) and is, therefore, contraindicated for use in critically ill patients. Growth hormone is also contraindicated in patients with PWS who have upper airway obstructions or severe respiratory impairment and obesity (Growth Hormone Research Society, 2001).

Growth hormone's anabolic and lipolytic effects have made it attractive as a performance enhancement drug among athletes. Illicit hGH usage has been anecdotally reported for the last 20 years. Detection of rhGH abuse is now possible due to the development of assays which rely on detecting changed ratios of exogenous rhGH (22 kDa only) and endogenous hGH (22 kDa, 20 kDa, and other forms). Screening for rhGH abuse, based on the new ratio assays, was included in the 2006 Olympic games for the first time (McHugh et al., 2005).

## CONCLUDING REMARKS

The abundant supply of hGH, made possible by recombinant DNA technology, has allowed enormous advances to be made in understanding the basic structure, function and physiology of hGH over the past 20 years. As a result of those advances, recombinant hGH has been developed into a safe and efficacious therapy for a variety of growth and metabolic disorders in children and adults. Continuing basic research in GH and IGF-1 biology, genomics and GH-related diseases, and continuing clinical studies in inflammatory bowel disease, burn treatment, congestive heart failure and cystic fibrosis hold promise for additional future uses for this versatile hormone.

## REFERENCES

Allen DB, Carrel AL (2004). Growth hormone therapy for Prader–Willi syndrome: a critical appraisal. J Ped Endocrinol Metab 17:1297–306.

Baumann G (1991). Growth hormone heterogeneity: Genes, isohormones, variants and binding proteins. Endoc. Rev 12:424–49.

Boguszewski CL (2003). Molecular heterogeneity of human GH: from basic research to clinical implications. J Endocrinol Invest 26:274–88.

Bouillon R (1991). Growth hormone and bone. Horm Res 36 (Suppl 1): 49–55.

Brook CGD, Hindmarsh PC (1992). The somatotropic axis in puberty. Endocrinol Metab Clin N Am 21:767–82.

Burgess E, Wanke C (2005). Use of recombinant human growth hormone in HIV-associated lipodystrophy. Curr Opin Infect Dis 18:17–24.

Cameron DP, Burger HG, Catt KJ, et al. (1972). Metabolic clearance of human growth hormone in patients with hepatic and renal failure, and in the isolated perfused pig liver. Metab 21:895–904.

Carroll PV, van den Berghe G (2001). Safety aspects of pharmacological GH therapy in adults. Growth Horm IGF Res 11:166–72.

Casanueva F (1992). Physiology of growth hormone secretion and action. Endocrin. Metab Clin N Am 21:483–517.

Colao A, Vitale G, Pivonello R, et al. (2004). The heart: an end-organ of GH action. Eur J Endocrinol 151:S93–101.

Fisker S (2006). Physiology and pathophysiology of growth hormone binding protein: methodological and clinical aspects. Growth Horm IGF Res 16:1–28.

Giustina A, Veldhuis JD (1998). Pathophysiology of the neuroregulation of growth hormone secretion in experimental animals and in the human. Endocrinol Rev 19(6):717–97.

Goeddel DV, Heyreker HL, Hozumi T, et al. (1979). Direct expression in Escherichia coli of a DNA sequence coding for human growth hormone. Nature 281:544–8.

Greenbaum LA, Del Rio M, Bamgbola F, et al. (2004) Rationale for growth hormone therapy in children with chronic kidney disease. Adv Chronic Kidney Dis 11(4): 377–86.

Growth Hormone Research Society (2001). Critical evaluation of the safety of recombinant human growth hormone administration: statement from the Growth Hormone Research Society. J Clin Endocrinol Metab 86(15): 1868–70.

Hansen TK (2002). Pharmacokinetics and acute lipolytic actions of growth hormone: impact of age, body composition, binding proteins and other hormones. Growth Horm IGF Res 12:342–58.

Hardin DS (2004). GH improves growth and clinical status in children with cystic fibrosis—a review of published studies. Eur J Endocrinol 151:S81–5.

Harris M, Hofman PL, Cutfield WS (2004). Growth hormone treatment in children. Pediatr Drugs 6(2):93–106.

Harvey S (1995). Growth hormone metabolism. In: Harvey S, Scanes CG, Daughaday WH, eds. Growth Hormone. Boca Raton, FL: CRC Press, Inc, 285–301.

Herington AC, Ymer S, Stevenson J (1986). Identification and characterization of specific binding proteins for growth hormone in normal human sera. J Clin Invest 77:1817–23.

Herndon DN, Tompkins RG (2004). Support of the metabolic response to burn injury. Lancet 363:1895–902.

Herrington J, Carter-Su C (2001). Signaling pathways activated by the growth hormone receptor. Trends Endocrinol Metab 12(6):252–7.

Hintz RL, Rosenfeld RG, Wilson DM, et al. (1982). Biosynthetic methionyl human growth hormone is biologically active in adult man. Lancet 1:1276–9.

Iglesias P, Diez JJ (1999). Clinical applications of recombinant human growth hormone in adults. Expert Opin Pharmacother 1(1):97–107.

Isaksson OG, Ohlsson C, Bengtsson B, et al. (2000). GH and bone-experimental and clinical studies. Endocrin J 47 (Suppl):S9–16.

Jeevanandam M, Ali MR. Holaday NJ, et al. (1995). Adjuvant recombinant human hormone normalizes plasma amino acids in parenterally fed trauma patients. J Parenter Enteral Nutr 19:137–44.

Jorgensen JOL (1991). Human growth hormone replacement therapy: pharmacological and clinical aspects. Endocrinol Rev 12:189–207.

Keating GM, Wellington K (2004). Somatropin (Zorbtive™) in short bowel syndrome. Drugs 64(12):1375–81.

Kojima M, Hosoda H, Matsuo H, et al. (2001). Ghrelin: discovery of the natural endogenous ligand for the growth hormone secretagogue receptor. Trends Endocrinol Metab 12(3):118–26.

Laursen T (2004). Clinical pharmacological aspects of growth hormone administration. Growth Horm IGF Res 14:16–44.

Le Roith D, Adamo M, Werner H, Roberts Jr CT (1991). Insulin-like growth factors and their receptors as growth regulators in normal physiology and pathologic states. Trends Endocrinol Metab 2: 134–9.

Lewis UJ, Sinhda YN, Lewis GP (2000). Structure and properties of members of the hGH family: a review. Endocr J 47:S1–8.

Martial JA, Hallewell RA, Baxter JD (1979). Human growth hormone: complementary DNA cloning and expression in bacteria. Science 205:602–7.

Mauras N, Attie KM, Reiter EO, et al. (2000). High dose recombinant human growth hormone (GH) treatment of GH-deficient patients in puberty increases near-final height: a randomized, multicenter trial. J Clin Endocrinol Metab 85:3653–60.

McHugh CM, Park RT, Sonksen PH, et al. (2005). Challenges in detecting the abuse of growth hormone in sport. Clin Chem 51(9):1587–93.

Mertani HC, Delehaye-Zervas MC, Martini JF, et al. (1995). Localization of growth hormone receptor messenger RNA in human tissues. Endocrine 3:135–42.

Owens D, Srivastava MC, Tompkins CV, et al. (1973). Studies on the metabolic clearance rate, apparent distribution space and plasma half-disappearance time of unlabelled human growth hormone in normal subjects and in patients with liver disease, renal disease, thyroid disease and diabetes mellitus. Europ J Clin Invest 3:284–94.

Pasquino AM (2004). Turner syndrome and GH treatment: the state of the art. J Endocrinol Invest 27:1072–5.

Piwien-Pilipuk G, Huo JS, Schwartz J (2002). Growth hormone signal transduction. J Ped Endocrinol Metab 15:771–86.

Ponting GA, Halliday D, Teale JD, et al. (1988). Postoperative positive nitrogen balance with intravenous hyponutrition and growth hormone. Lancet 1:438–40.

Raben MS (1958). Treatment of a pituitary dwarf with human growth hormone. J Clin Endocrinol Metab 18:901–3.

Rappaport R (2004). Growth and growth hormone in children born small for gestational age. Growth Horm IGF Res 14:S3–6.

Simpson H, Savine R, Sonksen P, et al. (2002). Growth hormone replacement therapy for adults: into the new millennium. Growth Horm IGF Res 12:1–33.

Sklar CA, Mertens AC, Mitby P, et al. (2002). Risk of disease recurrence and second neoplasms in survivors of children cancer treated with growth hormone: a report from the Childhood Cancer Survivor Study. J Clin Endocrinol Metab 87(7):3136–41.

Slonim AE, Bulone L, Damore MB, et al. (2000). A preliminary study of growth hormone therapy for Crohn's disease. New Engl J Med 342:1633–7.

Society (2001). Critical evaluation of the safety of recombinant human growth hormone administration: Statement from the Growth Hormone Research Society. J Clin Endocrinol Metab 86(5):1868–70.

Strobl JS, Thomas MJ (1994). Human growth hormone. Pharm Rev 46:1–34.

Takala J, Ruokonen E, Webster NR, et al. (1999). Increased mortality associated with growth hormone treatment in critically ill adults. New Engl J Med 341 (11):785–92.

Theiss AL, Fruchtman S, Lund PK (2004). Growth factors in inflammatory bowel disease. The actions and interactions of growth hormone and insulin-like growth factor-I. Inflamm Bowel Dis 10(6):871–80.

Voerman BJ, Strack van Schijndel RJM, Goreneveld ABJ, et al. (1995). Effects of human growth hormone in critically ill non-septic patients: results from a prospective, randomized, placebo-controlled trial. Crit Care Med 23:665–73.

Wells JA, Cunningham BC, Fuh G, et al. (1993). The molecular basis for growth hormone-receptor interactions. Rec Prog Horm Res 48:253–75.

## FURTHER READING

Boguszewski CL (2003). Molecular heterogeneity of human GH: from basic research to clinical implications. J Endocrinol Invest 26:274–88.

Fisker S (2006). Physiology and pathophysiology of growth hormone binding protein: Methodological and clinical aspects. Growth Horm IGF Res 16:1–28.

Giustina A, Veldhuis JD (1998). Pathophysiology of the neuroregulation of growth hormone secretion in experimental animals and in the human. Endocrinol Rev 19(6):717–97.

Harvey S, Scanes CG, Daughaday WH, eds. (1995). Growth Hormone. Boca Raton, FL: CRC Press, Inc.

Harris M, Hofman PL, Cutfield WS (2004). Growth hormone treatment in children. Pediatr Drugs 6 (2):93–106.

Laursen T (2004). Clinical pharmacological aspects of growth hormone administration. Growth Horm IGF Res 14:16–44.

Simpson H, Savine R, Sonksen P, et al. (2002). Growth hormone replacement therapy for adults: into the new millennium. Growth Horm IGF Res 12:1–33.

# Recombinant Coagulation Factors and Thrombolytic Agents

*Nishit B. Modi*
*ALZA Corporation, Mountain View, California, U.S.A.*

### PHARMACOTHERAPY INFORMATION

Further information on the applied pharmacotherapy with recombinant coagulation factors and thrombolytic agents can be found in the  following frequently used textbooks:

- **Applied Therapeutics: The Clinical Use of Drugs** (*Koda-Kimble, MA et al., Eds.*), *8th edition, Lippincott Williams & Wilkins, Baltimore 2005* : Chapters 18, 55.
- **Pharmacotherapy: A Pathophysiologic Approach** (*DiPiro, JT, et al., Eds.*), *6th edition, McGraw-Hill, New York 2005* : Chapters 16, 45, 100.
- **Textbook of Therapeutics: Drug and Disease Management** (*Helms, RA, et al., Eds.*), *8th edition, Lippincott Williams & Wilkins, Baltimore 2006* : Chapters 24, 33, 44.

## INTRODUCTION

Coagulation and fibrinogenolysis exist in a mutually compensatory or balanced state. Endogenous regulatory mechanisms ensure that the processes of hemostasis and blood coagulation at a site of injury, and the subsequent fibrinolysis of the blood clot, are localized and well controlled. This ensures a rapid and efficient hemostatic response at a site of injury while avoiding thrombogenic events at sites distant from the site of injury, or the hemostatic response persisting beyond its physiologic need. This chapter will focus on recombinant products that are available to facilitate coagulation and for thrombolysis.

Blood coagulation has been divided into the extrinsic (tissue factor dependent) and intrinsic pathways that converge to the common pathway, leading to the generation of thrombin (Fig. 1). More recently, a revised cell-based model of coagulation has been proposed (Hoffman and Monroe, 2005). This cell-based model emphasizes the interaction of clotting factors with cell surfaces, and appears to explain some of the unresolved issues with the cascade model (Hoffman, 2003).

Normally hemostasis is a highly efficient and tightly regulated process to ensure that it occurs quickly and is localized. Abnormalities that result in a delay in blood coagulation are associated with a bleeding tendency termed hemophilia. Hemophilia is an X chromosome-linked recessive disorder. The incidence of hemophilia is estimated at 5 to 6 people per 100,000 males. Hemophilia A (classical hemophilia) patients have decreased, defective, or absent production of factor VIII, whereas patients with hemophilia B lack factor IX. Factor XI deficiency (originally termed hemophilia C) is less common and in most cases is a mild bleeding disorder. The availability of recombinant coagulation factors has been a major advance in the area of hemophilia, providing the promise of unlimited supply, ease of use, improved safety, and reducing the risk of infections transmitted by transfusion.

## FACTOR VIII

Factor VIII (antihemophilia factor) is a plasma protein that functions as a cofactor by increasing the maximum catabolic capacity ($V_{max}$) in the activation of factor X by factor IXa in the presence of calcium ions and negatively charged phospholipid (Jackson and Nemerson, 1980). The congenital absence of factor VIII is termed hemophilia A and afflicts approximately 1 in 10,000 males (Antonarakis et al., 1987).

### Structure

Factor VIII is synthesized as a single-chain polypeptide of 2332 amino acids (Eaton et al., 1987). Shortly after synthesis, cleavage occurs, and most plasma factor VIII circulates as an 80-kDa light chain associated with a series of 210-kDa heavy chains in a metal ion-dependent complex. There are 25 potential N-linked glycosylation sites and 22 cysteines (Vehar et al., 1984a).

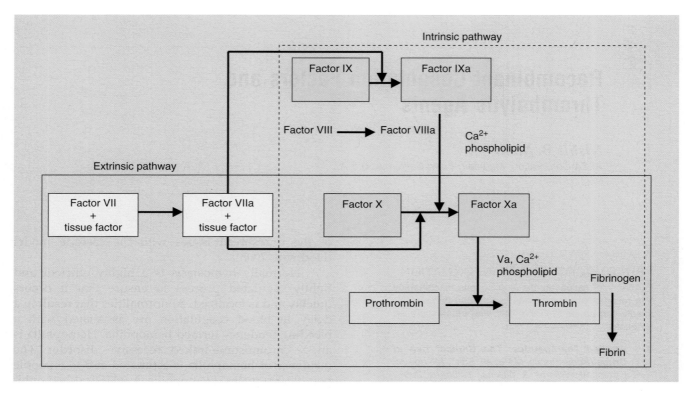

**Figure 1** ■ Schematic representation of fibrinolytic pathway.

*Pharmacology*

The concentration of factor VIII in plasma is about 200 ng/mL (Hoyer, 1981). It is not known where factor VIII is synthesized although evidence suggests that several different tissues, including the spleen, liver, and kidney, may play a role. Factor VIII is normally covalently associated with a 50-fold excess of von Willebrand factor. Von Willebrand factor protects factor VIII from proteolytic cleavage and allows concentration at sites of hemostasis. Circulating von Willebrand factor is bound by exposed subendothelium and activated platelets at sites of injury, which allows localization of von Willebrand factor and factor VIII.

Factor VIII circulates in the body as a large precursor polypeptide devoid of coagulant activity. Cleavage by thrombin at Arg372-Ser373, Arg740-Ser741, and Arg1689-Ser1690 results in procoagulant function (Vehar et al., 1984a). While cleavage at Arg740 is not essential for coagulant activity, cleavage at the other two sites is necessary. Although factor VIII is synthesized as a single-chain polypeptide, the single-chain polypeptide is cleaved shortly after synthesis. Most of the factor VIII in plasma exists as an 80-kDa light chain and a series of heavy chains. Factor VIII circulates as a heterodimer of the 80-kDa light chain and a variable (90–210 kDa) heavy chain in a metal ion-dependent complex.

■ **Recombinant Factor VIII**

Recombinant factor VIII (rFVIII) is available from three sources: Baxter Hyland, Bayer Corporation, and Wyeth. rFVIII products may be divided into three classes based on the use of human or mammalian-derived raw materials (Table 1). rFVIII from Baxter Hyland (Advate®, Recombinate®) and Wyeth (Refacto®) is produced using transfected Chinese hamster ovary (CHO) cells, whereas that from Bayer (Kogenate®) is produced using transfected baby hamster kidney cells. A major difference between rFVIII from Bayer and Baxter Hyland is the presence of a Gal 1->3Gal carbohydrate moiety in the Baxter product (Hironaka et al., 1992). The recombinant product from Baxter and Bayer consists of full-length factor VIII which, like plasma-derived factor VIII, consists of a dimer of the 80-kDa light chain and a heterogeneous heavy chain of 90 to 210 kDa (Schwartz et al., 1990). The Wyeth product (moroctocog alfa, ReFacto®) is a deletion mutant in which the heavy chain lacks nearly the entire B-domain, which is not needed for clotting activity (Roddie and Ludlam, 1997). After proteolytic cleavage by thrombin, the activated B-domain-depleted molecule is essentially identical to the activated full-length native rFVIII.

| Product (manufacturer) | Viral inactivation procedure(s) | Purity/specific activity (IU factor VIII activity/mg total protein) |
|---|---|---|
| **First generation**: | | |
| Recombinate (Baxter/Immuno, Inc.) human albumin as stabilizer | Immunoaffinity, ion exchange chromatography<br>Bovine serum albumin used in culture medium for CHO cells | >4,000 IU/mg |
| **Second generation (human albumin-free final formulations)**: | | |
| Kogenate FS (Bayer, Inc)<br>Helixate FS (Bayer for ZLB Behring, Inc.)<br>Sucrose as stabilizer | Immunoaffinity chromatography<br>Ion exchange<br>Solvent detergent (TNBP/polysorbate 80)<br>Ultrafiltration | > 4,000 IU/mg |
| Refacto (Wyeth, Inc.) B-domain deleted<br>Sucrose as stabilizer | Ion exchange<br>Solvent detergent (TNBP/Triton X-100)<br>Nanofiltration | >11,200–15,500 IU/mg measured via chromogenic assay technique |
| **Third generation (no human or animal protein used in culture medium or manufacturing process; does contain trace amounts of murine monoclonal antibody protein)**: | | |
| Advate (Baxter/Immuno, Inc.)<br>Trehalose as stabilizer | Immunoaffinity chromatography<br>Ion exchange<br>Solvent detergent (TNBP/polysorbate 80) | >4,000–10,000 IU/mg |

*Source*: Adapted from Kessler, 2005.

**Table 1** ■ Summary of factor VIII concentrates available in the United States.

## Pharmaceutical Considerations

Advate® recombinant antihemophilic factor-plasma/albumin free method (rAHF-PFM, Baxter) is formulated as a sterile, non-pyrogenic, lyophilized cake for intravenous injection and is provided in single-dose vials, containing nominally 250, 500, 1000, or 1500 international units (IU). Biological potency is determined using an in vitro assay that employs a factor VIII concentrate standard that is referenced to the World Health Organization (WHO) International Standard for factor VIII:C concentrates. The specific activity is 4000 to 10,000 IU per milligram of protein. The final product contains no preservative nor added human or animal components in the formulation. Recombinant antihemophilic factor is administered only by intravenous infusion following reconstitution with 5 mL sterile water for injection. The product contains mannitol, trehalose, sodium, histidine, Tris, calcium, polysorbate 80, and glutathione. Plastic syringes must be used since the protein can adhere to glass syringes.

rFVIII (Kogenate®, Bayer; Recombinate®, Baxter; Refacto®, Wyeth) is supplied as sterile, single-dose vials containing 250 to 1000 IU of factor VIII. The preparation is lyophilized and stabilized with human albumin (Kogenate® and Recombinate®) or polysorbate 80 (Refacto®). Recently a reformulated product, Kogenate® FS (Bayer), has become available. This product is similar to its predecessor Kogenate Antihemophilic Factor but incorporates a revised purification and formulation process that eliminates addition of human albumin as a stabilizer, instead using histidine. The products contain no preservatives and should be stored at 2°C to 8°C. The lyophilized powder may be stored at room temperature (up to 25°C) for up to 3 months without loss of biological activity. Freezing should be avoided. Factor VIII should be reconstituted with the diluent provided. The reconstituted product must be administered intravenously by direct syringe injection or drip infusion within 3 hours of reconstitution.

## Clinical Usage

rFVIII (Kogenate® and Kogenate® FS, Bayer Corporation; Recombinate and Advate, Baxter; ReFacto, Wyeth) is indicated in hemophilia A (classical hemophilia) for the prevention and control of bleeding episodes.

The pharmacokinetics of plasma derived and rFVIII are summarized in Table 2. The increase in factor VIII concentration is dose proportional and the disposition is similar following single and chronic dosing. The mean biological half-life was similar for recombinant and plasma-derived factor VIII.

The incidence of inhibitors to recombinant and plasma-derived factor VIII in previously untreated patients is similar, about 20% and 10% to 15%,

| Pharmacokinetic parameter | rFVIII | B-domain deleted rFVIII | pdFVIII | rFIX | PdFIX |
|---|---|---|---|---|---|
| Area under the curve, AUC (IU·h/dL) | NR[a] | NR | NR | 548 | 928 |
| Maximum concentration, $C_{max}$ (IU/dL) | 172 | 120 | 102–120 | 39 | 62 |
| Clearance, CL (mL/h/kg) | 3.1±1.2 | 3.2 | 2.9–3.9 | NR | NR |
| Mean residence time, MRT (h) | NR | 16 | 16 | 25 | 23 |
| Volume of distribution, $V_{ss}$ (mL/kg) | 62±18[b] | 45 | 43–70 | NR | NR |
| Half-life, $t_{1/2}$ (h) | 15–17 | 11 | 11–17 | 17–18 | 15–18 |
| In vivo recovery (IU/dL per IU/kg) | 2.4 | 2.4 | 2.4–2.5 | 0.8–0.9 | 1.1–1.7 |

[a] Not reported.
[b] $V_{area}$.
Source: Adapted from Shapiro et al., 2005.

**Table 2** ■ Clinical pharmacokinetic profile of rFVIII or rFIX following intravenous administration of 50 IU/kg.

respectively (McMillan et al., 1988; Lusher et al., 1993). The risk of developing antibodies to rFVIII correlates with severity of disease and the intensity of exposure to factor VIII (Lusher et al., 1993).

Dosage of rFVIII (in IU) must be individualized to the needs of the patient, the severity of the deficiency and of the hemorrhage, the presence of inhibitors, and to the desired increase in factor VIII activity (in IU/dL, or percentage of normal). The in vivo percent elevation in factor VIII level may be estimated as follows (Abildgaard et al., 1966):

Dosage required (IU) = Body wt (kg) × Desired increase in factor VIII (%) × 0.5 IU/kg %

### Safety Concerns
Trace amounts of mouse or hamster protein may be present in rFVIII as contaminants from the expression system. Therefore, caution should be exercised when administering rFVIII to individuals with known hypersensitivity to plasma-derived antihemophilic factor, or with hypersensitivity to biological preparations with trace amounts of murine or hamster proteins.

## FACTOR VIIA

Development of recombinant factor VIIa was motivated by the fact that a small fraction of patients with hemophilia (15–20% of patients with hemophilia A and 2–5% of patients with hemophilia B) develop antibodies (inhibitors) to factor VIII or factor IX. High titers of inhibitors make it impossible to give sufficient coagulation factor to overcome the inhibitor, and therapy is ineffective or is associated with unacceptable side effects. Factor VIIa can be valuable in these instances since in the absence of tissue factor, factor VII has very low proteolytic activity.

### Structure
Factor VII is a vitamin K-dependent glycosylated serine protease proenzyme that is synthesized in the liver. It has 406 amino acids and the molecular weight is ~50 kDa. The protein is not functionally active unless it is γ-carboxylated. There are two sites of N-linked glycosylation on factor VII. Factor VII is synthesized as a proenzyme that becomes activated and cleaved upon hydrolysis of Arg-152 and Ile-153.

### ■ Recombinant Factor VIIa
Recombinant factor VII is expressed in baby hamster kidney cells as a single-chain form and is spontaneously activated to factor VIIa during purification. Characterization of the protein indicates that it is very similar to plasma-derived factor VIIa with regard to amino acid sequence, carbohydrate composition, and γ-carboxylation (Thim et al., 1988).

### Pharmacokinetics and Pharmacodynamics
The single-dose pharmacokinetics of recombinant factor VIIa were investigated in 15 patients with hemophilia with severe factor VIII or factor IX deficiency (Lindley et al., 1994). Table 3 summarizes the pharmacokinetics from this study. Following an intravenous dose of 17.5, 35, and 70 µg/kg, the plasma clearance was 30.3, 32.5, and 36.1 mL/h/kg, respectively. The pharmacokinetics were linear and no difference in clearance was noted between non-

| Dose (µg/kg) | 17.5 | 35 | 70 |
|---|---|---|---|
| $C_{max}$ (U/ml) | 4.92 | 10.8 | 19.6 |
| CL (ml/h/kg) | 30.3 | 32.5 | 36.1 |
| $t_{1/2}$ (h) | 2.6 | 2.7 | 2.8 |
| MRT (h) | 3.3 | 3.3 | 3.4 |
| $V_{ss}$ (ml/kg) | 98.1 | 110 | 120 |
| Recovery (%) | 50.1 | 49.0 | 42.6 |

Note: $C_{max}$ values are presented in IU/mL based on a specific activity of 21–25 IU/µg.
Source: From Lindley et al., 1994.

**Table 3** ■ Clinical pharmacokinetic profile of recombinant factor VIIa.

bleeding and bleeding episodes. Median clearance was 31.0 mL/h in non-bleeding episodes and 32.6 mL/h in bleeding episodes. The median half-life was 2.9 hours in non-bleeding episodes and 2.3 hours in bleeding episodes. There was considerable inter-individual variability whereas intraindividual variability appears to be lower.

Based on preclinical studies in dogs, a concentration of >8 U/mL should result in immediate hemostasis, whereas a concentration of 4 U/mL seems to be below the hemostatic level (Hedner, 1996). Based on the results of several pharmacokinetic/pharmacodynamics studies, it is necessary to maintain plasma levels above 5 to 6 U/mL for adequate hemostasis. This may be done by administering sufficiently high initial concentrations to ensure this, or by maintaining a strict 2-hour dosing interval following doses of 70 to 90 μg/kg (Hedner, 1996).

### Pharmaceutical Considerations

NovoSeven® (Novo Nordisk) is supplied as a white lyophilized powder in single-use glass vials formulated with sodium chloride, calcium chloride dihydrate, glycylglycine, polysorbate 80, and mannitol. The pH is adjusted to 5.3 to 6.3. The product does not contain any stabilizing protein. Before reconstitution, NovoSeven should be stored refrigerated (2–8°C/ 36–46°F) avoiding exposure to direct sunlight.

NovoSeven® should be reconstituted with sterile water for injection, USP (2.2 mL for the 1.2-mg vial and 8.5 mL for the 4.8-mg vial). After reconstitution with the appropriate volume of diluent, each vial contains approximately 0.6 mg/mL. Following reconstitution, NovoSeven® may be stored refrigerated or at room temperature for up to 3 hours. NovoSeven® is intended for intravenous bolus injection and should not be mixed with infusion solutions.

### Clinical Usage

Recombinant factor VIIa (NovoSeven®) is indicated for the treatment of bleeding episodes or the prevention of bleeding in surgical intervention or invasive procedures in patients with hemophilia A or B with inhibitors to factor VIII or factor IX. It is also indicated for treatment of bleeding episodes or the prevention of bleeding in surgical intervention or invasive procedures in patients with congenital factor VII deficiency. The recommended dose of recombinant factor VIIa for patients with hemophilia A or B with inhibitors is 90 μg/kg every 2 hours by bolus infusion until hemostasis is achieved or until treatment is judged to be inadequate. The minimum effective dose has not been established. Doses between 35 and 120 μg/kg have been used successfully in clinical trials. Both the dose and administration interval may be adjusted based on the severity and degree of hemostasis.

A randomized, double-blind study investigating 35 and 70 μg/kg recombinant factor VIIa in 84 patients with hemophilia A or B with or without inhibitors found both doses were ~70% effective (Lusher et al., 1998a). A randomized study evaluating doses of 35 and 90 μg/kg in hemophilia patients with inhibitors undergoing elective surgery showed that the higher dose was more effective than the lower dose (Shapiro et al., 1988).

### Safety

Based on the clinical safety database of 1939 treatment episodes in 298 patients with hemophilia A or B with inhibitors, adverse events reported at rates of more than 2% of patients treated included fever, hemorrhage, decreased fibrinogen, hemarthrosis, and hypertension.

Recombinant factor VIIa (NovoSeven®) should not be administered to patients with known hypersensitivity to recombinant factor VIIa or any of the components of recombinant factor VIIa. Recombinant factor VIIa is contraindicated in patients with known hypersensitivity to mouse, hamster, or bovine proteins.

## FACTOR IX

Factor IX is activated by factor VII/tissue factor complex in the extrinsic pathway and by factor XIa in the intrinsic pathway (Fig. 1). Activated factor IX, in combination with activated factor VIII, activates factor X, resulting in the conversion of prothrombin to thrombin. Thrombin then converts fibrinogen to fibrin, forming a blood clot at a site of hemorrhage.

### ■ Recombinant Factor IX

Recombinant coagulation factor IX (BeneFix®, Wyeth) is produced in a CHO cell line. The transfected cell line secretes recombinant factor IX in the culture medium from which the protein is purified via several chromatographic steps. Recombinant factor IX is a 415 amino acid glycoprotein with a molecular weight of ~55 kDa.

While plasma-derived factor IX carries a Thr/ Ala dimorphism at position 148, the primary amino acid sequence of recombinant factor IX is identical to the Ala148 allelic form. As a result of post-translational modifications, recombinant and plasma-derived factor IX differ in a number of respects (White et al., 1997). First, plasma-derived factor IX carries 12 γ-carboxyglutamic acid (Gla) residues in its amino-terminal Gla-domain, whereas 40% of recombinant factor IX is undercarboxylated, lacking γ-carboxylation at Glu40. Other differences between recombinant and plasma-derived factor IX are in the activation peptide region (residues 146–180), which is cleaved off upon factor IX activation. These include the lack of sulfation at Tyr155, and of phosphorylation at Ser158, as well as different N-linked glycosylation patterns at Asn157 and Asn167.

The potency of recombinant factor IX is determined in IUs using an in vitro clotting assay. One international unit is the amount of factor IX activity present in a milliliter of pooled normal human plasma. The specific activity of BeneFix® is greater than or equal to 200 IU/mg protein.

### Pharmacology

In Beagle dogs, administration of recombinant factor IX once daily for 14 days at doses of 50, 100, or 200 IU/kg showed a dose-proportional increase in maximum concentration ($C_{max}$) and area under the curve (AUC). The elimination half-life ranged between 10.9 and 15.8 hours and was independent of dose (McCarthy et al., 1995). In addition, the pharmacokinetics were similar between Days 1 and 7. Pharmacokinetic and pharmacodynamic studies have indicated that increases in recombinant factor IX plasma concentrations are correlated ($r = 0.86$) with factor IX activity as measured by a clotting assay (Schaub et al., 1998). Comparison of recombinant factor IX and plasma-derived factor IX in a dog model of hemophilia B indicated that while plasma-derived factor IX had a higher AUC and $C_{max}$ compared with recombinant factor IX, the efficacy of the two products was similar (Keith et al., 1995).

### Pharmaceutical Considerations

Recombinant factor IX (BeneFix®) is supplied as a sterile, non-pyrogenic, lyophilized powder in single-use vials containing nominally 250, 500, or 1000 IU per vial. The approved shelf life is 36 months at 2°C to 8°C. The product has been stored at room temperature (25°C) for up to 12 months. Freezing should be avoided to prevent damage to the diluent vial.

Recombinant factor IX should be reconstituted with the sterile water for injection (diluent) provided. After reconstitution, BeneFix® should be injected intravenously over several minutes. The product does not contain a preservative and should be used within 3 hours of reconstitution.

### Clinical Usage

BeneFix® is indicated for the control and prevention of hemorrhagic episodes in patients with hemophilia B, including control and prevention of bleeding in surgical settings.

The pharmacokinetics of recombinant factor IX and of plasma-derived factor IX are summarized in Table 2. The in vivo recovery using BeneFix® was 28% less than the recovery using highly purified plasma-derived factor IX, whereas there was no difference in the biological half-life. Factor IX clotting activity is highly correlated ($r = 0.97$) with plasma concentrations of recombinant factor IX (White et al., 1998).

The dosage and duration of substitution treatment depends on the severity of factor IX deficiency, the location and extent of bleeding, the clinical condition, patient age, and the desired recovery in factor IX. The dose of BeneFix® should be based on the empirical finding that 1 IU of factor IX per kilogram is expected, on average, to increase the circulating level of factor IX by $0.8 \pm 0.2$ IU/dL (range 0.4–1.4).

Higher doses of factor IX may be necessary in patients with inhibitors. If the expected levels of factor IX are not attained, or if bleeding is not controlled, biological testing may be merited to determine if factor IX inhibitors are present.

### Safety

Since BeneFix® is produced in a CHO cell line, it may be contraindicated in patients with known history of hypersensitivity to hamster protein and other constituents in the preparation. During uncontrolled open-label clinical studies with recombinant factor VII, adverse events reported in more than 2% of patients included nausea, taste perversion, injection site reaction, injection site pain, headache, dizziness, allergic rhinitis, rash, hives, flushing, fever, and shaking.

## RECOMBINANT THROMBOLYTIC AGENTS

### ■ Tissue-Type Plasminogen Activator

Deposition of fibrin and platelets in the vasculature leads to thromboembolic diseases that are responsible for considerable mortality and morbidity. Early thrombolytic therapy can decrease mortality and improve coronary artery patency in patients with acute myocardial infarction (AMI). During fibrinolysis, the inactive zymogen plasminogen is enzymatically converted to the active moiety, plasmin, which in turn digests the insoluble fibrin matrix of a thrombus to soluble fibrin degradation products. Tissue-type plasminogen activator (t-PA) exhibits fibrin-specific plasminogen activation with minimal systemic fibrinogenolysis. The relative absence of systemic fibrinogenolysis with t-PA means that there are fewer systemic side effects compared to other plasminogen activators. Mean t-PA antigen concentrations at rest in humans are approximately 5 μg/mL and can increase 1.5- to 2-fold in venous occlusion (Holvoet et al., 1987).

## Structure

Native t-PA is a serine protease synthesized by vascular endothelial cells as a single-chain polypeptide of 527 amino acids with a molecular mass of 64 kDa (Pennica et al., 1983). Approximately 6% to 8% of the molecular mass consists of carbohydrate. A schematic of the primary structure of human t-PA is shown in Figure 2. There are 17 disulfide bridges and an additional free cysteine at position 83, and 4 putative N-linked glycosylation sites recognized by the consensus sequence Asn-X-Ser/Thr at residues 117, 184, 218, and 448 (Pennica et al., 1983). In addition, the presence of a fucose attached to Thr61 via an O-glycosidic linkage has been reported (Harris et al., 1991). Two forms of t-PA that differ by the absence or presence of a carbohydrate at Asp184 have been characterized (Bennett, 1983): Type I t-PA is glycosylated at asparagine 117, 184, and 448; whereas

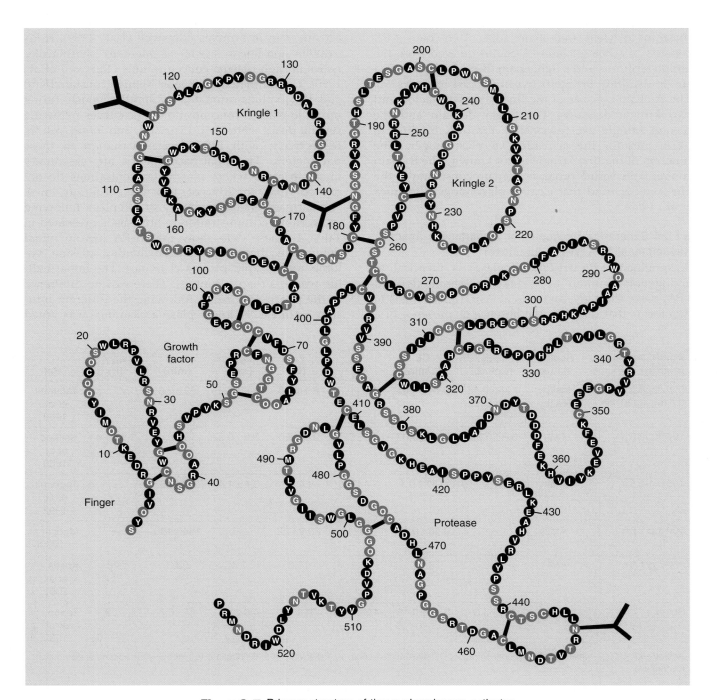

**Figure 2** ■ Primary structure of tissue-plasminogen activator.

Type II t-PA lacks a glycosylation at asparagine 184. The asparagine at amino acid 218 is normally not occupied in either form of t-PA (Vehar et al., 1984b). Asparagine 117 contains a high-mannose oligosaccharide whereas Asn184 and Asn448 are of the complex carbohydrate type (Spellman et al., 1989). Complex N-linked glycan structures contain a disaccharide Gal (1,4)GlcNac and terminate in sialic acid residues, while an oligomannose (high mannose)-type glycan contains only mannose in the outer arms.

During fibrinolysis, the single-chain t-PA polypeptide is cleaved between Arg275 and Ile276 by plasmin to yield two-chain t-PA. Two-chain t-PA consists of a heavy chain (A-chain) derived from the amino terminus and a light chain (B-chain) linked by a single disulfide bridge between Cys264 and Cys395. The A-chain consists of the finger, growth factor, and two kringle domains. The finger domain and the second kringle are responsible for t-PA binding to fibrin and for the activation of plasminogen. The function of the first kringle is not known. The B-chain contains the serine protease domain consisting of the His-Asp-Ser triad that cleaves plasminogen (Pennica et al., 1983).

## ■ First Generation Recombinant Thrombolytic Agents: Recombinant t-PA (rt-PA; Alteplase)

Recombinant t-PA (rt-PA; alteplase) is identical to endogenous human t-PA. Like melanoma-derived t-PA, rt-PA lacks glycosylation at Asn218 and exists in two forms that differ by the absence or presence of a

carbohydrate at residue Asn184 (Vehar et al., 1986). Type II t-PA has a slightly higher specific activity in vitro compared with Type I t-PA (Einarsson et al., 1985).

### Pharmacokinetics of rt-PA

The pharmacokinetics of rt-PA have been studied in mice, rats, rabbits, primates, and humans. After intravenous administration, the plasma concentrations decline rapidly with an initial dominant half-life of less than 5 minutes in all species. Plasma clearance ranges from 27 mL/min in rabbits (Hotchkiss et al., 1988) to 29 mL/min in monkeys (Baughman, 1987), to 620 mL/min in humans (Tanswell et al., 1989). rt-PA exhibits non-linear (Michaelis–Menten) pharmacokinetics at high plasma concentrations (Tanswell et al., 1990). The estimated Michaelis–Menten constant (Km) and $V_{max}$ values estimated by simultaneously fitting multiple plasma concentration–time curves following several doses were 12 to 15 μg/mL and 3.7 μg/mL/h, respectively, with little species variation in these parameters. The pharmacokinetics are essentially linear in cases where plasma concentrations do not exceed 10% to 20% of Km (i.e., 1.5–3 μg/mL). A pharmacokinetic summary of alteplase following intravenous administration in humans is presented in Table 4. These data show that rt-PA has an initial volume of distribution approximating plasma volume, and a rapid plasma clearance. The initial half-life was less than 5 minutes. There was no difference in the pharmacokinetics following the different infusion regimens. A lower plasma clearance was noted

| Administration regimen | Health status | $C_{max}$ (μg/mL) | CL (L/min) | $V_1$ (L) | $V_{ss}$ (L) | $t_{1/2}\alpha$ (min) | $t_{1/2}\beta$ (min) | $t_{1/2}\gamma$ (h) | Ref. |
|---|---|---|---|---|---|---|---|---|---|
| 0.25 mg/kg/30 min
0.5 mg/kg/30 min | Healthy
Healthy | 0.96±0.18
1.8±0.25 | 0.64±0.05 | 4.6±0.3 | 8.1±0.8 | 4.4±0.2 | 39±2.6 | – | Tanswell et al., 1989 |
| 100 mg/2.5 h | AMI | 3.3±0.95 | 0.38±0.07 | 2.8±0.9 | 9.3±5.0 | 3.6±0.9 | 15±5.4 | 3.7±1.4 | Seifried et al., 1989 |
| 100 mg/1.5 h | AMI | 4±1 | 0.57±0.1 | 3.4±1.5 | 8.4±5 | 3.4±1.4 | 72±68 | – | Tanswell et al., 1992 |
| 100 mg/1.5 h | AMI | – | 0.45±0.17 | 7.2±4 | 28.9±22 | – | 144±100 | – | Modi et al., 2000 |
| 100 mg/1.5 h | AMI | – | 0.39 | 6.7 | 17.3 | 7.4 | 22.3 | 228 | Kostis et al., 2002 |
| Bolus | AMI | 9.8±3.6 | 0.48±0.15 | 4.5±1.3 | 31±18 | 4.8±1.0 | 17±6.3 | 9.1±3.1 | Tebbe et al, 1989. |

*Abbreviations*: $C_{max}$, maximum plasma concentration; CL, plasma clearance; $V_1$, initial volume of distribution; $V_{ss}$, steady-state volume of distribution; $t_{1/2}$, half-life.

**Table 4** ■ Pharmacokinetic parameters (mean±SD) for alteplase antigen following intravenous administration in healthy volunteers and patients with AMI.

following intravenous bolus injection, possibly suggesting saturation of clearance mechanisms.

The primary route of alteplase clearance is via receptor-mediated clearance mechanisms in the liver. Three cell types in the liver are responsible for the clearance of t-PA: parenchymal cells, endothelial cells, and Kupffer cells. Kupffer cells and endothelial cells mediate t-PA clearance via the mannose receptor. Parenchymal cells clear t-PA via a carbohydrate-independent, receptor-mediated mechanism. Data suggest that this carbohydrate-independent clearance is mediated by the low-density lipoprotein receptor-related protein (Bu et al., 1993).

## Clinical Usage

Recombinant human t-PA (alteplase t-PA) is indicated for use in the management of AMI in adults for the improvement of ventricular function following AMI, reduction of the incidence of congestive heart failure, reduction of mortality associated with AMI, and for the management of acute massive pulmonary embolism in adults. It is also indicated for the management of acute ischemic stroke if therapy is initiated within 3 hours after the onset of stroke symptoms and after exclusion of intracranial hemorrhage by cranial computerized tomography (CT) scan.

Two dose regimens, the 90-minute accelerated regimen and the 3-hour regimen have been studied in patients experiencing AMI; controlled studies comparing the clinical outcome of the two regimens have not been conducted. For the accelerated regimen, the recommended dose is based on patient weight, not to exceed 100 mg alteplase. For patients weighing more than 67 kg, the recommended dose regimen is 100 mg as a 15-mg intravenous bolus injection, followed by 50 mg infused over 30 minutes, and then 35 mg infused over the next 60 minutes. For patients weighing no more than 67 kg, the recommended dose regimen is a 15-mg intravenous bolus injection, followed by 0.75 mg/kg infused over 30 minutes not to exceed 50 mg, and then 0.5 mg/kg over the next 60 minutes not to exceed 35 mg.

For the 3-hour regimen, the recommended dose is 100 mg administered as 60 mg in the first hour (6–10 mg as a bolus), and 20 mg over each of the second and third hours. For patients weighing less than 65 kg, the dose is 1.25 mg/kg over 3 hours. Infarct artery-related patency rates of 70% to 77% are achieved at 90 minutes with this 3-hour regimen (Vestraete et al., 1985). Patency grades of blood flow in the infarct-related artery are defined by the Thrombolysis in Myocardial Infarction (TIMI) scale and are assessed angiographically with TIMI Grade 0 representing no flow; Grade 1, minimal flow; Grade 2, sluggish flow; and Grade 3, complete or full, brisk flow.

The efficacy of the accelerated 90-minute regimen was demonstrated in an international, multicenter trial, Global Utilization of Streptokinase and Tissue Plasminogen Activator for Occluded Coronary Arteries (GUSTO), that enrolled approximately 41,000 patients (The GUSTO Investigators, 1993a,b). The GUSTO trial demonstrated a higher infarct-related artery patency rate at 90 minutes in the group treated with rt-PA with heparin compared with streptokinase with either intravenous or subcutaneous heparin. The patency in the alteplase group was 81.3% compared with 53.5% to 59.0% in the streptokinase groups. In addition, the alteplase group had a reduced mortality (an additional 10 lives saved per 10,000 patients treated). The intracranial hemorrhage rate was approximately 1%.

In a multicenter, open-label study in 461 patients with AMI randomized to receive 100 mg alteplase over 90 minutes or two 50-mg bolus doses 30 minutes apart, the 90-minute angiographic patency rate was 74.5% for the double bolus group and 81.4% in the infusion group ($p = 0.08$). The 30-day mortality rates were 4.5% in the bolus group and 1.7% in the infusion group (not significantly different) (Bleich et al., 1998). Similarly, the Continuous Infusion Versus Double-Bolus Administration of Alteplase (COBALT) trial in 7,169 patients with AMI showed a higher incidence of 30-day mortality in the double bolus alteplase group (7.98%) compared with the accelerated-infusion group (7.53%). There was also a slightly higher incidence of intracranial hemorrhage in the double bolus group (COBALT Investigators, 1997).

For acute ischemic stroke, the recommended dose is 0.9 mg/kg not to exceed 90 mg infused over 60 minutes, with 10% of the total dose administered as an initial intravenous bolus over 1 minute. The safety and efficacy of this regimen with concomitant use of heparin and aspirin during the first 24 hours has not been investigated.

The recommended dose for treatment of pulmonary embolism is 100 mg administered by intravenous infusion over 2 hours. Heparin therapy should be instituted or reinstituted near the end of or immediately following alteplase infusion when the partial thromboplastin time or thrombin time returns to twice normal or less.

## Safety Concerns

Since thrombolytic therapy increases the risk of bleeding, alteplase is contraindicated in patients with a history of cerebrovascular accidents, or patients who have any kind of active internal bleeding, intracranial neoplasm, arteriovenous malformation, or aneurism or who have had recent intracranial or intraspinal surgery or trauma.

## Pharmaceutical Considerations

Recombinant human t-PA (Alteplase; Activase®, Genentech, Inc; Actilyse®, Boehringer Ingelheim) is supplied as a sterile, white to off-white lyophilized powder. rt-PA is practically insoluble in water, and arginine is included in the formulation to increase aqueous solubility. Phosphoric acid and/or sodium hydroxide may be used to adjust the pH. The sterile lyophilized powder should be stored at controlled room temperatures not to exceed 30°C, or refrigerated at 2°C to 8°C, and it should be protected from excessive light.

The powder is reconstituted by adding the accompanying sterile water for injection, USP to the vial, resulting in a colorless to pale yellow transparent solution containing 1 mg/mL rt-PA, with a pH of approximately 7.3 and an osmolality of approximately 215 mOs/kg. rt-PA is stable in solution over a pH range of 5 to 7.5. Since the reconstituted solution does not contain any preservatives, it should be used within 8 hours of preparation and should be refrigerated before use. The solution is incompatible with bacteriostatic water for injection. Other solutions such as sterile water for injection or preservative-containing solutions should not be used for further dilution. The 1-mg/mL solution can be diluted further with an equal volume of 0.9% sodium chloride for injection, USP or 5% dextrose injection, USP to yield a solution with a concentration of 0.5 mg/mL. This solution is compatible with glass bottles and polyvinyl chloride bags.

## ■ Second Generation Recombinant Thrombolytic Agents

The rapid clearance of rt-PA from the circulation by the liver necessitates administration as an intravenous infusion. Although alteplase provides more rapid thrombolysis and superior patency compared with streptokinase and urokinase, at therapeutic doses, there is some fibrinogenolysis and the administration scheme is relatively complicated. Thus, there is room for further improvements in efficacy and safety. Considerable non-clinical and clinical research has been underway to identify rt-PA variants that are fibrin specific and that have a simpler administration regimen compared with alteplase. Several reviews (e.g., Higgins and Bennett, 1990) have outlined the progress of efforts to develop second-generation thrombolytic agents. Strategies that have been used to develop t-PA variants have included domain deletions, glycosylation changes, or site-directed amino acid substitutions. A number of these second-generation thrombolytic agents are currently in late-stage clinical trials or have been approved for marketing.

## ■ Reteplase

Reteplase is a 355-amino acid deletion variant of t-PA, consisting of the protease and kringle 2 domains of human t-PA. It is expressed in *Escherichia coli* cells as a single chain, non-glycosylated, 39.6-kDa peptide.

## Pharmacology

Like alteplase, reteplase is a fibrin-specific activator of plasminogen. In vitro, the plasminogenolytic activity of reteplase is 2- to 3.8-fold lower than alteplase on a molar basis (Kohnert et al., 1993), which may be attributed to the absence of the finger domain in reteplase. Reteplase had a similar in vitro maximal efficacy ($E_{max}$) compared with alteplase, however, the molar concentration required to produce 50% clot lysis ($EC_{50}$) was 6.4-fold higher for reteplase than for alteplase (Martin et al., 1993). The data also suggested that in vitro, reteplase has a lower thrombolytic potency in lysing aged and platelet-rich clots compared with alteplase.

A summary of the pharmacokinetics of reteplase in humans is presented in Table 5.

## Clinical Usage

Reteplase (Retavase®, PDL) is indicated for use in the management of AMI in adults for the improvement of ventricular function following AMI, the reduction of the incidence of congestive heart failure, and the reduction of mortality associated with AMI.

The potency of reteplase is expressed in units using a reference standard that is specific for reteplase and is not comparable with units used for other thrombolytic agents. Reteplase is administered as a double bolus injection regimen consisting of 10 U each. Each bolus is administered as an intravenous injection of 2 minutes via an intravenous line in which no other medications are being administered simultaneously. The second bolus injection is given 30 minutes after the first. Heparin and reteplase are incompatible when combined in solution, and should not be administered simultaneously through the same intravenous line. If reteplase is administered through an intravenous line containing heparin, normal saline or 5% dextrose solution should be flushed through the intravenous line before and following reteplase.

The International Joint Efficacy Comparison of Thrombolytics (INJECT) trial evaluated the effects of reteplase (10 + 10 U) and streptokinase (1.6 million Units over 60 minutes) on 35-day mortality in 6010 AMI patients in a double-blind randomized fashion. The 35-day mortality was 9.0% for patients treated with reteplase and 9.5% for those treated with streptokinase with no difference between the two groups. The incidence of stroke was also similar between the groups, however, more patients treated with reteplase experienced hemorrhagic strokes.

Two open-label angiographic studies (Reteplase Angiographic Phase II International Dose-finding study (RAPID 1) and Reteplase versus Alteplase

| Dose | n | $C_{max}$ | CL (L/h) | $t_{1/2}\alpha$ (min) | $t_{1/2}\beta$ (h) | Ref. |
|------|---|-----------|----------|-----------------------|--------------------|------|
| **Reteplase[a]** | | | | | | |
| 10 U | 4 | 4620 | 6.24 | 19.2 | 6.3 | Sefried et al., 1992 |
| 15 U | 9 | 5060 | 8.34 | 18.8 | 6.3 | Sefried et al., 1992 |
| 15 U | 9 | 5170 | 8.70 | 21.4 | 5.0 | Grünewald et al., 1997 |
| 10 U + 5 U | 7 | 3610 | 9.12 | 16.3 | 5.4 | Grünewald et al., 1997 |
| 10 U + 10 U | 8 | 3370 | 6.90 | 17.0 | 5.5 | Grünewald et al., 1997 |
| **Tenecteplase[b]** | | | | | | |
| 30 mg | 48 | 10.0 | 98.5 | 21.5 | 1.93 | Modi et al., 2000 |
| 40 mg | 31 | 10.9 | 119 | 23.8 | 2.15 | Modi et al., 2000 |
| 50 mg | 20 | 15.2 | 99.9 | 20.1 | 1.50 | Modi et al., 2000 |
| **Lanatoplase** | | | | | | |
| 15 kU/kg | 4 | - | 3.42 | 36 | 12 | Kostis et al., 2002 |
| 30 kU/kg | 2 | - | 3.12 | 31 | 7.4 | Kostis et al., 2002 |
| 60 kU/kg | 8 | - | 3.42 | 32 | 8.7 | Kostis et al., 2002 |
| 120 kU/kg | 8 | - | 2.4 | 47 | 10.5 | Kostis et al., 2002 |

Note: $C_{max}$ values are reported in [a]U/mL or [b]ng/ml.

**Table 5** ■ Pharmacokinetic parameters for second-generation thrombolytic agents.

Patency Investigation During myocardial infarction (RAPID 2)) have compared reteplase with alteplase. In RAPID 1 patients were treated with reteplase (10 + 10 U, 15 U, or 10 + 5 U) or the standard alteplase regimen (100 mg over 3 hours) within 6 hours of symptoms. Ninety-minute TIMI grade 3 flow was seen in 63% of patients in the 10 + 10 U reteplase group and 49% of the patients in the standard regimen alteplase group.

RAPID 2 was an open-label, randomized trial in 320 patients comparing 10 + 10 U reteplase and accelerated alteplase within 12 hours of symptom onset. Percentages of patients with TIMI grade 3 flow at 90 minutes were 59.9% in the reteplase group and 45.2% in the alteplase group. There was no significant difference in the 35-day mortality between the two groups. Neither trial was powered to compare the efficacy or safety with respect to mortality or incidence of stroke.

The more favorable results for reteplase compared with alteplase noted in smaller trials were not replicated in a large, randomized, double-blind trial. In the GUSTO-III trial, 15,059 patients were randomized in a 2:1 fashion to receive reteplase in 2 bolus doses of 10 U 30 minutes apart or up to 100 mg alteplase infused over 90 minutes. The 30-day mortality rates were 7.47% for reteplase and 7.24% for alteplase (The Global Use of Strategies to Open Occluded Coronary Arteries (GUSTO III) Investigators, 1997). The stroke rate was 1.64% for reteplase and 1.79% for alteplase ($p = 0.50$). Reteplase, while easier to administer than accelerated alteplase, did not demonstrate any survival advantage.

### Safety Concerns

As with other thrombolytic agents, reteplase is contraindicated in cases of active internal bleeding, history of cerebrovascular accident, recent intracranial or intraspinal surgery or trauma, intracranial neoplasm, arteriovenous malformation, or aneurism, in cases of known bleeding diathesis, and in severe uncontrolled hypertension.

### Pharmaceutical Considerations

Reteplase is supplied as a sterile, white, lyophilized powder for intravenous injection after reconstitution with sterile water for injection, USP supplied as part of the kit. Following reconstitution, the pH of the solution is 6.0. Reteplase contains no antibacterial preservatives and should be reconstituted immediately before use. The solution should be used within 4 hours when stored at 2°C to 30°C (36–86°F).

### ■ Tenecteplase

Tenecteplase (TNKase™, Genentech, Inc.) is a t-PA variant that has amino acid substitutions in three regions of t-PA. Replacement of threonine at amino acid 103 by asparagine (T103N) incorporates a complex oligosaccharide carbohydrate structure at this position. Replacement of arginine at position 117 by glutamine (N117Q) results in removal of the high mannose carbohydrate present at this site. A tetra-alanine substitution at positions 496 through 499 (KHRR496-499AAAA) contributes to increased fibrin specificity. These three design modifications result in a thrombolytic that, compared to the parent t-PA molecule, is approximately 10- to 14-fold more fibrin specific, is 80-fold more resistant to local inactivation, and has an 8-fold slower clearance in rabbits (Keyt et al., 1994). Allometric scaling of pharmacokinetic data in animals predicted that tenecteplase would have a 5-fold slower plasma clearance compared with alteplase (McCluskey et al., 1997).

*Pharmacology*

Like alteplase, tenecteplase has Type I and Type II glycoforms. Type I has three carbohydrate structures at asparagine 103, 184, and 448; and Type II lacks the carbohydrate at asparagine 184. Carbohydrate structures on tenecteplase are all of the complex oligosaccharide type with no high mannose structures. For this reason, the rapid mannose receptor-mediated clearance observed for alteplase does not occur with tenecteplase. Rather, tenecteplase is thought to be cleared by galactose receptors present in liver sinusoidal cells.

Enzymatic removal of terminal sialic acid from tenecteplase has been shown to increase the clearance in rabbits and is likely due to increased exposure of underlying galactose sugars. This desialylation effect is more profound with tenecteplase than with alteplase and is probably due to the predominant mannose receptor-mediated clearance for alteplase. A second possible clearance pathway for tenecteplase is a non-carbohydrate mediated mechanism via the low-density lipoprotein receptor-related protein (LRP) that is also a clearance pathway for alteplase (Camani et al., 1998).

The thrombolytic potency of tenecteplase was 5- to 10-fold greater than alteplase in animal models of coronary artery thrombosis (Benedict et al., 1995) and embolic stroke (Thomas et al., 1994). The slower clearance of tenecteplase results in a longer exposure of the clot to the thrombolytic agent, which likely offsets the slightly lower activity. The higher fibrin specificity of tenecteplase results in lower systemic activation of plasminogen and an observed conservation of fibrinogen.

*Clinical Usage*

Tenecteplase is indicated for the reduction of mortality associated with AMI. The recommended total dose of tenecteplase should not exceed 50 mg and is based on patient weight according to the following weight-adjusted dosing table (Wang-Clow et al., 2001):

| Patient weight (kg) | Tenecteplase dose (mg) |
|---|---|
| <60 | 30 |
| ≥60 to <70 | 35 |
| ≥70 to <80 | 40 |
| ≥80 to <90 | 45 |
| ≥90 | 50 |

Treatment should be initiated as soon as possible after the onset of AMI symptoms. Tenecteplase is contraindicated in patients with known bleeding diathesis or active internal bleeding, history of cerebrovascular accident, recent intracranial or intraspinal surgery or trauma, intracranial neoplasm, arteriovenous malformation, aneurysm, or severe uncontrolled hypertension due to an increased risk of bleeding.

The clinical pharmacokinetics of tenecteplase have been examined in two studies (TIMI 10A and TIMI 10B). TIMI 10A was a Phase I pilot safety study in patients with AMI. Pharmacokinetic data were obtained in 82 patients following intravenous bolus doses of 5 to 50 mg. Tenecteplase plasma concentrations decreased in a biphasic manner with an initial half-life of 11 to 20 minutes and a terminal half-life of 41 to 138 minutes. Mean plasma clearance of tenecteplase ranged from 125 to 216 mL/min and decreased with increasing dose (Modi et al., 1998).

TIMI 10B was a dose-finding Phase II efficacy study comparing 30-, 40- and 50-mg doses of bolus tenecteplase to 100 mg alteplase administered via the accelerated infusion regimen. The pharmacokinetic data from TIMI 10B are summarized in Table 5. Tenecteplase plasma clearance was approximately 100 mL/min compared to 453 mL/min for accelerated alteplase. In contrast to TIMI 10A, no dose-dependent decrease in plasma clearance was noted in TIMI 10B, likely as a result of the narrower dose range examined. Additionally, the plasma clearances noted in TIMI 10B were slightly lower than those noted in TIMI 10A at comparable doses (Modi et al., 2000). The 30-, 40- and 50-mg doses in TIMI 10B produced TIMI grade 3 flow in 54.3%, 62.8%, and 65.8% of the patients, respectively. TIMI grade 3 flow was seen in 62.7% of patients in the accelerated alteplase group, not significantly different from that in the 40-mg tenecteplase group. An additional finding of this dose-finding efficacy trial was that dose-adjusted dosing is important in achieving optimal reperfusion (Cannon et al., 1998). In addition, tenecteplase resulted in a lower change from baseline in systemic coagulation factors compared with alteplase.

The safety and efficacy of tenecteplase were studied in a large double-blind randomized trial

(Assessment of the Safety and Efficacy of a New Thrombolytic (ASSENT-2)). This trial in 16,949 AMI patients showed that the 30-day mortality rates for single bolus tenecteplase and accelerated alteplase were almost identical (6.18% for tenecteplase and 6.15% for alteplase) (Assessment of the Safety and Efficacy of a New Thrombolytic (ASSENT-2) Investigators, 1999). Intracranial hemorrhage rates were similar in both groups (0.9%), but fewer noncerebral hemorrhages and a lower need for blood transfusion were noted in the tenecteplase group. In conclusion, tenecteplase and 90-minute alteplase are equivalent in terms of mortality and rates of intracranial hemorrhage. The single-bolus regimen for tenecteplase may facilitate thrombolytic therapy.

### Pharmaceutical Considerations

Tenecteplase is supplied as a sterile, white to off-white, lyophilized powder in a 50-mg vial under a partial vacuum. It should be stored at controlled room temperature not to exceed 30°C (86°F) or it should be stored refrigerated at 2°C to 8°C (36–46°F). Tenecteplase is intended for intravenous bolus injection following reconstitution with sterile water for injection. Each vial nominally contains 52.5 mg tenecteplase (comprising a 5% overfill), 0.55 g L-arginine, 0.17 g phosphoric acid, and 4.3 mg polysorbate 20. Biological potency of tenecteplase is determined by an in vitro clot lysis assay and is expressed in tenecteplase-specific activity units. The specific activity of tenecteplase has been defined as 200 U/mg protein.

### ■ Lanoteplase

Lanoteplase is currently in development and published information is limited at this time. Lanoteplase is a t-PA variant in which the fibronectin fingerlike and epidermal growth factor domains have been removed (Collen et al., 1988). In addition, an asparagine to glutamine substitution at amino acid 117 provides reduced clearance (Hansen et al., 1988). Lanoteplase has enhanced fibrinolytic activity in the presence of fibrin-related plasminogen, and it is more fibrin specific compared with streptokinase and urokinase. The pharmacokinetics of lanoteplase in AMI patients are summarized in Table 5.

The Intravenous nPA for Treatment of Infarcting Myocardium Early (InTIME) study was a multicenter, double-blind, randomized, double placebo, dose-ranging study in 613 patients comparing 4 doses of lanoteplase with accelerated alteplase. Patients were randomized to receive intravenous bolus doses of 15, 30, 60, or 120 kU/kg (not to exceed 12,000 kU) of lanoteplase or accelerated alteplase (den Heijer et al., 1998). A statistically significant increase in the proportion of patients with TIMI grade 3 flow at 60 minutes was noted with increasing lanoteplase

dose ($p < 0.001$). Patients given the highest lanoteplase dose appeared to have a higher rate of TIMI grade 3 flow at 90 minutes compared with alteplase (57% vs. 46%), although this may be a result of the unusually low TIMI grade 3 flow in the alteplase arm of this small study. There was no difference in the 30-day composite endpoint of death, heart failure, major bleeding, or non-fatal infarction (Ross, 1999).

A larger randomized, multicenter equivalence trial (InTIME II) in 15,078 patients compared the safety and efficacy of 120 kU/kg lanoteplase with that of accelerated alteplase (Ferguson, 1999). Patients were randomized in a 2:1 fashion to the lanoteplase arm or the alteplase arm. The primary endpoint of the study was 30-day mortality with an incidence of 6.7% for lanoteplase and 6.6% for alteplase. The difference in the incidence of stroke was not statistically significantly different between the treatment groups (1.89% for lanoteplase and 1.52% for alteplase). Intracranial hemorrhage was significantly more frequent in the lanoteplase arm than in the alteplase arm (1.13% vs. 0.62%).

## CONCLUSIONS

Recombinant technology has brought about significant advances in the treatment of coagulation disorders and in the availability of thrombolytic agents for the treatment of thrombotic disorders.

## REFERENCES

Abildgaard CF, Simone JV, Corrigan JJ, et al. (1966). Treatment of hemophilia with glycine-precipitated Factor VIII. New Eng J Med 275:471–75.

Antonarakis SE, Youssoufian H, Kazazian Jr HH (1987). Molecular genetics of hemophilia A in man (Factor VIII deficiency). Mol Biol Med 4:81–94.

Assessment of the Safety and Efficacy of a New Thrombolytic (ASSENT-2) Investigators (1999). Single-bolus tenecteplase compared with front-loaded alteplase in acute myocardial infarction: The ASSENT-2 double-blind randomized trial. Lancet 354:716–22.

Baughman RA (1987). Pharmacokinetics of tissue plasminogen activator. In: Sobel B, Collen, D, Grossbard E, eds. Tissue Plasminogen Activator in Thrombolytic Therapy New York: Marcel Dekker, 41–53.

Benedict CR, Refino CJ, Keyt BA, et al. (1995). New variant of human tissue plasminogen activator (tPA) with enhanced efficacy and lower incidence of bleeding compared with recombinant human tPA. Circulation 92:3032–40.

Bennett WF (1983). Two forms of tissue-type plasminogen activator (tPA) differ at a single specific glycosylation site. Thromb Haemost 50:106.

Bleich SD, Adgey AAJ, McMechan SR, Love TW (1998). An angiographic assessment of alteplase: Double-bolus and front-loaded infusion regimens in myocardial infraction. Am Heart J 136:74–8.

Bu G, Maksymovitch EA, Schwartz AL (1993). Receptor-mediated endocytosis of tissue-type plasminogen activator by low density lipoprotein receptor-related protein on human hepatoma HepG2 cells. J Biol Chem 268:13002–9.

Camani C, Gavin O, Bertossa C, Samatani E, Kruithof EK (1998). Studies on the effect of fucosylated and non-fucosylated finger/growth factor constructs on the clearance of tissue type plasminogen activator mediated by the low-density lipoprotein-receptor related protein. Eur J Biochem 251:804–11.

Cannon CP, Gibson CM, McCabe CH, et al. (1998). TNK-tissue plasminogen activator compared with front-loaded alteplase in acute myocardial infarction. Circulation 98:2805–14.

Collen D, Stassen JM, Larsen GR (1988). Pharmacokinetics and thrombolytic properties of deletion mutants of human tissue-type plasminogen activator in rabbits. Blood 71:216–9.

The Continuous Infusion Versus Double-Bolus Administration of Alteplase (COBALT) Investigators (1997). A comparison of continuous infusion and alteplase with double-bolus administration for acute myocardial infarction. New Engl J Med 337:1124–30.

Eaton DL, Hass PE, Riddle L, et al. (1987). Characterization of recombinant human Factor VIII. J Biol Chem 262:3285–90.

Einarsson M, Brandt J, Kaplan L (1985). Large-scale purification of human tissue-type plasminogen activator using monoclonal antibodies. Biochim Biophys Acta 830:1–10.

Ferguson JJ (1999). Meeting highlights. Highlights of the 48th scientific sessions of the American College of Cardiology. Circulation 100:570–5.

The Global Use of Strategies to Open Occluded Coronary Arteries (GUSTO) Investigators (1993a). An international randomized trial comparing four thrombolytic strategies for acute myocardial infarction. New Engl J Med 329:673–82.

The Global Use of Strategies to Open Occluded Coronary Arteries (GUSTO) Investigators (1993b). The effects of tissue plasminogen activator, streptokinase, or both on coronary-artery patency, ventricular function, and survival after acute myocardial infarction. New Eng J Med 329:1615–22.

The Global Use of Strategies to Open Occluded Coronary Arteries (GUSTO III) Investigators (1997). A comparison of reteplase with alteplase for acute myocardial infarction. New Engl J Med 337:1118–23.

Grünewald M, Müller M, Ellbrück D, et al. (1997). Double- versus single-bolus thrombolysis with reteplase for acute myocardial infarction: a pharmacokinetic and pharmacodynamic study. Fibrinol Proteol 11:137–45.

Harris RJ, Leonard CK, Guzzetta AW, Spellman MW (1991). Tissue plasminogen activator has an O-linked fucose attached to Threonine-61 in the epidermal growth factor domain. Biochemistry 30:2311–4.

Hedner U (1996). Dosing and monitoring NovoSeven® treatment. Haemostasis 216(Suppl 1):102–8.

Hansen L, Blue Y, Barone K, Collen D, Larsen GR (1988). Functional effects of asparagine-linked oligosaccharide on natural and variant human tissue-type plasminogen activator. J Biol Chem 263:15713–9.

Higgins DL, Bennett WF (1990). Tissue plasminogen activator: the biochemistry and pharmacology of variants produced by mutagenesis. Annu Rev Pharmacol Toxicol 30:91–121.

Hironaka T, Furukawa K, Esmon PC, et al. (1992). Comparative study of the sugar chains of factor VIII purified from human plasma and from the culture media of recombinant baby hamster kidney cells. J Biol Chem 267:8012–20.

Hoffman M (2003) A cell-based model of coagulation and the role of factor VIIa. Blood Rev 17:S1–5.

Hoffman M, Monroe DM (2005). Rethinking the coagulation cascade. Current Hematol Rep 4:391–6.

Holvoet P, Boes J, Collen D (1987). Measurement of free, one-chain tissue-type plasminogen activator in human plasma with an enzyme-linked immunosorbent assay based on an active site-specific murine monoclonal antibody. Blood 69:284–9.

Hotchkiss A, Refino CJ, Leonard CK, et al. (1988). The influence of carbohydrate structure on the clearance of recombinant tissue-type plasminogen activator. Thromb Haemost 60:255–61.

Hoyer LW (1981). The Factor VIII complex: Structure and function. Blood 58:1–13.

Jackson CM, Nemerson Y (1980). Blood coagulation. Ann Rev Biochem 49:767–811.

Keith JC, Ferranti, Misra B, et al. (1995). Evaluation of recombinant human factor IX: Pharmacokinetic studies in the rat and dog. Thromb Haemost 73:101–5.

Kessler CM (2005). New perspectives in hemophilia treatment. Hematology. American Society of Hematology Education Program book, pp 429–35.

Keyt BA, Paoni NF, Refino CJ, et al. (1994). A faster-acting and more potent form of tissue plasminogen activator. Proc Natl Acad Sci (USA) 91:3670–4.

Kohnert U, Horsch B, Fischer S (1993). A variant of tissue plasminogen activator (t-PA) comprised of the kringle 2 and the protease domain shows a significant difference in the in vitro rate of plasmin formation as compared to the recombinant human t-PA from transformed Chinese hamster ovary cells. Fibrinolysis 7:365–72.

Kostis JB, Dockens RC, Thadani U, et al. (2002). Comparison of pharmacokinetics of lanoteplase and alteplase during acute myocardial infarction. Clin Pharmacokinet 41:445–52.

Lindley CM, Sawyer WT, Macik G, et al. (1994). Pharmacokinetics and pharmacodynamics of recombinant factor VIIa. Clin Pharmacol Ther 55:638–48.

Lusher JM, Arkin S, Abildgaard CF, Schwartz RS, and The Kogenate Previously Untreated Patient Study Group (1993). Recombinant Factor VIII for the treatment of previously untreated patients with hemophilia A. New Engl J Med 328:453–9.

Lusher J, Ingerslev J, Roberts H, Hedner U (1998a). Clinical experience with recombinant factor VIIa. Blood Coag Fibrinol 9:119–28.

Lusher JM, Roberts HR, Davignon G, et al. (1998b). A randomized, double-blind comparison of two dosage levels of recombinant factor VIIa in the treatment of joint, muscle and mucocutaneous haemorrhages in person with haemophilia A and B, with and without inhibitors. RFVII Study Group. Haemophilia, 4: 790–8.

Martin U, Sponer G, Strein K (1993). Differential fibrinolytic properties of the recombinant plasminogen activator BM 06.022 in human plasma and blood clot systems in vitro. Blood Coag Fibrinolysis 4:235–42.

McCarthy KP, Timony GA, DeCoste MT, et al. (1995). Pharmacokinetics of recombinant factor IX in beagle dogs. Thromb Haemost 73:1016.

McCarthy KP, Brinkhous KM, Stewart PF, et al. (1997). The pharmacokinetics of fully γ-carboxylated factor IX and factor IX lacking γ–carboxylation at Glu-40 are similar in the hemophilia beagle dog. XVI Congress of the International Society of Thrombosis and Haemostasis, June 8–10, Florence, Italy.

McCluskey ER, Keyt BA, Refino CJ, et al. (1997). Biochemistry, pharmacology, and initial clinical experience with TNK-tPA in New therapeutic agents. In: Sasahara AA, Loscalzo, eds. Thrombosis and Thrombolysis.. New York: Marcel Dekker, 475–593.

McMillan CW, Shapiro SS, Whitehurst D, Hoyer LW, Rao AV, Lazerson J (1988). The natural history of factor VIII:C inhibitors in patients with hemophilia A: a natural cooperative study. II. Observations on the initial development of factor VIII:C inhibitor. Blood 71:344–8.

Modi NB, Eppler S, Breed J, Cannon CP, Braunwald E, Love T (1998). Pharmacokinetics of a slower clearing tissue plasminogen activator variant, TNK-tPA, in patients with acute myocardial infarction. Thromb Haemost 79:134–9.

Modi NB, Fox NL, Clow F-W, et al. (2000). Pharmacokinetics and pharmacodynamics of tenecteplase: Results from a Phase II study in patients with acute myocardial infarction. J Clin Pharmacol 40:508–15.

Pennica D, Holmes WE, Kohr WJ, et al.. (1983). Cloning and expression of human tissue-type plasminogen activator cDNA in *E. coli*. Science 301:214–21.

Roddie PH, Ludlam CA (1997). Recombinant coagulation factors. Blood Rev 11:169–77.

Ross AM (1999). New plasminogen activators: A clinical review. Clin Cardiol 22:165–71.

Schaub R, Garzone P, Bouchard P, et al. (1998). Preclinical students of recombinant factor IX. Semin Hematol 2 (Suppl 2) 28–32.

Schwartz RS, Abildgaard CF, Aledort LM, et al. (1990). Human recombinant DNA-derived antihemophilic factor (Factor VIII) in the treatment of hemophilia A. New Engl J Med 323:1800–5.

Seifried E, Tanswell P, Ellbrück D, Haerer W, Schmidt A (1989). Pharmacokinetics and haemostatic status during consecutive infusions of recombinant tissue-type plasminogen activator in patients with acute myocardial infarction. Thromb Haemost 61:497–501.

Shapiro A, Gilchrist GS, Hoots WK, Gastineau DA (1988). Prospective randomized trial of two doses of rFVII (Novoseven) in hemophilic patients with inhibitors undergoing surgery. J Thromb Haemost 80:773–8.

Shapiro AD, Korth-Bradley J, Poon MC (2005). Use of pharmacokinetics in the coagulation factor treatment of patients with haemophilia. Haemophilia 11:571–82.

Spellman MW, Basa LJ, Leonard CK, et al. (1989). Carbohydrate structures of human tissue plasminogen activator expressed in Chinese Hamster Ovary cells. J Biol Chem 264:14100–111.

Tanswell P, Seifried E, Su Pcaf, Feuerer W, Rijken DC (1989). Pharmacokinetics and systemic effects of tissue-type plasminogen activator in normal subjects. Clin Pharmacol Ther 46:155–62.

Tanswell P, Heinzel G, Greischel A, Krause J (1990). Nonlinear pharmacokinetics of tissue-type plasminogen activator in three animal species and isolated perfused rat liver. J Pharmacol Exp Ther 255:318–24.

Tanswell P, Tebbe U, Neuhaus K-L, Gläsle-Schwarz L, Wojcik J, Seifried E (1992). Pharmacokinetics and fibrin specificity of alteplase during accelerated infusions in acute myocardial infarction. J Am Coll Cardiol 19:1071–5.

Tebbe U, Tanswell P, Seifried E, Feuerer W, Scholz K-H, Herrmann KS (1989). Single-bolus injection of recombinant tissue-type plasminogen activator in acute myocardial infarction. Am J Cardiol 64:448–53.

Thim L, Bjoern S, Christensen M, et al. (1988) Amino acid sequence and posttranslational modifications of human factor VIIa from plasma and transfected baby hamster kidney cells. Biochemistry 27:7785–93.

Thomas GR, Thibodeaux H, Errett CJ, et al. (1994). A long-half-life and fibrin-specific form of tissue plasminogen activator in rabbit models of embolic stroke and peripheral bleeding. Stroke 25:2072–8.

van Griensven JMT, Huisman LGM, Stuurman T, et al. (1996). Effects of increased liver blood flow on the kinetics and dynamics of recombinant tissue-type plasminogen activator. Clin Pharmacol Ther 60:504–11.

Vehar GA, Keyt BA, Eaton D, et al. (1984a). Structure of human Factor VIII. Nature 312:337–42.

Vehar GA, Kohr WJ, Bennett WF, et al. (1984b). Characterization studies on human melanoma cell tissue plasminogen activator. Bio/Tech 2:1051–7.

Vehar GA, Spellman MW, Keyt BA, et al. (1986). Characterization studies of human tissue-type plasminogen activator produced using recombinant DNA technology. Cold Spring Harbor Symp Quant Biol 51:551–62.

Verstraete M, Bernard R, Bory M, Brower RW, Collen D, et al. (1985). Randomized trial of intravenous streptokinase in acute myocardial infarction. Report from the European Cooperative Study Group for recombinant tissue-type plasminogen activator. Lancet 1:842.

Wang-Clow F, Fox NL, Cannon CP, et al. (2001). Determination of a weight-adjusted dose of TNK-tissue plasminogen activator. Am Heart J 141:33–40.

White GC, Beeb A, Nielsen B (1997). Recombinant Factor IX. Thromb. Haemostasis 78:261–5.

White G, Shapiro A, Ragni M, et al. (1998). Clinical evaluation of recombinant factor IX. Semin Hematol 2(Suppl 2):33–8.

# 15

# Monoclonal Antibodies: From Structure to Therapeutic Application

*Banmeet Anand, Rong Deng, Frank-Peter Theil, Jing Li,*
*Shasha Jumbe, Thomas Gelzleichter, Paul Fielder,*
*Amita Joshi, and Saraswati Kenkare-Mitra*
Genentech, Inc., South San Francisco, California, U.S.A.

## INTRODUCTION

The exciting field of therapeutic monoclonal antibodies (mAbs) had its origins as Milstein and Koehler presented their murine hybridoma technology in 1975 (Kohler and Milstein, 1975). This technology provides a reproducible method for producing monoclonal antibodies with unique target selectivity in almost unlimited quantities. In 1984, both scientists received the Nobel Prize for their scientific breakthrough, and their work was viewed as a key milestone in the history of mAbs as therapeutic modalities and their other applications. Although it took some time until the first therapeutic mAb got market authorization from the FDA in 1986 (Orthoclone OKT3, Chapter 17), monoclonal antibodies are now the standard of care in several disease areas. In particular, in the areas of oncology (Chapter 16), transplantation (Chapter 17) and inflammatory diseases (Chapter 18) patients now have novel life-changing treatment alternatives for diseases which had very limited or non-existent medical treatment options before the emergence of mAbs. To date more than twenty mAbs, and mAb derivatives including fusion proteins and mAb fragments are available for different therapies (Table 1): nine mAbs and two immunoconjugates in oncology; six mAbs and three Fc (Fragment crystallization)-fusion proteins in inflammation; three mAbs in transplantation; one mAb fragment for the cardiovascular area). Technological evolutions have subsequently allowed much wider application of mAbs via the ability to generate mouse/human chimeric, humanized and fully human mAbs from the pure murine origin. In particular, the reduction of the xenogenic portion of the mAb structure decreased the immunogenic potential of the murine mAbs thus allowing their wider application. mAbs are generally very safe drugs because of their target selectivity, thus avoiding unnecessary exposure to and consequently activity in non-target organs. This is particularly apparent in the field of oncology, where mAbs like rituximab, trastuzumab and bevacizumab can offer a more favorable level of efficacy/safety ratios compared to common chemotherapeutic treatment regimens for some hematological and solid tumors.

The dynamic utilization of these biotechnological methods resulted not only in new drugs, but it also triggered the development of an entirely new business model for drug research and development with hundreds of newly formed and rapidly growing biotech companies. Furthermore, the ability to selectively target disease-related molecules resulted in a new scientific area of molecular targeted medicine, where the development of novel mAbs probably contributed substantially to setting new standards for a successful drug research and development process. The term translational medicine was developed to cover the biochemical, biological, (patho)physiological understanding and using this knowledge to find intervening options to treat diseases. During this process, biomarkers (e.g., genetic expression levels of marker genes, protein expression of target proteins, molecular imaging) are used to get the best possible understanding of the biological activities of drugs in a qualitative and most importantly quantitative sense, which encompasses essentially also the entire field of pharmacokinetics/pharmacodynamics (PK/PD). The application of those scientific methods together with the principle of molecular targeted medicine combined with the favorable PK and safety of mAbs might at least partly explain why biotechnologically derived products have substantially higher success rates to become marketed therapy compared to chemically-derived small molecule drugs.

The present chapter tries to address the following questions: What are the structural elements of mAbs? How do mAbs turn functional differences into different

| Name | Therapeutic area | Type | Antibody isotype | Target Receptor | Target Type | PK Behavior | PK Half-life | PK Clearance |
|---|---|---|---|---|---|---|---|---|
| Abciximab | Cardiovascular | Fragment | Chimeric Fab: mVar-hIgG1 | CD41 | | Linear | 0.29 days (Kleiman et al., 1995) | NA |
| Abatacept | Inflammation | Fusion protein | Extracellular domain of hCTLA-4+hinge of hFc | CD80/CD86 | | Linear | 13.1 days (Hervey and Keam, 2006) | 0.22 mL/h/kg (Hervey and Keam, 2006) |
| Adalimumab | Inflammation | mAb | hIgG1 | TNFα | Soluble and cell bound | Linear | 14.7–19.3 days (Weisman et al., 2003) | 9–12 mL/h (Weisman et al., 2003) |
| Alefacept | Inflammation | Fusion protein | LFA-3/ hIgG1(Fc) | CD2 | | Nonlinear | 11.3 days (Alefacept, 2003) | 18 mL/h(Alefacept, 2003) |
| Alemtuzumab | Oncology | mAb | rCDR-hIgG1 | CD52 | Soluble | Nonlinear | 12 days (Morris et al., 2003) | NA |
| Basiliximab | Transplantation | mAb | Chimeric: mVar-hIgG1 | CD25 | | NR | 4.1 days (Kovarik et al., 2001) | 75 mL/h (Kovarik et al., 2001) |
| Bevacizumab | Oncology | mAb | hIgG1 | VEGF | Soluble | Linear | 20 days (Avastin, 2004) | 0.207–0.262 L/day (Avastin, 2004) |
| Cetuximab | Oncology | mAb | Chimeric: mVar-hIgG1 | EGFR | Soluble | Nonlinear | 4.8 days (Erbitux, 2004) | 0.02–0.08 L/h/m² (Erbitux, 2004) |
| Daclizumab | Transplantation | mAb | Hyperchimeric: mCDRhIgG1 | CD25 | | Linear | 20 days (Zenapax, 2005) | 15 mL/h (Zenapax, 2005) |
| Efalizumab | Inflammation | mAb | mCDR-hIgG1 | CD11a | Cell bound internalized | Nonlinear | NR[a] | NR |
| Etanercept | Inflammation | Fusion protein | TNF-receptor/ hIgG1(Fc) | TNFα | Soluble and cell bound | Linear | 4 days (Lee et al., 2003) | 120 mL/h (Lee et al., 2003) |
| Gemtuzumab | Oncology | mAb-ADC | mCDR-hIgG4 | CD33 | Cell bound internalized | Nonlinear | 1.9–2.5 days (Dowell et al., 2001) | 265 mL/h (Dowell et al., 2001) |

| | Clinical indication | Format | Isotype | Antigen target | Soluble/cell bound | PK | Half-life | Clearance |
|---|---|---|---|---|---|---|---|---|
| Ibritumomab tiuxetan | Oncology | mAb | Murine IgG1 | CD20 | Cell bound stable | NR | NA | NA |
| Infliximab | Inflammation | mAb | Chimeric: mVar-hIgG1 | TNFα | Soluble and cell bound | Linear | 7.7–9.5 days (Cornillie et al., 2001; Remicade 2006) | NA |
| Muromonab-CD3 | Transplantation | mAb | Murine IgG2α | CD3 | | NR | 0.75 days (Hooks et al., 1991) | NA |
| Natalizumab | Inflammation | mAb | humanized IgG4κ | α4β1 and α4β7 integrins | | NR | 11 days (Tysabri, 2006) | 16 mL/h (Tysabri, 2006) |
| Omalizumab | Inflammation | mAb | mCDR-hIgG1 | IgE | Soluble | Linear | 26 days (Xolair, 2006) | 2.4 mL/kg/day (Xolair, 2006) |
| Palivizumab | Antiviral | mAb | mCDR-hIgG1 | RSV | | NR | 20 days (Synagis, 2004) | NR |
| Panitumumab | Oncology | mAb | hIgG2 | EGFR | Soluble | NA | NA | NA |
| Ranibizumab | Macular degeneration | Fragment | hIgG1κ | VEGF | Soluble | NA | 9 days[a] (Lucentis, 2006) | NA |
| Rituximab | Inflammation | mAb | Chimeric: mVar-hIgG1 | CD20 | Cell-bound stable | Linear | 19 days (Rituxan, 2006) | 10 mL/h (Rituxan, 2006) |
| Tositumomab | Oncology | mAb-radiolabeled | Murine IgG2α | CD20 | Cell bound stable | Nonlinear | NA | 68.2 mL/h (Bexxar, 2003) |
| Trastuzumab | Oncology | mAb | mCDR-hIgG1 | Her2 | Cell bound shed | Nonlinear | 1.7–12 days[b] (Herceptin, 2006) | 16–41 mL/h (Tokuda et al., 1999) |

[a]Dose dependent pharmacokinetics.
[b]Vitreous elimination half-life.

*Abbreviations:* CD, cluster of differentiation; CDR, complementarity determining region; CTLA, cytotoxic T-lymphocyte-associated antigen; EGFR, epidermal growth factor receptor; Fab, antigen-binding fragment; Fc, constant fragment; Ig, immunoglobulin; LFA-1, lymphocyte function-associated antigen; mAb, monoclonal antibody; mVar, murine variable; RSV, respiratory syncytial virus; TNF, tumor necrosis factor; VEGF, vascular endothelial growth factor; NA, information not found; NR, not reported.

**Table 1** ▪ The pharmacological properties of the approved therapeutic antibodies, antibody isotype, antigen target, clinical indication, and PK parameters.

functional activities? And how is a mAb protein turned from a potential clinical drug candidate into a therapeutic drug by using a translational medicine framework? In this sense, this chapter provides a general introduction to the Chapters 16, 17 and 18, where the currently marketed mAbs and mAb derivatives are discussed in the context of their therapeutic applications. To illustrate the application of PK/PD principles in the development process, efalizumab (anti-CD11a, Raptiva), a mAb marketed as anti-psoriasis drug in the United States and European Union, was chosen and will be used across the different parts of this chapter.

## ANTIBODY STRUCTURE AND CLASSES

Antibodies (Abs), immunoglobulin (Ig) are roughly Y-shaped molecules or combinations of such molecules. There are five major classes of Ig's: IgG, IgA, IgD, IgE, and IgM. Table 2 summarizes the characteristics of these molecules, particularly their structure (monomer, dimer, pentamer, or hexamer), molecular weight (ranging from ~150 kDa to ~1150 kDa), functions (e.g., activate complement, $Fc\gamma R$ binding). Among these classes, IgGs and their derivatives form the framework for the development of therapeutic antibodies. Figure 1 depicts the general structure of an IgG with its structural components as well as a conformational structure of efalizumab (anti-CD11a, Raptiva®). An IgG molecule has four peptide chains, including two identical heavy (H) chains (~50–55 kDa) and two identical light (L) chains (25 kDa), which are linked via disulfide (S-S) bonds at the hinge region. The first ~110 amino acids of both chains form the variable regions ($V_H$ and $V_L$), and are also the antigen binding regions. Each V domain contains three short stretches of peptide with hypervariable sequences (HV1, HV2, and HV3), known as complementarity determining regions (CDRs), i.e., the region that binds the antigen. The remaining sequences of each light chain consist of a single constant domain ($C_L$). The remainder of each heavy chain contains three constant regions ($C_{H1}$, $C_{H2}$, and $C_{H3}$). Constant regions are responsible for effector recognition and binding. IgG can be further divided into four subclasses (IgG1, IgG2, IgG3, and IgG4). The differences among these subclasses are also summarized in Table 2.

### ■ Murine, Chimeric, Humanized and Fully Humanized mAbs

With the advancement of technology early murine mAbs have been engineered further to chimeric (mouse CDR human Fc), humanized and fully human mAbs (Fig. 2). Murine mAbs, chimeric mAbs, humanized mAbs and fully humanized mAbs have 0%, ~60% to ~70%, ~90% to ~95% and ~100% sequences

that are similar to human mAbs, respectively. Decreasing the xenogenic portion of the mAb potentially reduces the immunogenic risks of generating anti-therapeutic antibodies (ATAs). The first therapeutic mAbs were murine mAbs produced via hybridomas, however, these murine antibodies easily elicited formation of neutralizing human anti-mouse antibodies (HAMA) (Kuus-Reichel et al., 1994). Muromonab-CD3 (Orthoclone OKT3), a first generation mAb of murine origin, has shown efficacy in the treatment of acute transplant rejection and was the first mAb licensed for use in humans. It is reported that 50% of the patients who received OKT3 produced HAMA after the first dose. HAMA interfered with OKT3's binding to T-cells, thus decreasing the therapeutic efficacy of the mAb (Norman et al., 1993). Later, molecular cloning and the expression of the variable region genes of IgGs have facilitated the generation of engineered antibodies. A second generation of mAbs, chimeric mAbs consist of human constant regions and mouse variable regions. The antigen specificity of chimeric mAb is the same as the parental mouse antibodies; however, the human Fc region renders a longer in vivo half-life than the parent murine mAb and similar effector functions as the human Ab. Currently, there are five chimeric antibodies and fragments on the market (abciximab, basiliximab, cetuximab, infliximab, and rituximab). These antibodies can still induce human anti-chimeric antibodies (HACA). For example, about 61% of patients who received infliximab had HACA response associated with shorter duration of therapeutic efficacy and increased risk of infusion reactions (Baert et al., 2003). The development of ATA is currently not predictable, as 6 of 17 patients with systemic lupus erythematosus receiving rituximab developed high-titer HACA (Looney et al., 2004), whereas only 1 of 166 lymphoma patients developed HACA (McLaughlin et al., 1998). Humanized mAbs contain significant portions of human sequence except the CDR which is still of murine origin. There are 10 marketed humanized antibodies on the market (alemtuzumab, bevacizumab, daclizumab, efalizumab, gemtuzumab, natalizumab, omalizumab, palivizumab, ranibizumab and trastuzumab). The incidence rate of anti-drug antibody [i.e., human anti-human antibody (HAHA)] was greatly decreased for these humanized mAbs. Trastuzumab has a reported HAHA incidence rate of only 0.1% (1 of 903 cases) (Herceptin, 2006), but daclizumab had a HAHA rate as high as 34% (Zenapax, 2005). Another way to achieve biocompatibility of mAbs is to develop fully humanized antibodies, which can be produced by two approaches: through phage display library and by using transgenic XenoMouse® with human heavy and light chain gene fragments (Weiner, 2006).

| Property | IgA | | IgG | | | | IgM | IgD | IgE |
|---|---|---|---|---|---|---|---|---|---|
| | IgA1 | IgA2 | IgG1 | IgG2 | IgG3 | IgG4 | | | |
| Serum concentration in adult (mg/mL) | 1.4–4.2 | 0.2–0.5 | 5–12 | 2–6 | 0.5–1 | 0.2–1 | 0.25–3.1 | 0.03–0.4. | 0.0001–0.0002 |
| Molecular form | Monomers (m), dimer (d) | | Monomer | | | | Pentamer (p), hexamer (h) | Monomer | Monomer |
| Functional valency | 2 or 4 | | 2 | | | | 10 (p) or 12 (h) | 2 | 2 |
| Molecular weight (kDa) | 160 (m), 300 (d) | 160 (m), 350 (d) | 150 | 150 | 160 | 150 | 950 (p) | 175 | 190 |
| Serum half-life (days) | 5–7 | 4–6 | 21–24 | 21–24 | 7–8 | 21–24 | 5–10 | 2–8 | 1–5 |
| % total Ig in adult serum | 11–14 | 1–4 | 45–53 | 11–15 | 3–6 | 1–4 | 10 | 0.2 | 0.0004 |
| Function — Activate classical complement pathway | – | – | + | +/– | ++ | – | +++ | – | – |
| Activate alternative complement pathway | + | – | – | – | – | – | – | – | – |
| Cross placenta | – | | + | +/– | + | + | – | – | – |
| Present on membrane of mature B cell | – | – | ++ | – | – | – | + | + | – |
| Bind to Fc receptors of phagocytes | – | – | ++ | +/– | ++ | + | ? | – | – |
| Mucosal transport | ++ | ++ | – | – | – | – | + | – | – |
| Induces mast-cell degranulation | – | – | – | – | – | – | – | – | + |
| Biological properties | Secretory Ig, binds to polymeric Ig receptor | | Placental transfer, secondary antibody for most response to pathogen, binds macrophage and other phagocytic cells by Fcγ receptor | | | | Primary antibody response, some binding to polymeric Ig receptor, some binding to phagocytes | Mature B-cell marker | Allergy and parasite reactivity, binds FcεR on mast cells and basophils |

*Source:* From Goldsby et al., 1999; Kolar and Capra, 2003.

**Table 2** ■ Important properties of endogenous immunoglobulin subclass.

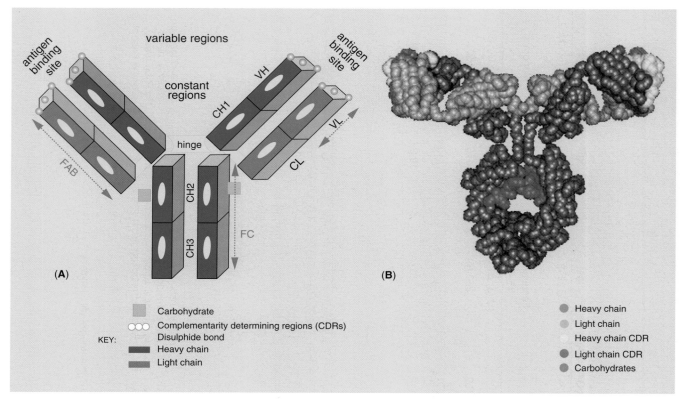

**Figure 1** ■ (**A**) IgG1 antibody structure. Antigen is bound via the variable range of the antibody, whereas the Fc part of the IgG determines the mode of action (also called effector function). *Abbreviations*: H-chain, Heavy chain consisting of VH, CH1, CH2, CH3; L-chain, light chain consisting of VL, CL; VH, VL, variable light and heavy chain; CHn, CL, constant light and heavy chain; Fv, variable fraction; Fc, crystallizable fraction; Fab, antigen-binding fraction. (**B**) Example efalizumab (anti-CD11a), Raptiva. (See art for key.)

Adalimumab is the first licensed fully humanized mAb generated by the phage display library. Adalimumab was approved in 2002 and 2007 for the treatment of rheumatoid arthritis and Crohn's disease, respectively (Humira, 2007). However, despite its fully human Ab structure, the incidence of HAHA was about 5% (58 of 1062 patients) in three randomized clinical trials with adalimumab (Cohenuram and Saif, 2007; Humira, 2007). Panitumumab is the first approved fully humanized monoclonal antibody generated by using transgenic mouse technology. No HAHA responses have been reported yet in clinical trials after chronic dosing with panitumumab to date (Vectibix, 2006; Cohenuram and Saif, 2007). Of note, typically ATAs are measured using ELISA assays and the reported incidence rates of ATAs for a given mAb can be influenced by the sensitivity and specificity of the assay. Additionally, the observed incidence of antibody positivity in an assay may be also influenced by several other factors including sample handling, timing of sample collection, concomitant medications, and underlying disease. For these reasons, comparison of the incidence of a specific mAb with the incidence of antibodies to other products may be misleading.

## ■ Key Structural Components of MAbs

Proteolytic digestion of antibodies releases different fragments termed Fv (Fragment variable), Fab (Fragment antigen binding) and Fc. These different forms have been reviewed by others (Wang, et al., 2007). These fragments can also be generated by recombinant engineering. Treatment with papain generates two identical Fab's and one Fc. Pepsin treatment generates a F(ab')2 fragment and several smaller fragments. Reduction of F(ab')2 will produce two Fab's. The Fv fragment consists of the heavy chain variable domain ($V_H$) and the light chain variable domain ($V_L$) held together by strong non-covalent interaction. Stabilization of the Fv fragment by a peptide linker generates a single chain Fv (scFv).

## ■ Modifying Fc Structures

The Fc regions of mAbs play a critical role not only in their function but also in their disposition in the body. Monoclonal antibodies elicit effector functions [antibody-dependent cellular cytotoxicity (ADCC) and complement-dependent cytotoxicity (CDC)] following interaction between their Fc regions and different Fcγ receptors and complement fixation (C1q, C3b). The

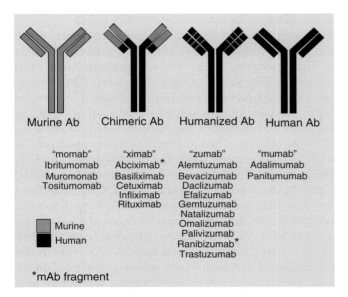

**Figure 2** ■ Different generations of therapeutic antibodies.

CH2 domain or the hinge region joining CH1 and CH2 have been identified as the crucial regions for binding to FcγR (Presta et al., 2002). Engineered mAbs with enhanced or decreased ADCC and CDC activity have been produced by manipulation of the critical Fc regions. Umana et al. (1999) engineered an anti-neuroblastomal IgG1 with enhanced ADCC activity compared with wild-type (WT). Shields et al. (2001) demonstrated that selected IgG1 variants with improving binding to FcγRIIIA showed an enhancement in ADCC for peripheral blood monocyte cells or natural killer cells. These findings indicate that Fc-engineered antibodies may have important applications for improving therapeutic efficacy. It was found that the FcγRIIIA gene dimorphism generates two allotypes: FcγRIIIa-158V and FcγRIIIa-158F and the polymorphism in FcγRIIIA is associated with favorable clinical response following rituximab

administration in non-Hodgkin's lymphoma patients (Cartron et al., 2004; Dall'Ozzo et al., 2004). Currently, several anti-CD20 mAbs with increased binding affinity to FcγRIIIA are in clinical trials. The efficacy of antibody-interleukin-2 fusion protein (Ab-IL-2) was improved by reducing its interaction with Fcγ receptors (Gillies et al., 1999). In addition, the Fc portion of mAbs also binds to the FcRn receptor (FcRn- named based on discovery in neonatal rats as neonatal Fc receptor), an Fc receptor belonging to the major histocompatibility complex structure, which is involved in IgG transport and clearance (Junghans, 1997). Engineered mAbs with a decreased or increased FcRn binding affinity have been investigated for the potential of modifying the PK behavior of mAb (see section "Antibody clearance" for detail).

### ■ Antibody Derivatives [F(ab')2, Fab, Antibody Drug Conjugates (ADC)] and Fusion Proteins

The fragments of antibodies (Fab, F(ab')2, and scFv) have a shorter half-life compared with the full-sized corresponding antibodies. scFv can be further engineered into a bivalent dimer (diabody) (~60 kDa, or trimer: triabody ~90 kDa). Two diabodies can be further linked together to generate bispecific tandem diabody (tandab). Figure 3 illustrates the structure of different antibody fragments. Of note, abciximab and ranibizumab are two Fab fragments approved by FDA. Abciximab is a chimeric Fab used for keeping blood from clotting and it exhibits a half-life of 20 to 30 minutes in serum and 4 hours in platelets (Schror and Weber, 2003). Ranibizumab, which is administrated via an intravitreal injection, was approved for the treatment of macular degeneration in 2006 and exhibits a vitreous elimination half-life of 9 days (Albrecht and DeNardo, 2006).

The half-life of Fc fragments is more similar to that of full sized IgGs (Lobo et al., 2004). Therefore, Fc portions of IgGs have been used to form fusions with

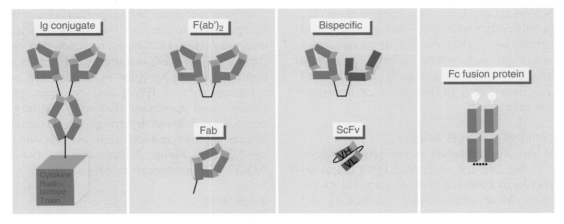

**Figure 3** ■ Schematic representation of antibody derivatives [F(ab')2, Fab, ScFv, and antibody conjugates] and Fc fusion proteins.

molecules such as cytokines, growth factor enzymes or the ligand-binding region of receptor or adhesion molecules to improve their half-life and stability. Alefacept, abatacept, and etanercept are three Fc-fusion proteins on the market. Etanercept, a dimeric fusion molecule consisting of the TNF-α receptor fused to the Fc region of human IgG1, has a half-life of approximately 70 to 100 hours (Zhou, 2005), which is much longer than the TNF-α receptor itself (30 minutes to 2 hours) (Watanabe et al., 1988).

Antibodies and antibody fragments can also be linked covalently with toxic drugs or radioisotopes to form immunoconjugates or ADC. In each case, the Ab is used as a delivery mechanism to selectively target the toxic drugs to tumors. An example is gemtuzumab, an anti-CD33 mAb linked with a chemotherapy drug ozogamicin. Ozogamicin itself has very significant side effects. It is hypothesized that by virtue of targeting ozogamicin is mainly delivered to cells expressing the CD33 protein with reduced exposure to normal cells. This leads to an improved therapeutic window. The current radioimmunotherapy agents licensed by the FDA are ibritumomab/ [131]I-tiuxetan and tositumomab/[131]I-tositumomab for lymphoma. Both of the above intact mAbs bind CD-20 and carry a potent beta particle-emitting radioisotope ([90]Y for ibritumomab/tiuxetan and [131]I for tositumomab).

## HOW ANTIBODIES FUNCTION AS THERAPEUTICS

The pharmacological effects of antibodies are first initiated by the specific interaction between antibody and antigen. Monoclonal antibodies generally exhibit exquisite specificity for the target antigen. The binding site on the antigen called the epitope can be linear or conformational, and may comprise continuous or discontinuous amino acid sequences. The epitope is the primary determinant of the antibody's modulatory functions and depending on the epitope, the antibody may exert antagonist or agonist effects, or it may be non-modulatory. The epitope may also influence the antibody's ability to induce ADCC and CDC. Monoclonal antibodies exert their pharmacological effects via multiple mechanisms that include direct modulation of the target antigen, CDC and ADCC, and delivery of a radionuclide or immunotoxin to target cells.

### ■ Direct Modulation of Target Antigen
Examples of direct modulation of the target antigen include anti-TNFα, anti-IgE and anti-CD11a therapies that are involved in blocking and/or removal of the target antigen. Most monoclonal antibodies act through multiple mechanisms and may exhibit cooperativity with concurrent therapies.

### ■ Complement-Dependent Cytotoxicity (CDC)
The complement system is an important part of the innate (i.e., non-adaptive) immune system. It consists of many enzymes that form a cascade with each enzyme acting as a catalyst for the next. CDC results from interaction of cell-bound monoclonal antibodies with proteins of the complement system. CDC is initiated by binding of the complement protein, C1q, to the Fc domain. The IgG1 and IgG3 isotypes have the highest CDC activity, while the IgG4 isotype lacks C1q binding and complement activation (Presta, 2002). Upon binding to immune complexes, C1q undergoes a conformational change and the resulting activated complex initiates an enzymatic cascade involving complement proteins C2 to C9 and several other factors. This cascade spreads rapidly and ends in the formation of the membrane attack complex (MAC), which inserts into the membrane of the target and causes osmotic disruption and lysis of the target. Figure 4 illustrates the mechanism for CDC with rituximab (a chimeric antibody, which targets the CD20 antigen) as an example.

### ■ Antibody-Dependent Cellular Cytotoxicity (ADCC)
ADCC is a mechanism of cell-mediated immunity whereby an effector cell of the immune system actively lyses a target cell that has been bound by specific antibodies. It is one of the mechanisms through which antibodies, as part of the humoral immune response, can act to limit and contain infection. Classical ADCC is mediated by natural killer (NK) cells, monocytes or macrophages but an alternate ADCC is used by eosinophils to kill certain parasitic worms known as helminths. ADCC is part of the adaptive immune response due to its dependence on a prior antibody response. The typical ADCC involves activation of NK cells, monocytes or macrophages and is dependent on the recognition of antibody-coated infected cells by Fc receptors on the surface of these cells. The Fc receptors recognize the Fc portion of antibodies such as IgG, which bind to the surface of a pathogen-infected target cell. The Fc receptor that exists on the surface of NK cell is called CD16 or FcγRIII. Once bound to the Fc receptor of IgG the NK cell releases cytokines such as IFN-γ, and cytotoxic granules like perforin and granzyme that enter the target cell and promote cell death by triggering apoptosis. This is similar to, but independent of, responses by cytotoxic T-cells. Figure 5 illustrates the mechanism for ADCC with rituximab as an example.

### ■ Apoptosis
Monoclonal antibodies achieve their therapeutic effect through various mechanisms. In addition to the above

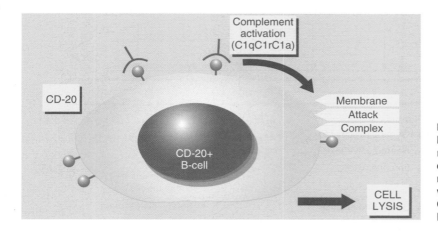

**Figure 4** ■ An example of CDC, using a B-cell lymphoma model, where the monoclonal antibody, rituximab binds to the receptor and initiates the complement system, also known as the "complement cascade." The end result is a MAC, which leads to cell lysis and death. *Abbreviations*: CDC, complement-dependent cytotoxicity; MAC, membrane attack complex.

mentioned effector functions they can have direct effects in producing apoptosis or programmed cell death. It is characterized by nuclear DNA degradation, nuclear degeneration and condensation, and phagocytosis of the cell remains.

## TRANSLATIONAL MEDICINE/DEVELOPMENT PROCESS

The connection between basic and clinical sciences is an essential part of translational medicine, the purpose of which is to translate the knowledge obtained from basic science into practical therapeutic applications for patients. This knowledge transfer is also often refered to as "bench-to-bedside" transition of scientific advancements into clinical applications. This framework of translational medicine is applied during the discovery and drug development process

of a specific antibody against a certain disease. It includes major steps such as identifying an important and viable pathophysiological target antigen to modify the disease in a beneficial way, producing mAbs with structural elements providing optimal PK, testing the mAb in non-clinical safety and efficacy models, and finally clinical studies in patients. An overview of the development phases for a molecule and various activities in the PK/PD/toxicology areas is outlined in Figure 6. Furthermore the critical components of the entire development process of mAbs from a PK/PD perspective are explained in details in the following sections.

### ■ Preclinical Safety Assessment of mAbs

Preclinical safety assessment of mAbs offers unique challenges as many of the classical evaluations employed for small molecules are not appropriate for protein therapeutics in general and mAbs in particular. For example, in vitro genotoxicology tests such as the Ames and chromosome aberration assays are generally not conducted for mAbs given their limited interaction with nuclear material and the lack of appropriate receptor/target expression in these systems. As mAb binding tends to be highly species-specific, suitable animal models are often limited to non-human primates and for this reason, many common in vivo models such as rodent carcinogenesis bioassays and some safety pharmacology bioassays are not viable for mAb therapeutic candidates. For general toxicology studies, cynomolgus and rhesus monkeys are most commonly employed and offer many advantages given their close phylogenetic relationship with humans; however, due to logistics, animal availability, and costs, group sizes tend to be much smaller than typically used for lower species thus limiting statistical power. In some cases, alternative models are employed to enable studies in rodents. Rather than directly testing the therapeutic

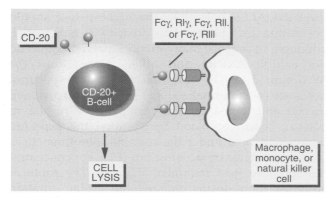

**Figure 5** ■ An example of ADCC. In this situation rituximab targets the CD20 antigen. This antigen is expressed on a significant number of B-cell malignancies. The Fc fragment of the monoclonal antibody binds the Fc receptors found on monocytes, macrophages, and NK cells. These cells in turn engulf the bound tumor cell and destroy it. NK cells secrete cytokines that lead to cell death, and they also recruit B cells. *Abbreviations*: ADCC, antibody-dependent cellular cytotoxicity; NK, natural killer.

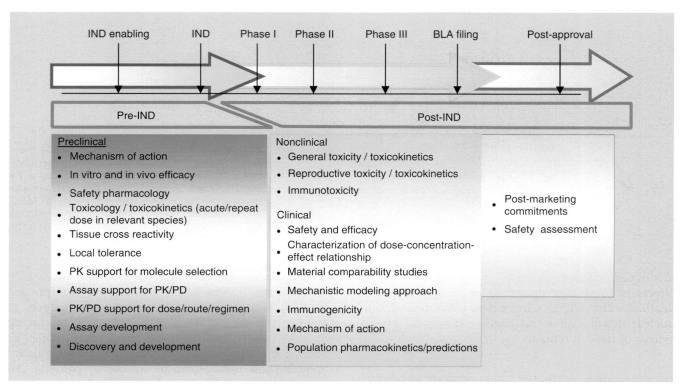

**Figure 6** ▪ Flowchart depicting PK/PD/toxicology study requirements during preclinical and clinical drug product development. *Abbreviations*: BLA, biologics license application; IND, investigational new drug application; PD, pharmacodynamic; PK, pharmacokinetic.

candidate, analogous monoclonal antibodies that can bind to target epitopes in lower species (e.g., mice) can be engineered and used as a surrogate mAb for safety evaluation (Clarke et al., 2004). Often the antibody framework amino acid sequence is modified to reduce antigenicity thus enabling longer-term studies (Albrecht and DeNardo, 2006; Weiner, 2006; Cohenuram and Saif, 2007). Another approach is to use transgenic models that express the human receptor/target of interest (Bugelski et al., 2000); although, results must be interpreted with caution as transgenic models often have altered physiology and typically lack historical background data for the model. To address development issues that are specific to monoclonal antibodies and other protein therapeutics the International Conference of Harmonization (ICH) has developed guidelines specific to the preclinical evaluation of biotechnology-derived pharmaceuticals (ICH, 1997a).

For general safety studies, species selection is an important consideration given the exquisite species-specificity often encountered with mAbs. Model selection needs to be justified based on appropriate expression of the target epitope, appropriate binding affinity with the therapeutic candidate, and appropriate biologic activity in the test system. To aid in the interpretation of results, tissue cross reactivity studies offer the ability to compare drug localization in both

animal and human tissues. For mAb therapeutic candidates, a range of three or more dose levels are typically selected to attain pharmacologically relevant serum concentrations, to approximate levels anticipated in the clinic, and to provide information at doses higher than anticipated in the clinic. For most indications, it is important to include dose levels that allow identification of a no observable adverse effect level (NOAEL). If feasible, the highest dose should fall within the range where toxicity is anticipated; although, in practice many monoclonal antibodies do not exhibit toxicity and other factors limit the maximum dose. To best reflect human exposures, doses are often normalized and selected to match and exceed anticipated human therapeutic exposure in plasma, serum or blood based upon the exposure parameters, area under the concentration-time curve (AUC), maximum concentrations ($C_{max}$) or concentration prior to next treatment ($C_{trough}$). The route of administration, dosing regimen and dosing duration should be selected to best model the anticipated use in clinical trials (ICH, 1997b).

To adequately interpret non-clinical study results it is important to characterize ATA responses. For human mAbs, ATA responses are particularly prominent in lower species but also evident in non-human primates albeit to a lesser degree, making these species more viable for chronic toxicity studies. ATAs can impact drug activity in a variety of ways. Neutralizing ATAs are those that bind to the therapeutic in a manner that prevents activity, often by inhibiting direct binding to the target epitope. Non-neutralizing antibodies may also indirectly impact drug activity, for example rapid clearance of drug-ATA complexes can effectively reduce serum drug concentrations. In situations where prominent ATA responses are expected, administration of high dose multiples of the anticipated clinical dose may overcome these issues by maintaining sufficient circulating concentrations of active drug. To properly interpret study results it is important to characterize ATA incidence and magnitude as the occurrence of ATA responses could mask toxicities. Alternatively, robust ATA responses may induce significant signs of toxicity such as infusion-related anaphylaxis that may not be predictive of human outcome where ATA formation is likely to be less of an issue. If ATA formation is clearly impacting circulating drug levels, ATA positive individuals are often removed from consideration when evaluating PK parameters to better reflect the anticipated PK in human populations.

## ■ Pharmacokinetics

A thorough and rigorous PK program in the early learning phase of preclinical drug development can provide a linkage between drug discovery and preclinical development. PK information can be linked to PD by mathematical modeling, which allows characterizing the time course of the effect intensity resulting from a certain dosing regimen. Antibodies often exhibit PK properties that are much more complex than those typically associated with small-molecule drugs (Meibohm and Derendorf, 2002). In the following sections we have summarized the basic characteristics of antibody PK.

The PK of antibodies is very different from small molecules. Table 3 summarizes the PK differences between small molecule drugs and therapeutic antibodies regarding PK. Precise sensitive and accurate bioanalytical methods are essential for PK interpretation. However, for mAbs, the immunoassays and bioassay methodologies are often less specific as compared to assays used for small molecule drugs (e.g., LC/MS/MS). Monoclonal antibodies are handled by the body very differently than small molecules. In

| Small molecule drugs | Monoclonal antibodies | | | | |
|---|---|---|---|---|---|
| | Target is soluble antigen with low endogenous level | Target is soluble antigen with high endogenous level | Target is cell-bound antigen | Target is cell-bound antigen that is internalized and down-regulated | Target is cell-/tissue-bound antigen that can be shed |
| PK usually independent of PD | PK often independent of PD | PK often dependent of PD | | | |
| Binding generally non-specific (can affect multiple enzymes) | Binding very specific for target protein or antigen | | | | |
| Usually linear PK Non-linear PK problematic | Linear PK | Non-linear PK | | | |
| Relatively short $t_{1/2}$ | Long $t_{1/2}$ | Low dose: short $t_{1/2}$ High dose: long $t_{1/2}$ | | | |
| Not always orally available | Need parenteral dosing. SC or IM is possible | | | | |
| Metabolism by P450s or other enzymes | Metabolism by non-specific clearance mechanisms; no P450s involved | Metabolism by specific and non-specific clearance mechanisms. No P450s involved | | | |
| Renal clearance often important | mAbs: No renal clearance of intact antibody. May be cleared by damaged kidneys. Antibody fragment might be eliminated by renal clearance | | | | |
| Binding to tissues, high Vd | Distribution usually limited to blood and extracellular space | | | | |

*Abbreviations*: PK, pharmacokinetic; PD, pharmacodynamic.
*Source*: Lobo et al., 2004; Roskos et al., 2004; Mould and Sweeney, 2007.

**Table 3** ■ Comparison of the pharmacokinetics of small molecule drugs and monoclonal antibodies.

contrast to small molecule drugs, the typical metabolic enzymes and transporter proteins such as cytochrome P450, multi-drug resistance efflux pumps are not involved in the disposition of mAbs. Consequently, drug-drug interaction at the level of these drug metabolizing enzymes and transporters are not complicating factors in the drug development process of mAbs and do not need to be addressed by in vitro and in vivo studies. Intact mAbs cannot be cleared by normal kidneys because of the large molecular weight; however, renal clearance processes can play an important role in the elimination of molecules of smaller molecular weight such as Fabs and chemically derived small molecule drugs. The different **A**bsorption, **D**istribution, **M**etabolism and **E**limination (ADME) processes comprising PK of mAbs will be discussed separately to address their individual specificities.

## Absorption

Monoclonal antibodies are not administrated orally because of their limited gastrointestinal stability, low lipophilicity, and size all of which result in insufficient resistance against the hostile proteolytic gastrointestinal milieu and very limited permeation through the lipophilic intestinal wall. Therefore, intravenous administration is still the most frequently used route, which allows for immediate systemic delivery of large volume of drug product and provides complete systemic availability. Of note, 6 of over 20 FDA approved antibody therapies listed in Table 1 are administered by extravascular route [adalimumab (SC), efalizumab (SC), omalizumab (SC), alefacept (IM), palivizumab (IM), ranibizumab [intravitreal injection (ITV)]. The absorption mechanisms of SC or IM administration are poorly understood. However, it is believed that the absorption of mAbs after IM or SC is likely via lymphatic drainage due to their large molecular weight, leading to a slow absorption rate (see Chapter 5). The bioavailability for antibodies after SC or IM administration has been reported to be around 50% to 100% with maximal plasma concentrations observed 1 to 8 days following administration (Lobo et al., 2004). For example, following an IM injection, the bioavailability of alefacept was ~60% in healthy male volunteers; its $C_{max}$ was 3-fold (0.96 vs. 3.1 μg/mL) lower and its $T_{max}$ was 30 times longer (86 vs. 2.8 hours) than a 30-minute IV infusion (Vaishnaw and TenHoor, 2002). Interestingly differences in PK have also been observed between different sites of IM dosing. PAmAb, a fully human mAb against Bacillus anthracis protective antigen, has a significantly different PK between IM-GM (gluteus maximus site) and IM-VL (vastus lateralis site) injection in healthy volunteers (Subramanian et al., 2005). The bioavailability of PAmAb is 50–54% for IM-GM injection and 71% to 85% for IM-VL injection (Subramanian et al., 2005). Of note, mAbs appear to have greater bioavailability after SC administration in monkeys than in humans. The mean bioavailability of adalimumab is around 64% with $C_{max}$ of 4.7±1.6 μg/mL and $T_{max}$ of 131± 56 hours after a single 40 mg SC administration in healthy adult subjects (Humira, 2007). The mean bioavailability of omalizumab is around 62% and peak serum concentration was observed at 7 to 8 days after a single SC dose in patients with asthma (Xolair, 2006). Humanized monoclonal anti-interleukin-5 was reported to have completed absorption (118% ± 1.16%) in monkeys following SC administrations (Zia-Amirhosseini et al., 1999). A similar finding was also observed for adalimumab after single SC administration in monkeys (96%).

## Distribution

After reaching the bloodstream, mAbs undergo biphasic disposition from serum, beginning with a rapid distribution phase. The distribution volume of the rapid distribution compartment is relatively small in the range of the plasma volume. It is reported that the volume of the central compartment (Vc) is about 2 to 3 L and the steady state volume of distribution (Vss) is around 3.5 to 7 L for mAbs in humans (Lobo et al., 2004; Roskos et al., 2004). The small Vc and Vss for mAbs indicate that the distribution of mAbs is restricted to the blood and extracellular spaces or target tissues, which is in agreement with their hydrophilic nature thus limiting the access to the lipophilic tissue compartments and their large molecular weight. Small volumes of distributions are consistent with relatively small tissue: blood ratios for most antibodies typically ranging from 0.1 to 0.5 (Baxter et al., 1994; Berger et al., 2005). For example, the tissue: blood concentration ratios for a murine IgG1 mAb against the human ovarian cancer antigen CA125 in mice at 24 hours after injection is 0.44, 0.39, 0.48, 0.34, 0.10, and 0.13 for the spleen, liver, lung, kidney, stomach and muscle, respectively (Berger et al., 2005). Brain and cerebrospinal fluid are anatomically protected by blood-tissue barriers. Therefore, both compartments are very limited distribution compartments for Abs hindering the access for therapeutic mAbs. For example endogenous IgG levels in CSF were shown to be in the range of only 0.1 to 1% of their respective serum levels (Wurster and Haas, 1994). However, it has been repeatedly pointed out that the reported Vss obtained by traditional non-compartmental or compartmental analysis may be not correct for some mAbs with high extent of catabolism within tissue (Tang et al., 2004; Lobo et al., 2004; Straughn, 2006). The rate and extent of antibody distribution will be dependent on the kinetics of antibody extravasation within tissue, distribution within tissue, and elimination from tissue. Convection, diffusion, transcytosis, binding and catabolism are important determining factors for antibody distribution (Lobo et al., 2004). Therefore, the Vss might be substantially greater than the plasma volume in particular for those mAbs demonstrating high binding affinity in the tissue. Effects of the presence of specific receptors (i.e., antigen sink) on the distribution for mAb have been reported by different research groups (Danilov et al., 2001; Kairemo et al., 2001). Danilov et al. (2001) found that anti-PECAM-1 (CD31) mAbs show tissue:blood concentration ratios of 13.1, 10.9, and 5.96 for the lung, liver, and spleen, respectively, in rats at 2 hours after injection. Therefore, the true Vss of the anti-PECAM-1 is likely to be 15-fold greater than plasma volume.

Another complexity, which needs to be considered, is that the distribution via interaction with target proteins (e.g., cell surface proteins) and subsequent internalization of the antigen-mAb complex might be dose-dependent. For the murine analog mAb of efalizumab (M17) (Coffey et al., 2005), a pronounced dose-dependent distribution was demonstrated by comparing tissue:blood concentration ratios for liver, spleen, bone marrow, and lymph node after a tracer dose of radiolabeled M17 and a high dose treatment. The tracer dose of M17 resulted into substantially higher tissue:blood concentration ratios of 6.4, 2.8, 1.6, and 1.3 for the lung, spleen, bone marrow and lymph node, respectively, in mice at 72 hours after injection. Whereas, the saturation of the target antigen at the high dose level reduced the tissue distribution to the target independent distribution and resulted consequently into substantially lower tissue:blood concentration ratios (less than one).

FcRn may play an important role in the transport of IgGs from plasma to the interstitial fluid of tissue. However, the effects of FcRn on the mAbs' tissue distribution have not been fully understood. Ferl et al. (2005) reported that a physiologically based pharmacokinetic (PBPK) model, including the kinetic interaction between the mAb and the FcRn within intracellular compartments, could describe the biodistribution of an anti-CEA mAb in a variety of tissue compartments such as plasma, lung, spleen, tumor, skin, muscle, kidney, heart, bone and liver. FcRn was also reported to mediate the IgG across the placental barriers (Junghans, 1997) and the vectorial transport of IgG into the lumen of intestine (Dickinson et al., 1999) and lung (Spiekermann et al., 2002).

## Antibody Clearance

Antibodies are mainly cleared by catabolism and broken down into peptide fragments and amino acids which can be recycled-used as energy supply or for new protein synthesis. Due to small molecular weight

of antibodies fragments (e.g., Fab and Fv), elimination of these fragments is faster than intact IgGs, and they can be filtered through glomerus and reabsorbed and/or metabolized by proximal tubular cells of the nephron (Lobo et al., 2004). Murine monoclonal anti-digoxin Fab, F(ab')2 and IgG1 have half-lives of 0.41, 0.70 and 8.10 hr in rats, respectively (Bazin-Redureau et al., 1997). Several studies reported that the kidney is the major route for the catabolism of Fab and elimination of unchanged Fab (Druet et al., 1978; McClurkan et al., 1993).

IgGs have a half-life of approximately 21 days with clearance values of about 3 to 5 mL/day/kg in the clinically used dose range resulting in linear PK. The exception is IgG3, which has only a half-life of 7 days. The half-life of IgGs is much longer than other Igs (IgA 6 days, IgE 2.5 days, IgM 5 days, IgD 3 days). Recent reports have demonstrated that the FcRn receptor is a prime determinant of the disposition of IgG antibodies (Ghetie et al., 1996; Junghans and Anderson, 1996; Junghans, 1997). FcRn, which protects IgG from catabolism and contributes to the long plasma half-life of IgG, was first postulated by Brambell in 1964 (Brambell et al., 1964) and cloned in the late 1980s (Simister and Mostov, 1989a,b). FcRn is a heterodimer comprising of a $\beta_2$m light chain and a MHC class-I like heavy chain. The receptor is ubiquitously expressed in cells and tissues. Several studies have shown that IgG clearance in $\beta_2$m knockout mice (Ghetie et al., 1996; Junghans and Anderson, 1996) and FcRn-heavy chain knockout mice (Roopenian et al., 2003) is increased 10- to 15-fold, with no changes in the elimination of other Igs. Figure 7 illustrates how the FcRn protects IgG from catabolism and contributes to its long half-life. The FcRn binds to IgG in a pH dependent manner: binding to IgG at acidic pH (6.0) at endosome and releasing IgG at physiological pH (7.4). The unbound IgG proceeds to the lysosome and undergoes proteolysis.

It is demonstrated that IgG half-life is dependent on its affinity to FcRn. The shorter half-life of IgG3 was attributed to its low binding affinity to the FcRn (Junghans, 1997; Medesan et al., 1997). Murine mAbs have serum half-lives of 1 to 2 days in human. The shorter half-life of murine antibodies in human is due to their low binding affinity to the human FcRn receptor. It is reported that human FcRn binds to human, rabbit, and guinea pig IgG, but not to rat, mouse, sheep and bovine IgG; however, mouse FcRn binds to IgG from all of these species (Ober et al., 2001). Interesting, human IgG1 has greater affinity to murine FcRn (Petkova et al., 2006), which indicates potential limitations of using mice as preclinical models for human IgG1 PK evaluations. Ward's group confirmed that an engineered human IgG1 had

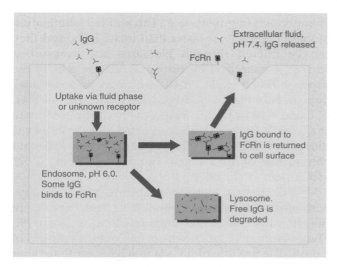

**Figure 7** ■ Schematic disposition pathway of IgG antibodies via interaction with FcRn in endosomes. 1. IgGs enter cells by receptor mediated endocytosis by binding of the Fc part to FcRn. 2. The intracellular vesicles (endosomes) can fuse with lysosome containing proteases. 3. Proteases can degrade non-bound IgG molecules, whereas IgG bound to FcRn is protected. 4. The intact IgG bound to FcRn is transported back to the cell surface and released back to the extracellular fluid.

disparate properties in murine and human systems (Vaccaro et al., 2006). Engineered IgGs with higher affinity to FcRn have a 2- to 3-fold longer half-life compared with WT in mice and monkeys (Hinton et al., 2006; Petkova et al., 2006). Two engineered human IgG1 mutants with enhanced binding affinity to human FcRn show a considerably extended half-life compared with wild-type in hFcRn transgenic mice ($4.35 \pm 0.53$, $3.85 \pm 0.55$ days vs. $1.72 \pm 0.08$ days) (Petkova et al., 2006). Hinton et al. (2006) found that the half-life of IgG1 FcRn mutants with increasing binding affinity to human FcRn at pH 6.0 is about 2.5-fold longer than the WT Ab in monkey ($838 \pm 187$ hours vs. $336 \pm 34$ hours).

Dose-proportional, linear clearance has been observed for mAbs against soluble antigens with low endogenous levels (such as TNF-$\alpha$, IFN-$\alpha$, VEGF and IL-5). For example, linear PK has been observed for a humanized mAb directed to human interleukin-5 following intravenous administration over a 6000-fold dose range (0.05–300 mg/kg) in monkeys (Zia-Amirhosseini et al., 1999). The clearance of rhuMAb against vascular endothelial growth factor after IV dosing (2–50 mg/kg) ranged from 4.81 to 5.59 mL/day/kg and did not depend on dose (Lin et al., 1999). The mean total serum clearance and the estimated mean terminal half-life of adalimumab was reported to range from 0.012 to 0.017 L/h, 10.0 to 13.6 days, respectively, for a five cohorts clinical trial (0.5–10 mg/kg), with an overall mean half-life of 12 days (den Broeder et al., 2002). However, mAbs against soluble

antigens with high endogenous levels (such as IgE) exhibit non-linear PK. The PK of omalizumab, an antibody against IgE, are linear only at doses greater than 0.5 mg/kg (Petkova et al., 2006; Xolair, 2006).

Elimination of mAbs may also be impacted by interaction with the targeted cell-bound antigen, and this phenomenon was demonstrated by dose-dependent clearance and half-life. At low dose, mAbs show a shorter half-life and a faster clearance due to receptor-mediated elimination. With increasing doses, receptors become saturated; the half-life gradually increases to a constant; and the clearance gradually decreases to a constant. The binding affinity ($K_d$), antigen density and antigen turn-over rate may influence the receptor-mediated elimination. Koon et al. (2006) found a strong inverse correlation between CD25+ cells expression and apparent daclizumab (a mAb specifically binding to CD25) half-life. It has been shown that the PK of murine anti-human CD3 antibodies may be determined by the disappearance of target antigen (Meijer et al., 2002). In monkeys and mice, clearance of SGN-40, a humanized monoclonal anti-CD40 antibody, was much faster at low dose, suggesting non-linear PK (Kelley et al., 2006). In addition, Ng et al. (2006) demonstrated that anti-CD4 monoclonal antibody had ~ 5-fold faster CL at 1 mg/kg dose compared with 10 mg/kg dose ($7.8 \pm 0.6$ vs. $37.4 \pm 2.4$ mL/day/kg) in healthy volunteers. They also found that receptor-mediated CL contributed to 8.69%, 27.1%, and 41.7% of total CL when the dose was 1, 5, and 10 mg/kg, respectively.

In addition to FcRn and antigen-antibody interaction, other factors may also contribute to mAb elimination (Lobo et al., 2004; Roskos et al., 2004; Tabrizi et al., 2006):

*Immunogenicity of antibody:* The elimination of mAbs in humans often increases with increasing level of immunogenicity (Ternant and Paintaud, 2005; Tabrizi et al., 2006).

*The degree and the nature of antibody glycosylation:* The study conducted by Newkirk et al. (1996) shows that the state of glycosylation of IgG affects the half-life in mice, and that by removing the terminal sugars (sialic acid and galactose), the antibody (IgG2a) will remain in circulation significantly longer. However, a recent study demonstrated that a humanized anti-A$\beta$ mAb with different glycans in the Fc region had the same clearance in mice (Huang et al., 2006).

*Susceptibility of antibody to proteolysis:* Gillies et al. (2002) improved the circulating half-life of antibody-interleukin 2 immunocytokine 2-fold compared with wild-type (1.0 hour vs. 0.54 hour) by increasing the resistance to intracellular degradation.

*Effector function:* Effector function, such as interactions with FcγR, could also regulate elimination and PK of mAbs (Mahmood and Green, 2005). Mutation of the binding site of FcγR has dramatic effects on the clearance of the Ab-IL-2 fusion protein (Gillies et al., 1999).

*Concomitant medications:* Methotrexate reduced adalimumab apparent clearance after single dose and multiple dosing by 29% and 44%, respectively in patients with rheumatoid arthritis (Humira, 2007). In addition, azathioprine and mycophenolate mofetil were reported to reduce clearance of basiliximab by approximately 22% and 51%, respectively (Simulect, 2005). These interactions could be explained by the effects of small molecule drugs on the expression of Fcγ receptors. It has been found that methotrexate have the impact on the expression profiles of FcγRI on monocytes significantly in rheumatoid arthritis patients (Bunescu et al., 2004).

*Demographics:* Body weight, age, disease state, and other factors can also change mAb PK (Mould and Sweeney, 2007) (see discussion on "Population PK").

## ■ Prediction of Human PK/PD Based on Preclinical Information

Prior to first human studies, several preclinical in vivo and in vitro experiments are performed to understand the PK of potential new drugs as well as their safety and efficacy in animal models. However, the ultimate goal is at all times to predict how these preclinical results on PK, safety and efficacy translate into a given patient population. Therefore, predictions of human PK, safety and efficacy are the focus of early drug development acknowledging the similarities and differences between preclinical models and the respective patient populations (see section "Preclinical Safety Assessment of mAbs").

Over the years, many theories and different approaches have been proposed and used for scaling preclinical data to clinical data. Figure 8 illustrates the prediction of human PK/PD based on preclinical information. Allometric scaling is the simplest and most widely used method (see Chapter 5), which is based on the power law relationship between body size and physiological and anatomical parameters. This can be described by equation: $Y = a \cdot BW^b$, where $Y$ is the PK parameter (such as CL, V); BW is the body weight; $a$ is the coefficient; $b$ is the exponent of the allometric equations. Maximum life potential, brain weight, and two-term power equation have been proposed as correction factors to improve the prediction for CL. The accuracy of prediction of PK parameters by allometric scaling is dependent on many factors, such as species, experimental design, analytical errors, and others (Mahmood, 2005; Tang

and Mayersohn, 2005). However, there are only few reports on PK predictions using allometric scaling for mAbs. Lin et al. (1999) projected the CL of bevacizumab in human as ~2.4 mL/day/kg based on simple allometric scaling principles. Also Kelley et al. (2006) used simple allometry to predict the CL of the anti-CD40 mAb of about 12 mL/day/kg in humans. For these two examples, the human clearance was confirmed to be in agreement with the preclinical prediction by allometry.

Another approach for interspecies scaling is physiologically based pharmacokinetic (PBPK) modeling, which establishes the animal PK based on preclincial in vitro and in vivo data in the first step. In the second step, the model is then scaled to humans by using human physiological information such as blood flow, tissue volumes as well as potentially some additional human in vitro data. Although PBPK modeling provides a mechanism based evaluation of drug disposition, this approach is costly, mathematically complex and time consuming. Therefore in drug development and discovery, PBPK models are not as widely used compared to allometry. However, for mAb interspecies scaling, PBPK modeling allows to explore some physiological factors by simulation technology which can not be incorporated into empirical allometric scaling methods, such as the binding affinity, binding kinetics and non-linear PK. Baxter et al. (1995) used PBPK models to predict PK of mAb against carcinoembryonic antigen in human in different tissues including tumor compartments. It also has been shown that a PBPK model including FcRn components worked very well to describe the PK of an intact mAb and its Fab in different tissues in mice, with or without tumor (Ferl et al., 2005).

In addition, species-invariant time method (Mahmood, 2005) and non-linear mixed-effect modeling (Martin-Jimenez and Riviere, 2002; Jolling et al., 2005) have been used for interspecies scaling for small molecules. Species-invariant time method, also called Dedrick approach, was first described in 1973 (Dedrick, 1973). Physiological time, the time required to complete a species independent physiological event, can be obtained by transformation of chronological time into a species invariant time (equivalent time, kallynochrons, apolysichron, and dienetichrons). In the case that PK follows allometric principles the transformation of chronological to physiological time should provide superimposed concentration-time profiles for all species. In his pioneering work Dedrick demonstrated this for methotrexate as model compound (Dedrick, 1973).

Interspecies allometric scaling can also be performed using a population approaches (non-linear mixed effect modeling techniques). Allometric coefficients and exponents as well as the variability from

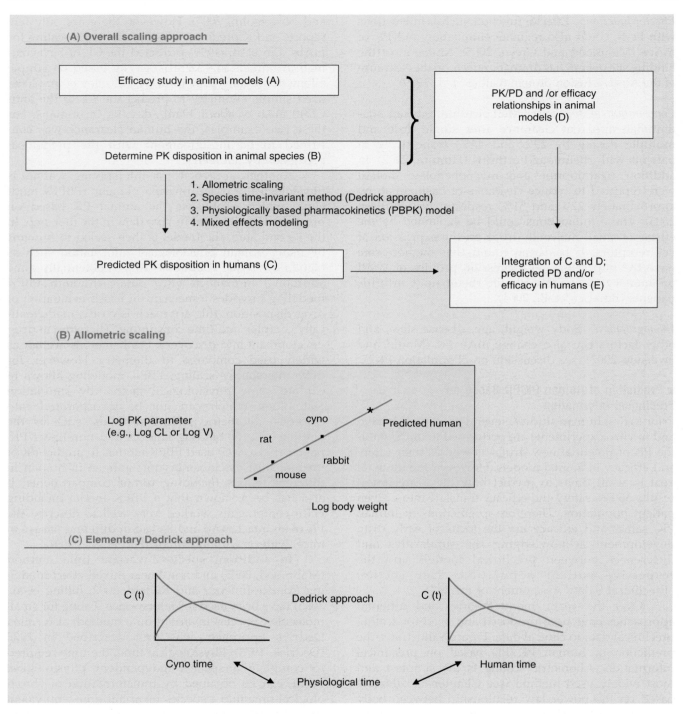

**Figure 8** ■ PK/PD scaling approach from preclinical studies to humans. **(A)** Overall scaling approach. **(B)** Allometric scaling. **(C)** Elementary Dedrick approach. *Abbreviations*: Cyno, Cynomolgus monkey; PK, pharmacokinetic; PD, pharmacodynamic.

inter-animals, intra-animals and inter-species and random errors can be estimated in one single step by using this approach.

Due to the complexity of PD, any extrapolation to human requires more complex considerations than for PK. Through PK/PD modeling and integration the interspecies scaling of PK, the PD in human may be predicted if the PK/PD relationship is assumed to be the same between the animal models and humans. For example, a PK/PD model was first developed to optimize the dosing regimen of the mAb against EGF/r3 using tumor bearing nude mice as an animal model of human disease (Duconge et al., 2004). This PK/PD model was then integrated with allometric scaling to calculate the dosage schedule required in a potential clinical trial to achieve a certain effect (Duconge et al., 2004).

In summary, species differences in antigen density, antigen–antibody binding, and antigen kinetics, differences in FcRn binding between species, the immunogenicity and other factors need to be considered during PK/PD scaling of mAbs from animals to humans.

## ■ PK/PD in Clinical Development of Antibody Therapeutics

Several new developments have taken place in the antibody therapeutics in the last years. The emphasis in the field has grown and is obvious by the fact that many of the companies are now involved in building antibody product based collaborations. Drug development has traditionally been performed in sequential phases, divided into preclinical as well as clinical phases I-IV. During the development phases of the molecules, the safety and PK/PD characteristics are established in order to narrow down on the compound selected for development and its dosing regimen. This information-gathering process has recently been characterized as two successive learning-confirming cycles (Sheiner, 1997; Sheiner and Wakefield, 1999).

The first cycle (Phases I and IIa) comprises learning about the dose that is tolerated in healthy subjects and confirming that this dose has some measurable benefits in the targeted patients. An affirmative answer at this first cycle provides the justification for a larger and more costly second learn-confirm cycle (Phases IIb and III), where the learning step is focused on how to use the drug benefit/risk ratio, whereas the confirm step is aimed at demonstrating acceptable benefit/risk in a large patient population (Meibohm and Derendorf, 2002). In the following sections we have provided a case study with efalizumab as an approved therapeutic antibody to understand the various steps during the development of antibodies for various indications.

A summary of the overall PK/PD data from multiple studies within the efalizumab (Raptiva®) clinical development program and an integrated overview of how these data were used for development and the selection of the approved dosage of efalizumab for psoriasis will be discussed in detail. Psoriasis is a chronic skin disease characterized by abnormal keratinocyte differentiation and hyperproliferation and by an aberrant inflammatory process in the dermis and epidermis. T-cell infiltration and activation in the skin and subsequent T-cell-mediated processes have been implicated in the pathogenesis of psoriasis (Krueger, 2002).

Efalizumab is a subcutaneously (SC) administered recombinant humanized monoclonal IgG1

antibody that has received approval for the treatment of patients with psoriasis in more than 30 countries, including the United States and the European Union (Raptiva, 2004). Efalizumab is a targeted inhibitor of T-cell interactions (Werther et al., 1996). An extensive preclinical research program was conducted to study the safety and mechanism of action (MOA) of efalizumab. Multiple clinical studies have also been conducted to investigate the efficacy, safety, PK, PD, and MOA of efalizumab in patients with psoriasis.

### Pre-Phase I Studies

In the process of developing therapeutic antibodies integrated understanding of the (PK/PD) concepts provide a highly promising tool. A thorough and rigorous preclinical program in the early learning phase of preclinical drug development can provide a linkage between drug discovery and preclinical development. As it sets the stage for any further development activities, the obtained information at this point is key to subsequent steps (Meibohm and Derendorf, 2002). At the preclinical stage, potential applications might comprise the evaluation of in vivo potency and intrinsic activity, the identification of bio-/surrogate markers, understanding the MOA as well as dosage form/regimen selection and optimization. A few of these specific aims are described below with information on efalizumab as an example.

### Identification of MOA and PD Biomarkers

The identification of appropriate PD endpoints is crucial to the process of drug development. Thus, biomarkers are usually tested early during exploratory preclinical development for their potential use as PD or surrogate endpoints.

Through an extensive preclinical research program, the MOA and PD biomarkers for efalizumab have been established. Efalizumab binds to CD11a, the α-subunit of leukocyte function antigen-1 (LFA-1), which is expressed on all leukocytes, and decreases cell surface expression of CD11a. Efalizumab inhibits the binding of LFA-1 to intercellular adhesion molecule-1 (ICAM-1), thereby inhibiting the adhesion of leukocytes to other cell types. Interaction between LFA-1 and ICAM-1 contributes to the initiation and maintenance of multiple processes, including activation of T lymphocytes, adhesion of T-lymphocytes to endothelial cells, and migration of T-lymphocytes to sites of inflammation, including skin. Consistent with the proposed MOA for efalizumab, in vitro experiments have demonstrated that efalizumab binds strongly to human lymphocytes with a $K_d$ of approximately 110 ng/mL (Werther et al., 1996; Dedrick et al., 2002) and blocks the interaction of human T-lymphocytes with tissue-specific cells such as keratinocytes in a concentration-dependent manner.

Upon understanding the MOA, PD effects relevant to the MOA of efalizumab are usually measured in order to identify the efficacious dosage of antibody therapeutics. As saturation of CD11a binding sites by efalizumab has been shown to increase while T-cell activation is increasingly inhibited, maximum saturation of CD11a binding sites occurs at efalizumab concentrations >10 µg/mL, resulting in maximum T-cell inhibition (Werther et al., 1996; Dedrick et al., 2002). Therefore, CD11a expression and saturation have been chosen as relevant PD markers for this molecule.

### Role of Surrogate Molecules

The role of surrogate molecules in assessing ADME of therapeutic antibodies is important as the antigen specificity limits ADME studies of humanized monoclonal antibodies in rodents. In the development of therapeutic antibodies various molecules may be used to provide a comprehensive view of their PK/PD properties. Studies with surrogates might lead to important information regarding safety, mechanism of action, disposition of the drug, tissue distribution and receptor pharmacology, which might be too cumbersome and expensive to conduct in non-human primates. Surrogates (mouse/rat) provide a means to gaining knowledge of PK and PD in a preclinical rodent model thus allowing rational dose optimization in the clinic. Therefore in the case of efalizumab to complete a more comprehensive safety assessment, a chimeric rat anti-mouse CD11a antibody, muM17, was

developed and evaluated as a species-specific surrogate molecule for efalizumab. muM17 binds mouse CD11a with specificity and affinity similar to those of efalizumab to human. In addition, muM17 in mice was demonstrated to have similar pharmacological activities as that of efalizumab in human (Nakakura et al., 1993; Clarke et al., 2004). Representative PK profiles of efalizumab and muM17 in various species are depicted in Figure 9 to help understand the species differences in the PK behavior of molecules.

### PK of Efalizumab

A brief overview of efalizumab non-clinical PK/PD results is provided in the following sections to summarize the key observations that led to decisions in designing the subsequent clinical programs. The ADME program consisted of PK, PD (CD11a down-modulation and saturation), and toxicokinetic data from PK, PD, and toxicology studies with efalizumab in chimpanzees and with muM17 in mice. The use of efalizumab in the chimpanzee and muM17 in mice for PK and PD and safety studies was supported by in vitro activity assessments. The non-clinical data were used for PK and PD characterization, PD-based dose selection, and toxicokinetic support for confirming exposure in toxicology studies. Together, these data have supported both the design of the non-clinical program and its relevance to the clinical program.

The observed PD as well as the mechanism of action of efalizumab and muM17 are attributed to their binding to CD11a present on cells and tissues. The binding affinities of efalizumab to human and

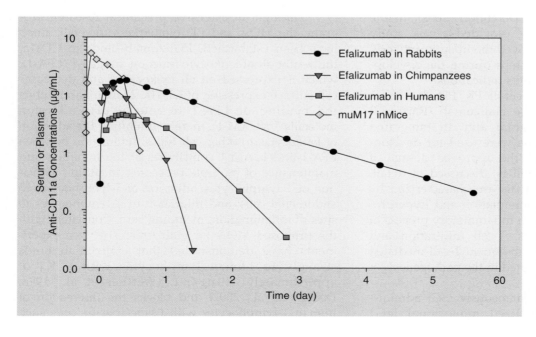

**Figure 9** ▪ Anti-CD11a molecules comparative PK profiles in humans, chimpanzees, rabbits and mice following SC dose. Due to the species differences in binding, the pharmacokinetics of efalizumab are non-linear (i.e., dose-dependent) in humans and chimpanzees while being linear in rabbits (non-binding species). muM17, on the other hand, binds to the mouse anti-CD11a and exhibits dose-dependent pharmacokinetics in mice.

chimpanzee CD11a on CD3 lymphocytes are comparable confirming the use of chimpanzees as a valid nonclinical model for humans. CD11a expression has been observed to be greatly reduced on T-lymphocytes in chimpanzees and mice treated with efalizumab and muM17, respectively. Expression of CD11a is restored as efalizumab and muM17 are eliminated from the plasma. The bioavailability of efalizumab in chimpanzees and muM17 in mice after an SC dose was dose-dependent and ranged from 35% to 48% and 63% to 89% in chimpanzees and mice, respectively. Binding to CD11a serves as a major pathway for clearance of these molecules, which leads to non-linear PK depending on the relative amounts of CD11a and efalizumab or muM17 (Coffey et al., 2005).

The disposition of efalizumab and the mouse surrogate muM17 is mainly determined by the combination of both specific interactions with the ligand-CD11a and by their IgG1 framework and is discussed in detail as follows. The factors controlling the disposition of these antibodies are shown in Figure 10 and include the following:

1. The binding of the free antibody with its ligand CD11a present on both circulating lymphocytes and tissues leads to its removal from circulation. Data suggests that anti-CD11a antibodies are internalized by purified T-cells and upon internalization, the antibodies appeared to be targeted to lysosomes and cleared from within the cells in a time-dependent manner. CD11a-mediated internalization and lysosomal targeting of efalizumab

may constitute one pathway by which this antibody is cleared in vivo (Coffey et al., 2005).
2. Binding to CD11a is both specific and saturable as demonstrated by the dose dependent clearance of efalizumab in chimpanzees and humans or muM17 in mice.
3. Because of its IgG1 framework, free or unbound efalizumab or muM17 levels are also likely to be influenced by:
    a. recycling and circulation following binding to and internalization by the neonatal Fc receptor (FcRn),
    b. non-specific uptake and clearance by tissues,
    c. binding via its Fc framework to Fc receptors present on hepatic sinusoidal endothelial cells.

The disposition of efalizumab is governed by the species specificity and affinity of the antibody for its ligand CD11a, the amount of CD11a in the system, and the administered dose.

Based on the safety studies, efalizumab was generally well tolerated in chimpanzees at doses up to 40 mg/kg/week IV for 6 months, providing an exposure ratio of 339-fold based on cumulative dose and 174-fold based on the cumulative AUC, compared with a clinical dose of 1 mg/kg/wk. The surrogate antibody muM17 was also well tolerated in mice at doses up to 30 mg/kg/week SC. In summary efalizumab was considered to have an excellent non-clinical safety profile thereby supporting the use in adult patients.

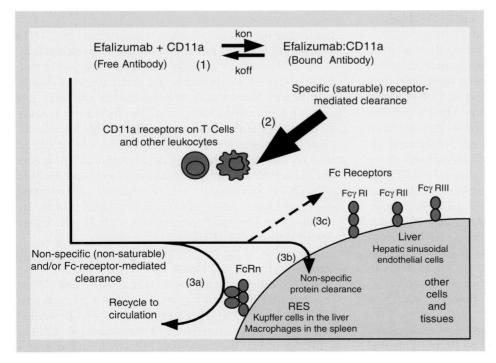

**Figure 10** Clearance pathways for efalizumab.

## Clinical Program of Efalizumab: PK/PD Studies, Assessment of Dose, Route, and Regimen

The drug development process at the clinical stage provides several opportunities for integration of PK/PD concepts. Clinical Phase I dose escalation studies provide, from a PK/PD standpoint, the unique chance to evaluate the dose-concentration-effect relationship for therapeutic and toxic effects over a wide range of doses up to or even beyond the maximum tolerated dose under controlled conditions (Meredith et al., 1991). PK/PD evaluations at this stage of drug development can provide crucial information regarding the potency and tolerability of the drug in vivo and the verification and suitability of the PK/PD concept established during preclinical studies.

Efalizumab PK and PD data are available from 10 studies in which more than 1700 patients with psoriasis received IV or SC efalizumab. In the Phase I studies, PK and PD parameters were characterized by extensive sampling during treatment; in the Phase III trials, steady-state trough levels were measured once or twice during the first 12-week treatment period for all the studies and during extended treatment periods for some studies. Several early Phase I and II trials have examined IV injection of efalizumab and dose-ranging findings from these trials have served as the basis for SC dosing levels used in several subsequent phase I and all Phase III trials.

### Administration of Efalizumab

The PK of monoclonal antibodies varies greatly, depending primarily on their affinity for and the distribution of their target antigen (Lobo et al., 2004). Efalizumab exhibits concentration-dependent non-linear PK after administration of single IV doses of 0.03, 0.1, 0.3, 0.6, 1.0, 2.0, 3.0, and 10.0 mg/kg in a Phase I study. This non-linearity is directly related to specific and saturable binding of efalizumab to its cell surface receptor, CD11a, and has been described by a PK/PD model developed by Bauer et al. (1999) which is discussed in the following sections. The PK profiles of efalizumab following single IV doses with observed data and model predicted fit are presented in Figure 11. Mean clearance (CL) decreased from 380 mL/kg/d to 6.6 mL/kg/d for doses of 0.03 mg/kg to 10 mg/kg, respectively. The volume of distribution of the central compartment (Vc) of efalizumab was 110 mL/kg at 0.03 mg/kg (approximately twice the plasma volume) and decreased to 58 mL/kg at 10 mg/kg (approximately equal to plasma volume), consistent with saturable binding of efalizumab to CD11a in the vascular compartment. Because of efalizumab's non-linear PK, its half-life (t1/2) is dose-dependent.

In a Phase II study of efalizumab, it was shown that at a weekly dosage of 0.1 mg/kg IV, patients did

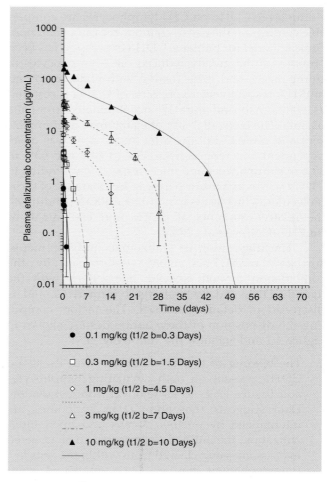

**Figure 11** ▪ Plasma concentration *versus* time profile for efalizumab following single IV doses in psoriasis patients.

not maintain maximal down modulation of CD11a expression and did not maintain maximal saturation. Also at the end of 8 weeks of efalizumab treatment, 0.1 mg/kg/wk IV, patients did not have statistically significant histological improvement and did not achieve a full clinical response. The minimum weekly IV dosage of efalizumab tested that produced histological improvements in skin biopsies was 0.3 mg/kg/wk and this dosage resulted in submaximal saturation of CD11a binding sites but maximal down-modulation of CD11a expression. Improvements in patients' psoriasis were also observed, as determined by histology and by the Psoriasis area and severity index (PASI) (Papp et al., 2001).

### Determination of SC Doses

Although efficacy was observed in Phase I and Phase II studies with 0.3 mg/kg/wk IV efalizumab, dosages of 0.6 mg/kg/wk and greater (given for 7 to 12 weeks) provided more consistent T lymphocyte CD11a saturation and the maximal PD effect. At dosages

≤0.3 mg/kg/wk, large between subject variability was observed, whereas at dosages of 0.6 or 1.0 mg/kg/wk, patients experienced better improvement in PASI scores, with lower between-patient variability in CD11a saturation and down-modulation. Therefore, this dosage was used to estimate an appropriate minimum SC dose of 1 mg/kg/week (based on a 50% bioavailability) that would induce similar changes in PASI, PD measures, and histology. The safety, PK, and PD of a range of SC efalizumab doses (0.5–4.0 mg/kg/wk administered for 8–12 weeks) were evaluated initially in 2 Phase I studies (Gottlieb et al., 2003). To establish whether a higher SC dosage might produce better results, several Phase III clinical trials assessed a 2.0 mg/kg/wk SC dosage in addition to the 1.0 mg/kg/wk dosage. A dose of 1.0 mg/kg/wk SC efalizumab was selected as it produced sufficient trough levels in patients to maintain the maximal down-modulation of CD11a expression and binding-site saturation between weekly doses (Joshi et al., 2006). Figure 12 depicts the serum efalizumab levels, CD11a expression, and available CD11a binding sites on T-lymphocytes (mean ± SD) after subcutaneous administration of 1 mg/kg efalizumab.

### SC Administration of Efalizumab

The PK of SC efalizumab has been well characterized following multiple SC doses of 1.0 and 2.0 mg/kg/wk (Mortensen et al., 2005; Joshi et al., 2006). A Phase I study that collected steady-state PK and PD data for 12 weekly SC doses of 1.0 and 2.0 mg/kg in psoriasis patients, provided most of the pharmacologic data relevant to the marketed product. Although peak serum concentration after the last dose ($C_{max}$) was observed to be higher for the 2.0 mg/kg/wk (30.9 µg/

mL) than for the 1.0 mg/kg/wk dosage (12.4 µg/mL), no additional changes in PD effects were observed at the higher dosages (Mortensen et al., 2005). Following a dose of 1.0 mg/kg/wk, serum efalizumab concentrations were adequate to induce maximal down-modulation of CD11a expression and a reduction in free CD11a binding sites on T-lymphocytes (Fig. 13). Steady state serum efalizumab levels were reached more quickly with the 1.0 mg/kg/wk dosage at 4 weeks compared with the 2.0 mg/kg/wk dosage at 8 weeks (Mortensen et al., 2005), which is in agreement with the average effective half-life for SC efalizumab 1.0 mg/kg/wk of 5.5 days (Boxenbaum and Battle, 1995). The bioavailability was estimated at approximately 50%. Population PK analyses indicated that body weight was the most significant covariate affecting efalizumab SC clearance, thus supporting body weight-based dosing for efalizumab (Sun et al., 2005).

### ■ Mechanistic Modeling Approaches

In clinical drug development, PK/PD modeling approaches can be applied as analytical tools for identifying and characterizing the dose-response relationships of drugs and the mechanisms and modulating factors involved. Additionally, they may be used as predictive tools for exploring various dosage regimens as well as for optimizing further clinical trial designs, which might allow one to perform fewer, more focused studies with improved efficiency and cost effectiveness. The PK/PD database established during the preclinical and clinical learning phases in the development process and supplemented by population data analysis provides the backbone for these assessments.

PK/PD modeling has been used to characterize efalizumab plasma concentrations and CD11a expression on CD3-positive lymphocytes in chimpanzees and in subjects with psoriasis (Bauer et al., 1999). As the PK data revealed that CL of efalizumab was not constant across dose levels, one of the models described by Bauer et al. (1999) incorporated a Michaelis–Menten clearance term into the PK equations and utilized an indirect-response relationship to describe CD11a turnover. However in the above model the exposure-response relationship of efalizumab was not addressed and another report expanded on the developed receptor-mediated PK and PD model by incorporating data from five Phase I and II studies to develop a PK–PD-efficacy (E) model to further increase the understanding of efalizumab interaction with CD11a on T-cells and consequent reduction in severity of psoriasis (Ng et al., 2005). A general outline of the mechanistic modeling approach for various molecules is presented alongside the model for efalizumab in Figure 14A. The description

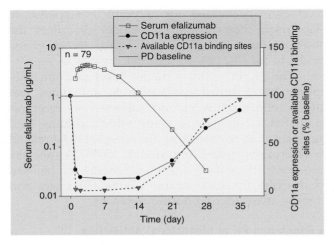

**Figure 12** ■ PK/PD profile following efalizumab in humans (1 mg/kg SC). *Abbreviations*: PK, pharmacokinetic; PD, pharmacodynamic.

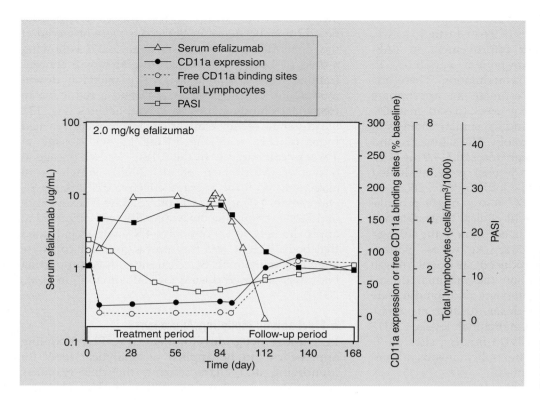

**Figure 13** ■ Serum efalizumab, CD11a expression, and free CD11a binding sites on T lymphocytes, absolute lymphocyte counts, and Psoriasis PASI score (mean) following 1.0 mg/kg/wk SC efalizumab for 12 weeks and 12 weeks post treatment. *Abbreviation*: PASI, Psoriasis area and severity index.

of the PK–PD-efficacy model of efalizumab in psoriasis patients is described below and is schematically represented in Figure 14B. Details on parameters utilized in the model can be found in the paper by Ng et al. (2005).

## PK Analysis

A first-order absorption, two-compartment model with both linear and Michaelis-Menten elimination was used to describe the plasma efalizumab concentration data. This model is schematically represented in Figure 14B (iv).

## PD Analysis

A receptor-mediated PD model previously developed was used to describe the dynamic interaction of efalizumab to CD11a, resulting in the removal of efalizumab from the circulation and reduction of cell surface CD11a (Bauer, Dedrick et al., 1999). This model is schematically represented in Figure 14B (v).

## Efficacy Analysis

The severity of the disease has been assessed by the PASI score that is assumed to be directly related to the psoriasis skin production. The rate of psoriasis skin production was then modeled to be directly proportional to the amount of free surface CD11a on T-cells, which is offset by the rate of skin healing [Fig. 14B (vi)].

## Model Results

Upon evaluation and development, the model was used to fit the PK/PD/efficacy data simultaneously. The plasma concentration-time profile of efalizumab was reasonably described by use of the first-order absorption, two-compartment model with Michaelis–Menten elimination from the central compartment. In addition, the PD model described the observed CD11a-time data from all the studies reasonably well. In the efficacy model an additional CD11a-independent component to psoriasis skin production accounted for incomplete response to efalizumab therapy and the model described the observed data well. Figure 15 depicts the fit of the model to the PK/PD/efficacy data.

The PK–PD-efficacy model developed for efalizumab has a broad application to antibodies that target cell-bound receptors, subjected to receptor-mediated clearance, and for which coating and modulation of the receptors are expected to be related to clinical response (Mould et al., 1999). Despite the non-linear PK of these agents, the model can be used to describe the time course of the PD effect and efficacy after different dosing regimens.

## ■ Population PK of Monoclonal Antibodies

Compared to small molecule drugs, monoclonal antibodies typically exhibit less inter- and intra-subject variability of the standard PK parameters

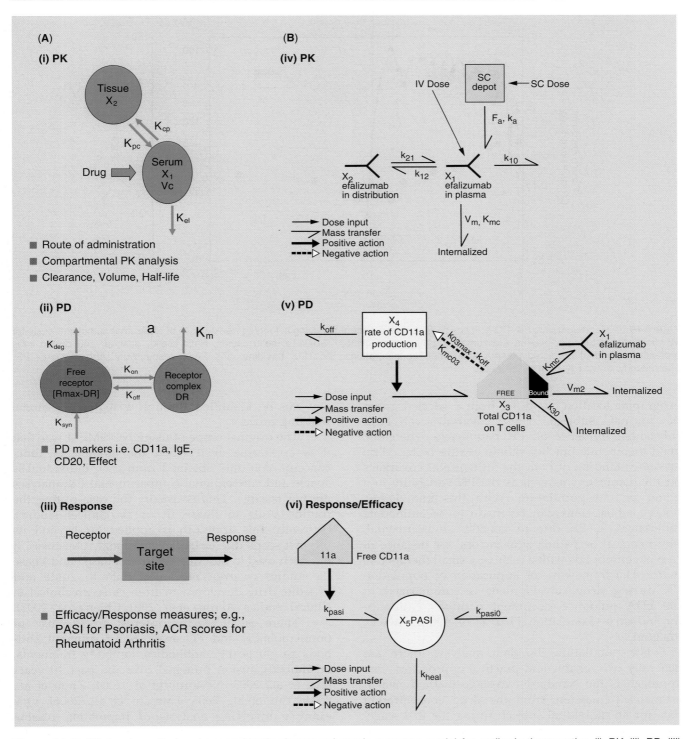

**Figure 14** ■ **(A)** A schematic for pharmacokinetic-pharmacodynamic-response model for antibody therapeutics (i) PK (ii) PD (iii) Response. **(B)**. Schematic representation of PK–PD-efficacy model of efalizumab in psoriasis patients. (iv) First-order absorption, two-compartment PK model with linear and non-linear elimination from the central compartment. (v) PD model with negative feedback mechanism. (vi) Efficacy model with CD11a-dependent and -independent pathway. *Abbreviations*: PK, pharmacokinetic; PD, pharmacodynamic; PASI, psoriasis area and severity index.

such as volume of distribution and clearance. However, it is possible that certain pathophysiological conditions may result into substantially increased intra- and inter-patient variability. In addition, patients are usually not very homogeneous; patients vary in sex, age, body weight; they may have concomitant disease and may be receiving multiple drug treatments. Even the diet, lifestyle, ethnicity, and

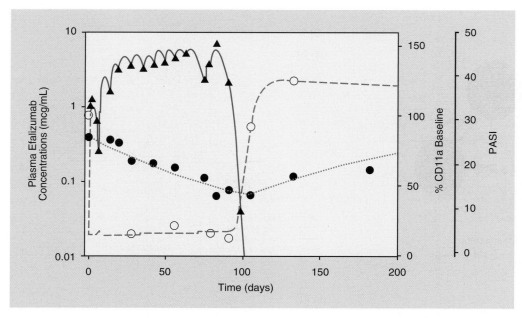

**Figure 15** ■ Representative PK–PD-efficacy profiles from a patient receiving a 1 mg/kg weekly dose of efalizumab subcutaneously for 12 weeks. Solid triangle, plasma efalizumab (μg/mL); open circles, %CD11a; solid circles, PASI. Solid, dashed, and dotted lines represent individual predicted plasma efalizumab concentrations, %CD11a baseline, and PASI, respectively. *Abbreviations*: PD, pharmacodynamic; PK, pharmacokinetic.

geographic location can differ from a selected group of "normal" subjects. These covariates can have substantial influence on PK parameters. Therefore, good therapeutic practice should always be based on an understanding of both the influence of covariates on PK parameters as well as the PK variability in a given patient population. With this knowledge, dosage adjustments can be made to accommodate differences in PK due to genetic, environmental, physiological or pathological factors, for instance in case of compounds with a relatively small therapeutic index. The framework of application of population PK during drug development is summarized in the FDA guidance document entitled "Guidance for Industry—Population Pharmacokinetics" (www. fda.gov).

For population PK data analysis, there are generally two reliable and practical approaches. One approach is the standard two-stage method, which estimates parameters from the drug concentration data for an individual subject during the first stage. The estimates from all subjects are then combined to obtain a population mean and variability estimates for the parameters of interest. The method works well when sufficient drug concentration-time data are available for each individual patient. A second approach, the non-linear mixed effect modeling (NONMEM) attempts to fit the data and partition the unpredictable differences between theoretical and observed values into random error terms. The influence of fixed effect (i.e., age, sex, body weight,

etc) can be identified through a regression model building process.

The original scope of using NONMEM was that it is applicable even when the amount of time-concentration data obtained from each individual is sparse and conventional compartmental PK analyses are not feasible. This is usually the case during the routine visits in Phase III or IV clinical studies. Currently, this approach is applied far beyond its original scope due to its flexibility and robustness. It has been used to describe data-rich Phase I and Phase IIa studies or even preclinical data to guide and expedite drug development from early preclinical to clinical studies (Aarons et al., 2001; Chien et al., 2005).

There is increasing interest in the use of population PK and PD analyses for different antibody products (i.e., antibodies, antibody fragments, or antibody fusion proteins) over the past 10 years (Lee et al., 2003; Nestorov et al., 2004; Zhou et al., 2004; Yim et al., 2005; Hayashi et al., 2006). One example involving analysis of population plasma concentration data involved a dimeric fusion protein, etanercept (Enbrel®). A one-compartment first-order absorption and elimination population PK model with interindividual and interoccasion variability on clearance, volume of distribution, and absorption rate constant, with covariates of sex and race on apparent clearance and body weight on clearance and volume of distribution, was developed for etanercept in rheumatoid arthritis adult patients (Lee et al., 2003). The population PK model for etanercept was further applied to pediatric patients with juvenile rheumatoid arthritis and established the basis of the 0.8 mg/kg once-weekly regimen in pediatric patients with juvenile rheumatoid arthritis (Yim et al., 2005). Unaltered etanercept PK with concurrent methotrexate in patients with rheumatoid arthritis has been demonstrated in a Phase IIIb study using population PK modeling approach (Zhou et al., 2004). Thus, no etanercept dose adjustment is needed for patients taking concurrent methotrexate. A simulation exercise of using the final population PK model of subcutaneously administered etanercept in patients with psoriasis indicated that the two different dosing regimens (50 mg every week vs. 25 mg every other week) provide a similar steady-state exposure (Nestorov et al., 2004). Therefore, their respective efficacy and safety profiles are likely to be similar as well.

An added feature is the development of a population model involving both PK and PD. Population PK/PD modeling has been used to characterize drug PK and PD with models ranging from simple empirical PK/PD models to advanced mechanistic models by using drug-receptor binding principles or other physiologically based principles. A mechanism-based population PK and PD binding model was developed for a recombinant DNA-derived humanized IgG1 monoclonal antibody, omalizumab (Xolair®) (Hayashi et al., 2006). Clearance and volume of distribution for omalizumab varied with body weight, whereas clearance and rate of production of IgE were predicted accurately by baseline IgE and overall, these covariates explained much of the inter-individual variability. Furthermore, this mechanism-based population PK/PD model enabled the estimation of not only omalizumab disposition, but also the binding with its target, IgE, and the rate of production, distribution and elimination of IgE.

Population PK/PD analysis can capture uncertainty and the expected variability in PK/PD data generated in preclinical studies or early phases of clinical development. Understanding the associated PK or PD variability and performing clinical trial simulation by incorporating the uncertainty from the existing PK/PD data allows projecting a plausible range of doses for future clinical studies and final practical uses.

## FUTURE PERSPECTIVE

The success of monoclonal antibodies as new therapeutic agents in several disease areas such as oncology, inflammatory diseases, autoimmune diseases and transplantation has triggered growing scientific, therapeutic and business interest in the mAb technology. The market for therapeutic mAbs is one of the most dynamic sectors within the pharmaceutical industry. Further growth is expected by developing mAbs towards other surface protein targets, which are not covered yet by marketed mAbs. Particularly, the technological advancement in the area of immunoconjugates and mAb fragments may overcome some of the limitations of mAbs by providing highly potent drugs selectively to effect compartments and to extend the distribution of the active moiety, which are typically not reached by mAbs. In particular immunoconjugates hold great promise for selective drug delivery of potent drugs with unfavorable own selectivity to target cells (e.g., highly potent cytotoxic drugs). Several of such immunoconjugates are under development to target different tumor types and are expected to reach the market in the next years. Modification of the mAb structure allows adjusting the properties according to therapeutic needs (e.g., adjusting half-life, increasing volume of distribution, changing clearance pathways). By using modified mAb derivatives, optimized therapeutic agents might become available. So far this technology has been successfully used for two antibody fragments marketed in inflammatory disease and anti-angiogenesis (abciximab, ranibizumab).

A particular challenge in drug development will be the combination therapy with different mAbs targeting different target antigens at the same time in order to use synergistic or additive effects of mAbs. The complex biochemical, pathophysiological dynamics of the disease states will require new and challenging PK/PD model development to understand the combined activities of the mAb combinations with regard to safety and efficacy.

mAbs have become very attractive therapeutics and will continue to be a focus area of drug discovery and development.

## REFERENCES

Alefacept (2003). Alefacept (Amevive) (prescribing information). Cambridge, MA: Biogen Inc.

Avastin (2004). Avastin (Bevacizumab) (prescribing information). South San Francisco, CA: Genentech, Inc.

Baert F, Noman M, Vermeire S, et al. (2003). Influence of immunogenicity on the long-term efficacy of infliximab in Crohn's disease. N Engl J Med 348 (7):601–8.

Bauer RJ, Dedrick RL, White ML, et al. (1999). Population pharmacokinetics and pharmacodynamics of the anti-CD11a antibody hu1124 in human subjects with psoriasis. J Pharmacokinet Biopharm 27(4):397–420.

Baxter LT, Zhu H, Mackensen DG, et al. (1995). Biodistribution of monoclonal antibodies: scale-up from mouse to human using a physiologically based pharmacokinetic model. Cancer Res 55(20):4611–22.

Baxter LT, Zhu H, Mackensen DG, Jain RK. (1994). Physiologically based pharmacokinetic model for specific and nonspecific monoclonal antibodies and fragments in normal tissues and human tumor xenografts in nude mice. Cancer Res 54(6):1517–28.

Bazin-Redureau MI, Renard CB, Scherrmann JM. (1997). Pharmacokinetics of heterologous and homologous immunoglobulin G, F(ab')2 and Fab after intravenous administration in the rat. J Pharm Pharmacol 49 (3):277–81.

Berger MA, Masters GR, Singleton J, et al. (2005). Pharmacokinetics, biodistribution, and radioimmunotherapy with monoclonal antibody 776.1 in a murine model of human ovarian cancer. Cancer Biother Radiopharm 20(6):589–602.

Bexxar (2003). Bexxar (Tositumomab) (prescribing information). Seattle, WA: Corixa Corp and Philadelphia, PA: GlaxoSmithKline.

Boxenbaum H, Battle M. (1995). Effective half-life in clinical pharmacology. J Clin Pharmacol 35(8):763–6.

Brambell F, Hemmings W, Morris I. (1964). A theoretical model of gamma-globulin catabolism. Nature 203:1352–1355.

Bugelski PJ, Herzyk DJ, Rehm S, et al. (2000). Preclinical development of keliximab, a Primatized anti-CD4 monoclonal antibody, in human CD4 transgenic mice: characterization of the model and safety studies. Hum Exp Toxicol 19(4):230–43.

Bunescu A, Seideman P, Lenkei R, et al. (2004). Enhanced Fcgamma receptor I, alphaMbeta2 integrin receptor expression by monocytes and neutrophils in rheumatoid arthritis: interaction with platelets. J Rheumatol 31(12):2347–55.

Cartron G, Watier H, Golay J, Solal-Celigny P. (2004). From the bench to the bedside: ways to improve rituximab efficacy. Blood 104(9):2635–42.

Clarke J, Leach W, Pippig S, et al. (2004). Evaluation of a surrogate antibody for preclinical safety testing of an anti-CD11a monoclonal antibody. Regul Toxicol Pharmacol 40(3):219–26.

Coffey GP, Fox JA, Pippig S, et al. (2005). Tissue distribution and receptor-mediated clearance of anti-CD11a antibody in mice. Drug Metab Dispos 33(5):623–9.

Cohenuram M, Saif MW. (2007). Panitumumab the first fully human monoclonal antibody: from the bench to the clinic. Anticancer Drugs 18(1):7–15.

Cornillie F, Shealy D, D'Haens G, et al. (2001). Infliximab induces potent anti-inflammatory and local immunomodulatory activity but no systemic immune suppression in patients with Crohn's disease. Aliment Pharmacol Ther 15(4):463–73.

Dall'Ozzo S, Tartas S, Paintaud G, et al. (2004). Rituximab-dependent cytotoxicity by natural killer cells: influence of FCGR3A polymorphism on the concentration-effect relationship. Cancer Res 64 (13):4664–9.

Danilov SM, Gavrilyuk VD, Franke FE, et al. (2001). Lung uptake of antibodies to endothelial antigens: key determinants of vascular immunotargeting. Am J Physiol Lung Cell Mol Physiol 280(6):L1335–47.

Dedrick RL. (1973). Animal scale-up. J Pharmacokinet Biopharm 1(5):435–61.

Dedrick RL, Walicke P, Garovoy M. (2002). Anti-adhesion antibodies efalizumab, a humanized anti-CD11a monoclonal antibody. Transpl Immunol 9(2–4):181–6.

den Broeder A, van de Putte L, Rau R, et al. (2002). A single dose, placebo controlled study of the fully human anti-tumor necrosis factor-alpha antibody adalimumab (D2E7) in patients with rheumatoid arthritis. J Rheumatol 29(11):2288–98.

Dickinson BL, Badizadegan K, Wu Z, et al. (1999). Bidirectional FcRn-dependent IgG transport in a polarized human intestinal epithelial cell line. J Clin Invest 104(7):903–11.

Dowell JA, Korth-Bradley J, Liu H, et al. (2001). Pharmacokinetics of gemtuzumab ozogamicin, an antibody-targeted chemotherapy agent for the treatment of patients with acute myeloid leukemia in first relapse. J Clin Pharmacol 41(11):1206–14.

Druet P, Bariety J, Laliberte F, et al. (1978). Distribution of heterologous antiperoxidase antibodies and their fragments in the superficial renal cortex of normal Wistar-Munich rat: an ultrastructural study. Lab Invest 39(6):623–31.

Duconge J Castillo R, Crombet T, et al. (2004). Integrated pharmacokinetic-pharmacodynamic modeling and allometric scaling for optimizing the dosage regimen of the monoclonal ior EGF/r3 antibody. Eur J Pharm Sci 21(2–3):261–70.

Erbitux (2004). Erbitux (Cetuximab) (prescribing information). Branchburg, NJ: Imclone Systems Incorporated and Princeton, NJ: Bristol-Myers Squibb Company.

Ferl GZ, Wu AM, DiStefano JJ. III. (2005). A predictive model of therapeutic monoclonal antibody dynamics and regulation by the neonatal Fc receptor (FcRn). Ann Biomed Eng 33(11):1640–52.

Ghetie V, Hubbard JG, Kim JK, et al. (1996). Abnormally short serum half-lives of IgG in beta 2-microglobulin-deficient mice. Eur J Immunol 26(3):690–6.

Gillies SD, Lan Y, Lo KM, et al. (1999). Improving the efficacy of antibody-interleukin 2 fusion proteins by reducing their interaction with Fc receptors. Cancer Res 59(9):2159–66.

Gillies SD, Lo KM, Burger C, et al. (2002). Improved circulating half-life and efficacy of an antibody-interleukin 2 immunocytokine based on reduced intracellular proteolysis. Clin Cancer Res 8(1):210–16.

Goldsby RA, Kindt TJ, Osborine BA. (1999). Immunoglobulins: Structure and Function Kuby Immunology. 4th ed. New York: W.H. Freeman and Company.

Gottlieb AB, Miller B, Lowe N, et al. (2003). Subcutaneously administered efalizumab (anti-CD11a) improves signs and symptoms of moderate to severe plaque psoriasis. J Cutan Med Surg 7(3):198–207.

Hayashi N, Tsukamoto Y, Sallas WM, Lowe PJ. (2007). A mechanism-based binding model for the population pharmacokinetics and pharmacodynamics of omalizumab. Br J Clin Pharmacol 63(5):548–61.

Herceptin (2006). Herceptin (Trastuzumab) (prescribing information). South San Francisco, CA, USA.

Hervey PS, Keam SJ. (2006). Abatacept. BioDrugs 20 (1):53–61; discussion 62.

Hinton PR, Xiong JM, Johlfs MG, et al. (2006). An engineered human IgG1 antibody with longer serum half-life. J Immunol 176(1):346–56.

Hooks MA, Wade CS, Millikan WJ, Jr. (1991). Muromonab CD-3: a review of its pharmacology, pharmacokinetics, and clinical use in transplantation. Pharmacotherapy 11(1):26–37.

Huang L, Biolsi S, Bales KR, Kuchibhotla U. (2006). Impact of variable domain glycosylation on antibody clearance: an LC/MS characterization. Anal Biochem 349 (2):197–207.

Humira (2007). Humira (Adalimumab) (prescribing information). Chicago, IL, USA.

ICH (1997a). ICH Harmonized Tripartite Guideline S6: Preclinical Safety Evaluation of Biotechnology-Derived Pharmaceuticals.

ICH (1997b). ICH Harmonized Tripartite Guideline M3: Nonclinical Safety Studies for the Conduct of Human Clinical Trials for Pharmaceuticals.

Jolling K, Perez Ruixo JJ, Hemeryck A, et al. (2005). Mixed-effects modelling of the interspecies pharmacokinetic scaling of pegylated human erythropoietin. Eur J Pharm Sci 24(5):465–75.

Joshi A, Bauer R, Kuebler P, et al. (2006). An overview of the pharmacokinetics and pharmacodynamics of efalizumab: a monoclonal antibody approved for use in psoriasis. J Clin Pharmacol 46(1):10–20.

Junghans RP. (1997). Finally! The Brambell receptor (FcRB). Mediator of transmission of immunity and protection from catabolism for IgG. Immunol Res 16(1):29–57.

Junghans RP, Anderson CL. (1996). The protection receptor for IgG catabolism is the beta2-microglobulin-containing neonatal intestinal transport receptor. Proc Natl Acad Sci USA 93(11):5512–16.

Kairemo KJ, Lappalainen AK, Kaapa E, et al. (2001). In vivo detection of intervertebral disk injury using a radiolabeled monoclonal antibody against keratan sulfate. J Nucl Med 42(3):476–82.

Kelley SK, Gelzleichter T, Xie D, et al. (2006). Preclinical pharmacokinetics, pharmacodynamics, and activity of a humanized anti-CD40 antibody (SGN-40) in rodents and non-human primates. Br J Pharmacol 148 (8):1116–23.

Kleiman NS, Raizner AE, Jordan R, et al. (1995). Differential inhibition of platelet aggregation induced by adenosine diphosphate or a thrombin receptor-activating peptide in patients treated with bolus chimeric 7E3 Fab: implications for inhibition of the internal pool of GPIIb/IIIa receptors. J Am Coll Cardiol 26(7):1665–71.

Kohler G, Milstein C. (1975). Continuous cultures of fused cells secreting antibody of predefined specificity. Nature 256(5517):495–7.

Kolar GR, Capra JD. (2003). In: Paul WE, ed. Immunoglobulins: Structure and Function Fundamental Immunology. 5th ed. Philadephia, PA: Lippincott Williams & Wilkins.

Koon HB, Severy P, Hagg DS, et al. (2006). Antileukemic effect of daclizumab in CD25 high-expressing leukemias and impact of tumor burden on antibody dosing. Leuk Res 30(2):190–203.

Kovarik JM, Nashan B, Neuhaus P, et al. (2001). A population pharmacokinetic screen to identify demographic-clinical covariates of basiliximab in liver transplantation. Clin Pharmacol Ther 69(4):201–9.

Krueger JG. (2002). The immunologic basis for the treatment of psoriasis with new biologic agents. J Am Acad Dermatol 46(1):1–23; quiz 23–6.

Kuus-Reichel K, Grauer LS, Karavodin LM, et al. (1994). Will immunogenicity limit the use, efficacy, and future development of therapeutic monoclonal antibodies? Clin Diagn Lab Immunol 1(4):365–72.

Lee H, Kimko HC, Rogge M, et al. (2003). Population pharmacokinetic and pharmacodynamic modeling of etanercept using logistic regression analysis. Clin Pharmacol Ther 73(4):348–65.

Lin YS, Nguyen C, Mendoza JL, et al. (1999). Preclinical pharmacokinetics, interspecies scaling, and tissue distribution of a humanized monoclonal antibody against vascular endothelial growth factor. J Pharmacol Exp Ther 288(1):371–8.

Lobo ED, Hansen RJ, Balthasar JP. (2004). Antibody pharmacokinetics and pharmacodynamics. J Pharm Sci 93(11):2645–68.

Looney RJ, Anolik JH, Campbell D, et al. (2004). B cell depletion as a novel treatment for systemic lupus erythematosus: a phase I/II dose-escalation trial of rituximab. Arthritis Rheum 50(8):2580–9.

Lucentis (2006). Lucentis (Ranibizumab) (prescribing information). South San Francisco, CA, USA.

Mahmood I. (2005a). Interspecies Pharmacokinetics Scaling. Rockville: Pine House Publishers.

Mahmood I. (2005b). Prediction of concentration-time profiles in humans. In: Interspecies Pharmacokinetics Scaling. Rockville: Pine House Publishers:219–41.

Mahmood I, Green MD. (2005). Pharmacokinetic and pharmacodynamic considerations in the development of therapeutic proteins. Clin Pharmacokinet 44 (4):331–47.

Martin-Jimenez T. Riviere JE. (2002). Mixed-effects modeling of the interspecies pharmacokinetic scaling of oxytetracycline. J Pharm Sci 91(2):331–41.

McClurkan MB, Valentine JL, Arnold L, Owens SM. (1993). Disposition of a monoclonal anti-phencyclidine Fab fragment of immunoglobulin G in rats. J Pharmacol Exp Ther 266(3):1439–45.

McLaughlin P, Grillo-Lopez AJ, Link BK, et al. (1998). Rituximab chimeric anti-CD20 monoclonal antibody therapy for relapsed indolent lymphoma: half of patients respond to a four-dose treatment program. J Clin Oncol 16(8):2825–33.

Medesan C, Matesoi D, Radu C, et al. (1997). Delineation of the amino acid residues involved in transcytosis and catabolism of mouse IgG1. J Immunol 158(5):2211–17.

Meibohm B, Derendorf H. (2002). Pharmacokinetic/pharmacodynamic studies in drug product development. J Pharm Sci 91(1):18–31.

Meijer RT, Koopmans RP, ten Berge IJ, Schellekens PT. (2002). Pharmacokinetics of murine anti-human CD3 antibodies in man are determined by the disappearance of target antigen. J Pharmacol Exp Ther 300 (1):346–53.

Meredith PA, Elliott HL, Donnelly R, Reid JL. (1991). Dose-response clarification in early drug development. J Hypertens Suppl 9(6):S356–7.

Morris EC, Rebello P, Thomson KJ, et al. (2003). Pharmacokinetics of alemtuzumab used for in vivo and in vitro T-cell depletion in allogeneic transplantations: relevance for early adoptive immunotherapy and infectious complications. Blood 102(1):404–6.

Mortensen DL, Walicke PA, Wang X, et al. (2005). Pharmacokinetics and pharmacodynamics of multiple weekly subcutaneous efalizumab doses in patients with plaque psoriasis. J Clin Pharmacol 45(3):286–98.

Mould DR, Davis CB, Minthorn EA, et al. (1999). A population pharmacokinetic-pharmacodynamic analysis of single doses of cleneloximab in patients with rheumatoid arthritis. Clin Pharmacol Ther 66 (3):246–57.

Mould DR, Sweeney KR. (2007). The pharmacokinetics and pharmacodynamics of monoclonal antibodies–mechanistic modeling applied to drug development. Curr Opin Drug Discov Devel 10(1):84–96.

Nakakura EK, McCabe SM, Zheng B, et al. (1993). Potent and effective prolongation by anti-LFA-1 monoclonal antibody monotherapy of non-primarily vascularized heart allograft survival in mice without T cell depletion. Transplantation 55(2):412–17.

Nestorov I, Zitnik R, Ludden T. (2004). Population pharmacokinetic modeling of subcutaneously administered etanercept in patients with psoriasis. J Pharmacokinet Pharmacodyn 31(6):463–90.

Newkirk MM, Novick J, Stevenson MM, et al. (1996). Differential clearance of glycoforms of IgG in normal and autoimmune-prone mice. Clin Exp Immunol 106 (2):259–64.

Ng CM, Joshi A, Dedrick RL, et al. (2005). Pharmacokinetic-pharmacodynamic-efficacy analysis of efalizumab in patients with moderate to severe psoriasis. Pharm Res 22(7):1088–100.

Ng CM, Stefanich E, Anand BS, et al. (2006). Pharmacokinetics/pharmacodynamics of nondepleting anti-CD4 monoclonal antibody (TRX1) in healthy human volunteers. Pharm Res 23(1):95–103.

Norman DJ, Chatenoud L, Cohen D, et al. (1993). Consensus statement regarding OKT3-induced cytokine-release syndrome and human antimouse antibodies. Transplant Proc 25(2 Suppl 1):89–92.

Ober RJ, Radu CG, Ghetie V, Ward ES. (2001). Differences in promiscuity for antibody-FcRn interactions across species: implications for therapeutic antibodies. Int Immunol 13(12):1551–9.

Papp K, Bissonnette R, Krueger JG., et al. (2001). The treatment of moderate to severe psoriasis with a new anti-CD11a monoclonal antibody. J Am Acad Dermatol 45(5):665–74.

Petkova SB, Akilesh S, Sproule TJ, et al. (2006). Enhanced half-life of genetically engineered human IgG1 antibodies in a humanized FcRn mouse model: potential application in humorally mediated autoimmune disease. Int Immunol 18(12):1759–69.

Presta LG. (2002). Engineering antibodies for therapy. Curr Pharm Biotechnol 3(3):237–56.

Presta LG, Shields RL, Namenuk AK, et al. (2002). Engineering therapeutic antibodies for improved function. Biochem Soc Trans 30(4):487–90.

Raptiva (2004). Raptiva (Efalizumab) (prescribing information). South San Francisco, CA: Genentech, Inc.

Remicade (2006). Remicade (Infliximab) (prescribing information). Malvenr, PA: Centocor Inc.

Rituxan (2006). Rituxan (Rituximab) (prescribing information). South San Francisco, CA, USA: Genentech Inc. and Cambridge, MA: Biogen Inc.

Roopenian DC, Christianson GJ, Sproule TJ, et al. (2003). The MHC class I-like IgG receptor controls perinatal IgG transport, IgG homeostasis, and fate of IgG-Fc-coupled drugs. J Immunol 170(7):3528–33.

Roskos LK, Davis CG, Schwab GM. (2004). The clinical pharmacology of therapeutic monoclonal antibodies. Drug Develop Res 61(3):108–20.

Schror K, Weber AA. (2003). Comparative pharmacology of GP IIb/IIIa antagonists. J Thromb Thrombolysis 15 (2):71–80.

Sheiner L, Wakefield, J. (1999). Population modelling in drug development. Stat Methods Med Res 8 (3):183–93.

Sheiner LB. (1997). Learning versus confirming in clinical drug development. Clin Pharmacol Ther 61(3):275–91.

Shields RL, Namenuk AK, Hong K, et al. (2001). High resolution mapping of the binding site on human IgG1 for Fc gamma RI, Fc gamma RII, Fc gamma RIII, and FcRn and design of IgG1 variants with improved binding to the Fc gamma R. J Biol Chem 276 (9):6591–604.

Simister NE, Mostov KE. (1989a). Cloning and expression of the neonatal rat intestinal Fc receptor, a major histocompatibility complex class I antigen homolog. Cold Spring Harb Symp Quant Biol 54(Pt 1):571–80.

Simister NE, Mostov KE. (1989b). An Fc receptor structurally related to MHC class I antigens. Nature 337 (6203):184–7.

Simulect (2005). Simulect (Basiliximab) (prescribing information). East Hanover, NJ, USA.

Spiekermann GM, Finn PW, Ward ES, et al. (2002). Receptor-mediated immunoglobulin G transport across mucosal barriers in adult life: functional expression of FcRn in the mammalian lung. J Exp Med 196(3):303–10.

Straughn AB. (2006). Limitations of noncompartmental pharmacokinetic analysis of biotech drugs. In: Meibohm B, ed. Pharmacokinetics and Pharmacodynamics of Biotech Drugs. Weinheim: Wiley, 181–8.

Subramanian GM, Cronin PW, Poley G, et al. (2005). A phase 1 study of PAmAb, a fully human monoclonal antibody against Bacillus anthracis protective antigen, in healthy volunteers. Clin Infect Dis 41(1):12–20.

Sun YN, Lu JF, Joshi A, et al. (2005). Population pharmacokinetics of efalizumab (humanized monoclonal anti-CD11a antibody) following long-term subcutaneous weekly dosing in psoriasis subjects. J Clin Pharmacol 45(4):468–76.

Synagis (2004). Synagis (Palivizumab) (prescribing information). Gaithersburg, MD: MedImmune, Inc. and Columbus, OH: Abbott Laboratories Inc.

Tabrizi MA, Tseng CM, Roskos LK. (2006). Elimination mechanisms of therapeutic monoclonal antibodies. Drug Discov Today 11(1–2):81–8.

Tang H, Mayersohn M. (2005). Accuracy of allometrically predicted pharmacokinetic parameters in humans: role of species selection. Drug Metab Dispos 33(9):1288–93.

Tang L, Persky AM, Hochhaus G, Meibohm B. (2004). Pharmacokinetic aspects of biotechnology products. J Pharma Sci 93(9): 2184–204.

Ternant D, Paintaud G. (2005). Pharmacokinetics and concentration-effect relationships of therapeutic monoclonal antibodies and fusion proteins. Expert Opin Biol Ther 5(Suppl 1):S37–47.

Tokuda Y, Watanabe T, Omuro Y, et al. (1999). Dose escalation and pharmacokinetic study of a humanized anti-HER2 monoclonal antibody in patients with HER2/neu-overexpressing metastatic breast cancer. Br J Cancer 81(8):1419–25.

Tysabri (2006). Tysabri (Natalizumab) (prescribing information). San Diego, CA: Elan Pharmaceuticals Inc. and Cambridge, MA: Biogen Idec Inc.

Umana P, Jean-Mairet J, Moudry R, et al. (1999). Engineered glycoforms of an antineuroblastoma IgG1 with optimized antibody-dependent cellular cytotoxic activity. Nat Biotechnol 17(2):176–80.

Vaccaro C, Bawdon R, Wanjie S, et al. (2006). Divergent activities of an engineered antibody in murine and human systems have implications for therapeutic antibodies. Proc Natl Acad Sci USA 103(49):18709–14.

Vaishnaw AK, TenHoor CN. (2002). Pharmacokinetics, biologic activity, and tolerability of alefacept by intravenous and intramuscular administration. J Pharmacokinet Pharmacodyn 29(5–6):415–26.

Wang W, Singh S, Zeng DL, et al. (2007). Antibody structure, instability, and formulation. J Pharm Sci 96(1):1–26.

Watanabe N, Kuriyama H, Sone H, et al. (1988). Continuous internalization of tumor necrosis factor receptors in a human myosarcoma cell line. J Biol Chem 263 (21):10262–6.

Weiner LM. (2006). Fully human therapeutic monoclonal antibodies. J Immunother 29(1):1–9.

Weisman MH, Moreland LW, Furst DE, et al. (2003). Efficacy, pharmacokinetic, and safety assessment of adalimumab, a fully human anti-tumor necrosis factor-alpha monoclonal antibody, in adults with rheumatoid arthritis receiving concomitant methotrexate: a pilot study. Clin Ther 25(6):1700–21.

Werther WA, Gonzalez TN, O'Connor SJ, et al. (1996). Humanization of an anti-lymphocyte function-associated antigen (LFA)-1 monoclonal antibody and reengineering of the humanized antibody for binding to rhesus LFA-1. J Immunol 157(11):4986–95.

Wurster U, Haas J. (1994). Passage of intravenous immunoglobulin and interaction with the CNS. J Neurol Neurosurg Psychiatry 57(Suppl):21–5.

Xolair (2006). Xolair (Omalizumab) (prescribing information). South San Francisco, CA, USA: Genentech Inc. and East Hanover, NJ, USA: Novartis.

Yim D S, Zhou H, Buckwalter M, et al. (2005). Population pharmacokinetic analysis and simulation of the time-concentration profile of etanercept in pediatric patients with juvenile rheumatoid arthritis. J Clin Pharmacol 45(3):246–56.

Zenapax (2005). Zenapax (Daclizumab) (prescribing information). Nutley, NJ, USA.

Zhou H. (2005). Clinical pharmacokinetics of etanercept: a fully humanized soluble recombinant tumor necrosis factor receptor fusion protein. J Clin Pharmacol 45 (5):490–7.

Zhou H, Mayer PR, Wajdula J, Fatenejad S. (2004). Unaltered etanercept pharmacokinetics with concurrent methotrexate in patients with rheumatoid arthritis. J Clin Pharmacol 44(11):1235–43.

Zia-Amirhosseini, P, Minthorn E, Benincosa LJ, et al. (1999). Pharmacokinetics and pharmacodynamics of SB-240563, a humanized monoclonal antibody directed to human interleukin-5, in monkeys. J Pharmacol Exp Ther 291(3):1060–7.

# Monoclonal Antibodies in Cancer

*John C. Kuth*
*Medical College of Georgia Health, Inc., Augusta, Georgia, U.S.A.*

*Terreia S. Jones*
*Department of Clinical Pharmacy, University of Tennessee College of Pharmacy, Memphis, Tennessee, U.S.A.*

*Jennifer Hanje*
*The Ohio State University Medical Center and James Cancer Hospital, Columbus, Ohio, U.S.A.*

*Susannah E. Motl Moroney*
*Roche Laboratories Inc., Nutley, New Jersey, U.S.A.*

---

## PHARMACOTHERAPY INFORMATION

Further information on the applied pharmacotherapy with monoclonal antibodies in cancer can be found in the following frequently used textbooks:

- **Applied Therapeutics: The Clinical Use of Drugs** (Koda-Kimble, MA, et al., Eds.), 8th edition, Lippincott Williams & Wilkins, Baltimore 2005: Chapters 88, 89, 90.
- **Pharmacotherapy: A Pathophysiologic Approach** (DiPiro, JT, et al., Eds.), 6th edition, McGraw-Hill, New York 2005: Chapters 124, 125, 127, 129, 131, 132.
- **Textbook of Therapeutics: Drug and Disease Management** (Helms, RA, et al., Eds.), 8th edition, Lippincott Williams & Wilkins, Baltimore 2006: Chapters 93, 94, 95, 96, 98.

## INTRODUCTION

Cancer is the second-leading cause of death in the United States with one of every four deaths attributable to cancer (Jemal et al., 2006). However, when mortality rates were considered on the basis of age, cancer began to surpass heart disease as the leading cause of death for persons younger than 85 years starting in 1999 (Jemal et al., 2006). Survival rates have improved only modestly over the last several decades (e.g., 5 year relative survival rates from 1995 to 2001 were 65% compared to 50% from 1974 to 1976) with most survival advances occurring through earlier detection of cancer rather than through treatment advances (American Cancer Society, 2006). New treatments that can exploit intrinsic differences between normal and neoplastic cells are needed to offer patients additional options besides traditional treatment modalities of surgery, radiation, and chemotherapy (Zangmeister-Wittke, 2005). Therapeutic monoclonal antibodies represent a new type of treatment that can be used to improve overall survival, increase the time to progression, and delay the time to recurrence of many oncologic diseases. These drugs will provide many treatment alternatives for cancer patients.

Because of the high incidence, morbidity, and mortality rates associated with cancer, staying abreast of emerging therapeutic innovations in cancer care are paramount for health care professionals and scientists, both professionally and personally. This chapter summarizes pertinent points about the currently approved oncologic monoclonal antibodies in the United States. Antibodies are organized based on their target [i.e., CD cell, epidermal growth factor receptor (EGFR), and vascular endothelial growth factor (VEGF) receptor]. Table 1 summarizes the current FDA approved monoclonal antibodies for cancer indications, year of approval, their origin and target, and appropriate indications that will be discussed (Adams and Weiner, 2005).

## CLASSES OF MONOCLONAL ANTIBODIES: CD ANTIGENS

### ■ Alemtuzumab

#### Pharmacology and Mechanism of Action

Alemtuzumab is an unconjugated, humanized, $IgG_1$ kappa monoclonal antibody (MAb) directed against the 21–28 kDa cell surface glycoprotein CD52 (Frampton and Wagstaff, 2003). Most lymphocytes (including 95% of B- and T-cells at various stages of differentiation), monocytes, natural killer cells,

| FDA-approved monoclonal antibodies in cancer: generic name (Trade) | Approval year | Origin | Target | Indication |
|---|---|---|---|---|
| **CD cells** | | | | |
| Alemtuzumab (Campath-1H) | 2001 | Humanized | CD-52 | B-cell CLL |
| Gemtuzumab (Mylotarg®) | 2000 | Humanized | CD-33 | Acute myeloid leukemia |
| Rituximab (Rituxan®) | 1997 | Chimeric | CD-20 | NHL |
| Yttrium-90 ($^{90}$Y) ibritumomab tiuxetan (Zevalin®) | 2002 | Murine | CD-20 | B-cell NHL |
| Iodine-131 ($^{131}$I) tositumomab (Bexxar®) | 2003 | Murine | CD-20 | NHL |
| **Epidermal growth factor receptor (EGFR)** | | | | |
| Cetuximab (Erbitux®) | 2004 | Chimeric | EGFR | CRC, SCCHN |
| Panitumumab (Vectibix®) | 2006 | Human | EGFR | CRC |
| Trastuzumab (Herceptin®) | 1998 | Humanized | HER2/neu | Breast cancer |
| **Vascular endothelial growth factor (VEGF)** | | | | |
| Bevacizumab (Avastin®) | 2004 | Humanized | VEGF | NSCLC, CRC |

*Abbreviations*: CLL, chronic lymphocytic leukemia; colorectal cancer CRC; EGFR, endothelial growth factor receptor and epidermal growth factor receptor; non-Hodgkin's lymphoma NHL; NSCLC, nonsmall cell lung cancer; SCCHN, squamous cell carcinoma of the head and neck; VEGF, vascular endothelial growth factor.

**Table 1** ▇ FDA approved monoclonal antibodies in cancer.

macrophages and eosinophils, as well as cells lining the distal epididymis, vas deferens, and seminal vesicles in the male reproductive tract express CD52; however, it is not found on erythrocytes, platelets, or stem cells (Lui and O'Brien, 2004; O'Brien et al., 2005). In addition, while CD52 is highly expressed in some forms of chronic lymphocytic leukemia (CLL), non-Hodgkin lymphoma (NHL), and acute lymphoblastic leukemia (ALL), it is not shed or internalized, making it an excellent therapeutic target (Lui and O'Brien, 2004). Recent studies have found that malignant CD52 expression occurs in not only CLL, low-grade lymphomas, and T-cell malignancies, but also some cases of myeloid, monocytic, and ALL; thus, use of alemtuzumab is expanding to a variety of disease states (O'Brien et al., 2005). The compound exerts its effect by binding to CD52 antigenic sites and stimulating cross-linking by antibodies, which promotes antibody-dependent cellular cytotoxicity and direct cellular apoptosis via natural killer activity as shown in Figure 1 (Greenwood et al., 1994; O'Brien et al., 2005).

*Pharmacokinetics*

Pharmacokinetic parameters of alemtuzumab have been investigated in a phase I dose-escalation trial. Patients with B-cell CLL and NHL were given alemtuzumab once weekly for a maximum of 12 weeks, and plasma levels were obtained. Patients who received higher doses exhibited higher values for maximum plasma concentration ($C_{max}$) as well as area under the curve (AUC), demonstrating dose-dependent proportionality. The median half-life ($t_{1/2}$) was approximately 12 days (Berlex, 2005). A subsequent pharmacokinetic analysis was conducted in CLL patients who received 30 mg intravenous alemtuzumab thrice weekly. While much interpatient variability was observed, patients exhibited a trend of gradually rising plasma concentrations during initial therapy, which continued until steady-state was achieved. This typically occurred after 6 weeks. Authors noted that the rise in alemtuzumab concentrations corresponded to a simultaneous decline in circulating CD52-positive malignant lymphocytes (Berlex, 2005).

In addition to intravenous administration, alemtuzumab has been given via the subcutaneous route (Hale et al., 2004). In one comparative study, 30 patients with relapsed CLL received intravenous alemtuzumab 30 mg thrice weekly, while 20 patients received similar doses subcutaneously. The authors noted that over time, maximal trough concentrations progressed to similar levels in both groups; however, accumulation of antibody in the blood was slower in the subcutaneous group, with these patients requiring slightly higher cumulative doses to achieve similar concentrations. In this study, the mean steady-state volume of distribution ($V_d$) among both groups of patients during initial treatment was 0.185 L/kg, which expanded to 0.252 L/kg during the terminal phase. This for a MAb comparatively large $V_d$ is consistent with the notion that alemtuzumab distributes beyond the plasma compartment to encompass an extravascular lymphocytic compartment. Mean terminal half-life was 6.1 days in this population; however, clearance appeared to correlate with

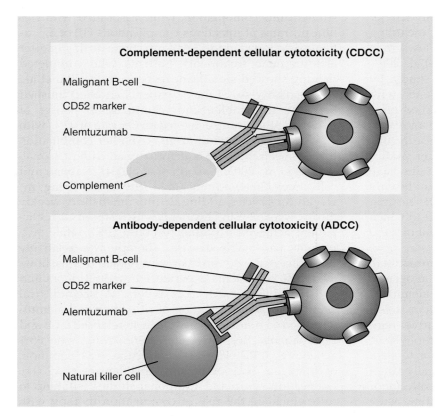

**Figure 1** ▪ Alemtuzumab mechanism of action. Diagram showing alemtuzumab bound to the CD52 surface marker on chronic lymphocytic leukemia cells where it triggers complement-dependent cytotoxicity and natural killer cell action. *Source*: From the Association of the British Pharmaceutical Industry.

antigenic burden (Hale et al., 2004). Patients with undetectable CLL cells exhibited a single elimination phase with a longer half-life, whereas patients with bulkier tumors cleared alemtuzumab more rapidly. Authors concluded that the prevailing factor influencing alemtuzumab pharmacokinetic parameters appears to be CD52 concentration, which accounts for a great deal of interpatient variability. Thus, alemtuzumab exhibits target-mediated drug disposition (see Chapter 5), and it is unsuitable to classify the pharmacokinetic parameters of alemtuzumab into a simple pharmacokinetic model (Hale et al., 2004).

### Indications and Clinical Efficacy

While it is utilized in a variety of disease states, alemtuzumab is FDA-approved for use in B-cell CLL patients who have been treated with alkylating agents and failed fludarabine therapy. Three major studies have assessed alemtuzumab in this population (Osterborg et al., 1997; Keating et al., 2002a; Rai et al., 2002b). An international collaboration of centers in the United States and Europe published the largest of these studies. Ninety-two fludarabine-resistant patients, of whom 76% had Rai stage III or IV disease, were treated with 12 weeks of intravenous alemtuzumab (Keating et al., 2002a). The overall response (OR) rate was 33%, with 2% achieving a complete response (CR). Median survival was

16 months. Patients with bulky lymphadenopathy were less likely to respond, possibly indicating poor tumor penetration of alemtuzumab (Keating et al., 2002a; Lui and O'Brien, 2004). Toxicity was moderate and consisted mainly of infectious problems and infusion reactions. Rai and colleagues (2002b) supported these findings with a study evaluating 24 poor-prognosis, fludarabine-resistant CLL patients. After approximately 16 weeks of treatment with alemtuzumab (target dose 30 mg three times weekly), the OR rate was 33%. Median time to progression was 19.6 months.

Because of the high incidence of infusion-related reactions encountered with alemtuzumab intravenous infusion, subcutaneous administration has been explored as a potential alternative. A pivotal trial evaluated subcutaneous alemtuzumab as first-line therapy in 41 patients with advanced, previously untreated CLL (Lundin et al., 2002). An OR rate of 87% was seen, with 19% CR. While injection site reactions were seen in 90% patients, these were grades 1–2 in severity, and typically disappeared with continued treatment (often within 2 weeks). The more severe infusion reactions encountered with intravenous dosing, such as dyspnea, hypotension, and nausea were absent; however, some patients did experience fever and rigors (Lundin et al., 2002; Mavromatis and Cheson, 2003).

Alemtuzumab has demonstrated some activity in other hematologic malignancies as well, including T-Cell prolymphocytic leukemia (PLL) and low-grade lymphomas (Pawson et al., 1997; Dearden et al., 2001; Keating et al., 2002b). An encouraging study by Pawson et al. (1997) evaluated 15 patients with refractory T-cell PLL, most of whom had failed prior treatment with pentostatin. The response rate was 73%, with 60% patients achieving CR. These results have been subsequently investigated in other studies with T-cell lymphoma patients; response rates have consistently remained above 50%, even in heavily pretreated populations (Dearden et al., 2001; Keating et al., 2002b). It remains to be seen the extent to which alemtuzumab will play a role in the treatment of these disease states.

Another important application for alemtuzumab includes its use in CLL patients undergoing allogeneic stem cell transplant (SCT). In this setting, alemtuzumab has been effectively utilized in various roles, including nonmyeloablative SCT preparative regimens, graft-versus-host disease (GvHD) prophylaxis, and in vitro purging of T-lymphocytes prior to stem cell infusion. Because of its ability to specifically target CD52 antigen, alemtuzumab may deplete both donor and recipient T-lymphocytes, thus preventing acute and chronic GvHD while sparing the graft-versus-leukemia effect (Giralt, 2006). Studies have evaluated the addition of alemtuzumab to standard nonmyeloablative preparative regimens such as BEAM (Cull et al., 2000; Kottaridis et al., 2000; Faulkner et al., 2004). Faulkner and colleagues (2004) evaluated 65 patients with lymphoproliferative disorders undergoing reduced-intensity allogeneic SCT in a multicenter study. Authors reported that 97% of patients achieved donor engraftment, with a low incidence of acute GVHD (grades 1–2 in 17%). Disease progression was the major cause of treatment-related failure; however, the incidence was low and corresponded to histologic grade of lymphoma (relapse risk was 10% at 2 years for low-grade lymphomas, but 68% at 2 years for high-grade NHL and mantle cell lymphomas). Overall, the regimen was well tolerated, and transplant-related mortality was similar to other reports of BEAM conditioning regimens for autologous transplants (7.6%) (Cull et al., 2000; Kottaridis et al., 2000). Authors concluded that alemtuzumab appears to be a safe and effective addition to the reduced-intensity SCT regimen.

Combination therapy with alemtuzumab has recently been explored; one study evaluated six patients with refractory disease who were treated with fludarabine and alemtuzumab concurrently (Kennedy et al., 2002). Five patients responded, with one patient achieving a CR. Additionally, sequential therapy with fludarabine followed by alemtuzumab has been studied; this combination, while associated with significant rates of infectious complications (12 of 57 patients developed grade 3 or 4 infections during or after alemtuzumab treatment), patients who completed therapy showed significant response rates (Rai et al., 2002a). Thirty-six of the 57 patients enrolled finished both the fludarabine and alemtuzumab phases of treatment; this group achieved an OR rate of 92%, with 42% CR (Dearden et al., 2001). Another combination that has been explored is alemtuzumab with rituximab (Faderl et al., 2003; Nabhan et al., 2004). Nabhan and colleagues (2004) administered rituximab 375 mg/m² weekly for 4 cycles, adding alemtuzumab thrice weekly during weeks 2–5 in 12 patients with relapsed CLL. One patient achieved a partial response (PR), while 90% patients had stable disease. Therapy was relatively well-tolerated, with no treatment-related deaths; however, 75% of patients experienced grade 2 rigors and 33% exhibited grade 3/4 fevers. A second trial evaluating the combination of rituximab and alemtuzumab used a similar schedule in 48 relapsed CLL and PLL patients. Response rates were strong, with 65% achieving a PR. However, infection was common, occurring in 56% of patients (Nabhan et al., 2004). Longer follow-up and additional studies will help to fully elucidate the role of combination therapy with alemtuzumab, further addressing the issue of additive myelosuppression and infectious risk with this agent. Selected clinical studies of alemtuzumab are summarized in Table 2.

### Safety Concerns

The most common adverse effects associated with alemtuzumab consist of infusion-related reactions, infectious complications, and hematologic toxicities. Infusion reactions are quite widespread, seen in approximately 90% of patients receiving drug intravenously in a large trial by Keating et al. (2002a). Rigors, fever, nausea, vomiting, and rash are often seen with initial infusions; however, these typically decrease with subsequent drug exposure (Greenwood et al., 1994). Rarely, hypotension and dyspnea are encountered (Lui and O'Brien, 2004). Premedication with acetaminophen and antihistamines is recommended to reduce this possibility. Subcutaneous administration of alemtuzumab also significantly lessens the risk of infusion-related adverse reactions (Bowen et al., 1997; Montillo et al., 2006). Unfortunately, subcutaneous administration is associated with transient local skin reactions in most patients (Lundin et al., 2002). Another substantial adverse effect commonly associated with alemtuzumab is infection; lymphocyte counts drop rapidly after treatment, resulting in a severe and prolonged lymphopenia. This profound T-cell depletion leads to an increased risk of opportunistic infections, particularly cytomegalovirus reactivation. Additionally, *Herpes*

| Investigators | Disease(s), no. of patients | Alemtuzumab dosing regimen | CR/PR (%) | Median overall survival | Significant adverse events (grade 3/4) |
|---|---|---|---|---|---|
| Keating et al. (2002a) | Relapsed/refractory B-cell CLL, n = 93 | 3 mg IV until tolerated, then 10 mg IV until tolerated, then 30 mg IV thrice weekly for up to 12 weeks | CR 2% PR 31% | 16 months | Infection 26.9% |
| Rai et al. (2002b) | B or T-cell CLL after failing fludarabine, n = 24 | 10 mg IV until tolerated, then 30 mg IV thrice weekly for up to 16 weeks | PR 33% | 35.8 months | Neutropenia 20.8% Infection 41.7% |
| Osterborg et al. (1997) | Relapsed/refractory CLL, n = 29 | 3 mg IV escalated as tolerated, to 30 mg IV thrice weekly for up to 12 weeks | CR 4% PR 38% | Median response duration = 12 months | Neutropenia 41% Thrombocytopenia 27% Hypotension 3% Infection 17% |
| Lundin et al. (2002) | Primary B-cell CLL, n = 41 | 3 mg SC escalated to 10 mg SC and 30 mg SC as tolerated then 30 mg SC thrice weekly for 18 weeks maximum | CR 19% PR 68% | Not reached yet; 8–44 + months | Neutropenia 21% Pain at injection site 7% Thrombocytopenia 5% Infection 12% |
| Pawson et al. (1997) | Relapsed T-cell PLL, n = 15 | 10 mg IV escalated to 30 mg IV thrice weekly as tolerated[a] | CR 60% PR 13% | Not reached yet | Hematologic 27% Infection 33% |
| Ferrajoli et al. (2003) | Relapsed lymphoproliferative disorders, including CLL, T-cell PLL, n = 78 | 3 mg IV escalated to 10 mg IV and 30 mg IV as tolerated, then 30 mg IV thrice weekly for 12 weeks maximum | CR 13% PR 22% | 12 months | Neutropenia 27% Thrombocytopenia 32% Dyspnea 7% |
| McCune et al. (2002) | Relapsed/refractory CLL or PLL, n = 23 | 3 mg IV escalated to 10 mg IV and 30 mg IV as tolerated, then 30 mg IV thrice weekly for 12 weeks maximum | CR 35% PR 18% | N/A | Neutropenia 9% Thrombocytopenia 9% Infection 9% |

[a] One patient received subcutaneous alemtuzumab.

*Abbreviations*: CR, complete response; PR, partial response.

**Table 2**  Selected clinical trials with alemtuzumab (campath-1H).

*simplex* virus infection, *Pneumocystic carinii* pneumonia, candidiasis, and septicemia have all been reported (Keating et al., 2002a). These often manifest between 3 and 8 weeks from treatment, during the T-lymphocyte count nadir (Osterborg et al., 2006). Currently, prophylaxis with antibacterial and antiviral medications is strongly recommended in order to prevent these complications. Myelosuppression, on the other hand, consisting of anemia, neutropenia, and thrombocytopenia, is typically moderate and transient, with grade 4 neutropenia occurring in about 20% of cases but neutropenic fever less commonly (Keating et al., 2002a; Lui and O'Brien, 2004; Osterborg et al., 2006).

Rarely, cardiac toxicity has been reported with alemtuzumab, consisting of atrial fibrillation and left ventricular dysfunction (Lenihan et al., 2004). These case reports have occurred in patients with mycosis fungoides/Sezary syndrome, and authors suggested that

patients with T-cell malignancies may be at increased risk of cardiac toxicity from alemtuzumab. However, other reports have found no link between alemtuzumab and cardiac toxicity in patients with mycosis fungoides/Sezary syndrome (Lundin et al., 2005).

### Pharmaceutical Considerations: Formulation, Other Routes of Administration, Dosing Regimens

Alemtuzumab treatment should be administered according to a dose-escalation schedule. Prior to each dose, appropriate premedication, consisting of acetaminophen and an antihistamine such as diphenhydramine, should be given to help prevent infusion reactions. Corticosteroids, such as hydrocortisone, may be used to treat severe infusion-related events. An initial dose of 3 mg should be given as a 2-hr IV infusion daily; once this dose is tolerated (infusion-related toxicities are ≤ grade 2), the dose should be increased to 10 mg IV over 2 hr; once the 10 mg dose is tolerated (infusion-related toxicities are $\leq$ grade 2), the maintenance dose of 30 mg IV over 2 hr may be initiated. This dose should be given thrice weekly. Single doses of greater than 30 mg and weekly doses exceeding 90 mg are not recommended, due to the risk of severe pancytopenia (Berlex, 2005). Alemtuzumab has also been administered via the subcutaneous route (Lundin et al., 2002).

Alemtuzumab is commercially formulated in a single-use clear glass ampule containing 30 mg of alemtuzumab in 3 mL of solution. The ampule should be inspected for particulate matter prior to use. Aseptic technique should be employed to withdraw the appropriate amount of drug from the ampule into a syringe. Drug should be filtered with a sterile, low-protein binding, nonfiber releasing 5 μm filter prior to dilution. This should be further diluted with 100 ml of either sterile 0.9% sodium chloride for injection or 5% dextrose in water solution. The resultant solution should be protected from light, and should be stored under refrigeration (2 to 8°C). Stability of this product is 8 hr once diluted. Alemtuzumab should be infused through an intravenous line that does not contain any other drug substances (Berlex, 2005).

## ■ Gemtuzumab

### Pharmacology and Mechanism of Action

Gemtuzumab ozogamicin (GO) was one of the first commercially available bispecific monoclonal antibodies. This recombinant, humanized, $IgG_4$ MAb to cell surface marker CD33 is covalently bonded by a bifunctional linker to the potent cytotoxic antibiotic, calicheamicin (see Chapter 4). Immature and mature myeloid cells, as well as erythroid, megakaryocytic, and multipotent progenitor cells express the 67-kDa glycosylated transmembrane protein CD33. In addition, this protein is expressed on the surface of most leukemic blast cells found in acute myelogenous leukemia (AML) (greater than 90% of patients) as well as myelodysplastic syndromes (MDS) (Van der Velden et al., 2001; Cersosimo, 2003b). However, CD33 is not expressed on stem cells, nor is it expressed outside of the hematopoietic system, making it an excellent therapeutic target. The cytotoxic antibiotic calicheamicin is a natural antineoplastic compound derived from *Micromonospora echinospora*. It is made up of two molecules of the enediyne antitumor antibiotic n-acetyl-γ-calicheamicin dimethyl hydrazine (Sievers et al., 1999). This compound, along with its metabolites, has antineoplastic activity that is thousand times more potent than doxorubicin (Giles et al., 2003).

GO exerts its clinical effects through direct binding to the CD33 antigen. Following a standard 9 mg/m² infusion, CD33 antigenic sites are maximally saturated within 3 hr (Van der Velden et al., 2001). Endocytosis quickly follows, resulting in rapid internalization of the antibody-antigen complex. Additional expression of new CD33 antigenic sites occurs after internalization of the GO molecule, leading to further accumulation and increased concentration of intracellular GO (Van der Velden et al., 2001). Once inside the cell, GO is directed to lysosomes which cleave the molecule via acid hydrolysis, liberating the calicheamicin compound. Calicheamicin then binds to double-stranded DNA helixes in the minor groove, causing site-specific double strand cleavage at oligopyrimidine-oligopurine tracts (Zein, 1998; Giles et al., 2003). Induction of apoptosis is observed after approximately 72–96 hr (Van der Velden et al., 2001). In addition to direct induction of apoptosis from calicheamicin, antibody-dependent cell-mediated cytotoxicity and complement-mediated cytotoxicity also stimulate leukemic cell death.

### Pharmacokinetics/Pharmacodynamics

Clinical studies investigating the pharmacokinetic parameters of GO have been conducted in adults with AML in first relapse (Dowell et al., 2001; Korth-Bradley, 2001). Initial phase I pharmacokinetic trials found that a dose of 9 mg/m² fully saturated CD33 sites in all patients regardless of disease burden. Phase II studies confirmed the efficacy of GO in refractory AML patients, and helped consolidate the treatment schedule of two 9 mg/m² infusions separated by approximately 14 days. Measurements of serial plasma concentrations have confirmed a distinct difference in pharmacokinetic parameters between the first and second doses, largely thought to be due to a decline in circulating leukemic blast cells that express CD33. A study conducted by Dowell and colleagues in 59 adult patients with relapsed AML found that maximum plasma concentrations ($C_{max}$) of both MAb and calicheamicin typically occurred shortly after the end of the 2 hr infusion; additionally, $C_{max}$ values were generally higher after the second dose (Dowell et al., 2001). Values for $V_d$ changed as well, averaging approximately 20.9 L after the first dose and only 9.9 L after the second (Dowell et al., 2001). This decrease in $V_d$ is likely also due to a decline in the number of circulating cells expressing CD33. In addition, the relatively low distribution volumes suggest that GO does not distribute beyond the plasma compartment, but rather remains bound to CD33 antigenic sites within the vascular space. This has been confirmed by radiolabeled studies, which demonstrates that organs with a large blood pool, such as the spleen and liver, are primarily responsible for uptake and distribution of the antibody

(Scheinberg et al., 1991; Caron et al., 1994). Another pharmacokinetic evaluation of GO by Korth-Bradley and colleagues (2001) compared the kinetic parameters of GO in different populations. Although a great deal of interpatient variability was observed, the authors concluded that there were no significant differences in $C_{max}$, time to $C_{max}$, AUC, clearance, or $V_d$ between males and females, nor were there any significant differences between those over 60 and those under 60 years of age. Clearance of GO from the plasma occurs mainly through uptake by CD33-positive cells and subsequent internalization, and is therefore influenced by antigen concentration. Elimination half-life of the drug is fairly long, and increases upon second exposure. Median half-life of the antibody component is 72.4 hr after the first dose and 93.7 hr after the second, while the median half-life of the calicheamicin component is 45.1 hr after the first dose and 61.1 hr after the second (Cersosimo, 2003b). Accumulation between doses was not found to be significant, as evidenced by concentrations equivalent to 1% of $C_{max}$ measured just prior to the second dose (Dowell et al., 2001b).

## Indications and Clinical Efficacy

Results of a phase I study evaluating dose range, pharmacokinetics, and safety of GO in adults with CD33-positive relapsed AML showed that two doses of 9 mg/m$^2$ resulted in >75% saturation of CD33 antigen on peripheral blood mononuclear cells (Nabhan and Tallman, 2002). Subsequently, a series of three phase II trials utilizing the 9 mg/m$^2$ dose were conducted to evaluate the efficacy of the compound. Initially, 142 patients with untreated, relapsed AML were enrolled. The data were compiled and published in one report (Sievers et al., 2001). The FDA granted approval of GO based on this analysis, but stated that approval was contingent upon ongoing studies to further clarify the role of GO in recurrent AML (Bross et al., 2001; Cersosimo, 2003b). Three years later, a final report summarizing the results of these studies was published by Larson and colleagues. This study corroborated the findings of the initial data summary (Larson et al., 2005). In total, 277 patients were evaluated. Seventy-one patients (26%) achieved CR, with 35 (13%) fully recovering platelets and 36 (13%) achieving CRp (CR without full platelet recovery >100,000/L). Median relapse-free survival was 5.2 months for all patients (6.4 months for patients in CR); overall survival was 4.9 months (12.6 months for patients achieving remission). Toxicities consisting of fever, rigors, hypotension, and other infusion-related events were common (grade 3 or 4 infusion reactions occurred in 34% of patients after the first dose, but only 12% after the second dose). Other significant grades 3 and 4 adverse

events were similar to previous reports, and included thrombocytopenia (99%), neutropenia (97%), and infections (25%) (McGavin and Spencer, 2001; Cersosimo, 2003b). The most clinically significant adverse event noted by investigators was hepatotoxicity, which typically manifested as hyperbilirubinemia (29% grade 3 or 4) and liver enzyme elevations (18% and 9% for AST and ALT, respectively). These generally appeared within a few days of exposure and were reversible without medical intervention. However, 16 episodes of veno-occlusive disease of the liver (VOD) were reported from 299 administered courses (5%). Other phase II trials have shown similar results (Table 3).

GO has been evaluated in combination with other chemotherapeutic agents (Table 3). Various investigators have explored the utility of GO at different doses and with different agents, including cytarabine, daunorubicin, topotecan, idarubicin, cyclosporine, and fludarabine (Cortes et al., 2002; Estey et al., 2002a,b; Tsimberidou et al., 2003; Piccaluga et al., 2004b). One study utilized the combination of GO with fludarabine, cytarabine, and cyclosporine for treatment of patients with relapsed or refractory AML. The response rate of 30% (CR 28%, CRp 6%) was superior to the typical response rates seen with other regimens in refractory AML (17–20%) (Tsimberidou et al., 2003; Tsimberidou et al., 2005). However, hyperbilirubinemia was reported in 44% of patients, and 9% developed VOD (Bearman, 2000; Tsimberidou et al., 2005). While some combination regimens have shown high response rates, toxicity has remained a significant concern. The exact role of GO in combination with other chemotherapeutic agents requires further investigation.

Significant activity has been demonstrated with the use of GO in the treatment of acute promyelocytic leukemia (APL) (Estey et al., 2002a; Lo-Coco et al., 2004). Cells isolated from APL patients frequently express CD33, and are therefore an effective target for GO (Tsimberidou et al., 2005). A study by Lo-Coco and colleagues (2004) evaluated GO as single-agent therapy in patients with advanced stages of APL, and found that after two doses were administered, 91% patients attained a molecular remission (MR); after three doses were administered, essentially 100% of 13 patients achieved MR. Only 1 patient (6%) developed clinically significant hepatotoxicity (grade 3), and this patient had received stem cell transplantation and had chronic GvHD during therapy (Lo-Coco et al., 2004). Combination therapy for APL has also been studied; Estey and colleagues (2002a) administered GO with tretinoin in newly diagnosed APL patients, and found a response rate of 84%. Therapy was relatively well tolerated, and no patients developed VOD. The authors concluded that GO appears to

| Investigators | Diseases, no. of patients | Mono- vs. combi therapy | Regimen | CR + CRp | Median survival (all patients) | Median survival (CR +CRp patients) | Significant adverse effects (grade 3/4) |
|---|---|---|---|---|---|---|---|
| Larson et al. (2002) | AML in first relapse, $n = 101$ | Mono | GO 9 mg/m$^2$ q14d × 2 doses | 13% + 15% = **28%** | 5.4 months | 14.5 months + 11.8 months | Hematologic 99% Hyperbilirubinemia 24% Transaminase elevation 15% |
| Roboz et al. (2002) | Refractory or relapsed AML; new AML with poor cytogenetics, CML blast crisis, $n = 43$ | Mono | GO 9 mg/m$^2$ q14d × 2 doses | 9% + 5% = **14%** | NA | NA; Average response duration = 4.2 months | Hematologic 95% Infection 84% Hepatic 21% Bleeding 12% |
| Piccaluga et al. (2004a) | AML patients unable to receive standard chemotherapy, $n = 24$ | Mono | GO 6 or 9 mg/m$^2$ q14d × 2–3 doses | 13% + 8% = **21%** | 2 months | 6 months | Hematologic 100% Hyperbilirubinemia 4% Transaminase elevation 4% Bleeding 25% |
| Lo-Coco et al. (2004) | Molecularly relapsed APL, $n = 16$ | Mono | GO 6 mg/m$^2$ q14d × 2–3 doses | MR 91% | MR duration 3–31 months | NA | Hematologic 100% Hepatic 6% |
| Nabhan et al. (2005) | Previously untreated AML patients >65 years old, $n = 12$ | Mono | Induction: GO 9 mg/m$^2$ q14d × 2 doses Consolidation: GO 6 mg/m$^2$ × 1 dose Maintenance: GO 3 mg/m$^2$ q4wk × 4 doses | CR 27% | NA | 7.6 months | Hematologic 100% Hepatic 0% Cardiac 25% Pulmonary 25% Hypotension 25% |
| Larson et al. (2005) | AML in first relapse, $n = 277$ | Mono | GO 9 mg/m$^2$ q14d × 2 doses | 13% + 13% = **26%** | 4.9 months | 5.2 months | Infusion reactions 30% Neutropenia 98% Thrombocytopenia 99% Bleeding 13% Hyperbilirubinemia 29% VOD 5% |

| Study | Patient population | Mono/Combi | Regimen | Response | | | Toxicities |
|---|---|---|---|---|---|---|---|
| Amadori et al. (2005) | AML patients unable to receive standard chemotherapy, n = 40 | Mono | GO 9 mg/m² q14d × 2 doses | 10% + 7% = **17%** | 4.3 months | 11.4 months (pts 61–75 years old); 1.0 month (pts >75 years old) | Infusion reactions 12% / Cardiac 7% / Elevated bilirubin/transaminases 10% / Febrile neutropenia 52% |
| Cortes et al. (2002) | Refractory AML, n = 27 | Combi | GO 9 mg/m² d1, cytarabine 1 g/m² days 1–5, topotecan 1.25 mg/m²CIV days 1–5 | **12%** | 8.2 weeks | N/A; 1 of 2 pts in CR still alive at 50 weeks follow-up | Hematologic 100% / Hepatic 29% / Nausea/vomiting 18% |
| Tsimberidou et al. (2003) | Primary resistant or relapsed AML, n = 32 | Combi | GO 4.5 mg/m² IV day 1; fludarabine 15 mg/m² q12h × 10 doses days 2–6; cytarabine 0.5 g/m² q12h × 10 doses days 2–6; cyclosporine 6 mg/kg IV × 1, then 16 mg/kg CIV days 1 and 2 | 28% + 6% = **34%** | 5.3 months | 9 months | Hematologic 100% / Hyperbilirubinemia 44% / VOD 9% / Nausea/vomiting 12% |
| Piccaluga et al. (2004b) | Primary or refractory AML, n = 9 | Combi | GO 6 mg/m² day 1, 4 mg/m² day 8 + cytarabine 100 mg/m²CIV days 1–7 | **55%** | 6 months | Not yet reached, 3 pts still alive at time of publication | Hematologic 100% / Bleeding 44% / Neutropenic fever 33% / Hepatic 22% |
| Estey et al. (2002a) | Primary APL, n = 19 | Combi | GO 9 mg/m² day 1 or day 5[a] + ATRA 45 mg/m²/day until CR + idarubicin 12 mg/m²/day × 3 days[b] | **84%** | Not yet reached; 12 of 19 pts are PCR (−) at 12 months | Not yet reached; 12 of 19 pts are PCR (−) at 12 months | Bleeding 10% / Multiorgan failure 5% |

[a] GO was administered day 1 if admission WBC >10,000/μL; day 5 if WBC <10,000/μL.
[b] Only 3 patients who presented with WBC >30,000/μL received idarubicin. *Abbreviations:* ATO, arsenic trioxide 0.15 mg/kg/day; ATRA, tretinoin 45 mg/m²/day; CR, complete response; CRp, complete response except for platelet recovery >100,000/μL; MR, molecular remission; PCR, polymerase chain reaction; GO, gemtuzumzb ozogamicin.

**Table 3** ■ Selected clinical trials with gemtuzumab.

demonstrate activity in and be feasible for the treatment of APL.

## Safety Concerns

GO is associated with a variety of adverse effects, the most common of which are infusion-related reactions, hepatotoxicity, and myelosuppression (Giles et al., 2003). Myelosuppression is profound and prolonged, occurring in 99–100% of patients; counts typically nadir at 7–14 days and recover within 28–35 days (Giles et al., 2003). In some cases, recovery may take even longer, and platelets may never return to normal values. Infusion-related events, including fever, rigors, hypotension, dyspnea, nausea, emesis, and headache are common as well; however, these are typically mild in severity, and risk decreases after initial exposure (Larson et al., 2005; Tsimberidou et al., 2005). Premedication with corticosteroids and diphenhydramine may reduce this complication. Hepatotoxicity associated with GO therapy is another recognized adverse effect. Hyperbilirubinemia and transaminase elevations are often mild and reversible without medication, occurring within 8 days of drug exposure and lasting approximately 20 days (Giles et al., 2003). However, a more concerning manifestation of hepatotoxicity is VOD. This seems to be more common when GO is used in combination with other chemotherapeutic agents, or after SCT (Giles et al., 2003). When GO is utilized in the approved single-agent manner, VOD incidence is approximately 1–5%. However, when GO is used in combination therapy, VOD risk increases to 5–12%. Age, gender, underlying disease, preexisting renal or hepatic function, alcoholism and hepatitis history do not predict which patients will develop VOD (Giles et al., 2003). It has been postulated that premedication with acetaminophen could increase the risk of VOD; interference with glutathione oxidation-reduction reactions by acetaminophen could leave sinusoidal endothelial cells susceptible to attack by calicheamicin-generated free radicals, thus increasing the risk of toxicity. Until the exact mechanism of VOD is elucidated, some clinicians advocate the avoidance of premedication with acetaminophen prior to GO treatment (Gordon, 2001; Cersosimo, 2003b). VOD remains a significant concern with GO therapy, and more data are needed to determine the risks and benefits of treatment with this agent.

## Pharmaceutical Considerations: Formulation, Other Routes of Administration, Dosing Regimens

GO is indicated for the treatment of CD33-positive AML in first relapse for patients ≥ 60 years of age who are not candidates for other chemotherapy. The recommended dose is 9 mg/m$^2$ IV over 2 hr repeated after 14 days for a total of two doses (Wyeth, 2006).

GO is commercially formulated as a lyophilized powder for injection in 5 mg amber vials. The contents of each vial should be stored under refrigeration (2°C to 8°C) and protected from light. After reconstitution with 5 mL sterile water for injection, the appropriate amount of drug should be drawn up and further diluted with 100 mL of sterile 0.9% sodium chloride for injection. This product should be protected from light with the addition of a UV-protectant bag. Infusions should be administered over 2 hr through an intravenous line that is equipped with a low-protein-binding 1.2 μm terminal filter. This medication can be infused peripherally or centrally. Patients should also receive appropriate premedication with diphenhydramine prior to receiving GO (Wyeth, 2006).

## ■ Rituximab, Yttrium-90 ($^{90}$Y) Ibritumomab Tiuxetan, Iodine-131 ($^{131}$I) Tositumomab

### Pharmacology and Mechanism of Action

Rituximab (Rituxan®) was approved for use in 1997 and was the first MAb approved for the treatment of cancer. It is a chimeric MAb that binds to the antigen CD20 (cluster of differentiation 20), which is found on B-lymphocytes (B-cells). Rituximab is approved in the United States for the following indications: treatment of relapsed or refractory, B-cell CD20-positive, low grade or follicular NHL; first-line treatment of follicular or diffuse large B-cell (DLBCL) CD20-positive NHL in combination with chemotherapy; treatment of low grade, CD20-positive B-cell NHL in patients achieving a response or stable disease to first-line chemotherapy; and, in combination with methotrexate for the treatment of moderate to severe rheumatoid arthritis (Genentech, 2006c). This last indication speaks to the many present and future nononcology uses of this MAb. However, the non-oncology uses will not be discussed here.

The antigen CD20 is found on all normal B-cells and most malignant B-cells (Maloney et al., 1994). CD20 is the human B-lymphocyte-restricted differentiation antigen, Bp35, and is a hydrophobic transmembrane protein (ASHP, 2002). CD20 is involved with cell cycle initiation regulation and differentiation by activation of B-cells from the GO (resting) phase to the G1 (gap 1) phase, and CD20 has also been shown to operate as a calcium ion channel (Golay et al., 1985; Maloney et al., 1994; Kanzaki et al., 1997; Maloney et al., 1997a; Genentech, 2006c). Rituximab is thought to mediate death of CD20 positive tumor cells through several mechanisms, as shown in Figure 2. Specifically, antibody-dependent cell-mediated cytotoxicity, direct effects via CD20 ligation, and complement-mediated lysis are all believed to play a role (Maloney et al., 1997b; Genentech, 2006c).

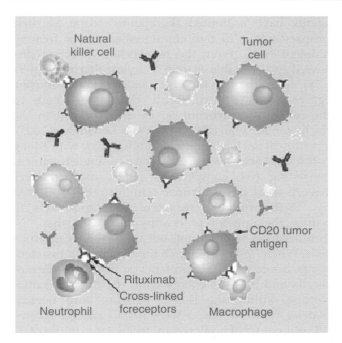

**Figure 2** ■ Rituximab mechanism of action. *Source*: From Point Therapeutics.

## Pharmacokinetics/Pharmacodynamics

The pharmacokinetics of rituximab were studied in patients with NHL. They were given a dose of $375 \, mg/m^2$ IV weekly for 4 weeks. The mean serum half-life increased throughout the study (76.3 hr after the first week to 205.8 hr after the fourth week). This increase is thought to occur secondary to depletion of the CD20 antigen. Without an antigen to bind to, rituximab's clearance will be reduced. After 4 weeks of treatment, rituximab may be detectable in a patient's serum for up to six months.

After 8 weeks of weekly rituximab infusions using the same dose, the mean maximum concentration was found to increase from 243 µg/mL after the first infusion to 550 µg/mL after the eighth infusion (Genentech, 2006c).

As mentioned above, depletion of B-cells, via the CD20 antigen, can be extensive and prolonged. In one study of 166 patients, B-cells were depleted within the first three doses of rituximab and the depletion was maintained throughout 6 to 9 months in the majority of patients. B-cell levels should return to normal levels by twelve months after the last dose of rituximab (Genentech, 2006c).

When B-cells become activated, they turn into plasma cells and secrete immune globulins. Therefore, depletion of immune globulins has also been examined. Statistically significant reductions in IgG, IgM, and IgA have been observed. However, in the majority of cases, the levels remain in the normal range (Genentech, 2006c).

## Indications and Clinical Efficacy

Rituximab has been studied as a single agent in many trials of low-, intermediate-, and high-grade lymphomas. A review of low-grade lymphoma studies using single agent rituximab shows the ranges of OR rate, which is the CR rate plus the PR rate, and CR to be 27–73% and 0–23%, respectively (Cersosimo, 2003a). A review of intermediate- and high-grade lymphomas using single agent rituximab show the ranges of OR and CR to be 14–73% and 0–44%, respectively (Cersosimo, 2003a).

Perhaps the most studied chemotherapy used in combination with rituximab is the CHOP regimen of cyclophosphamide, doxorubicin, vincristine, and prednisone. CHOP had been considered the gold standard for treatment of DLBCL until the combination trials became published in the late 1990s and early 2000s. A major study released in 2002 compared the addition of rituximab to CHOP versus CHOP alone in elderly patients with DLBCL (Coiffier et al., 2002). It demonstrated the combination provided statistically significant increases in CR, event-free survival, and overall survival, without increasing treatment-related toxicity. A review of rituximab in combination with chemotherapy regimens (mostly CHOP or CHOP-related regimens) show the ranges of OR and CR to be 29–100% and 11–85%, respectively (Cersosimo, 2003a).

Rituximab is also used in conjunction with a MAb designed with a conjugated radionuclide. This radioimmunotherapy allows radiation to be delivered directly to the tumor site and limits the radiation exposure and adverse effects to healthy tissues. Yttrium-90 ($^{90}$Y) ibritumomab tiuxetan (Zevalin®) was the first radioimmunoconjugated MAb approved by the FDA for treatment of relapsed or refractory follicular, low-grade, or transformed NHL. Rituximab is used in the $^{90}$Y ibritumomab tiuxetan therapeutic regimen to clear the peripheral blood of CD20 found on normal B-cells. This facilitates better binding of the $^{90}$Y ibritumomab tiuxetan to the CD20 antigen located on the tumor cells. Another radioimmunoconjugated MAb, iodine-131 ($^{131}$I) tositumomab (Bexxar®), utilizes a similar therapeutic regimen, however, tositumomab is used to clear the peripheral blood of CD20 instead of rituximab.

To date, there have been no head-to-head trials comparing these two radioimmunotherapies. However, $^{90}$Y-ibritumomab tiuxetan was compared to rituximab in a randomized controlled, phase III trial for rituximab-naïve patients with relapsed or refractory low-grade, follicular, or transformed B-cell NHL (Witzig et al., 2002). $^{90}$Y-ibritumomab tiuxetan was shown to produce a statistically significant increase in CR (30% vs. 16%) and OR (80% vs. 56%, $p = .002$). In spite of this, the study did not demonstrate a difference in time to progression.

## Safety Concerns

Adverse effects of MAbs can generally be determined by examining their international nonproprietary names (INN) and becoming familiar with their mechanisms of action. Because rituximab is a chimeric MAb and contains mouse protein, infusion-related events would be expected. In fact, infusion-related reactions, such as fever, chills, and myalgias, along with hypersensitivity reactions, such as bronchospasm, hypotension, and angioedema, have occurred during rituximab infusions. Patients are more likely to experience these reactions when receiving their first infusion of rituximab. The incidence decreases with subsequent infusions. Premedication with diphenhydramine and acetaminophen are recommended for all infusions.

Rituximab's package labeling contains a black box warning regarding three reactions: fatal infusion reactions, tumor lysis syndrome (TLS), and severe mucocutaneous reactions. The majority of fatal infusion reactions occur in relation to the first infusion. At any time an infusion reaction is expected, the rituximab infusion should be discontinued immediately. TLS has been reported to occur in patients with NHL who have received concomitant cisplatin and have had a high tumor burden. It may result in acute renal failure or death. Severe mucocutaneous reactions, such as Stevens-Johnson syndrome and toxic epidermal necrolysis have occurred within 1 to 13 weeks after receiving rituximab. Patients who experience a severe mucocutaneous reaction should not receive rituximab in the future (Genentech, 2006c).

## Pharmaceutical Considerations: Formulation, Other Routes of Administration, Dosing Regimens

Administration of rituximab should only be by IV infusion. The first infusion should be started at 50 mg/hr and titrated up to a maximum of 400 mg/hr through increasing increments of 50 mg/hr every 30 min. If the patient tolerated the first infusion, subsequent infusions may be titrated faster. It is recommended to start subsequent infusions at 100 mg/hr, increase by 100 mg/hr every 30 min (if tolerated), up to a maximum of 400 mg/hr (Genentech, 2006c).

## Radioimmunotherapy

Due to the limited scope of this chapter, the two conjugated MAbs, Yttrium-90 ($^{90}$Y) ibritumomab tiuxetan and iodine-131 ($^{131}$I) tositumomab, have only briefly been mentioned in the context of clinical efficacy section involving rituximab therapy. These agents have a limited therapeutic scope as their primary use is in radioimmunotherapy for treating indolent NHL. From the nomenclature section discussed earlier in this chapter, it is clear that Yttrium-90 ($^{90}$Y) ibritumomab tiuxetan comprises the murine IgG$_1$ MAb ibritumomab that is linked to the radioisotope yttrium-90 by stable chelation via the linker, tiuxetan (Hagenbeek and Lewington, 2005). Ytrrium-90 is a beta-emitter of high energy with a long half-life (64 hr). The drug is given as a single treatment consisting two components given approximately 1 week apart (i.e., rituximab administration followed by $^{90}$Y-ibritumomab tiuxetan. Rituximab acts to reduce the number of healthy B-cells so that $^{90}$Y-ibritumomab tiuxetan will not destroy noncancerous cells. When $^{90}$Y-ibritumomab tiuxetan is administered, it attaches to the CD20 proteins on the cell surface of B-cells and releases energy from the ytrrium radioisotope, killing the B-cell. Patients with normal platelet function (i.e., $>150 \times 10^9$/L) should receive 0.4 mCi per kg of body weight up to a maximum of 32 mCi. Those with a platelet count between 100 and $149 \times 10^9$/L should receive a reduced dose of 0.3 mCi/kg, which has been shown to have equal efficacy to higher doses (Hagenbeek and Lewington, 2005). The main safety concerns include myelosuppression with nadirs reached in 4–8 weeks after administration of therapy.

Iodine-131 tositumomab is another conjugated MAb that acts in a similar mechanism to $^{90}$Y-ibritumomab tiuxetan although it emits both beta and gamma radiation. Specifically, it binds to the CD20 antigen found on B-cells to kill them via two mechanisms; 1) activating an immune host response to B-cells and 2) causing apoptosis in B-cells to which it is bound as shown in Figure 3 (Biodrugs, 2003; GlaxoSmithKline, 2006).

## CLASSES OF MONOCLONAL ANTIBODIES: VASCULAR ENDOTHELIAL GROWTH FACTOR INHIBITORS

Angiogenesis inhibitors have been in clinical development for decades, based on the theory by Folkman that the development of new blood vessels (i.e., angiogenesis) must occur for tumor growth beyond 1–2 mm$^3$(Folkman, 1971, 1995; Miller, 2002). As tumors enlarge, the centers become hypoxic and stimulate angiogenic growth factors, as shown in Figure 4. VEGF is thought to be one of the most potent growth factors and has been shown to induce neovascularization for malignant cells in an autocrine fashion (Gordon et al., 2001). High levels of VEGF have also been correlated with poor prognosis, disease recurrence, and metastases in a variety of neoplasms.

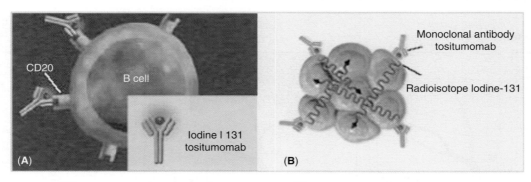

**Figure 3** ▪ Iodine-131 ($^{131}$I) tositumomab mechanism of action. (**A**) $^{131}$I-tositumomab binds to the CD20 antigen on normal and malignant B lymphocytes. (**B**) "Cross-fire" effect of Iodine-131 in $^{131}$I-tositumomab will cause damage to tumor cells as well as adjacent normal tissue. *Source*: From GlaxoSmithKline.

## ▪ Bevacizumab

### Pharmacology and Mechanism of Action

Bevacizumab (Avastin®) is currently the only FDA approved VEGF inhibitor available. It is a humanized MAb that consists of a normal human IgG$_1$ (93%) and the VEGF binding residues from a murine neutralizing antibody (7%) (Gordon et al., 2001; Yang et al., 2003). Bevacizumab is produced in a system containing Chinese hamster ovary mammalian cell expression and a gentamicin-containing nutrient medium (Genentech, 2006a).

In vivo and in vitro studies have shown that bevacizumab inhibits the biologic activities of VEGF and does not allow any VEGF isoforms to bind to its receptors (Margolin et al., 2001). This halts tumor growth, as shown in Figure 4. Preclinical trials in animal models have demonstrated the suppression and stabilization of multiple tumor lines through bevacizumab administration.

Bevacizumab has demonstrated both cytostatic and cytotoxic effects in clinical trials (Cobleigh et al., 2003). Specifically, objective responses, a reduction in tumor growth, an increase in time to tumor progression, and an increase in overall survival have been documented in various solid tumor states (Yang et al., 2002, 2003; Kabbinavar et al., 2003).

### Pharmacokinetics/Pharmacodynamics

After a single dose of bevacizumab (0.1–10 mg/kg), the maximum concentration ($C_{max}$) ranges from 2.80 to 284 μg/mL, showing a dose-response increase (Gordon et al., 2001). AUC values range from 31 to 87 μg/mL for a 0.3 mg/kg dose up to 2,480–6,010 μg/mL for a 10 mg/kg dose (Gordon et al., 2001). Multidosing studies have demonstrated an accumulation ratio of 2.8 when 10 mg/kg of bevacizumab is administered every 14 days (Gordon et al., 2001). Steady state concentrations are reached in approximately 100 days (Genentech, 2006a).

Bevacizumab demonstrates linear kinetics over a dosing range of 3–10 mg/kg, a limited volume of distribution, and a low clearance (Gordon et al., 2001). The volume of distribution is 45.7 mL/kg or 3260 mL (Gaudreault, 2001) with a serum half-life of approximately 13–21 days (Gordon et al., 2001; Margolin et al., 2001). Clearance appears to vary based on gender, tumor burden, body weight, and albumin levels (Gaudreault, 2001; Genentech, 2006a). Males have a higher clearance (CL) and larger volume of distribution ($V_d$) compared to females (CL: 0.262 L/day vs. 0.207 L/day, $V_d$: 3.25 L vs. 2.66 L, respectively) after body weight adjustments (Genentech, 2006a). Patients with higher tumor burdens have a higher clearance compared to those with lower burdens (CL: 0.249 L/day vs. 0.199 L/day) (Genentech, 2006a). Additionally, a 30% change in body weight results in an 18% change in clearance (Hsei et al., 2002). Finally, reduced albumin levels increase bevacizumab clearance (Gaudreault, 2001). Despite the differences seen in gender, tumor burden, weight and albumin levels, no significant differences are seen in response rate or toxic effects and no dosing modifications are needed.

Many malignant cell lines have been shown to produce VEGF (Gordon et al., 2001). High levels of free VEGF correlate with a poor prognosis and an increased risk of metastatic disease. Most laboratory assays measure total and free VEGF serum concentrations. An increase in the concentration of total VEGF serum concentration is observed during bevacizumab treatment (Gordon et al., 2001; Margolin et al., 2001; Yang et al., 2003). This may be due to decreased clearance of VEGF-bound inactive bevacizumab, as this laboratory assessment does not distinguish between free and bound VEGF. At single doses greater than 0.3 mg/kg, phase I studies demonstrated complete suppression of free serum VEGF that remained undetectable throughout the study (Gordon et al., 2001; Margolin et al., 2001). More recent investigations suggest that plasma VEGF levels

Normal tumor growth

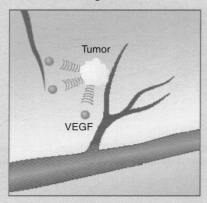
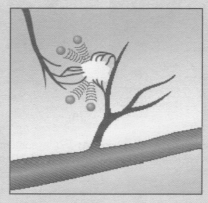
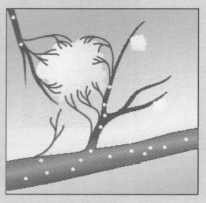

**(A)** When a growing tumor reaches a critical size (.5–2mm), it can no longer supply itself with nutrients and oxygen from nearby small blood vessels, In response, the tumor secretes proteins called vascular endothelial growth factor (VEGF) that attach to nearby blood vessels and stimulate growth towards the tumor allowing it to thrive.

Possible anti-VEGF mechanism of action

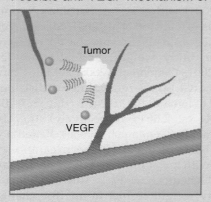
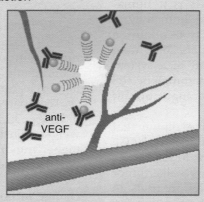
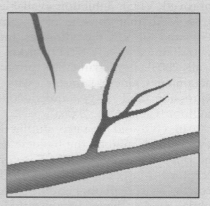

**(B)** Anti-VEGF, a monoclonal antibody specific for VEGF, blocks the signals from the tumor that prompt blood vessel growth. without nutrients and oxygen, the tumor stops growing.

**Figure 4** ■ Mechanism of action of vascular endothelial growth factor (VEGF) **(A)** and theorized mechanism of action of VEGF inhibitors **(B)**. *Source*: From the American Journal of Health-System Pharmacy and GlaxoSmithKline.

are more accurate to assess of circulating VEGF, but are not as widely available (Hsei et al., 2002).

Currently, there is no clear association between the dose of bevacizumab, disease stability, or toxicity. However, a phase I trial did note that bevacizumab patients with stable disease had slightly elevated baseline VEGF levels compared to bevacizumab patients demonstrating progressive disease (Gordon et al., 2001). The authors hypothesized that elevated baseline VEGF levels may indicate patients that may be better candidates for bevacizumab therapy.

### Indications and Clinical Efficacy
Bevacizumab is currently approved by the FDA for the first or second-line treatment of patients with metastatic carcinoma of the colon and rectum (in combination with intravenous 5-fluorouracil-based chemotherapy) and for the first-line treatment of locally advanced, recurrent, or metastatic nonsmall cell lung cancer (NSCLC) in combination with carboplatin and paclitaxel (Genentech, 2006a).

Bevacizumab, as an additive to standard chemotherapy, appears to significantly prolong overall survival in metastatic colorectal patients. Two multicentered, randomized phase III trials provided the bulk of efficacy and safety evidence leading to FDA's approval of bevacizumab as part of first- and second-line chemotherapy in metastatic colorectal cancer (CRC) patients. The first trial randomized 925 previously untreated patients to one of three arms: (*i*) irinotecan, 5 fluorouracil (5-FU), leucovorin (LV) (Saltz regimen), (*ii*) Saltz plus bevacizumab, or (*iii*) 5-FU, LV plus bevacizumab (Hurwitz et al., 2003). The Saltz plus bevacizumab arm demonstrated statistically significant advantages compared to the Saltz regimen alone in overall survival (20.3 vs. 15.6 months), progression-free survival (10.6 vs. 6.24 months), OR (45% vs. 35%), and duration of response (10.4 vs. 7.1 months) (Dearden et al., 2001). Grade 3/4 toxicities were similar between each arm. The second phase III trial, E3200, investigated oxaliplatin, 5-FU, LV (FOLFOX4) versus FOLFOX4 plus bevacizumab versus bevacizumab alone in 757 pretreated metastatic colorectal patients (Benson et al., 2003). Overall survival, time to progression, and OR all significantly favored bevacizumab plus FOLFOX4 vs. FOLFOX alone. Bevacizumab monotherapy was not effective in this patient population.

Bevacizumab has also shown promising results with combination chemotherapy in patients with advanced NSCLC. The addition of bevacizumab to paclitaxel plus carboplatin in the first-line treatment of advanced NSCLC significantly prolonged overall survival by >2 months in over 878 patients randomized to receive triplet therapy versus the paclitaxel and carboplatin combination (12.3 vs. 10.3 months, respectively) (Genentech, 2006a). However, it must be noted that patients with central tumors with a squamous histology were excluded as phase II data showed that these patients were more likely to develop hemoptysis (Devore et al., 2000; Kabbinavar et al., 2001; Novotny et al., 2001). Post hoc analyses did show that bevacizumab therapy was less effective in women, patients older than 65 years of age, and those with greater than 5% weight loss from the study's start (Genentech, 2006a).

Since angiogenesis is an important step in the proliferation of breast cancer cells (Cobleigh et al., 2003), bevacizumab has been investigated in two large scale phase III trials in women with breast cancer (Miller et al., 2002; Hillan et al., 2003; Miller, 2003). The first trial compared capecitabine monotherapy to capecitabine plus bevacizumab in 462 metastatic breast cancer patients. No statistically significant difference was found for the primary endpoint; time to disease progression (4.17 months for the control vs. 4.86 months for bevacizumab arm; hazards ratio: 0.98). However, the OR rate, a secondary endpoint, was favorable for the bevacizumab arm (19.8% vs. 9.1%). The second phase III trial is still ongoing and is investigating bevacizumab in locally recurrent breast cancer patients (Miller, 2003), as it is theorized that antiangiogenic therapy in less advanced patients may halt the spread of metastatic disease. A total of 722 locally recurrent or metastatic patients were randomized to receive paclitaxel alone or in combination with bevacizumab. Interim results show that a significant 5-month extension in time to progression is offered by the combination (11 months) compared to paclitaxel alone (6 months) (Lyseng-Williamson and Robinson, 2006).

## Safety Concerns

The most common adverse events in all clinical trials have been headache, nausea, vomiting, anorexia, stomatitis, constipation, upper respiratory infection, epistaxis, dyspnea, and proteinuria (Genentech, 2006a). No patients have developed antibodies to bevacizumab during clinical trials (Gordon et al., 2001).

The most serious adverse events associated with bevacizumab treatment include hypertensive crises, nephrotic syndrome, hemorrhage, gastrointestinal perforations, wound healing complications, and congestive heart failure (Genentech, 2006a).

The development of hypertension is hypothesized to occur through a decreased production of nitric oxide (NO) through VEGF receptor blockade (Cobleigh et al., 2003). The manufacturer recommends that patients treated with bevacizumab should have their blood pressure monitored every 2 to 3 weeks during treatment. During clinical trials, treatment of bevacizumab-associated hypertension included diurectics, calcium channel blockers, beta blockers, and angiotensin-converting enzyme inhibitors. Bevacizumab should be discontinued if patients develop hypertensive crises (Genentech, 2006a).

Proteinuria was an early concern in phase I and II trials, although it has not been associated with renal impairment. The manufacturer recommends monitoring for the development or worsening of proteinuria through serial urinalyses (Genentech, 2006a). Patients with a urine dipstick reading of 2 + or greater should be further evaluated. Nephrotic syndrome has been reported in 5/1032 (0.5%) bevacizumab patients (Genentech, 2006a). Bevacizumab should be discontinued in patients with nephrotic syndrome.

One area of concern with antiangiogenesis inhibitors is vascular dysfunction, as VEGF regulates vascular proliferation and permeability (Kilickap et al., 2003). The package insert contains a boxed warning regarding the risk of wound healing complications, hemorrhage, and gastrointestinal perforations (Genentech, 2006a). Bevacizumab has shown varying adverse effects on the vasculature including bleeding, thrombotic events, wound healing complications, and gastrointestinal perforations. Bevacizumab therapy should not be initiated within 28 days of major surgery and should be stopped prior to elective surgery. It is unknown how soon before elective surgery that therapy should be halted, but the manufacturer recommends that clinicians take into consideration the long half-life (i.e., 20 days) of bevacizumab (Genentech, 2006a).

A phase II trial comparing carboplatin, paclitaxel (CP) plus bevacizumab to CP alone in 99 Stage IIIb/IV

NSCLC patients uncovered life-threatening hemoptysis in 6 patients receiving bevacizumab (DeVore et al., 2000). This was fatal in four patients. A subset analysis identified squamous cell histology and central, cavitary, or necrotic tumors as risk factors (Novotny et al., 2001). To prevent further cases, patients with a previous history of hemoptysis should not receive bevacizumab (Gray et al., 2003; Sparano et al., 2004).

### Pharmaceutical Considerations: Formulation, Other Routes of Administration, Dosing Regimens

Bevacizumab should be administered as an IV infusion given after the completion of chemotherapy (Genentech, 2006a). After the infusion, the line should be flushed with 0.9% sodium chloride equal to the amount present in the intravenous tubing.

The initial dose should be given over 90 min. No premedications are required. If this is tolerated, the next infusion may be given over 60 min. Subsequent infusions may then be infused over 30 min. Less than 3% of patients had infusion reactions with initial bevacizumab regimens (Genentech, 2006a). Some institutions are now administering bevacizumab in a shorter amount of time based on lack of infusion reactions. Specifically, Memorial Sloan Kettering Cancer Center administers a 5 mg/kg dosage over 10 min, a 10 mg/kg dose over 20 min, and 15 mg/kg over 30 min (Saltz et al., 2006).

Preparation of bevacizumab includes withdrawing the necessary amount of bevacizumab for a 5 mg/kg dose and diluting it with 0.9% sodium chloride for injection for a total volume of 100 mL (Genentech, 2006a). Vials should be discarded within 8 hr after entry. Dextrose solutions should never be used as diluents or administered concomitantly. Both polyethylene and polyvinyl bags may be used for administration.

The FDA approved dosages are 5–10 mg/kg administered every 14 days for CRC and 15 mg/kg every 3 weeks for NSCLC (Genentech, 2006a).

## CLASSES OF MONOCLONAL ANTIBODIES: ENDOTHELIAL GROWTH FACTOR RECEPTOR (EGFR) INHIBITORS

EGFR or HER-1 and EGFR 2 or HER-2 are transmembrane glycoproteins constitutively expressed in many normal epithelial tissues including skin and hair follicle and are overexpressed in many cancers including the colon, rectum and breast. EGFR and HER-2 are members of the Erb family of receptors that play a role in normal cell growth and differentiation. HER-2 protein overexpression can occur in up to 30% of patients with metastatic breast cancer and is often associated with more aggressive disease, a faster

relapse time, and an overall poor prognosis (Folkman, 1971; Miller, 2002).

## ■ Trastuzumab

### Pharmacology and Mechanism of Action

Trastuzumab (Herceptin®) is a recombinant DNA-derived humanized MAb ($IgG_1$ kappa) that selectively binds to the extracellular domain of the human HER-2 receptor with high affinity. This receptor-antibody interaction, through a series of other cellular actions, induces autophosphorylation of the tyrosine kinase internal domain resulting in decreased tumorigenic potential and possibly reversal of chemoresistance as shown in Figure 5.

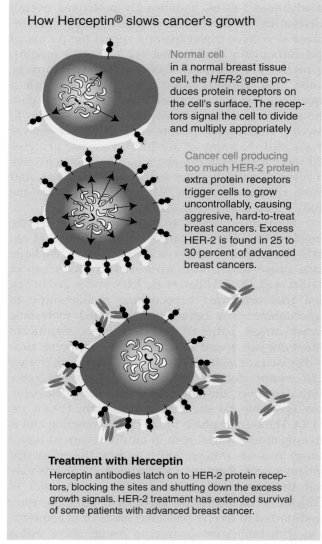

How Herceptin® slows cancer's growth

**Normal cell**
in a normal breast tissue cell, the *HER*-2 gene produces protein receptors on the cell's surface. The receptors signal the cell to divide and multiply appropriately

**Cancer cell producing too much HER-2 protein**
extra protein receptors trigger cells to grow uncontrollably, causing aggresive, hard-to-treat breast cancers. Excess HER-2 is found in 25 to 30 percent of advanced breast cancers.

**Treatment with Herceptin**
Herceptin antibodies latch on to HER-2 protein receptors, blocking the sites and shutting down the excess growth signals. HER-2 treatment has extended survival of some patients with advanced breast cancer.

**Figure 5** ■ Trastuzumab mechanism of action. *Source*: From the Dana-Farber Cancer Institute.

## Pharmacokinetics/Pharmacodynamics

Weekly administration of trastuzumab exhibits dose-dependent pharmacokinetics. When 10 and 500 mg doses (administered by short duration intravenous infusions) were studied in women with metastatic breast cancer the mean half-life increased and clearance decreased with the increased dose. The observed average half-life was 1.7 days for the 10 mg dose and 12 days for the 500 mg dose. However, in studies analyzing the commonly used regimen for trastuzumab of an initial loading dose of 4 mg/kg followed by a 2 mg/kg weekly maintenance dose, the mean half-life was 5.8 days. Studies also suggest that age and serum creatinine do not effect the disposition of trastuzumab. It is also important to note that when trastuzumab is administered in combination with paclitaxel, a 1.5-fold elevation in serum concentrations of trastuzumab is observed as compared to when trastuzumab is administered in combination with anthracycline and cyclophosphamide (AC).

## Indications and Clinical Efficacy

In both in vitro and in vivo studies trastuzumab was shown to inhibit the proliferation of human tumor cells that overexpress HER-2 (Hudziak et al., 1989; Baselga et al., 1998). Trastuzumab was approved by the FDA in September 1998 as a single agent for the treatment of patients having HER-2 overexpressing metastatic breast cancer and who had previously been treated with chemotherapy; in combination with paclitaxel in patients with HER-2 overexpressing metastatic breast cancer and had not received any prior chemotherapy (Genentech, 2006b). Trastuzumab has been found to have a 15% response rate in breast tumors overexpressing HER-2. However, this response rate increases to 25% when it is used in combination with chemotherapy.

The safety and efficacy of trastuzumab was determined in a multicenter, randomized, controlled clinical trial (H0648g) of 469 patients with HER2 overexpressing metastatic breast cancer who had not been treated for their metastatic disease (Slamon et al., 2001). Patients were randomized to receive either chemotherapy alone or chemotherapy plus trastuzumab. There were two chemotherapy subgroups. The first subgroup included patients who had previously been treated with an anthracycline in an adjuvant setting and thus received paclitaxel as chemotherapy in this study. The second subgroup included patients who had not received an anthracycline previously and received doxorubicin or epirubicin plus AC. Patients in the chemotherapy plus trastuzumab study arm had a significantly higher response rate, longer time to disease progression, a longer median duration of response, and a higher 1-year survival rate. Although

these results were observed in both chemotherapy subpopulations, the patients receiving paclitaxel plus trastuzumab had a greater effect than did patients receiving AC plus trastuzumab. In addition, a higher incidence of cardiac events occurred in the trastuzumab plus AC treatment group.

Another pivotal clinical trial (M77001) studied the combination of trastuzumab plus weekly or thrice weekly docetaxel in 188 patients who had no not been previously treated for their metastatic disease. After 24 months, a median overall survival of 31.2 months was observed for patients treated with trastuzumab plus docetaxel versus 22.7 months for patients treated with docetaxel alone (Marty et al., 2005). The outcome of these two trials has proven that trastuzumab plus a taxane is superior to a taxane alone and thus trastuzumab plus a taxane is now considered a standard of care for HER-2 positive metastatic breast cancer.

A multicenter, open-label, single arm clinical trial was conducted to assess the utility of trastuzumab as a single agent. This study enrolled 222 patients who had previously received one or more chemotherapy regimens for metastatic disease. Patients were treated with a trastuzumab loading dose of 4 mg/kg IV followed by 2 mg/kg IV weekly. A 14% response rate was observed (12% PR and 2% CR) in this study. As in the previous study, the degree of HER2 protein overexpression was a predictor of treatment response (Cobleigh et al., 1999). Preliminary results from other clinical trials looking at trastuzumab in combination with other chemotherapeutic agents include: trastuzumab plus vinorelbine shows data supporting a high response rate when used as first line therapy (84%) (Burstein et al., 2001); in combination with gemcitabine a response rate of 38% was observed (O'Shaughnessy et al., 2004); and in combination with capecitabine a response rate of up to 60% was observed (Schaller et al., 2005). All of these studies suggest that trastuzumab is as tolerable as in the pivotal trials.

## Safety Concerns

Trastuzumab has a black box warning for cardiomyopathy because of its potential to cause ventricular dysfunction and congestive heart failure. The severity and occurrence of cardiomyopathy was higher in patients who received anthracyclines and AC in combination with trastuzumab. Patients who require trastuzumab therapy must receive a full cardiac workup prior to the initiation of therapy and left ventricular function must be monitored during treatment. The most common adverse reaction is infusion reactions (usually mild to moderate), but rarely require discontinuation of therapy (Genentech,

2006b). Other adverse effects associated with trastuzumab are anemia and leukopenia, nausea/vomiting, diarrhea, and upper respiratory infections.

## Pharmaceutical Considerations: Formulation, Other Routes of Administration, Dosing Regimens

Trastuzumab is only available for IV administration. It is commercially available as a white to pale yellow, preservative-free, lyophilized powder containing 440 mg of trastuzumab packaged sterilely in a vial. The powder can be reconstituted with 20 mL of the supplied bacteriostatic water for injection. The recommended adult dosage is an initial loading dose of 4 mg/kg infused over 90 min followed by a weekly dose of 2 mg/kg infused over 90 min.

## ■ Cetuximab

### Pharmacology and Mechanism of Action

EGFR is an important marker in CRC because it is overexpressed in as much as 70% of CRC tumors and overexpression has been associated with decreased survival (Salomon et al., 1995). Cell signaling involving EGFR (or HER-2 as with trastuzumab) is associated with neoplastic cell proliferation, angiogenesis, and resistance to apoptosis, among other tumorigenic characteristics as shown in Figure 6 (Castillo et al., 2004). Typically, advanced CRC is treated with fluoropyrimidine, irinotecan, and

oxaliplatin, which have been shown to increase overall survival. However, once these drugs have been tried and are no longer effective, other treatment modalities including cetuximab have been found that can significantly prolong survival.

### Pharmacokinetics/Pharmacodynamics

Dose escalation studies have shown that cetuximab exhibits nonlinear pharmacokinetics. The area under the concentration time curve shows a much greater proportionate increase than would be expected when the dose was increased from 20 to 400 mg/m$^2$. In addition, the drug clearance decreased from 0.08 to 0.02 L/h/m$^2$ with 20 and 200 mg/m$^2$ doses. When doses greater than 200 mg/m$^2$ were analyzed the clearance appeared to plateau. It was also found that when males and females were compared, female patients had a 25% lower intrinsic cetuximab clearance. Steady-state levels were reached by week 3 of cetuximab infusions with a 114 hr mean half-life when the recommended regimen of 400 mg/m$^2$ (loading dose) followed by weekly 250 mg/m$^2$ was administered (Nolting et al., 2006).

### Indications and Clinical Efficacy

Cetuximab (Erbitux®) was approved by the FDA in February 2004 for chemoresistant CRC. However, several studies are ongoing to study the efficacy of cetuximab plus irinotecan or cetuximab plus an

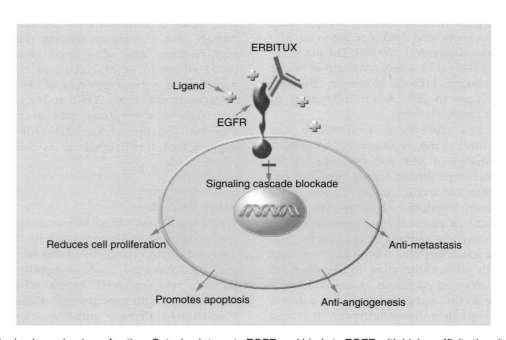

**Figure 6** ■ Cetuximab mechanism of action. Cetuximab targets EGFR and binds to EGFR with higher affinity than its natural ligands. Binding results in the internalization of the antibody receptor complex without activation of the intrinsic tyrosine kinase. Consequently, signal transduction through this cell pathway is blocked, which inhibits tumor growth and leads to apoptosis. Other mechanisms of action include the inhibition of the production of angiogenic factors and synergistic activity with both radiotherapy and chemotherapy. *Source*: From the Merck KGaA.

oxaliplatin-based chemotherapy regimen as first-line therapy. Cetuximab is a chimeric $IgG_1$ MAb composed of the Fv region of a murine anti-EGFR antibody with human IgG heavy and kappa light chain constant regions (Bristol Myers Squibb, 2006). This antibody binds specifically to the extracellular domain of the human EGFR with a high affinity resulting in inhibition of cell growth, induction of apoptosis, decreased matrix metalloproteinase, and VEGF production. Cetuximab is currently indicated for use in combination with irinotecan for EGFR expressing, metastatic CRC in patients refractory to irinotecan-based chemotherapy; and as a single agent in patients intolerable to irinotecan-based chemotherapy (Bristol Myers Squibb, 2006). As with trastuzumab, the clinical study design was based on the assumption that EGFR protein expression in the tumor of interest is required in order to observe a tumor response from cetuximab therapy. However, recent studies suggest there is no correlation between EGFR expression and tumor response to cetuximab therapy (Cunningham et al., 2004).

In the pivotal BOND trial, 329 patients with metastatic EGFR expressing chemo-refractory CRC were randomized to receive either cetuximab plus irinotecan or cetuximab alone (Cunningham et al., 2004). Both study arms received a $400\,mg/m^2$ loading dose followed by $250\,mg/m^2$ weekly until either the patient had intolerable toxicities or disease progression occurred. The OR rate in the two treatment arms was 22.9% in patients receiving combination therapy (irinotecan plus cetuximab) and 10.8% in the cetuximab monotherapy group. In addition, two prespecified subpopulations were analyzed; an irinotecan-oxaliplatin failure group (irinotecan refractory patients who had previously been treated with and failed an oxaliplatin containing regimen) and the irinotecan refractory group. The irinotecan-oxaliplatin failure subpopulation had a 23.8% response rate and a 2.9 month median time to disease progression for the cetuximab plus irinotecan study arm; and an 11.4% response rate and 1.5 month time to progression for the cetuximab monotherapy study arm. The irinotecan refractory subpopulation had a 25.8% and 14.5% response rate with a 4 month and 1.5 month time to progression for the cetuximab plus irinotecan and cetuximab monotherapy treatment groups, respectively. These data suggest that cetuximab plus chemotherapy will result in a higher tumor response rate than when cetuximab is given alone via overcoming irinotecan tumor resistance. There was no observed correlation between the level of the EGFR expression and response rate. Therefore, other genomic markers are needed to better define the correlation between EGFR inhibitors and tumor response rate.

A phase II study was conducted to assess the safety and efficacy of two monoclonal antibodies, cetuximab plus bevacizumab with or without irinotecan in irinotecan refractory CRC patients (Saltz et al., 2005). The cetuximab plus bevacizumab plus irinotecan resulted in a 37% response rate and 7.9 month time to progression as compared to 20% response rate and 5.6 month time to progression in the group that did not receive irinotecan. In addition, several small studies are assessing the utility of cetuximab as first line therapy in combination with other commonly used chemotherapy regimens (Hohler et al., 2004; Van Cutsem et al., 2004). The results of these studies seem very promising with a response rate ranging from 24% (patients receiving cetuximab and 5-fluorouracil/leucovorin/oxaliplatin, FUFOX) up to 81% (patients receiving cetuximab and an oxaliplatin-containing regimen).

*Safety Concerns*
Cetuximab has a black box warning for severe infusion reactions occurring in approximately 3% of patients most of which (90%) was associated with the first infusion (Segaert and Van Cutsem, 2005). The types of infusion reactions observed include rapid onset of airway obstruction, urticaria, and hypotension. Premedication with an $H_1$-antagonist is required to help minimize the degree of the hypersensitivity reactions. Other serious side effects associated with cetuximab include severe diarrhea (when given in combination with irinotecan), dehydration, fever, interstitial lung disease, dermatologic toxicities, kidney failure, and pulmonary embolus. One of the most common side effects of cetuximab is acneiform eruptions (a maculopapular rash occurring in >50% of patients), which are characteristic of EGFR blockade and is a result of the role of EGFR in the maintenance of skin integrity. Furthermore, a positive correlation has been made with tumor response to cetuximab and severity of the skin rash (Cunnigham et al., 2004; Segaert and Van Cutsem, 2005). Other common side effects include xerosis, diarrhea, nausea, abdominal pain, vomiting, and constipation. Cardiopulmonary arrest, mouth sores, severe radiation skin reactions, weight loss, dry mouth, and difficulty swallowing may occur when cetuximab is given in combination with radiation therapy.

*Pharmaceutical Considerations: Formulation, Other Routes of Administration, Dosing Regimens*
Cetuximab is only available for IV administration. It is commercially available in a 50 mL vial containing 100 mg of cetuximab (2 mg/mL) formulated in a sterile, preservative free, colorless, clear liquid. The recommended dose (in combination therapy or as monotherapy) is $400\,mg/m^2$ as a one time loading

dose infused intravenously over 120 min followed by a weekly maintenance dose of 250 mg/m$^2$ infused over 60 min. Premedication with an H$_1$ antagonist is recommended to circumvent infusion reactions. Patients who experience grade 1 or 2 infusion reactions require a decrease in the rate of infusion by 50%. Individuals who experience a grade 3 or 4 infusion reaction require permanent discontinuation of cetuximab therapy.

## ■ Panitumumab

### Pharmacology and Mechanism of Action

Panitumumab (Vectibix®) is the first fully human MAb inhibitor of EGFR in clinical use today. It is an IgG$_2$ kappa MAb that inhibits EGFR by binding to the extracelluar ligand-binding domain of the receptor (Cohenuram and Saif, 2007). As reviewed earlier, inhibition of EGFR is thought to inhibit neoplastic proliferation, metastatic spread, and produce apoptosis. Although panitumumab shares the same mechanism of action as cetuximab, the two monoclonal entities have two main differences. First, panitumumab is fully humanized, which theoretically should reduce the risk of immunogenicity. Second, in vitro studies have shown that panitumumab has a stronger affinity and specificity for EGFR compared to cetuximab (Cohenuram and Saif, 2007).

Similar to other EGFR inhibitors, in preclinical mouse models, low-dose panitumumab monotherapy was found to eliminate large tumors (i.e., 1.2 cm$^3$) in one study and completely eradicate up to 65% of inoculated mouse tumors in another study (Yang and Jia, 1999; Cohenuram and Saif, 2007). What many find noteworthy is that up to 9 months after treatment cessation, no tumor regrowth occurred (Yang and Jia, 1999). While elimination of tumors has been shown previously with these agents, the potential for complete eradication for monotherapy panitumumab in these preclinical studies is novel.

### Pharmacokinetics/Pharmacodynamics

Preclinical pharmacokinetic studies in Cynomolgus monkeys showed a rapid clearance at nonsaturating doses while a phase I pharmacokinetic study demonstrated low interindividual variability and both liner and saturable EGFR-mediated clearance (Roskos et al., 2002; Cohenuram and Saif, 2007). Phase II clinical trials to date have not shown any drug interactions with any chemotherapeutic agents, including irinotecan, LV, fluoruracil, paclitaxel, and carboplatin.

In terms of pharmacodynamics, one preclinical study demonstrated that the tumor growth inhibition of panitumumab was related to a threshold EGFR level, where xenografts that contained at least 17,000 receptors per cell were treatable with panitumumab, while those with less than 11,000 were not treatable (Yang et al., 2001). Similar to other EGFR inhibitors in clinical trials, increasing dose corresponded to an increasing frequency of an acneiform rash. Specifically in the phase I study performed by Rowinsky et al. (2004), patients that received 1, 1.5, 2, and 2.5 mg/kg weekly of panitumumab had 68, 95, 87, and 100% incidence of rash with its apex at 3 to 5 weeks after starting therapy. A post hoc analysis revealed that rash intensity trended toward a relationship with progression free survival in patients.

### Indications and Clinical Efficacy

Panitumumab was recently approved by the FDA (September 2006) for the treatment of EGFR expressing, metastatic CRC with disease progression on or following fluoropyridine, oxaliplatin, and irinotecan containing chemotherapy regimens (Amgen, 2006). In addition, studies have demonstrated efficacy toward other cancer types such as renal carcinoma and NSCLC.

Approval of panitumumab was based solely on the results of a clinical study containing 463 patients randomized to receive best supportive care alone (BSC) or BSC plus panitumumab (6 mg/kg intravenously) every 2 weeks (Berlin et al., 2004). All patients met the above mentioned FDA approved indication. The mean progression-free survival was 96 days for the panitumumab group and 60 days for the BSC alone group. Eight percent of patients in the treatment arm exhibited a PR and no observable response was observed in the control arm. There was no difference in overall survival between the two groups, although this may have been confounded by a significant proportion of patients from the BSC group that later crossed over to receive panitumumab.

Another study conducted using panitumumab as first-line therapy in combination with irinotecan, 5-fluorouracil, and leucovorin (IFL) showed a 47% response rate with disease stabilization in 32% of patients (Berlin et al., 2004). All individuals who responded developed a skin rash suggesting that the degree of skin toxicity is relative to tumor response to panitumumab therapy. In addition, studies analyzing the utility of panitumumab as monotherapy have shown an 11% response rate in chemorefractory CRC and a 33% disease stabilization (Saif and Cohenuram, 2006).

Results are eagerly awaited for the Panitumumab Advanced Colorectal Cancer Evaluation Study (PACCE) that is evaluating first-line therapy in metastastic CRC (Cohenuram and Saif, 2007). The first 800 patients enrolled will receive FOLFOX and bevacizumab with or without panitumumab while the next 200 patients will receive FOLFIRI and bevacizumab with or without panitumumab. The primary endpoint is progression free survival in the FOLFOX arm.

*Safety Concerns*

Panitumumab has a black box warning for severe dermatologic toxicities and infusion reactions (Amgen, 2006). Severe skin toxicities (grade 3 or higher) were reported in 12% of patients to include dermatosis acneiform, pruritus, erythema, rash, and skin exfoliation. Severe infusion reactions (occuring in 1% of patients) were also observed and include anaphylactic reactions, bronchospasms, fever, chills, and hypotension. However, the infusion reactions are infrequent (as compared to cetuximab) and no premedication is required (Saif and Cohenuram, 2006). Pulmonary fibrosis has also occurred with panitumumab therapy. The more common adverse reactions include abdominal pain, hypomagnesemia, acneiform eruption (occurring in greater than 70% of patients) and other skin rashes, paronychia, fatigue, nausea, vomiting, and diarrhea (Amgen, 2006).

*Pharmaceutical Considerations: Formulation, Other Routes of Administration, Dosing Regimens*

Panitumumab does not require a loading dose, unlike cetuximab, or premedications to prevent immunogenic reactions (Cohenuram and Saif, 2007). Pharmacokinetic studies determined that 2.5 mg/kg is the optimal weekly dose although additional studies suggest that 6 mg/kg every 2 weeks and 9 mg/kg every 3 weeks produce similar trough levels, making alternate dosing regimens a possibility (Rowinsky et al., 2004; Arends and Yang, 2005; Cohenuram and Saif, 2007). The FDA approved regimen is 6 mg/kg every 2 weeks administered IV over 1 hr (Amgen 2006). The drug must be filtered using a 0.22 μm in-line filter or 0.2 μm low protein-binding filter. No other medications should be added to panitumumab.

# REFERENCES

Adams GP, Weiner LM (2005). Monoclonal antibody therapy of cancer. Nat Biotechnol 23(9):1147–57.

Amadori S, Suciu S, Stasj R, et al. (2005). Gemtuzumab ozogamicin (Mylotarg) as single-agent treatment for frail patients 61 years of age and older with acute myeloid leukemia: final results of AML-15B, a phase 2 study of the European Organisation for Research and Treatment of Cancer and Gruppo Italiano Malattie Ematologiche dell-Adulto leukemia groups. Leukemia 19(10):1768–73.

American Cancer Society. Cancer facts and figures 2006. Atlanta: American Cancer Society <http://www.cancer.org/downloads/STT/CAFF2006PWSecured.pdf>; 2006 [Last accessed 12/01/2006].

Amgen. Vectibix (Panitumumab) prescribing information (2006). Thousand Oaks, CA: Amgen, Inc.

Arends R, Yang B (2005). Flexible dosing schedules of panitumumab (ABX-EGF) in cancer patients. Proc Am Soc Clin Oncol Abstract 3089.

ASHP. AHFSfirst™ Web [computer program]. Version 2.0. Bethesda, MD: American Society of Health-System Pharmacists; 2002.

Baselga J, Norton L, Albanell J, et al. (1998). Recombinant humanized anti-HER2 antibody enhances the antitumor activity of paclitaxel and doxorubicin against HER2/neu overexpressing human breast cancer xenografts. Cancer Res 58(13):2825–31.

Bearman SI (2000). Veno-occlusive disease of the liver. Curr Opin Oncol 12:103–9.

Benson AB, Catalano PJ, Meropol NJ, et al. (2003). Bevacizumab (anti-VEGF) plus FOLFOX4 in previously treated advanced colorectal cancer (advCRC): an interim toxicity analysis of the Eastern Cooperative Oncology Group (ECOG) study E32000. Proc Am Soc Clin Oncol Abstract #975.

Berlex. Campath-1H (alemtuzumab) prescribing information. Montvale, NJ: Berlex; 2005.

Berlin J, Malik I, Picus J, et al. (2004). Panitumumab therapy with irinotecan, 5-fluorouracil, and leucovorin (IFL) in patients with metastatic colorectal cancer. Ann Oncol 15(Suppl. 3):70 [abstract 265PD].

Biodrugs [No authors listed]. Iodine-131 tositumomab: (131) I-anti-B1 antibody, (131)I-tositumomab, anti-CD20 murine monoclonal antibody-I-131, B1, Bexxar, (131) I-anti-B1 antibody, iodine-131 tositumomab, iodine-131 anti-B1 antibody, tositumomab. Biodrugs 2003; 17 (4):290–5.

Bowen AL, Zomas A, Emmett E, et al. (1997). Subcutaneous CAMPATH-1H in fludarabine-resistant/relapsed chronic lymphocytic and B-prolymphocytic leukaemia. Br J Haematol 96(3):617–9.

Bristol Myers Squibb. Erbitux (Cetuximab) prescribing information. Princeton, NJ: Bristol Myers Squibb; 2006.

Bross PF, Beitz J, Chen G, et al. (2002). Approval summary: gemtuzumab ozogamicin in relapsed acute myeloid leukemia. Clin Cancer Res 2001; 7(6):1490–6 [Erratum in: Clin Cancer Res 8(1):300].

Burstein HJ, Kuter I, Campos SM, et al. (2001). Clinical activity of trastuzumab and vinorelbine in women with HER2-overexpressing metastatic breast cancer. J Clin Oncol 19(10):2722–30.

Caron PC, Jurcic JG, Scott AM, et al. (1994). A phase 1B trial of humanized monoclonal antibody M195 (anti-CD33) in myeloid leukemia: specific targeting without immunogenicity. Blood 83(7):1760–8.

Castillo L, Etienne-Grimaldi MC, Fischel JL, et al. (2004). Pharmacological background of EGFR targeting. Ann Oncol 15(7):1007–12.

Cersosimo RJ (2003a). Monoclonal antibodies in the treatment of cancer, part 1. Am J Health Syst Pharm 60(15):1531–48.

Cersosimo RJ (2003b). Monoclonal antibodies in the treatment of cancer, part 2. Am J Health Syst Pharm 60(16):1631–41.

Cobleigh MA, Langmuir VK, Sledge GW, et al. (2003). A phase I/II dose-escalation trial of bevacizumab in previously treated metastatic breast cancer. Semin Oncol 30(5 Suppl. 16):117–24.

Cobleigh MA, Vogel CL, Tripathy D, et al. (1999). Multinational study of the efficacy and safety of humanized anti-HER2 monoclonal antibody in women who have HER2-overexpressing metastatic breast cancer that has progressed after chemotherapy for metastatic disease. J Clin Oncol 17(9):2639–48.

Cohenuram M, Saif MW (2007). Panitumumab the first fully humanized monoclonal antibody: from bench to the clinic. Anticancer Drugs 18(1):7–15.

Coiffier B, Lepage E, Briere J, et al. (2002). CHOP chemotherapy plus rituximab compared with CHOP alone in elderly patients with diffuse large B-cell lymphoma. N Engl J Med 346(4):235–42.

Cortes J, Tsimberidou AM, Alvarez R, et al. (2002). Mylotarg combined with topotecan and cytarabine in patients with refractory acute mylogenous leukemia. Cancer Chemother Pharmacol 50(6):497–500.

Cull GM, Haynes AP, Byrne JL, et al. (2000). Preliminary experience of allogeneic stem cell transplantation for lymphoproliferative disorders using BEAM-CAMPATH conditioning: an effective regimen with low procedural-related toxicity. Br J Haematol 108(4):754–60.

Cunningham D, Humblet Y, Siena S, et al. (2004). Cetuximab monotherapy and cetuximab plus irinotecan in irinotecan-refractory metastatic colorectal cancer. N Engl J Med 351(4):337–45.

Dearden CE, Matutes E, Cazin B, et al. (2001). High remission rate in T-cell prolymphocytic leukemia with CAMPATH-1H. Blood 98(6):1721–6.

DeVore R, Fehrenbacker L, Herbst R, et al. (2000). A randomized phase II trial comparing RhuMAb VEGF (recombinant humanized monoclonal antibody to vascular endothelial cell growth factor) plus carboplatin/paclitaxel (CP) to CP alone in patients with stage IIIB/IV NSCLC. Proc Am Soc Clin Oncol Abstract #1896.

Dowell JA, Korth-Bradley J, Liu H, et al. (2001). Pharmacokinetics of gemtuzumab ozogamicin, an antibody-targeted chemotherapy agent for the treatment of patients with acute myeloid leukemia in first relapse. J Clin Pharmacol 41(11):1206–14.

Estey EH, Giles FJ, Beran M, et al. (2002a). Experience with gemtuzumab ozogamicin (mylotarg) and all-trans retinoic acid in untreated acute promyelocytic leukemia. Blood 99(11):4222–4.

Estey EH, Giles FJ, Beran M, et al. (2002b). Gemtuzumab ozogamicin with or without interleukin 11 in patients 65 years of age or older with untreated acute myeloid leukemia and high-risk myelodysplastic syndrome; comparison with idarubicin plus continuous-infusion, high-dose cytosine arabinoside. Blood 99:4343–9.

Faderl S, Thomas DA, O'Brien S, et al. (2003). Experience with alemtuzumab plus rituximab in patients with relapsed and refractory lymphoid malignancies. Blood 101(9):3413–5.

Faulkner RD, Craddock C, Byrne JL, et al. (2004). BEAM: alemtuzumab reduced intensity allogeneic stem cell transplantation for lymphoproliferative disease. GVHD, toxicity and survival in 65 patients. Blood 103(2):428–34.

Ferrajoli A, O'Brien SM, Cortes JE, et al. (2003). Phase II study of alemtuzumab in chronic lymphoproliferative disorders. Cancer 98(4):773–8.

Folkman J (1971). Tumor angiogenesis: therapeutic implications. N Engl J Med 285:1182–6.

Folkman J (1995). Clinical implications of research on angiogenesis. N Engl J Med 333:1757–63.

Frampton JE, Wagstaff AJ (2003). Alemtuzumab. Drugs 63 (12):1229–43.

Gaudreault J (2001). Pharmacokinetics (PK) of bevacizumab (BV) in colorectal cancer. Clin Pharmacol Ther 69 (2 Suppl):P25.

Genentech. Avastin (bevacizumab) prescribing information. San Francisco, CA: Genentech, Inc.; 2006a.

Genentech. Herceptin (trastuzumab) prescribing information. San Francisco, CA: Genentech, Inc.; 2006b.

Genentech. Rituxan (rituximab) prescribing information. San Francisco, CA: Genentech, Inc.; 2006c.

Giles F, Estey E, O'Brien S (2003). Gemtuzumab ozogamicin in the treatment of acute myeloid leukemia. Cancer 98(10):2095–104.

Giralt S (2006). The role of alemtuzumab in nonmyeloablative hematopoietic transplantation. Semin Oncol 33 (2 Suppl. 5):S36–43.

GlaxoSmithKline. Bexxar (tositumomab and [131]I tositumomab) prescribing information. Research Triangle Park, NC: GlaxoSmithKline; 2006 October.

Golay JT, Clark EA, Beverly PC (1985). The CD20 (Bp35) antigen is involved in activation of B cells from the G0 to the G1 phase of the cell cycle. J Immunol 135 (6):3795–801.

Gordon LI (2001). Gemtuzumab ozogamicin (Mylotarg) and hepatic veno-occlusive disease: take two acetaminophen. Bone Marrow Transplant 28:811–2.

Gordon MS, Margolin K, Talpaz G, et al. (2001). Phase I safety and pharmacokinetics study of recombinant human anti-vascular endothelial growth factor in patients with advanced cancer. J Clin Oncol 19 (3):843–50.

Gray R, Giantonio BJ, O'Dwyer PJ, et al. (2003). The safety of adding angiogenesis inhibition into treatment for colorectal, breast, and lung cancer: the Eastern Cooperative Oncology Group's (ECOG) experience with bevacizumab. Proc Am Soc Clin Oncol Abstract #825.

Greenwood J, Gorman SD, Routledge EG, et al. (1994). Engineering multiple-domain forms of the therapeutic antibody CAMPATH-1H: effects on complement lysis. Ther Immunol 1(5):247–55.

Hagenbeek A, Lewington V (2005). Report of a European consensus workshop to develop recommendations for the optimal use of (90)Y-ibritumomab tiuxetan (Zevalin) in lymphoma. Ann Oncol 16(5):786–92.

Hale G, Rebello P, Brettman LR, et al. (2004). Blood concentrations of alemtuzumab and antiglobulin responses in patients with chronic lymphocytic leukemia following intravenous or subcutaneous routes of administration. Blood 104(4):948–55.

Hillan KJ, Koeppen HK, Tobin P, et al. (2003). The role of VEGF expression in response to bevacizumab plus capecitabine in metastatic breast cancer (MBC). Proc Am Soc Clin Oncol Abstract #766.

Hohler T, Dittrich C, Lordick F, et al. (2004). A phase I/II study of cetuximab in combination with 5-fluorouracil/folinic acid plus weekly oxaliplatin in the first-line treatment of patients with metastatic colorectal cancer expressing epidermal growth factor receptor: preliminary results. Ann Oncol 15(Suppl. 3):2620a.

Hsei VC, Novotny W, Margolin K, et al. (2001). Population pharmacokinetic (PK) analysis of bevacizumab (BV) in cancer subjects. Proc Am Soc Clin Oncol Abstract #272.

Hudziak RM, Lewis GD, Winget M, et al. p185$^{HER2}$ (1989) monoclonal antibody has antiproliferative effects in vitro and sensitizes human breast tumor cells to tumor necrosis factor. Mol Cell Biol; 9(3):1165–72.

Hurwitz H, Fehrenbacher L, Cartwright T, et al. (2003). Bevacizumab (a monoclonal antibody to vascular endothelial growth factor) prolongs survival in first-line colorectal cancer (CRC): results of a phase III trial of bevacizumab in combination with bolus IFL (irinotecan, 5-fluorouracil, leucovorin) as first-line therapy in subjects with metastatic CRC. Proc Am Soc Clin Oncol Abstract #3646.

Jemal A, Siegel R, Ward E, et al. (2006). Cancer statistics, 2006. CA Cancer J Clin 56:106–30.

Kabbinavar F, Hurwitz H, Fehrenbacher L, et al. (2003). Phase II, randomized trial comparing bevacizumab plus fluorouracil (FU)/leucovorin (LV) with FU/LV alone in patients with metastatic colorectal cancer. J Clin Oncol 21(1):60–5.

Kabbinavar F, Johnson D, Langmuir VK, et al. (2001). Patterns of tumor progression during therapy with bevacizumab (BV) and chemotherapy (CT) for metastatic colorectal cancer (MCRC) and advanced non-small cell lung cancer. Proc Am Soc Clin Oncol Abstract #1105.

Kanzaki M, Lindorfer MA, Garrison JC, et al. (1997). Activation of the calcium-permeable cation channel CD20 by alpha subunits of the Gi protein. J Biol Chem 272(23):14733–9.

Keating MJ, Flinn I, Jain V, et al. (2002a). Therapeutic role of alemtuzumab (CAMPATH-1H) in patients who have failed fludarabine: results of a large international study. Blood 99(10):3554–61.

Keating MJ, Cazin B, Coutre S, et al. (2002b). Campath-1H treatment of T-cell prolymphocytic leukemia in patients for whom at least one prior chemotherapy regimen has failed. J Clin Oncol 20(1):205–13.

Kennedy B, Rawstron A, Carter C, et al. (2002). CAMPATH-1H and fludarabine in combination are highly active in refractory chronic lymphocytic leukemia. Blood 99 (6):2245–47.

Kilickap S, Abali H, Celik I (2003). Bevacizumab, bleeding, thrombosis, and warfarin. J Clin Oncol 21(18):3542–6.

Korth-Bradley JM, Dowell JA, King SP, et al. (2001). Mylotarg Study Group impact of age and gender on the pharmacokinetics of gemtuzumab ozogamicin. Pharmacotherapy 21(10):1175–80.

Kottaridis PD, Miligan DW, Chopra R, et al. (2000). In vivo CAMPATH-1H prevents graft-versus-host disease following nonmyeloablative stem cell transplantation. Blood 96(7):2419–25.

Larson RA, Boogaerts M, Estey E, et al. (2002). Antibody-targeted chemotherapy of older patients with acute myeloid leukemia in first relapse using mylotarg (gemtuzumab ozogamicin). Leukemia 16: 1627–36.

Larson RA, Sievers EL, Stadtmauer EA, et al. (2005). Final report of the efficacy and safety of gemtuzumab ozogamicin (Mylotarg) in patients with CD33-positive acute myeloid leukemia in first recurrence. Cancer. 104(7):1442–52.

Lenihan DJ, Alencar AJ, Yang D, et al. (2004). Cardiac toxicity of alemtuzumab in patients with mycosis fungoides/Sezary syndrome. Blood 104(3):655–8.

Lo-Coco F, Cimino G, Breccia M, et al. (2004). Gemtuzumab ozogamicin (mylotarg) as a single agent for molecularly relapsed acute promyelocytic leukemia. Blood 104(7):1995–9.

Lui NS, O'Brien S (2004). Monoclonal antibodies in the treatment of chronic lymphocytic leukemia. Med Oncol 21(4):297–304.

Lundin J, Kennedy B, Dearden C, et al. (2005). No cardiac toxicity associated with alemtuzumab therapy for mycosis fungoides/sezary syndrome. Blood 105(10): 4148–9.

Lundin J, Kimby E, Bjorkholm M, et al. (2002). Phase II trial of subcutaneous anti-CD52 monoclonal antibody alemtuzumab (CAMPATH-1H) as first-line treatment for patients with B-cell chronic lymphocytic leukemia (B-CLL). Blood 100:768–73.

Lyseng-Williamson KA, Robinson DM (2006). Spotlight on bevacizumab in advanced colorectal, breast cancer, and non-small cell lung cancer. BioDrugs 20(3):193–5.

Maloney DG, Grillo-Lopez AJ, Bodkin DJ, et al. (1997a) IDEC-C2B8: results of a phase I multiple-dose trial in patients with relapsed non-Hodgkin's lymphoma. J Clin Oncol 15(10):3266–74.

Maloney DG, Grillo-Lopez AJ, White CA, et al. (1997b). IDEC-C2B8 (Rituximab) anti-CD20 monoclonal antibody therapy in patients with relapsed low-grade non-Hodgkin's lymphoma. Blood 90(6):2188–95.

Maloney DG, Liles TM, Czerwinski DK, et al. (1994). Phase I clinical trial using escalating single-dose infusion of chimeric anti-CD20 monoclonal antibody (IDEC-C2B8) in patients with recurrent B-cell lymphoma. Blood 84(8):2457–66.

Margolin K, Gordon MS, Holmgren E, et al. (2001). Phase Ib trial of intravenous recombinant humanized monoclonal antibody to vascular endothelial growth factor in combination with chemotherapy in patients with advanced cancer: pharmacologic and long-term safety data. J Clin Oncol 19(3):851–6.

Marty M, Cognetti F, Maraninchi D, et al. (2005). Randomized phase II trial of the efficacy and safety of trastuzumab combined with docetaxel in patients with human epidermal growth factor receptor 2-positive metastatic breast cancer administered as first-line treatment: the M7001 Study Group. J Clin Oncol 23(19):4265–74.

Mavromatis B, Cheson BD (2003). Monoclonal antibody therapy of chronic lymphocytic leukemia. J Clin Oncol 21(9):1874–81.

McCune SL, Gockerman JP, Moore JO, et al. (2002). Alemtuzumab in relapsed or refractory chronic lymphocytic leukemia and prolymphocytic leukemia. Leuk Lymphoma 43(5):1007–11.

McGavin JK, Spencer CM (2001). Gemtuzumab ozogamicin: ADIS new drug profile. Drugs 61(9):1317–22.

Miller KD, Rugo HS, Cobleigh MA, et al. (2002). Phase III trial of capecitabine (Xeloda®) plus bevacizumab (Avastin®) versus capecitabine alone in women with metastatic breast cancer (MBC) previously treated with an anthracyclines and a taxane. Breast Cancer Res Treat 76:S37.

Miller KD (2003). E2100: a phase II trial of paclitaxel versus paclitaxel/bevacizumab for metastatic breast cancer. Clin Breast Cancer 3(6):421–2.

Miller KD (2002). Issues and challenges for antiangiogenic therapies. Breast Cancer Res 75:S45–50.

Montillo M, Tedeschi A, Miqueleiz S, et al. (2006). Alemtuzumab as consolidation after a response to fludarabine is effective in purging residual disease in patients with chronic lymphocytic leukemia. J Clin Oncol 24(15):2337–42.

Nabhan C, Patton D, Gordon L, et al. (2004). A pilot trial of rituximab and alemtuzumab combination therapy in patients with relapsed and/or refractory chronic lymphocytic leukemia (CLL). Leuk Lymphoma 45 (11):2269–73.

Nabhan C, Rundhaugen LM, Riley MB, et al. (2005). Phase II pilot trial of gemtuzumab ozogamicin (GO) as first line therapy in acute myeloid leukemia patients age 65 or older. Leuk Res 29(1):53–7.

Nabhan C, Tallman MS (2002). Early phase I/II trials with gemtuzumab ozogamicin (Mylotarg) in acute myeloid leukemia. Clin Lymphoma 2(Suppl. 1):S19–23.

Nolting A, Fox FE, Kovar A (2006). Clinical drug development of cetuximab, a monoclonal antibody. In: Meibohm B, editor. Pharmacokinetics and pharmacodynamics of biotech drugs. Weinheim: Wiley; p. 353–72.

Novotny W, Holmgren E, Griffing S, et al. (2001). Identification of squamous cell histology and central, cavitary tumors as possible risk factors for pulmonary hemorrhage (PH) in patients with advanced NSCLC receiving bevacizumab (BV). Proc Am Soc Clin Oncol Abstract # 1318.

O'Brien S, Albitar M, Giles FJ (2005). Monoclonal antibodies in the treatment of leukemia. Curr Mol Med 5 (7):663–75.

O'Shaughnessy JA, Vukelja S, Marsland T, et al. (2004). Phase II study of trastuzumab plus gemcitabine in chemotherapy-pretreated patients with metastatic breast cancer. Clin Breast Cancer 5(2):142–7.

Osterborg A, Dyer MJS, Bunjes D, et al. (1997). Phase II multicenter study of human CD52 antibody in previously treated chronic lymphocytic leukemia. J Clin Oncol 15(4):1567–74.

Osterborg A, Karlsson C, Lundin J, et al. (2006). Strategies in the management of alemtuzumab-related side effects. Semin Oncol 33(2 Suppl. 5):S29–35.

Pawson R, Dyer MJS, Barge R, et al. (1997). Treatment of T-cell prolymphocytic leukemia with human CD52 antibody. J Clin Oncol 15(7):2667–72.

Piccaluga PP, Martinelli G, Rondoni M, et al. (2004a). Gemtuzumab ozogamicin for relapsed and refractory acute myeloid leukemia and myeloid sarcomas. Leuk Lymphoma 45(9):1791–5.

Piccaluga PP, Martinelli G, Rondoni M, et al. (2004b). First experience with gemtuzumab ozogamicin plus cytarabine as continuous infusion for elderly acute myeloid leukemia patients. Leuk Res 28(9):987–90.

Rai KR, Byrd JC, Peterson B, et al. (2002a). A phase II trial of fludarabine followed by alemtuzumab (CAMPATH-1H) in previously untreated chronic lymphocytic leukemia (CLL) patients with active disease; Cancer and Leukemia Group B (CALGB) Study 19901. Blood 100:205a (abstract 772).

Rai KR, Freter CE, Mercier RJ, et al. (2002b). Alemtuzumab in previously treated chronic lymphocytic leukemia patients who also had received fludarabine therapy. J Clin Oncol 20(18):3891–7.

Roboz GJ, Knovich MA, Bayer RL, et al. (2002). Efficacy and safety of gemtuzumab ozogamicin in patients with poor-prognosis acute myeloid leukemia. Leuk Lymphoma 43(10):1951–5.

Roskos L, Arends R, Lohner M, et al. (2002). Optimal dosing of panitumumab (ABX-EGF) in cancer patients. 18th UICC International Cancer Congress, June 30–July 5, Oslo, [abstract].

Rowinsky E, Schwartz GH, Gollob JA, et al. (2004). Safety, pharmacokinetics, and activity of ABX-EGF, a fully human anti-epidermal growth factor receptor monoclonal antibody in patients with metastatic renal cell carcinoma. J Clin Oncol 22(15):3003–15.

Saif MW and Cohenuram M (2006). Role of panitumumab in the management of metastatic colorectal cancer. Clin Colorectal Cancer 6(2):118–24.

Salomon DS, Brandt R, Ciardiello F, et al. (1995). Epidermal growth factor related peptides and their receptors in human malignancies. Crit Rev Oncol Hematol 19 (3):183–232.

Saltz LB, Chung KY, Timoney J, et al. (2006). Simplification of bevacizumab (bev) administration: do we need 90, 60, or even 30 minute infusion times? J Clin Oncol 24 (June 20 Suppl.):3542 [ASCO Annual Meeting Proceedings Part I. No. 18S].

Saltz LB, Lenz H, Hochster H, et al. (2005). Randomized phase II trial of cetuximab/bevacizumab/irinotecan (CBI) versus cetuximab/bevacizumab (CB) in irinotecan-refractory colorectal cancer. ASCO Annual Meeting Proceedings Abstract 169b.

Schaller G, Bangemann N, Weber J, et al. (2005). Efficacy and safety of trastuzumab plus capecitabine in a German multicenter phase II study of pre-treated metastatic breast cancer. J Clin Oncol 23:57s.

Scheinberg DA, Lovett D, Divgi CR, et al. (1991). A phase I monoclonal antibody M195 in acute myelogenous leukemia: specific bone marrow targeting and internalization of radionuclide. J Clin Oncol 9(3):478–90.

Segaert S, Van Cutsem E (2005). Clinical signs, pathophysiology and management of skin toxicity during therapy with epidermal growth factor receptor inhibitors. Ann Oncol 16(9):1425–33.

Sievers EL, Appelbaum FR, Spielberger RT, et al. (1999). Selective ablation of acute myeloid leukemia using antibody-targeted chemotherapy: a phase I study of an anti-CD33 calicheamicin immunoconjugate. Blood 93(11):3678–84.

Sievers EL, Larson RA, Stadtmauer EA, et al. (2001). Efficacy and safety of gemtuzumab ozogamicin in patients with CD33 positive acute myeloid leukemia in first relapse. J Clin Oncol 19(13):3244–54.

Slamon DJ, Lelland-Jones B, Shak S, et al. (2001). Use of chemotherapy plus a monoclonal antibody against HER2 for metastatic breast cancer that overexpresses HER2. N Engl J Med 344(11):783–92.

Sparano JA, Gray R, Giantonio B, et al. (2004). Evaluating angiogenesis agents in the clinic: the Eastern Cooperative Oncology Group portfolio of clinical trials. Clin Cancer Res 10:1206–11.

Tsimberidou A, Cortes J, Thomas D, et al. (2003). Gemtuzumab ozogamicin, fludarabine, cytarabine and cyclosporine combination regimen in patients with CD33 + primary resistant or relapsed acute myeloid leukemia. Leuk Res 27(10):893–7.

Tsimberidou A, Giles FJ, Estey E, et al. (2005). The role of gemtuzumab ozogamicin in acute leukemia therapy. Br J Haematol 132:398–409.

Van Cutsem E, Tabernero J, Diaz-Rubio E, et al. (2004). An international phase II study of cetuximab in combination with oxaliplatin/5-fluorouracil/folinic acid in the first-line treatment of patients with metastatic colorectal cancer expressing epidermal growth factor receptor. Ann Oncol 15(Suppl. 3):iii91. 339a.

Van der Velden VJ, te Marvelde JG, Hoogeveen PG, et al. (2001). Targeting of the CD33-calicheamicin immunoconjugate mylotarg (CMA-676) in acute myeloid leukemia: in vivo and in vitro saturation and internalization by leukemic and normal myeloid cells. Blood 97(10):3197–204.

Walport M (2006). Complement. In: Roitt I, Brostoff J, Male D, editors. Immunology. 4th ed. Barcelona, Spain: Mosby; p. 13.2–3.

Witzig TE, Gordon LI, Cabanillas F, et al. (2002). Randomized controlled trial of yttrium-90-labeled ibritumomab tiuxetan radioimmunotherapy versus rituximab immunotherapy for patients with relapsed or refractory low-grade follicular or transformed B-cell non-Hodgkin's lymphoma. J Clin Oncol 20 (10):2453–63.

Wyeth. Mylotarg (Gemtuzumab ozogamicin): prescribing information. Philadelphia, PA: Wyeth; 2006;

Yang JC, Haworth L, Sherry RM, et al. (2003). A randomized trial of bevacizumab, an anti-vascular endothelial growth factor antibody for metastatic renal cancer. N Engl J Med 349:427–34.

Yang JC, Haworth L, Steinberg SM, et al. (2002). A randomized double-blind placebo-controlled trial of bevacizumab (anti-VEGF antibody) demonstrating a prolongation in time to progression in patients with metastatic renal cancer. Proc Am Soc Clin Oncol Abstract #15.

Yang XD, Jia XC (1999). Eradication of established tumors by a fully human monoclonal antibody to the epidermal growth factor receptor without concomitant chemotherapy. Cancer Res 59(6):1236–43.

Yang XD, Xiao-Chi J, Corvalan JRF, et al. (2001). Development of ABX-EGF, a fully human anti-EGF receptor monoclonal antibody for cancer chemotherapy. Crit Rev Oncol Hematol 38(1):17–23.

Zangmeister-Wittke U (2005). Antibodies for targeted cancer therapy—technical aspects and clinical perspectives. Pathobiology 72(6):279–86.

Zein N, Sinha AM, McGahren WJ, et al. (1998). Calicheamicin gamma 1I: an antitumor antibiotic that cleaves double-stranded DNA site specifically. Science 240(4857):1198–201.

# 17

# Monoclonal Antibodies in Solid Organ Transplantation

*Nicole A. Weimert*
*Department of Pharmacy Services, Medical University of South Carolina, Charleston, South Carolina, U.S.A.*

*Rita R. Alloway*
*Department of Internal Medicine/Division of Nephrology, University of Cincinnati, Cincinnati, Ohio, U.S.A.*

## PHARMACOTHERAPY INFORMATION

Further information on the applied pharmacotherapy with monoclonal antibodies used in solid organ transplantation can be found in the following frequently used textbooks:

- **Applied Therapeutics: The Clinical Use of Drugs** (*Koda-Kimble, MA, et al., Eds.*), 8th edition, *Lippincott Williams & Wilkins, Baltimore 2005*: Chapter 35.
- **Pharmacotherapy: A Pathophysiologic Approach** (*DiPiro, JT, et al., Eds.*), 6th edition, *McGraw-Hill, New York 2005*: Chapters 84, 87, 134.
- **Textbook of Therapeutics: Drug and Disease Management** (*Helms, RA, et al., Eds.*), 8th edition, *Lippincott Williams & Wilkins, Baltimore 2006*: Chapter 27.

## INTRODUCTION

Administration of targeted immunosuppression, in the form of genetically engineered antibodies, is commonplace in solid organ transplantation. Polyclonal antibodies, such as rabbit anti-thymocyte globulin, offer global immunosuppression by targeting several cell surface antigens on B- and T-lymphocytes. However, secondary to their broad therapeutic targets, they are associated with infection, infusion related reactions, inter-batch variability, and post-transplant malignancy. Nevertheless, polyclonal antibodies are still commonly administered for induction and treatment of allograft rejection and offer an important role in current solid organ transplantation, which is beyond the scope of this chapter.

In an attempt to target solid organ transplant immunosuppression, monoclonal antibodies directed against key steps in specific immunologic pathways were introduced. The first agent, muromonab-CD3, was initially introduced in the early 1980s for the treatment of allograft rejection (Morris, 2004). The use of monoclonal antibodies has evolved and expanded over the past two decades and today are routinely included as part of the overall immunosuppression regimen. Both the innate and adaptive immune systems have multiple components and signal transduction pathways aimed at protecting the host from a foreign body, such as transplanted tissue. The ultimate goal of post-transplant immunosuppression is tolerance, a state in which the host immune system recognizes the foreign tissue but does not react to it. This goal has yet to be achieved under modern immunosuppression secondary to immune system redundancy as well as the toxicity of currently available agents. Therefore, monoclonal antibodies are used to provide targeted, immediate immunomodulation aimed at attenuating the overall immune response. Specifically, monoclonal antibodies have been used to (1) decrease the inherent immunoreactivity of the potential transplant recipient prior to engraftment, (2) induce global immunosuppression at the time of transplantation allowing for modified introduction of other immunosuppressive agents (calcineurin inhibitors or corticosteroids), (3) spare exposure to maintenance immunosuppressive agents, and (4) treat acute allograft rejection. Monoclonal antibody selection, as well as dose, is based on patient specific factors; such as, indication for transplantation, type of organ being transplanted, and the long-term immunosuppression objective. To understand the approach that the transplant clinician uses to determine which agent to administer and when, it is necessary to briefly describe how immunoreactivity can be predicted and review the immunological basis for the use and development of monoclonal antibodies in solid organ transplantation.

# IMMUNOLOGIC TARGETS: RATIONAL DEVELOPMENT/ USE OF MONOCLONAL ANTIBODIES IN ORGAN TRANSPLANT

The rational use of monoclonal antibodies in transplantation is focused on the prevention of host immune recognition of donor tissue. There are two ways in which allograft tissue can be immediately impaired secondary to the host immune response: complement-dependent antibody mediated cell lysis (antibody-mediated rejection) and T-cell-mediated parenchymal destruction leading to localized allograft inflammation and arteritis (cellular-mediated rejection) (Halloran, 2004). Pre-transplant screening for antibodies against donor tissues has significantly reduced the incidence and severity of antibody-mediated rejection. However, as will be discussed, preferential destruction of cells that produce these antibodies using monoclonal technology, such as rituximab, prior to transplant has become an option for recipients with preformed alloantibodies. Prevention and treatment of cellular-mediated rejection, therefore, is the main focus of maintenance immunosuppression and the rationale for use of monoclonal antibodies in the early post-transplant period. Cellular mediated rejection is characterized by initial recognition of donor tissue by T-cells. This leads to a complex signal transduction pathway traditionally described as three signals (Halloran, 2004):

- *Signal 1*: Donor antigens are presented to T-cells leading to activation
- *Signal 2*: CD80 and CD86 complex with CD28 on the T-cell surface activating signal transduction pathways (calcineurin, mitogen-activated protein kinase, protein kinase C, nuclear factor kappa B) which leads to further T-cell activation, cytokine release and expression of the interleukin-2 (IL-2) receptor (CD25)
- *Signal 3*: IL-2 and other growth factors cause the activation of the cell cycle and T-cell proliferation (Halloran, 2004)

Monoclonal antibodies have been developed against various targets within this pathway to prevent propagation and lymphocyte proliferation providing profound immunosuppression (Table 1). Monoclonal antibodies that were originally developed for treatment of various malignancies have also been employed as immunosuppressant agents in solid organ recipients. Use of these agents must be balanced with maintenance immunosuppression to minimize the patient's risk of infection or malignancy from over immunosuppression. Table 2 summarizes when and which monoclonal antibodies are currently used in solid organ transplantation.

## ■ Monoclonal Antibodies Administered Pre-Transplant

Immunologic barriers to solid organ transplantation are common. Improved management of end-stage organ disease has increased the number of potential organ recipients and produced a significant shortage of organs available for transplant in comparison to the growing demand. Therefore, clinicians have sought to transplant across previously contraindicated immunologic barriers. In addition, more patients are surviving through their first transplant and are now waiting for a subsequent transplant. Monoclonal antibodies are now being employed prior to transplant to desensitize the recipient's immune system. Desensitization is a strategy where immunosuppression is administered prior to transplant to prevent hyperacute or early rejection in patients who are known to have circulating antibodies against other

| Monoclonal antibody | Molecular weight (kDa) | Animal epitope | Molecular target | Target cells | Use |
|---|---|---|---|---|---|
| Alemtuzumab (Campath-1H®) | 150 | Murine/human | CD52 | Peripheral blood lymphocytes, natural killer cells, monocytes, macrophages, thymocytes | Induction antibody mediated rejection |
| Daclizumab (Zenapax®) | 14.4 | Murine/human | CD25 alpha subunit | IL2-dependent T-lymphocyte activation | Induction |
| Basiliximab (Simulect®) | 14.4 | Murine/human | CD25 alpha subunit | IL2-dependent T-lymphocyte activation | Induction |
| Muromonab-OKT3 (Orthoclone-OKT3®) | 75 | Murine | CD3 | T-lymphocytes (CD2, CD4, CD8) | Treatment of polyclonal antibody resistant cellular mediated rejection |
| Rituximab (Rituxan®) | 145 | Murine/human | CD20 | B-lymphocytes | Desensitization antibody mediated rejection |

**Table 1** ■ Use of monoclonal antibodies in solid organ transplantation.

|  | Hypertension | Hyperlipidemia | Hyperglycemia | Hematologic | Renal dysfunction | Dermatologic |
|---|---|---|---|---|---|---|
| Corticosteroids | + | ++ | ++ | — | — | ++ |
| Cyclosporine | +++ | +++ | ++ | + | +++ | ++ |
| Tacrolimus | +++ | +++ | +++ | +++ | +++ | ++ |
| Mycophenolate mofetil[a] | — | — | — | +++ | — | — |
| Rapamycin | ++ | +++ | — | +++ | + | +++ |

Note: Incidence based on manufacturer package insert clinical trial approval reports: +, <1%; ++,1 – 10%; +++, >10%.
[a]Adverse effects reported for mycophenolate mofetil (Cellcept®) are based on clinical trials using this agent in combination with cyclosporine or tacrolimus and corticosteroids; values modified to account for concurrent agents.

**Table 2** Complications of current maintenance immunosuppressants.

human antigens. This strategy is generally reserved for patients who are "highly sensitized" during their evaluation for transplant. Specifically, as a patient develops end-stage organ disease, their medical and immunologic profiles are characterized. Blood samples from these potential recipients are screened for the presence of antibodies against the major histocompatibility complexes (MHC) on the surface of other human cells, specifically human leukocyte antigens (HLA). Potential recipients who have received blood products, previous organ transplants, or have a history of pregnancy are at higher risk for the development of antibodies against HLA. In addition, all humans have pre-formed IgG and IgM antibodies against the major blood group antigens (A, B, AB, and A1) (Reid, 2005). These antibodies will recognize donor tissue and quickly destroy (hyperacute rejection) the implanted organ if the tissue contains previously recognized HLA within minutes to hours following transplant. Therefore, it is necessary to evaluate the presence of pre-formed circulating antibodies against HLA in the potential organ recipients. Some centers will implement desensitization which incorporates monoclonal antibodies prior to transplant to diminish the production of antibodies against a new organ, allowing for transplant across this immunologic barrier.

## ■ Monoclonal Antibodies Administered at the Time of Transplant

Current maintenance immunosuppression is aimed at various targets within the immune system to halt propagation of signal transduction pathway. Available agents, although effective, are associated with significant patient and allograft adverse effects which are associated with long-term exposure (Table 3). The leading cause of death in non-cardiac transplant recipients is a cardiovascular event. These cardiovascular events have been linked to long-term corticosteroid exposure. In addition, chronic administration of calcineurin inhibitors (cyclosporine and tacrolimus) is also associated with acute and chronic kidney dysfunction leading to hemodialysis or need for a kidney transplant. Monoclonal antibodies given at the time of transplant (induction) have been used to decrease the need for corticosteroids and allow for the delay or a reduction in the amount of calcineurin inhibitor used. Determination of the solid organ transplant recipient's immunologic risk at the time of transplant is necessary to determine which monoclonal antibody to use in order to minimize the risk of early acute rejection and graft loss. Recipients are stratified based on several donor, allograft and recipient variables to determine their immunologic risk. Patients at high risk for acute rejection or those in

| Organ | % Receiving induction | Alemtuzumab (%) | Basiliximab (%) | Daclizumab (%) | Muromonab (%) |
|---|---|---|---|---|---|
| Kidney | 72 | 7 | 20 | 10 | 0 |
| Pancreas | 80 | 43 | 15 | 5 | 0 |
| Heart | 47 | 0 | 10 | 15 | 4 |
| Lung | 50 | 3 | 23 | 15 | 0 |
| Liver | 11 | 2 | 6 | 5 | 0 |
| Intestine | 50 | 19 | 0 | 9 | 0 |

Source: Based on reported immunosuppression trends from 1994 to 2004, with data adapted from Meier-Kriesche et al., 2006.

**Table 3** Current trends of monoclonal antibody induction use in solid organ transplantation.

which maintenance immunosuppression is going to be minimized should receive a polyclonal or monoclonal antibody that provides cellular apoptosis, for example alemtuzumab or rabbit-antithymocyte globulin. Recipients at low risk for acute rejection may receive a monoclonal antibody which provides immunomodulation without lymphocyte depletion, such as basiliximab or daclizumab.

Several important pharmacokinetic parameters must be considered when these agents are administered to the various organ transplant recipients. The volume of distribution, biological half-life and total body clearance can differ significantly from a kidney transplant recipient to a heart transplant recipient. Clinicians must consider when to administer monoclonal antibodies in different transplant populations to maximize efficacy and minimize toxicity. For example, heart and liver transplant recipients tend to lose large volumes of blood around the time of transplant, therefore intraoperative administration may not be the optimal time to administer a monoclonal antibody since a large portion may be lost during surgery. Monoclonal antibodies are also removed by plasma exchange procedures, such as plasmapheresis, which may be performed during the perioperative period (Nojima et al., 2005).

### ■ Monoclonal Antibodies Administered Following Transplant

Monoclonal antibodies given following transplantation are used to treat allograft rejection. Administration of these agents is mainly reserved for severe allograft rejection in which the immunologic insult must be controlled quickly. Under normal homeostatic conditions the humoral immune system provides immediate control of infectious pathogens through secretion of antibodies. Cell mediated immunity, in addition to fighting infections, provides surveillance against the production of mutant cells capable of oncogenesis. Interruption of either of these immune systems through the use of monoclonal antibodies places these patients at significant risk for infection and malignancy. Careful post administration assessment of infection and post-transplant malignancy is commonplace.

## SPECIFIC AGENTS USED IN SOLID ORGAN TRANSPLANT

### ■ Muromonab

Muromonab was the first monoclonal antibody used in solid organ transplantation. Muromonab is a murine monoclonal antibody directed against human CD3 receptor, which is situated on the T-cell antigen receptor of mature T-cells, inducing apoptosis of the target cell (Bodziak, 2003; Wilde, 1996). Cells which display the CD3 receptor include CD2, CD4, and CD8 positive

lymphocytes (Ortho Biotech, 2004). Other investigators suggest that muromonab may also induce CD3 complex shedding, lymphocyte adhesion molecule expression causing peripheral endothelial adhesion, and cell mediated cytolysis (Wilde, 1996; Ortho Biotech, 2004 Buysmann et al., 1996; Magnussen and Moller, 1994; Wong et al., 1990). Muromonab is approved for the treatment of kidney allograft rejection and steroid resistant rejection in heart transplant recipients (Ortho Biotech, 2004). Muromonab was initially employed as an induction agent for kidney transplant recipients, in conjunction with cyclosporine, azathioprine, and corticosteroids. Muromonab administration at the time of transplant decreased the rate of acute rejection and prolonged the time to first acute rejection when compared to no induction (Kahana, 1989). Liver recipients with renal dysfunction at the time of transplant who received muromonab induction were able to avoid cyclosporine without an increased incidence of acute rejection and sustain renal function versus those who received cyclosporine (Mills, 1989). Therefore administration of muromonab enabled preservation of renal function in the setting of reduced calcineurin inhibitor exposure when compared to those who did not receive muromonab (Wilde, 1996). The use of muromonab as an induction agent is nearly extinct with the introduction of newer agents that have more favorable side effect profiles.

Today, muromonab is reserved for treatment of refractory rejection. Muromonab is extremely effective at halting most corticosteroid as well as polyclonal antibody resistant rejections. These rejections are treated with 5 mg of muromonab given daily for 7 to 14 days (Ortho Biotech, 2004). The dose and duration of therapy is often dependent on clinical or biopsy resolution of rejection or may be correlated with circulating CD3 cell concentrations in the serum.

Most patients who are exposed to muromonab will develop human against mouse antibodies (HAMA) following initial exposure. These IgG antibodies may lead to decreased efficacy of subsequent treatment courses, but pre-medication with corticosteroids or antiproliferative agents during initial therapy may reduce their development (Wilde, 1996). Following administration, in vitro data indicate that a serum concentration of 1000 µg/L is required to inhibit cytotoxic T-cell function (Wilde, 1996). In vivo concentrations near the in vivo threshold immediately (1 hour) following administration, but diminish significantly by 24 hours (Wilde, 1996). Steady-state concentrations of 900 ng/mL can be achieved after three doses, with a plasma elimination half life of 18 hours when used for treatment of rejection and 36 hours when used for induction (Wilde, 1996; Ortho Biotech, 2004).

Muromonab administration is associated with significant acute and chronic adverse effects.

Immediately following administration, patients will experience a characteristic OKT3 cytokine release syndrome. The etiology of this syndrome is characterized by the pharmacodynamic interaction the OKT3 molecule has at the CD3 receptor. Muromonab will stimulate the target cell following its interaction with the CD3 receptor prior to inducing cell death. Consequently, CD3 cell stimulation leads to cytokine production and release, which is compounded by acute cellular apoptosis leading to cell lysis and release of the intracellular contents. The cytokine release syndrome associated with muromonab manifests as high fever, chills, rigors, diarrhea, capillary leak and in some cases aseptic meningitis (Wilde, 1996). Capillary leak has been correlated with increased tumor necrosis factor release leading to an initial increase in cardiac output secondary to decreased peripheral vascular resistance, followed by a reduction in right heart filling pressures (pulmonary capillary wedge pressure) which leads to a decrease in stroke volume (Wilde, 1996). Sequelae of this cytokine release syndrome can occur immediately, within 30 to 60 minutes, and last up to 48 hours following administration (Ortho Biotech, 2004). This syndrome appears to be the most severe following the initial dose when the highest innoculum of cells is present in the patient's serum or when preformed antibodies against the mouse epitope exist. Subsequent doses appear to be better tolerated, though cytokine release syndrome has been reported after five doses, typically when the dose has been increased or the CD3 positive cell population has rebounded from previous dose baseline (Wilde, 1996). Pre-treatment against the effects of this cytokine release is necessary to minimize the host response. Specifically, corticosteroids are to prevent cellular response to cytokines, non-steroidal anti-inflammatory agents to prevent sequelae of the arachidonic acid cascade, acetaminophen to halt the effects of centrally acting prostaglandins, and diphenhydramine to attenuate the recipient's response to histamine.

In addition to immediate adverse effects, the potency of muromonab has been associated with a high incidence of post-transplant lymphoproliferative disease and viral infections. For all patients, the 10-year cumulative incidence of post-transplant lymphoproliferative disease is 1.6% (Opelz, 2004). Review of large transplant databases, revealed that deceased donor kidney transplant recipients who received muromonab for induction or treatment had a cumulative incidence of post-transplant lymphoproliferative disease that was 3 times higher than those who did not received muromonab or other T-cell depleting induction (Opelz, 2004). This observation may be multifactorial. It is well known that post-transplant lymphoproliferative disease may be induced secondary to Epstein-Barr viral B-cell

malignant transformation. Muromonab's potent inhibition of T-lymphocytes over a sustained period of time diminishes the immune system's normal surveillance and destruction of malignant cell lines, consequently leading to unopposed transformed B-cell proliferation and subsequent post-transplant lymphoma (Opelz, 2004).

Early use and development of muromonab in solid organ transplantation was beneficial for the novel development and use of newer monoclonal agents. The immunodepleting potency of muromonab, combined with the significant risk for malignancy, has reduced its use in modern transplantation. However, this agent is still a formidable option in the treatment of severe allograft rejection.

## ■ Interleukin-2 Receptor Antagonists

IL-2 antagonists were the next monoclonal antibodies to be used and were specifically developed for use in solid organ transplantation. As previously mentioned, monoclonal antibody use and development in solid organ transplantation is rational. The IL-2 receptor was targeted for several reasons. IL-2, the ligand for the IL-2 receptor, is a highly conserved protein, with only a single gene locus on chromosome 4 (Church, 2003). Animal IL-2 knockout models have decreased lymphocyte function at 2 to 4 weeks of age and early mortality at 6 to 9 weeks of age (Chen and Harrison, 2002). These models also display significantly diminished myelopoesis leading to severe anemia and global bone marrow failure (Chen and Harrison, 2002). This observation confirms the significant role that IL-2 and the IL-2 receptor complex play in immunity. The function and biological effect of IL-2 binding to the IL-2 receptor was first reported by Robb and Smith in 1981 (Robb and Smith in 1981). This in vitro study evaluated murine lymphocytes and found that the IL-2 receptor is only present on activated cells (CD4 + and CD8 +) (Church, 2003). Uchiyama and Waldmann (1981) reported one of the first monoclonal antibodies developed against activated human T-cells. This compound displayed in vitro preferential activity against activated T-cells, including terminally mature T-cells, but did exhibit activity against B-cells or monocytes (Uchiyama and Waldmann, 1981). Later it was determined that this antibody actually bound to the alpha subunit of the activated T-cell receptor, CD25 (Church, 2003). The actual T-cell receptor is made up of three subunits, alpha, beta, and gamma. When the beta and gamma subunits combine they can only be stimulated by high concentrations of IL-2, however, in conjunction with the alpha subunit the receptor shows high affinity for IL-2 and can be stimulated at very low concentrations. The expression of IL-2 and the IL-2 receptor alpha region are highly regulated at the DNA transcription level, and is induced following T-cell activation (Shibuya et al., 1990). The alpha subunit is continuously expressed during allograft rejection, T-cell mediated autoimmune diseases, and malignancies (Church, 2003). The beta and gamma subunit, however, has constitutive expression, resulting in low levels of expression in resting T-lymphocytes (Vincenti et al., 1997, 1998). There is no constitutive expression of IL-2 or the alpha receptor subunit (Shibuya et al., 1990; Noguchi et al., 1993). Both, the beta and gamma subunits, have similar molecular structures and are members of the cytokine receptor superfamily, but are structurally dissimilar to the alpha subunit (Noguchi et al., 1993). Therefore the alpha subunit (CD25) became a rational target for monoclonal development since it is only expressed on activated T-cells. Blockade of the CD25 receptor was to halt the activity of IL-2 thereby decreasing proliferation and clonal expansion of T-cells when activated by foreign donor antigens.

## Daclizumab

In 1997, daclizumab became the first anti-CD25 monoclonal antibody approved for use in the prevention of allograft rejection in kidney transplant recipients, when combined with cyclosporine and corticosteroids. Daclizumab was also the first "humanized" monoclonal antibody approved in the United States for human administration (Tsurushita and Kumar, 2005). The daclizumab molecule is a humanized IgG1 adapted from a mouse antibody against the alpha portion of the IL-2 receptor (Uchiyama and Waldmann, 1981). Daclizumab was developed as an alternative to the initial mouse antibody developed against the IL-2 receptor. The mouse antibody lead to the development of HAMA and inability to administer subsequent doses. Although daclizumab bound with one-third the affinity for the T-cell receptor site when compared to the original mouse molecule, it was still able to exhibit a high binding capacity ($Ka = 3 \times 10^9$ $M^{-1}$) (Tsurushita and Kumar, 2005; Queen et al., 1988). A daclizumab serum concentration of 1 µg/mL is required for 50% inhibition of antigen induced T-cell proliferation (Junghans et al., 1990) Early, phase I clinical trials in kidney transplant recipients, who received corticosteroids in combination with cyclosporine and azathioprine, used five doses of daclizumab (Vincenti et al., 1997). Pharmacokinetic studies revealed a mean serum half-life of 11.4 days, a steady-state volume of distribution of 5 L, and displayed weight dependent elimination. There was no change in the number of circulating CD3 positive cells following administration. Five doses of 1 mg per kg body weight given every other week were required to produce the serum

concentrations needed to achieve 90% inhibition of T-cell proliferation for 12 weeks. One patient did develop neutralizing antibodies against the daclizumab molecule after receiving weekly doses for 2 weeks. Saturation of the IL-2 receptor did not change. Intravenous doses were well tolerated with no infusion-related reactions. No infection or malignancies were reported up to 1 year following daclizumab administration. The authors concluded that daclizumab stayed within the intravascular space and doses should be based on patient weight at the time of transplant (Vincenti et al., 1997). Subsequent pre-marketing clinical trials confirmed these results and dosing schematic and were able to show that daclizimab administration reduced the incidence of acute rejection by 13% in low risk kidney transplant recipients (Vincenti et al., 1998). Following daclizumab's approval several trials have been conducted using various dosing regimens and immunosuppression combinations within various solid organ recipients. The exact number of doses or duration of therapy for each organ transplant recipient to achieve optimal therapy is currently unknown.

## Basiliximab

Basiliximab was developed as a more potent anti-IL-2 receptor antagonist when compared to daclizumab and may have several logistical advantages. Basiliximab, in combination with cyclosporine and corticosteroids, was approved for the prevention of acute allograft rejection in renal transplant recipients in May, 1998. Basiliximab is a murine/human (chimeric) monoclonal antibody directed against the alpha subunit of the IL-2 receptor on the surface of activated T-lymphocytes. The antibody is produced from genetically engineered mouse myeloma cells. The variable region of the purified monoclonal antibody is comprised of murine hypervariable region, RFT5, which selectively binds to the IL-2 receptor alpha region. The constant region is made up of human IgG1 and kappa light chains (Novartis Pharmaceuticals, 2005). Since the variable region is the only portion with a non-human epitope, there appears to be low antigenicity and increased circulating half-life associated with its administration (Amlot et al., 1995). Following administration, basiliximab rapidly binds to the alpha region of the IL-2 receptor and serves as a competitive antagonist against IL-2. The estimated receptor binding affinity (Ka) is $1 \times 10^{10}$ $M^{-1}$, which is three times more potent than daclizumab (Novartis Pharmaceuticals, 2005). Complete inhibition of the CD25 receptor occurs after the serum concentration of basiliximab exceeds 0.2 µg/mL and inhibition correlated with increasing dose (Novartis Pharmaceuticals, 2005; Kovarik et al., 1996). Initial dose finding studies of basiliximab were similar to daclizumab. Basiliximab, combined with cyclosporine and corticosteroids, was administered to adult kidney transplant recipients for the prevention of acute cellular rejection. Kovarik et al. (1997) performed a multicenter, open-label pharmacodynamic analysis evaluating basiliximab dose escalation in adult patients undergoing primary renal transplantation. Patients received a total of 40 or 60 mg of basiliximab in combination with cyclosporine, corticorticosteroids, and azathioprine. Thirty-two patients were evaluated and were primarily young (34±12 years), Caucasian (29/32) males (23/32). Basiliximab infusions were well tolerated with not changes in blood pressure, temperature, or hypersensitivity reactions. Thirty patients underwent pharmacokinetic evaluation. Basiliximab blood concentrations showed biphasic elimination with an average terminal half-life of 6.5 days. Significant intra- and interpatient variability in body weight or observed volume of distribution versus drug clearance was observed. This could not be corrected through body weight adjustment. Gender did not appear to influence the pharmacokinetic parameters of basiliximab, however, this cohort contained a small number of female recipients that may have limited the detection of a difference. Results also indicated that the combination of basiliximab with cyclosporine, corticosteroids, and azathioprine might be inadequate. A total of 22 patients had an acute rejection episode, 16 patients in the 40 mg groups and six in the 60 mg group. These rejections appeared within the first two weeks following transplantation, mean time to rejection 11 days. Also three patients experienced graft loss, two of these were immunologically mediated. There was no difference in the basiliximab serum concentration in the patients who experienced rejection versus those who did not. Authors concluded that increased cyclosporine concentrations, which would inhibit IL-2 production, within the first few days post-transplant may increase the efficacy of basiliximab when used for induction (Kovarik et al., 1996). The clinical efficacy of basiliximab has been confirmed in several prospective post-marketing trials. Currently, the recommended basiliximab dosing regimen is a total dose of 40 mg, with 20 mg administered 2 hours prior to transplanted organ reperfusion and a subsequent 20 mg dose on post-operative day 4.

IL-2 receptor antagonists are currently used in all solid organ transplant populations for induction (Table 3), but are only approved for use in kidney transplant recipients. Administration does not reduce the total number of circulating lymphocytes or the number of T-lymphocytes expressing other markers of activations, such as CD26, CD38, CD54, CD69 or HLA-DR (Chapman, 2003). Consequently, it is necessary that additional immunosuppressive agents, such

a calcineurin inhibitors and antiproliferative agents, be administered as soon as possible to decrease the risk of early acute rejection. The advantage of IL-2 receptor antagonists is that they confer a decreased risk of infusion related reactions, post-transplant infection and malignancy when compared to immunodepleting agents. The use of these agents has increased since the introduction of more potent maintenance immunosuppressant agents and they are now the agents of choice in kidney, lung, liver, and pancreas transplant recipients. Although these agents have been evaluated in organ recipients who are at high risk for acute rejection, they are mainly reserved for patients who are at low to moderate risk. Also, these agents are still being evaluated for use in immunosuppression protocols which withdraw or avoid corticosteroids or calcineurin inhibitors. There may be an increased risk of anti-idiotypic IgE anaphylactic reactions in patients who receive repeat courses of IL-2 receptor antagonists. Two published case reports describe patients who had been previously exposed to an IL-2 receptor antagonist and upon subsequent exposure developed dyspnea, chest tightness, rash and angioedema. However, in one case where basiliximab was the offending agent, daclizumab was successfully administered following a negative skin test. Therefore caution maybe warranted in patients who receive a dose of an IL-2 antagonist without concomitant corticosteroids following previous exposure in the past 6 months when circulating antibodies are expected to be present.

## ■ Alemtuzumab

Recently, alemtuzumab was introduced into solid organ transplantation. Alemtuzumab is a recombinant DNA-derived, humanized, rat IgG1κ monoclonal antibody targeting the 21 to 28 kDa cell surface protein glycoprotein CD52, which is produced in a Chinese hamster ovary suspension medium (Genzyme Corporation, 2005; Kneuchtle et al., 2004). Initially, the first anti-CD52 antibodies were developed from rat hybrid antibodies that were produced to lyse lymphocytes in the presence of complement (Morris, 2006). Campath-1M was the first agent developed. This molecule was a rat IgM antibody which produced little biological effect. In contrast, the rat IgG (Campath-1G) produced profound lymphopenia (Morris, 2006). In order to prevent the formation of antibodies against the rat IgG the molecule was humanized and called alemtuzumab or Campath-1H (Morris, 2006). The biologic effects of alemtuzumab are the same as Campath-1G, and include complement-mediated cell lysis, antibody-mediated cytotoxicity, and target cell apoptosis (Magliocca, 2006). The CD52 receptors accounts for 5% of lymphocyte surface antigens (Morris, 2006). Cells which express the CD52 antigen include T- and B-lymphocytes, natural killer cells, monocytes, and dendritic cells (Genzyme Corporation, 2005; Bloom et al., 2006). Following administration a marked decrease in circulating lymphocytes is observed. Use in the hematology population indicates that this effect is dose-dependent (see Chapter 16). However, single doses of 30 mg or two doses of 20 mg are currently used in the solid organ transplant population.

The plasma elimination half life after single doses is reported to be around 12 days and the molecule may be removed by post-transplant plasmapheresis (for more details see Chapter 16) (Magliocca, 2006). The biological activity of alemtuzumab, however, may last up to several months. One in vivo study of kidney transplant recipients aimed to observe the recovery and function of lymphocytes following administration of 40 mg of alemtuzumab (Bloom et al., 2006). Authors reported a 2 Log reduction in peripheral lymphocytes following administration. Absolute lymphocyte counts at 12 months remained marketly depleted, falling below 50% of their original baseline. Monocytes and B-lymphocytes were the first cell lines to recover at 3 to 12 months post-administration. T-lymphocytes returned to 50% of their baseline value by 36 months (Bloom et al., 2006).

Currently, alemtuzumab is only FDA approved for the treatment of B-cell chronic lymphocytic leukemia. The first report of alemtuzumab use in solid organ transplantation appeared in 1991. Friend et al. (1991) published a case series on the use of alemtuzumab to reverse acute rejection in renal transplant recipients. Shortly thereafter, Calne et al. (1999) issued the first report of alemtuzumab use as an induction agent. The authors reported the results of 31 consecutive renal transplant recipients. Patients received two 20 mg doses of alemtuzumab, the first dose was given in the operating room and the second dose was given on post-operative day 1. Patients were initiated on low dose cyclosporine monotherapy, with a goal trough range of 75 to 125 ng/mL. Three patients experienced corticosteroid responsive rejection (20%) and were maintained on corticosteroids and azathioprine following rejection. Allografts remained functional in 94% (29/31) of patients at 15 to 28 months post transplant (Calne et al., 1999).

Alemtuzumab is currently being used for induction and for treatment of rejection (Morris, 2006). In a recent review of immunosuppression trends in the United States, alemtuzumab use has markedly increase in the past 3 years, with use primarily limited to induction (Table 2). In 2004, alemtuzumab was the predominant agent used for induction in both pancreas and intestinal transplant recipients (Meier-Kriesche et al., 2006). Use in liver transplant has been limited, but

has appeared in a couple of published trials. Specific findings from these trials indicate that patients without hepatitis C were able to tolerate lower levels of calcineurin inhibitors which corresponded to lower serum creatinine levels at one year post transplant (Tzakis et al., 2004). In contrast, administration of alemtuzumab positively correlated with early recurrence of hepatitis C viral replication (Marcos et al., 2004). Alemtuzumab induction has allowed for early withdrawal of corticosteroids in several clinical trials, thereby decreasing long-term exposure which has been correlated with an increased incidence of cardiovascular disease, endocrine and metabolic side effects. However, early trials in which calcineurin inhibitor avoidance was initiated, the rate of early acute antibody-mediated rejection was 17% compared to 10% under traditional immunosuppression which included calcineurin inhibitors (Magliocca, 2006).

The infusion of alemtuzumab is well tolerated. In general, induction doses are administered immediately preceeding reperfusion of the transplanted allograft. Pre-treatment with corticosteroids, diphenhydramine and acetaminophen is generally advised to prevent sequelae from cellular apotosis. However, cytokine release associated with alemtuzumab is insignificant in comparison to other agents (Morris, 2006).

Currently, there are few published experiences detailing long-term outcomes in patients who received alemtuzumab induction (Magliocca, 2006). Initially clinicians were concerned that the profound lymphodepletion that was observed following administration would lead to a significant increase in the number of severe infections. Therefore, lymphocyte response to donor antigens following alemtuzumab administration was also evaluated in vitro (Bloom et al., 2006). Lymphocytes from patients treated with alemtuzumab were able to respond to donor antigens and cytokines. A small subset of patients, however, were hyporesponsive which is similar to the control patients observed in this study (Bloom et al., 2006). In addition, several reports detailing the use of alemtuzumab thus far suggest that both infection and malignancy rates are minimal when compared to other agents used for the same indication (Morris, 2006; Magliocca, 2006). At present, the most significant concern associated with alemtuzumab administration is an increased incidence of autoimmune diseases. The exact incidence and etiology of autoimmune diseases following alemtuzumab administration in solid organ transplant is currently unknown. Initial reports of autoimmune diseases associated with alemtuzumab administration came from the multiple sclerosis population. A single center observed the development of Grave's disease in 9 out of 27 patients who received alemtuzumab (Coles et al., 1999).

Thyroid function in all patients was normal prior to alemtuzumab and the mean time to development of autoimmune hyperthyroidism was 19 months (range 9 to 31 months) (Coles et al., 1999). Autoimmune hyperthyroidism was first reported in a kidney transplant recipient who received alemtuzumab induction 4 years earlier (Kirk et al., 2006). Watson et al. (2005) recently published a 5 years experience with alemtuzumab induction, in which they reported a 6% (2/33) incidence of autoimmune disease development following administration. One patient developed hyperthyroidism in the early post-transplant period and one patient developed hemolytic anemia which was refractory to corticosteroids. With the increased use of alemtuzumab in solid organ transplant the actual risk of autoimmune disease development may be more accurately assessed in the next decade.

### ■ Rituximab

Rituximab is a monoclonal antibody directed at the CD20 cell surface protein. Rituximab is currently FDA approved for the CD20 positive forms of Non-Hodgkin's lymphoma and refractory rheumatoid arthritis (see Chapters 16 and 18). The CD20 protein is expressed on all B-cells, from pre-B-cells to activated B-cells. This protein is not expressed on hematopoetic stem cells, plasma cells, or T-lymphocytes (Tobinai, 2003). The CD20 protein is a calcium channel and is responsible for B-cell proliferation and differentiation (Tobinai, 2003). Early monoclonal antibodies developed against CD20 revealed that antibody binding did not result in modulation of activity or shedding of the surface protein, making the development of a humanized anti-CD20 antibody rational (Tobinai, 2003). Rituximab was originally developed to treat B-cell lymphomas, as the vast majority of malignant B-cells express the CD20 receptor. Following continuously infused, high doses of engineered anti-CD20 monoclonal antibodies clearance of CD20 positive cells occurred within 4 hours of administration (Press et al., 1987). Circulating B-cell clearance was immediate; however, lymph node and bone marrow B-cell clearance was dose-dependent.

Rituximab was initially used in solid organ transplant recipients to treat post-transplant lymphoproliferative disorder (PTLD). Post-transplant lymphoproliferative disorder is a malignancy that develops following exposure to high levels of T-cell depleting immunosuppression (see the section "Immunologic Targets: Rational Development/Use of Monoclonal Antibodies in Organ Transplant"). Under normal physiologic conditions, both the humoral and cellular immune systems work in concert to fight infection. In addition, cytotoxic T-lymphocytes survey the body for malignant cells. Current immunosuppression and induction therapy is focused on decreasing communication and proliferation of T-lymphocytes which may lead to unopposed B-cell proliferation. Certain B-cells which are transfected with Ebstein Barr virus, or other viruses, may go onto unopposed cellular differentiation leading to PTLD. This disorder was first reported in two renal transplant recipients who developed "immunoblastic sarcomas" of the central nervous system (Matas et al., 1976). The incidence of post-transplant malignancy, specifically PTLD, increased as the number of solid organ transplants increased. Specific agents linked to the development of PTLD included OKT3 and rabbit anti-thymocyte globulin (Swinnen et al., 1990). The initial treatment for PTLD is a reduction in maintenance immunosuppression, to allow T-cell surveillance to resume and aid in the destruction of malignant cells. Rituximab was initially used in the 1990's to target B-cell specific forms of PTLD that did not involve the central nervous system (Faye et al., 1998; Cook et al., 1999; Davis, 2004). The molecular size of rituximab precludes its use for central nervous system tumors. Administration of rituximab in patients with peripheral lymphomas resulted in clearance of malignant B-cells for up to 12 months (Davis, 2004). Rituximab is currently used alone or in combination with chemotherapy for severe or refractory PTLD.

Rituximab has also been employed as a desensitizing agent (see the section "Monoclonal Antibodies Administered Pre-transplant") prior to solid organ transplant. Doses of 375 mg per $m^2$ administered prior to transplant enabled transplantation across ABO incompatible blood types and transplantation of highly sensitized patients. Often rituximab is given in combination with other immunosuppressants to halt the production of new B-lymphocytes and prevent the formation of new plasma cells. Desensitization protocols involve administration of pooled immunoglobulin followed by plasmapheresis to remove donor specific antibody complexes. Rituximab is administered following the course of plasmapheresis for two reasons: (*i*) rituximab is removed by plasmapheresis and (*ii*) rituximab only targets B-lymphocytes, not the plasma cells currently secreting antibody. Therefore, timing of administration is crucial to the success of the desensitization protocol.

Following transplant, rituximab is also used for the treatment of acute, refractory antibody-mediated rejection. Antibody-mediated rejection is characterized by host recognition of donor antigens followed by T-cell proliferation and antigen presentation to B-cells. B-cells then undergo clonal expansion and differentiation into mature plasma cells which secrete anti-donor antibody. This immune process may occur before or after transplantation. Often the presence of antibodies against donor tissue is discovered prior

| Monoclonal antibody | Dose[a] | US cost per course[b] (AWP) | European cost per course |
|---|---|---|---|
| Alemtuzumab | 30 mg × 1 | $ 5,524 | £ 270 |
| Basiliximab | 20 mg × 2 | $ 3,571 | £ 3,016 |
| Daclizumab | 75 mg × 2 | $ 14,800 | £ 1,338 |
| Muromonab | 5 mg × 7 | $ 6,935 | £ 619 |

[a] Based on 70 kg dosing weight, rounded to nearest vial size.
[b] Actual wholesale price (adapted from Murry L, ed. 2006 Redbook. Thomson PDR. Montvale, NJ, 2006).
[c] European cost calculations adapted from data presented in transplantation 2006; 81:1361–1367.

**Table 4** ■ Per-dose cost comparison among monoclonal antibodies currently used in solid organ transplantation.

to transplant, during final cross-match, thus preventing hyperacute rejection. Unfortunately, in some cases low levels of antibody or memory B-cells exist which can facilitate antibody-mediated rejection within the first several weeks following transplant. Rituximab, therefore, is used to induce apotosis of the B-cells producing or capable of producing antibodies against the allograft. Unfortunately, the CD20 receptor is absent on mature plasma cells, therefore, rituximab can only stop new B-cells from forming. Plasmapheresis is necessary to remove antibodies produced by secreting plasma cells. The optimal number of doses and length of therapy necessary to suppress antibody mediated rejection is unknown.

## CONCLUSION

Currently, there are three challenges remaining in solid organ transplant. The first challenge is optimizing patient specific immunosuppression based on risk factors for acute rejection. Monoclonal antibodies provide targeted immunosuppression, that when used in conjunction with specific maintenance immunosuppressants may allow more specific therapy. The second challenge is preventing over-immunosuppression which may lead to infection and malignancy. Although, monoclonal antibodies provide targeted therapy, the toxicity and potency must be balanced with over-immunosuppression. Consideration of the mechanism of action of both the monoclonal antibody and maintenance immunosuppression must be evaluated to ensure that appropriate antimicrobial prophylaxis and malignancy screening tools are utilized to minimize the patient's risk. Finally, increasing patient and graft survival through reducing the incidence of adverse effects associated with long-term exposure to maintenance immunosuppression, such as cardiovascular events or kidney dysfunction is necessary. Monoclonal, along with polyclonal antibodies, may allow for withdrawal or minimization of specific maintenance immunosuppressants that lead to the increased incidence of these long-term adverse effects. Oftentimes the use of specific monoclonal antibodies

in institutional protocols is driven by cost (Table 4) with careful consideration of the goal of therapy.

## REFERENCES

Amlot PL, Fernado ON, Griffin PJ, et al. (1995). Prolonged action of a chimeric interleukin-2 receptor (CD25) monoclonal antibody used in cadaveric renal transplantation. Transplantation 60:748–56.

Bloom DD, Fechner JH, Knechtle SJ. (2006). T-lymphocyte alloresponses of Campath-1H treated kidney transplant patients. Transplantation 81:81–7.

Bodziak KA. (2003). Minimizing the side effects of immunosuppression in kidney transplant recipients. Curr Opin Organ Transplant 8:160–6.

Buysmann S, Schellekens PT, van Kooyk Y, Figdor CG, ten Berge IJ. (1996). Activation and increased expression of adhesion molecules on peripheral blood lymphocytes is a mechanism for the immediate lymphocytopenia after administration of OKT3. Blood 87:404–11.

Calne R, Friend PJ, Jamieson NV, et al. (1999). Campath IH allows low-dose cyclosporine monotherapy in 31 cadaveric renal allograft recipients. Transplantation 68:1613–6.

Chapman TM. (2003). Basiliximab: a review of its use as induction therapy in renal transplantation. Drugs 63:2803–35.

Chen J, Harrison DE. (2002). Hematopoietic stem cell functional failure in interleukin-2-deficient mice. J Hematother Stem Cell Res 11:905–12.

Church AC. (2003). Clinical advances in therapies targeting the interleukin-2 receptor. Q J Med 96:91–102.

Coles AJ, Smith S, Coraddu F, et al. (1999). Pulsed monoclonal antibody treatment and autoimmune thyroid disease in multiple sclerosis. Lancet 354:1691–5.

Cook RC, Gascoyne RD, Fradet G, Levy RD. (1999). Treatment of post-transplant lymphoproliferative disease with rituximab monoclonal antibody after lung transplantation. Lancet 354:1698–9.

Davis JE. (2004). Treatment options for post-transplant lymphoproliferative disorder and other Epstein-Barr virus-associated malignancies. Tissue Antigens 63:285–92.

Faye A, Peuchmaur M, Mathieu-Boue A, Vilmer E. (1998). Anti-CD20 monoclonal antibody for post-transplant lymphoproliferative disorders. Lancet 352:1285.

Friend PJ, Hale G, Cobbold S, et al. (1991). Reversal of allograft rejection using the monoclonal antibody, Campath-1G. Transplant Proc 23:2253–4.

Genzyme Corporation: Alemtuzumab (Campath) Package Insert. (2005). Cambridge, MA: Genzyme Corporation.

Halloran PF. (2004). Immunosuppressive drugs for kidney transplantation. N Engl J Med 351:2715–29.

Junghans RP, Landolfi NF, Avdalovic NM, Schneider WP, Queen C. (1990). Anti-Tac-H, a humanized antibody to the interleukin 2 receptor with new features for immunotherapy in malignant and immune disorders. Cancer Res 50:1495–502.

Kahana L, Narvarte J, Ackermann J, et al. (1989). OKT3 prophylaxis versus conventional drug therapy: single-center perspective, part of a multicenter trial. Am J Kidney Dis 1989; 14:s5–s9.

Kirk AD, Swanson SJ, Mannon RB. (2006). Autoimmune thyroid disease after renal transplantation using depletional induction with alemtuzumab. Am J Transplant 6:1084–5.

Kneuchtle SJ, Pirsch JD, et al. (2004). Campath-1H in renal transplantation: the University of Wisconsin experience. Surgery 136:754–60.

Kovarik J, Cisterne JM, Mourad G, et al. (1997). Disposition of basiliximab, an interleukin-2 receptor antibody, in recipients of mismatched cadaver renal allografts. Transplantation 64:1701–5.

Kovarik JM, Sweny P, Fernado O, et al. (1996). Pharmacokinetics and immunosynamics of chimeric IL-2 receptor monoclonal antibody SDZ CHI 621 in renal allograft receipients. Transpl Int 9:S32–3.

Magliocca JF. (2006). The evolving role of alemtuzumab (Campath-1H) for immunosuppressive therpay in organ transplantation. Transpl Int 19:705–14.

Magnussen K, Moller B. (1994). CD3 antigen modulation in T-lymphocytes during OKT3 treatment. Transplant Proc 26:1731.

Marcos A, Fung JJ, Fontes P, et al. (2004). Use of alemtuzumab and tacrolimus monotherapy for cadaveric liver transplantation: with particular reference to hepatitis C virus. Transplantation 78:966–71.

Matas AJ, Rosai J, Simmoms RL, Najarian JS. (1976). Post-transplant malignant lymphoma. Distinctive morphologic features related to its pathogenesis. Am J Med 61:716–20.

Meier-Kriesche HU, Gruessner RWG, Fung JJ, Bustami RT, Barr ML, Leichtman AB. (2004). Immunosuppression: evolution in practice and trends, 1994–2004. Am J Transplant 6:1111–31.

Mills JM, McDiarmid SV, Hiatt JR, et al. (1989). Randomized prospective trial of OKT3 for early prophylaxis of rejection after liver transplantation. Transplantation 47:82–8.

Morris PJ. (2004). Transplantation—a medical miracle of the 20th century. N Engl J Med 351:2678–80.

Morris PJ. (2006). Alemtuzumab (Campath-1H): a systematic review in organ transplantation. Transplantation 81:1361–7.

Noguchi M, Cao X, Leonard WJ. (1993). Characterization of the human interleukin-2 receptor gamma gene. J Biol Chem 268:13601–8.

Nojima M, Nakao A, Itahana R, Kyo M, Hashimoto M, Shima H. (2005). Sequential blood level monitoring of basiliximab during multisession plasmapheresis in a kidney transplant recipient. Transplant Proc 37:875–8.

Novartis Pharmaceuticals: Basiliximab (Simulect) Package Insert. (2005). East Hanover, NJ: Novartis Pharmaceuticals Corporation.

Opelz G. (2004). Lymphomas after solid organ transplantation: a collaborative transplant study report. Am J Transplant 4:222–30.

Ortho Biotech: Muromonab (Orthoclone) Package Insert. (2004). Raritan, NJ: Ortho Biotech. Press OW, Ledbetter JA, Martin PJ, Zarling J, Kidd P, Thomas ED. (1987). Monoclonal antibody 1F5 (anti-CD20) serotherapy of human B cell lymphomas. Blood 69:584–1.

Queen C, Selick HE, Payne PW, et al. (1988). A humanized antibody that binds to the interleukin 2 receptor. Proc Natl Acad Sci USA 86:10029–33.

Reid ME. (2005). Human blood group antigens and antibodies. In: Hoffman R, Benz EJ, eds. Hematology: Basic Principles and Practice, 4th ed. Philadelphia, Pennsylvania, 2370–4.

Robb RJ, Smith KA. (1981). T cell growth factor receptors: quantitation, specific and biological relevance. J Exp Med 154:1455–74.

Shibuya H, Nakamura Y, Harada H, et al. (1990). The human interleukin-2 receptor beta-chain gene:genomic organization, promoter analysis and chromosomal assignment. Nucleic Acids Res 18:3697–703.

Swinnen LJ, Fisher SG, O'Sullivan EJ, et al. (1990). Increased incidence of lymphoproliferative disorder after immunosuppression with the monoclonal antibody OKT3 in cardiac-transplant recipients. N Engl J Med 323:1723–8.

Tobinai K. (2003). Rituximab and other emerging antibodies as molecular target-based therapy of lymphoma. Int J Clin Oncol 8:212–3.

Tsurushita N, Kumar S. (2005). Design of humanized antibodies: from anti-Tac to Zenapax. Methods 36:69–83.

Tzakis AG, Kato T, Nishida S, et al. (2004). Preliminary experience with alemtuzumab (Campath-1H) and low-dose tacrolimus immunosuppression in adult liver transplantation. Transplantation 77:1209–14.

Uchiyama T, Waldmann TA. (1981). A monoclonal antibody (anti-Tac) reactive with activated and functionally mature human T cells. J Immunol 126:1393–7.

Vincenti F, Light S, Bumgardner G, et al. (1998). Interleukin-2-receptor blockade with daclizumab to prevent acute rejection in renal transplantation. Daclizumab Triple Therapy Study Group. N Engl J Med 338:161–5.

Vincenti F, Birnbaum J, Garovoy M, et al. (1997). A phase I trial of humanized anti-interleukin 2 receptor antibody in renal transplantation. Transplantation 63:33–38.

Watson CJ, Friend PJ, Firth J, et al. (2005). Alemtuzumab (CAMPATH 1H) induction therapy in cadaveric kidney transplantation—efficacy and safety at five years. Am J Transplant 5:1347–533.

Wilde MI. (1996). Muromonab CD3: a reappraisal of its pharmacology and use of prophylaxis of solid organ transplant rejection. Drugs 51:866–87.

Wong JT, Ghobrial I, Colvin RB. (1990). The mechanism of anti-CD3 monoclonal antibodies. Mediation of cytolysis by inter-T cell bridging. Transplantation 50:683–9.

# 18

# Monoclonal Antibodies in Anti-inflammatory Therapy

*Jeffrey M. Harris and Peter Kuebler*
Genentech, Inc., South San Francisco, California, U.S.A.

*Michael A. Panzara*
Biogen-Idec, Inc., Cambridge, Massachusetts, U.S.A.

---

## PHARMACOTHERAPY INFORMATION

Further information on the applied pharmacotherapy with monoclonal antibodies targeted against inflammatory processes can be found in the following frequently used textbooks:

- **Applied Therapeutics: The Clinical Use of Drugs** (Koda-Kimble, MA, et al., Eds.), 8th edition, Lippincott Williams & Wilkins, Baltimore 2005: Chapters 23, 25, 28, 40, 43.
- **Pharmacotherapy: A Pathophysiologic Approach** (DiPiro, JT, et al., Eds.), 6thedition, McGraw-Hill, New York 2005: Chapter 26, 34, 47, 53, 85, 89, 93, 96, 100, 102.
- **Textbook of Therapeutics: Drug and Disease Management** (Helms, RA, et al., Eds.), 8th edition, Lippincott Williams & Wilkins,Baltimore 2006: Chapters 10, 33, 34, 46, 65, 68.

---

## INTRODUCTION

For decades corticosteroids and other immunomodulatory agents have been the cornerstone of therapy for inflammatory conditions. These other immunomodulatory agents are often referred to as disease-modifying anti-rheumatic drugs (DMARDs), which include not only anti-metabolites like methotrexate, azathioprine and leflunomide, but also gold salts, D-penicillamine, some "antimalarials" (chloroquine and hydroxychloroquine), as well as sulfasalazine. The successful development of targeted biologic agents, specifically monoclonal antibodies and recombinant receptor fusion proteins, as anti-inflammatory therapies for allergic and autoimmune diseases over the past decade has not only revolutionized options for patients with these disorders, but also begun to further elucidate the underlying pathology. Though at present there are only a handful of approved biologics for these chronic immunologic diseases, this area of pharmaceutical research and development is rapidly growing.

The currently approved targeted therapies for autoimmune disorders either block the tumor necrosis factor alpha (TNF-$\alpha$) or interleukin-1 (IL-1) pathway, block lymphocyte activation or migration, or directly deplete lymphocyte subsets. For allergic inflammatory conditions (allergic asthma), there is currently only one approved targeted therapy, omalizumab (Xolair®), which acts by neutralizing soluble immunoglobulin E (IgE). Although the potential risk-to-benefit ratio is always of central importance in making therapeutic decisions, the acceptable thresholds for potential safety risks is substantially different in these chronic inflammatory conditions as compared to more acutely life-threatening settings (like cancer and organ transplantation), where some of these types of immunomodulatory agents were first used. Besides the safety considerations, demonstration of therapeutic efficacy in these chronic inflammatory conditions also poses different challenges than for cancer or transplantation, because most of these disease courses wax and wane with episodic flares and spontaneous recoveries that complicate interpretation of efficacy in the short term. The hope for these newer therapies is that they will in fact provide safer and more tolerable therapeutic opportunities that can be used earlier in the course of disease to not only maintain control over the episodic disease flares, but also prevent the less reversible organ damage posed in the long-term from uncontrolled chronic inflammation.

There are already several agents with approvals for use in one or more specific forms of autoimmune arthritis including: rheumatoid arthritis (RA), juvenile rheumatoid arthritis (JRA), psoriatic arthritis (PsA), and ankylosing spondylitis (AS). Several agents are also now approved for use in one or more forms of inflammatory bowel disease, including fistulizing and/or non-fistulizing Crohn's disease (CD), and/or ulcerative colitis (UC). A few agents are approved for use in plaque psoriasis (PP) and only one targeted biologic treatment is approved for use in relapsing, remitting multiple sclerosis (RRMS). Also, as mentioned above, there is currently only one approved targeted agent for use in allergic asthma.

Though the list of indications continues to grow for these agents and newer agents every year, this chapter will focus on describing approved biologic therapies for only a few of the major inflammatory disease areas in order to provide a solid introduction, but without attempting to be exhaustive.

## ARTHRITIDES

Of all the autoimmune arthritides, RA is the most prevalent, affecting at least 1% of the general population in the United States. If not treated aggressively early in the course of disease RA can result in irreversible joint destruction, severe functional impairment and lead to a need for joint replacement surgery (Olsen and Stein, 2004). Although early intervention with steroids and DMARDs have helped demonstrate that the inflammatory course of RA can be interrupted and delayed, these therapies are not without significant side effects, and are not sufficient for many patients. For patients with safety issues or inadequate clinical efficacy with DMARDs, there are now many newer targeted options for treating RA including, anakinra (Kineret®), infliximab (Remicade®), etanercept (Enbrel®), adalimumab (Humira®), abatacept (Orencia®), and rituximab (Rituxan®) (Genovese, 2005).

The controlled clinical trials evaluating these agents in RA typically measure clinical efficacy over a 6 to 12 month period using a composite outcome like the one developed by and named after the American College of Rheumatology (ACR). For example, an ACR20 describes a 20 percent improvement from baseline on therapy in the number of tender and swollen joints plus a similar improvement in a composite of at least 3 out of 5 of the following: pain, patient's self global assessment, physician's global assessment, disability and a lab estimate of inflammation (erythrocyte sedimentation rate or C-reactive protein). A 50% or 70% improvement are termed ACR50 and ACR70, respectively. If a trial reports an ACR20 of 30% on active drug and 5% on placebo, that means the 30% of the patients receiving the active drug had a 20% improvement in the outcomes (as noted above) compared to only 5% of the patients receiving placebo. Product inserts also refer to "disease-modification," which is assessed in RA as a slowing in radiographic worsening of joint disease.

TNF-$\alpha$ is now recognized as a central inflammatory cytokine involved in endothelial permeability, upregulation of adhesion molecules and subsequent influx of leukocytes, activation of myeloid, granulocytic and lymphoid cell populations, induction of acute phase reactants from the liver and of proteolytic enzymes in tissues including cartilage and synovium. In addition both soluble and transmembrane forms of TNF-$\alpha$ are ubiquitous parts of cell death signaling pathways. Of the three approved anti-TNF therapies, one (etanercept) is a receptor-Fc fusion protein, whereas the other two (infliximab and adalimumab) are IgG$_1$ monoclonal antibodies. Although they have broadly similar efficacy and safety profiles in RA, there are significant differences in the three anti-TNF agents including their dosing characteristics, which are quite distinct (Furst et al., 2006).

### ■ Infliximab

Infliximab neutralizes biological activity of both soluble and transmembrane forms of TNF-$\alpha$, but does not neutralize TNF-$\beta$ (also known as lymphotoxin-$\alpha$), which utilizes the same receptors as TNF-$\alpha$. Infliximab is the only anti-TNF agent given intravenously, but has the longest potential dosing interval. It was also the first Food and Drug Administration (FDA) approved anti-TNF agent and has approvals in RA, PsA, AS, UC, adult and pediatric CD, and PP. For RA it is approved in combination with methotrexate "for reducing signs and symptoms, inhibiting the progression of structural damage and improving physical function in patients with moderately to severely active" disease. Pharmacokinetic studies in adults with single intravenous infusions of infliximab at 3 to 10 mg/kg showed linear kinetics, a median terminal half-life of 8.0 to 9.5 days, and the volume of distribution at steady state was independent of dose (i.e., primarily distributed within the vascular compartment). Multiple dose studies of IV infusions of infliximab at 3 to 10 mg/kg every 4 to 8 weeks showed no systemic accumulation, and after 8 weeks of maintenance dosing the median infliximab concentrations ranged from 0.5 to 6 μg/mL. Patients who developed anti-drug antibodies had increased drug clearance and undetectable (<0.1 μg/mL) serum trough concentrations at 8-week dosing intervals. No major differences in clearance or volume of distribution were observed in patient subsets defined by age, weight or gender, but it is unknown if these parameters are affected by impairment of renal or hepatic function.

The recommended dose of infliximab for RA is 3 mg/kg IV infusion given on an induction schedule at 0, 2, and 6 weeks followed by infusions every

8 weeks, though patients with incomplete responses may be given up to 10 mg/kg IV every 4 weeks. As a chimeric antibody infliximab is expected to have a higher rate of immunogenicity, and though the package insert mentions a rate of formation of anti-drug antibodies of approximately 10%. Higher rates are quoted in the literature and patients with anti-drug antibodies are more likely to have higher rates of drug clearance, reduced efficacy and a 2- to 3-fold increased incidence of infusion reactions. Other safety issues with infliximab include an increased risk of serious and opportunistic infections, malignancy, heart failure, and a significantly increased incidence of seroconversion for anti-nuclear (ANA) antibodies and anti-dsDNA antibodies. The label includes a black box warning and more specifics on infection and malignancy risks, and there is a contraindication for use of > 5 mg/kg dosing in patients with moderate to severe heart failure (St. Clair et al., 2002; package insert for Remicade, 2006).

## Etanercept

Etanercept is a dimeric soluble fusion protein composed of parts of the ligand binding regions of the p75 high-affinity type 2 TNF receptor (which binds both TNF-$\alpha$ and TNF-$\beta$ ) linked to parts of the IgG$_1$ Fc regions; it does not induce complement-mediated lysis of cells expressing TNF on their surface. Etanercept is FDA approved for use in patients with moderately to severely active RA (either used alone or in combination with methotrexate), as well as in polyarticular JRA, PsA, AS, and PP. For adult patients with RA, PsA, or AS the recommended dose of etanercept is 50 mg SC weekly, given either as one 50 mg injection or as two 25 mg injections on the same day or up to 4 days apart (package insert for Enbrel, 2006).

## Adalimumab

Adalimumab is a recombinant human IgG$_1$ monoclonal antibody to TNF-$\alpha$ that specifically blocks receptor binding of TNF-$\alpha$ (but not TNF-$\beta$); it also lyses cells expressing TNF-$\alpha$ on their surface in the presence of complement proteins. Adalimumab is currently FDA approved for use in patients with RA, PsA, and AS as a 40 mg dose SC every other week. It may be used in combination with glucocorticoids, salicylates, non-steroidal anti-inflammatory drugs (NSAIDs), analgesics, methotrexate or other DMARDs. In addition, an increased dosing frequency of 40 mg SC every week is on label for RA patients not receiving methotrexate in combination with adalimumab (package insert for Humira, 2006).

## Abatacept

Abatacept is indicated for use as monotherapy or in combination with DMARDs in patients with moderate to severe active rheumatoid arthritis who have had an inadequate response to DMARDs or TNF antagonists. Abatacept is a fusion protein consisting of the extracellular domain of human cytotoxic T-lymphocyte-associated antigen 4 and a modified Fc portion of IgG$_1$. Abatacept comes lyophilized and is administered after reconstitution in water by IV infusion over 30 minutes. The dose is weight-based such that patients weighing less than 60 kg receive 500 mg, patients weighing between 60 and 100 kg receive 750 mg, and patients weighing greater than 100 kg receive 1 gram. The dosing regimen consists of the first and second dose given 2 weeks apart followed my monthly dosing thereafter.

The interaction of CD80 and CD86 with CD28 is the costimulatory signal for full activation of T-lymphocytes. Abatacept is a costimulation modulator that binds CD80 and CD86 and blocks the interaction with CD28 inhibiting T-cell (T-lymphocyte) activation. The affinity of abatacept for its ligand is greater than the natural ligand CD28. Abatacept does not fix complement due to the modifications to the Fc portion of the molecule (Hervey and Keam, 2006).

In vitro studies demonstrated abatacept decreases T-cell proliferation and inhibits the production of TNF-$\alpha$, interferon-$\gamma$ (IFN$\gamma$), and IL-2 in one study and in IL-1$\beta$, IL-6 and matrix metalloproteinase-3 (MMP-3) in another. In the in vivo rat collagen-induced arthritis model, abatacept suppressed inflammation, decreased anti-collagen antibody production, and reduced antigen specific production of INF$\gamma$.

The pharmacokinetics after multiple doses of abatacept in RA patients was dose proportional between 2 and 10 mg/kg with steady-state achieved at 60 days. Steady-state clearance (mean) was 0.22 mL/hr/kg with mean peak and trough concentrations of 295 µg/mL and 24 µg/mL, respectively, with a half-life of 13.1 days (Hervey and Keam, 2006).

In clinical studies, abatacept treatment resulted in decreases of varying degrees in soluble interleukin-2 receptor (sIL-2r), IL6, MMP-3, C-reactive protein, TNF-$\alpha$ and rheumatoid factor. In a study of psoriasis patients, administration of abatacept reduced peak antibody titers associated with secondary immune responses (Abrams et al., 1999).

Anti-abatacept antibodies were detected in 1.7% (34/1993) patients overall. However, when assessed in discontinuing subjects in order to circumvent drug interference in the assay, 5.8% (9/154) had developed anti-abatacept antibodies. When anti-abatacept antibody positive subjects were assessed for neutralizing ability, 6/9 (67%) evaluable patients were shown to possess neutralizing antibodies.

In placebo controlled studies, ACR20, ACR50, and ACR70 scores (above placebo) ranged from 22% to 33%, 10% to 30%, and 6% to 23% depending on the duration of treatment and patient population. In the year long Abatacept in Inadequate Responders to Methotrexate (AIM) trial, treatment with abatacept inhibited the progression of radiographic evidence of structural joint damage as measured by Genant-modified Total Sharp Score (package insert for Orencia, 2006).

## ■ Rituximab

Rituximab in combination with methotrexate is indicated for the treatment of adult patients with moderate to severe rheumatoid arthritis who have had an inadequate response to one or more TNF antagonist therapies. Rituximab is a chimeric murine/human monoclonal antibody directed against the CD20 antigen found on the surface of B-lymphocytes. The antibody is an $IgG_1$ immunoglobulin containing murine light- and heavy-chain variable region sequences and human constant region sequences (see Chapter 16). Rituximab is given as two 1000 mg IV infusions separated by 2 weeks in combination with methotrexate. Glucocorticoids administered as methylprednisolone 100 mg IV or its equivalent 30 minutes prior to each infusion are recommended to reduce the incidence and severity of infusion reactions. After administration of the two 1000 mg doses of rituximab, the mean $C_{max}$ was 370 μg/mL. Mean volume of distribution was 4.3 L, mean systemic clearance was 0.01 L/h and mean terminal elimination half-life after the second dose was 19 days. Female patients with RA had a 37% lower clearance of rituximab than male patients, but this does not require dose adjustment.

Treatment of RA patients with rituximab results in nearly complete depletion of circulating B-cells within 2 weeks after receiving the first dose (Marin and Chan, 2006; Silverman, 2006). In clinical trials, the duration of B-cell depletion lasted for at least 6 months in the majority of patients with a gradual recovery thereafter. In a subset of patients (4%), B-cell depletion lasted for significantly longer. During treatment with rituximab, IgM, IgG, and IgA levels were reduced with the largest change in IgM. Mean immunoglobulin levels remained in the normal range with between 1% and 7% of subjects having individual values that fell below the lower limit of normal.

As with other RA treatments, rituximab treatment resulted in decreases in C-reactive protein, rheumatoid factor, and IL6. Additionally, reductions in serum amyloid protein (SAA), S100 A8/S100 A9 heterodimer complex (S100 A8/9) and anti-citrullinated peptide (anti-CCP). Efficacy of rituximab plus methotrexate at week 24 post first dose was significantly improved over placebo plus methotrexate, with 51% vs. 18% ACR20, 27% vs. 5% ACR50 and 12% vs. 1% ACR70. Development of anti-rituximab antibodies occurred in 5% of subjects (package insert for Rituxan,

2006). Use of corticosteroids to reduce the occurrence and severity of infusion reactions is recommended.

## PSORIASIS

Currently three biologic agents are approved for use in psoriasis: etanercept (Enbrel®), alefacept (Amevive®, which binds T and NK cells via CD2), and efalizumab (Raptiva®), the latter of which is further elaborated below.

## ■ Efalizumab

Efalizumab is indicated for the treatment of adult patients (>18 years of age) with moderate to severe plaque psoriasis. Efalizumab is a recombinant humanized $IgG_1$ isotype monoclonal antibody, which comes lyophilized and upon reconstitution will deliver 1.25 mL of a 100 mg/mL solution or 125 mg. The pH of the reconstituted product is 6.2. As is typical for protein therapeutics, the amount of active ingredient is larger than what is deliverable. This is due to properties of protein therapeutics in that due to viscosity or binding to vial after reconstitution, some drug product can not be withdrawn into a syringe for administration. Efalizumab must be reconstituted prior to administration and is dispensed with a single-use pre-filled syringe containing 1.3 mL of diluent. Efalizumab can be self-administered in the home by the patient.

The approved dose of efalizumab is 1 mg/kg/wk. This dose consistently resulted in the maximum effect on CD11a saturation and expression. In a comparison to the higher dose of 2 mg/kg/wk, there was no notable difference in the pharmacodynamics or efficacy profiles suggesting 1 mg/kg/wk is already at the top of the dose response curve. Efalizumab has not been tested in combination with other immunosuppressive medications such as methotrexate and cyclosporine.

The specificity of efalizumab is against the CD11a subunit of leukocyte function antigen-1 (LFA-1). LFA-1 consists of CD11a and CD18 and is primarily found on leukocytes but is also reported on activated platelets. Efalizumab exerts an immunosuppressive biologic effect by binding to CD11a thus interrupting the interaction of LFA-1 and its natural ligand intercellular adhesion molecule-1 (ICAM-1). In the absence of blockade by efalizumab, LFA-1/ICAM-1 binding stabilizes the immunological synapse necessary for an immune responses. The LFA-1/ICAM-1 interaction is also involved in the demargination of cells across the endothelium of blood vessels into tissues.

The effects of efalizumab have been extensively studied non-clinically in both in vitro and in vivo studies as well as in clinical trials. In vitro assays assessing T-cell activation showed efalizumab is able to block activation. Among the different cell types with LFA-1, the immunosuppressant effects on T-cells (CD4 and CD8 cells) have been the most extensively studied although efalizumab is known to attenuate primary immune responses to neoantigens.

Efalizumab pharmacokinetics have been well studied (Mortensen et al., 2005; Joshi et al., 2006). At the approved dose of 1 mg/kg, mean steady-state clearance was 24 mL/kg/day. Steady-state trough concentrations were approximately 9 µg/mL at the end of the approved 7-day dosing interval. Efalizumab is cleared through both receptor mediated and non-specific protein clearance mechanisms. The receptor-mediated clearance of efalizumab occurs through the binding of efalizumab to cell surface CD11a. The efalizumab-CD11a complex is then internalized and degraded (Coffey et al., 2004).

The primary pharmacodynamic marker for efalizumab is CD11a, the cell surface marker it targets. The amount of cell surface CD11a (CD11a expression) and saturation of CD11a binding sites on the cell surface were measured in clinical and non-clinical studies. Data from phase I/II studies with intravenous IV and SC administration of efalizumab were used to identify the optimal dose for psoriasis (Joshi et al., 2006). Treatment with efalizumab has been shown to blunt the secondary humoral immune response.

At doses of 1 mg/kg/wk SC, efalizumab consistently decreased the amount of CD11a on the surface of lymphocytes to <35% of baseline levels and saturated >95% of remaining cell surface CD11a. The effects on CD11a were not dose dependent beyond 1 mg/kg/wk suggesting this dose was at the top of the dose response curve. The maximal effect on CD11a occurs at concentrations between 1 and 3 µg/mL. The effects observed on CD11a were maintained throughout the dosing period but were reversible upon discontinuation.

In addition to CD11a expression and saturation, treatment related leukocytosis is a pharmacodynamic marker for efalizumab (Joshi et al., 2006). Consistent with the ability of efalizumab to inhibit LFA-1 mediated demargination, white blood cell counts increase during therapy with efalizumab. At the recommended dose of 1 mg/kg/wk, mean white blood cell counts increased 34% relative to baseline values. Among the leukocyte subsets, the increase in lymphocytes was the largest with a doubling of the baseline counts. Among the lymphocyte subsets tested, T-cells saw the greatest increase followed by B-cells then NK-cells. Similar to the effects on CD11a, the treatment related effects on absolute counts of circulating leukocytes and leukocyte subsets and lymphocyte subsets were reversible upon discontinuation of efalizumab.

In subjects who were evaluated, 6.3% (67/1063) developed anti-efalizumab antibodies. These were predominantly low-titer antibodies to efalizumab or other protein components of the drug product. Comparison of the incidence of antibodies to efalizumab relative to the incidence of antibodies to other products should be interpreted with caution due to ranges of sensitivity and specificity of this assay format across products.

The measure of response used in the pivotal trials of efalizumab was the Psoriasis Area and Severity Index (PASI) during the study. The PASI is a composite score that takes into consideration both the fraction of body surface area affected and the nature and severity of the psoriatic changes. After treatment with efalizumab, between 17% and 37% of subjects treated had a 75% reduction from their baseline PASI score (PASI-75) (package insert for Raptiva, 2006).

## MULTIPLE SCLEROSIS

### ■ Natalizumab

Natalizumab is a recombinant humanized IgG$_4$κ monoclonal antibody, is the first in a new class of selective adhesion molecule inhibitors and is used for the treatment of patients with relapsing forms of multiple sclerosis (MS) (package insert for Tysabri, 2006).

MS is a chronic inflammatory disease characterized by focal areas of nerve fiber and myelin destruction (lesions) within the central nervous system. The majority of individuals with MS develop a relapsing-remitting form of the disease (RRMS) (Weinshenker et al., 1989), which consists of episodic bouts of neurological deterioration, separated by periods of relative stability (Lublin and Reingold, 1996). Approximately 90% of untreated patients with RRMS develop a more progressive form of the disease (secondary progressive MS) (Weinshenker et al., 1989). There is no cure for MS; current therapies for RRMS modify the course of the disease by reducing the number of clinical relapses and slowing disability progression. Prior to the approval of natalizumab, available first-line therapies for patients with RRMS consisted of interferon-β (IFNβ) (Betaseron®), intramuscular (IM) IFNβ1a (Avonex®), and SC IFNβ1a (Rebif®) and glatiramer acetate (Copaxone®). These therapies reduce relapse rate by approximately 30% and slow disability progression by 12% to 37% (IFNβ Multiple Sclerosis Study Group, 1993; Jacobs et al., 1996; Johnson et al., 1995; PRISMS Study Group, 1998).

Natalizumab binds to the α$_4$ subunit of α$_4$β$_1$ (also known as very late antigen (VLA)-4) and α$_4$β$_7$ integrins, preventing its ability to interact with vascular-cell adhesion molecule-1 (VCAM-1; the endothelial receptor of $\alpha_4\beta_1$ integrin), mucosal addressin-cell adhesion molecule-1 (MadCAM-1; the endothelial receptor of $\alpha_4\beta_7$ integrin), fibronectin, osteopontin, and other extracellular matrix proteins. Natalizumab has also been studied for the potential treatment of CD (Sandborn et al., 2005) and rheumatoid arthritis. It is believed that natalizumab exerts its beneficial effects in MS by: (1) inhibiting the migration of immune cells into the central nervous system and (2) inhibiting interactions between $\beta_4$-integrin and its ligands, thereby possibly reducing immune cell activation and promoting apoptosis of lymphocytes (Rudick and Sandrock, 2004; Tchilian et al., 1997).

Following repeat IV administration of the approved dose of natalizumab (300 mg IV every 4 weeks) to patients with MS, the observed mean maximum serum concentration was $110\pm52$ g/mL, the mean average steady-state trough concentrations over the dosing period ranged from 23 to 29 g/mL, and the observed time to steady-state was approximately 24 weeks after every 4 weeks of dosing. The mean half-life was $11\pm4$ days, with a volume of distribution of $5.7\pm1.9$ L, and a clearance of $16\pm5$ mL/hour. Age and gender did not influence natalizumab pharmacokinetics (package insert for Tysabri 2006). Natalizumab increases the number of circulating leukocytes (lymphocytes, monocytes, basophils, and eosinophils, but not neutrophils) due to inhibition of transmigration out of the vascular space (package insert for Tysabri, 2006). Administration of natalizumab with IFNβ1a did not significantly alter the pharmacokinetic or pharmacodynamic profiles of natalizumab (Rudick and Sandrock, 2004; Vollmer et al., 2004).

The efficacy and safety of natalizumab were studied in two randomized, double-blind, placebo-controlled trials in patients with relapsing multiple sclerosis. The first study, the Natalizumab Safety and Efficacy in Relapsing Remitting Multiple Sclerosis (AFFIRM) study, evaluated natalizumab monotherapy. In AFFIRM, 942 patients were randomly assigned in a 2:1 ratio to receive natalizumab 300 mg ($n = 627$) or placebo ($n = 315$) administered as an IV infusion once every 4 weeks for up to 116 weeks (Polman et al., 2006). Compared with placebo, treatment with natalizumab significantly reduced the cumulative probability of sustained disability progression by 42% (HR 0.58, 95% CI 0.43, 0.77), the annualized rate of clinical relapse by 68% (0.23 vs. 0.73), and the risk of relapse by 59% (HR 0.41; 95% CI 0.34, 0.51) over 2 years (package insert for Tysabri, 2006; Polman et al., 2006). In addition, natalizumab reduced inflammatory activity and the accumulation of new lesions in the brain as shown by magnetic resonance imaging scans; the mean number of new or enlarging T2-hyperintense lesions was reduced by 83% and the mean number of

gadolinium-enhancing lesions by 92% in natalizumab-treated patients compared with placebo. The second study, the Safety and Efficacy of Natalizumab In Combination with Avonex (IFNβ1a) in Patients with Relapsing-Remitting MS study (SENTINEL), evaluated natalizumab in combination with IM IFNβ1a (Avonex®). In SENTINEL, 1,171 patients, who had experienced ≥1 relapse while receiving treatment with IFNβ1a 30 μg IM once weekly during the year prior to study entry, were randomly assigned to receive natalizumab 300 mg ($n = 589$) or placebo ($n = 582$) IV once every 4 weeks for up to 116 weeks; all patients continued treatment with IM IFNβ1a. Natalizumab significantly reduced the cumulative probability of sustained disability progression by 24% (HR 0.76, 95% CI: 0.61, 0.96), the annualized rate of clinical relapse by 55% (0.34 vs. 0.75), and the development of lesions over the effect produced by IFNβ1a alone (Rudick et al., 2006).

Natalizumab therapy was well tolerated in clinical trials. In the AFFIRM study, fatigue (27% natalizumab vs. 21% placebo) and allergic reaction (9% natalizumab vs. 4% placebo) were significantly ($P < 0.05$) more common in the natalizumab group than the placebo group (Polman et al. 2006). Serious adverse events occurred in 19% of patients in the natalizumab group and 24% in the placebo group ($P = 0.06$), with the most common being infection (3.2% vs. 2.6%), acute hypersensitivity reactions (1.1% vs. 0.3%), depression (1.0% for each group), and cholelithiasis (1.0% vs. 0.3%) (Polman et al., 2006). The incidence of infection was 79% in each treatment group; the rate of infection was 1.52 and 1.42 per patient-year in the natalizumab and placebo groups, respectively. Two deaths occurred in the natalizumab group (one due to malignant melanoma in a patient with a history of such and a new lesion at the time of the first natalizumab dose, and one due to alcohol intoxication).

Two cases of progressive multifocal leukoencephalopathy (PML) were reported in patients with MS treated with natalizumab in combination with IFNβ1a (Kleinschmidt-DeMasters and Tyler, 2005). A subsequent retrospective review of the natalizumab safety data identified an additional fatal case of PML in a patient with CD who had received eight infusions of natalizumab and had been previously diagnosed with astrocytoma (Van Assche et al., 2005). PML, which primarily affects individuals with suppressed immune systems, is an opportunistic infection of the brain that usually leads to death or severe disability. Symptoms of this rare disorder include mental deterioration, vision loss, speech disturbances, ataxia, paralysis, and, ultimately, coma. An evaluation of 3116 patients who received natalizumab in clinical trials of MS, CD, or rheumatoid arthritis found no new cases of PML (Yousry et al., 2006). Based on the results of this study (mean natalizumab exposure of 17.9 months), the estimated risk of PML associated with natalizumab is 1.0 in 1000 patients (95% CI 0.2, 2.8 per 1000) (Yousry et al., 2006).

Natalizumab is approved as monotherapy for the treatment of patients with relapsing forms of MS to delay the accumulation of physical disability and reduce the frequency of clinical exacerbations. Due to the increased risk of PML, natalizumab is generally recommended for patients who have had an inadequate response to, or are unable to tolerate, alternate MS therapies. Natalizumab is only available through a restricted distribution program (TOUCH™ Precribing Program (package insert for Tysabri, 2006). Under this program, only prescribers, pharmacies, and infusion centers enrolled in the program are able to prescribe, distribute, or infuse natalizumab. As part of TOUCH™), prescribers and patients are educated regarding the risk and symptoms of PML, and prescribers and infusion centers are instructed to withhold dosing immediately with any signs or symptoms suggestive of PML. As noted above, natalizumab is approved for use as monotherapy, as it is unknown whether the concomitant administration of natalizumab with other immunomodulatory agents increases PML risk (package insert for Tysabri, 2006).

## ALLERGIC ASTHMA

### ■ Omalizumab

Omalizumab (Xolair) is a recombinant humanized $IgG_1$ monoclonal antibody that selectively neutralizes soluble human IgE through binding at the same site utilized by the native high affinity receptor, Fc RI (Presta et al., 1994). Omalizumab is FDA approved for use by patients with allergic asthma inadequately controlled by inhaled corticosteroids, and is not only the first drug in this class of selective IgE inhibitors but also the first biologic therapy approved for asthma (package insert for Xolair, 2006).

Asthma is a syndrome of airway hyper-reactivity, which can result in potentially life-threatening bronchospasm. Bronchospastic exacerbations of asthma are triggered by noxious stimuli, most typically by airway inflammation resulting from either a viral respiratory infection or an aeroallergen (like dust mite, animal dander, pollen or mold). About 60% of asthmatics have allergic triggers of attacks.

IgE is a key intermediate in all forms of allergic disease because it is the interface between the inciting allergen and the resultant activation of effector cells (like mast cells and basophils), which can release histamine and other mediators of the allergic response. By directly neutralizing soluble IgE, omalizumab intervenes in this key intermediate step in the cascade of allergic inflammation and the resultant clinical exacerbation of allergic disease.

Doses of 150 to 375 mg of omalizumab are administered SC every 2 to 4 weeks using a table that adjusts target exposure based upon body weight and baseline levels of total IgE, aiming to achieve at least 0.016 mg/kg/IU in order to suppress free IgE levels below at least 50 ng/ml (package insert for Xolair, 2006; Hochhaus et al., 2003). With an average absolute bioavailability of 62% following a SC injection, peak serum concentrations of omalizumab are achieved after 7 to 8 days, with an apparent volume of distribution of $78 \pm 32$ mL/kg and linear PK at doses greater than 0.5 mg/kg. Following multiple doses SC, the serum omalizumab AUCs at steady state days 0 to 14 are up to 6-fold of those after the first dose. Omalizumab forms multiple stoichiometric complexes with IgE and is eliminated as complexes from the circulation via Fcγ receptors via the reticuloendothelial system at a rate generally faster than standard IgG clearance. It is also excreted in bile. Serum elimination half-life of omalizumab averaged 26 days, with apparent clearance averaging $2.4 \pm 1.1$ mL/kg/day; a doubling of body weight was noted to double apparent clearance. Serum free IgE levels decreased greater than 96% using the dosing table, with 98% of individuals having free IgE levels at or below 50 ng/mL by 3 months of multiple dosing per schedule. Because omalizumab forms complexes with IgE and these complexes has a slower elimination rate than free (unbound, monomeric) IgE, after omalizumab therapy there is an apparent increase in total IgE using standard laboratory tests which cannot distinguish bound from free IgE. Following discontinuation of omalizumab there is a slow (up to 12 months) washout of drug:IgE complexes without an apparent rebound increase in free IgE levels. No dose adjustment appears necessary for age (12–76 years), race, ethnicity, or gender (package insert for Xolair, 2006).

Pivotal safety and efficacy trials evaluated patients with moderate to severe persistent asthma per National Heart, Lung and Blood Institute criteria who were defined as having allergic-type asthma based upon a positive test to a perennial allergen. Total baseline IgE had to be between 30 and 700 IU/mL and body weight not more than 150 kg in order to use the dosing table.

Though some therapeutic effects on allergic and asthma symptoms, pulmonary function and need for concomitant medications were seen, omalizumab efficacy was based primarily on the reduction of asthma exacerbations, which were defined as a worsening of asthma that required treatment with systemic corticosteroids or a doubling of baseline inhaled corticosteroid dose.

Omalizumab was very well tolerated in the clinical trials, with only a slight increase in injection site reactions compared to controls. The incidence of anti-drug antibodies was reported as 1/1723 (<0.1%), which is an extremely low immunogenicity rate compared to nearly every other biologic therapy (package insert for Xolair, 2006).

Warnings were placed on the label regarding malignancy and anaphylaxis based on a numerically higher incidence of these events in the active vs. control groups. Malignant neoplasms were seen in 20 of 4127 (0.5%) of omalizumab-treated patients vs. 5 of 2236 (0.2%) of controls, with no specific pattern noted in terms of tumor types. Anaphylactoid reactions (with urticaria and throat and/or tongue edema) within 2 hours of the first or subsequent infusion of omalizumab were noted in 3 (<0.1%) patients without other identifiable allergic triggers (package insert for Xolair 2006). Therefore omalizumab is to be administered under appropriate medical observation with medications for the treatment of severe hypersensitivity reactions including anaphylaxis available.

## CONCLUSION

Decision making regarding how best to use these newer biological therapies may seem more like an art than a science. Considering the basics of therapeutics, one must always start by confirming the correct diagnosis (i.e., be sure the patient has RA and not gout or an infectious arthritis) and then individually assessing the patient's situation to decide with the patient what is the best choice for them at that time. Standard of care is to combine and escalate therapy based upon clinical presentation, starting for example in most RA patients with an NSAID and/or corticosteroids for controlling acute symptoms and then adding on DMARDs like methotrexate for more chronic control to slow disease progression (i.e., more pervasive and permanent joint involvement and longer term disability). The transition to DMARDs is accompanied by reduction and minimization of NSAID and steroid use, and close follow-up of side effects, active disease flares and chronic progression of disease. Similar escalation of therapy is also still typical in other disease areas with biologic therapies including use of omalizumab in asthma and natalizumab in MS. Though these therapies are expensive compared to more common "small molecule" therapies, they are also much more expensive to develop and manufacture than small molecule drugs. In the balance however, they appear to not only give targeted relief of symptoms with a better side effect profile than traditional medications, but may also offer an opportunity to modify the course of these diseases, as has been demonstrated in RA. It is for this hope of modifying the disease course, if not eventually curing or preventing the onset of disease altogether, that these therapies hold the greatest promise.

## REFERENCES

Abrams JR, Lebwohl MG, Guzzo CA, et al. (1999). CTLA4Ig-mediated blockade of T-cell costimulation in patients with psoriasis vulgaris. J Clin Invest 103(9):1243–52.

Coffey GP, Stefanich E, Palmieri S, et al. (2004). In vitro internalization, intracellular transport, and clearance of an anti-CD11a antibody (Raptiva) by human T-cells. J Pharmaco Exp Ther 310(3):896–904.

Furst DE, Breedveld FC, Kalden JR, et al. (2006). Updated consensus statement on biological agents for the treatment of rheumatic diseases. Ann Rheum Dis 65(Suppl3):2—15.

Genovese MC. (2005). Biologic therapies in clinical development for the treatment of rheumatoid arthritis. J Clin Rheum 11(3):S45–54.

Hervey PS, Keam SJ. (2006). Abatacept. Biodrugs 20(1):53–61.

Hochhaus G, Brookman L, Fox H, et al. (2003). Pharmacodynamics of omalizumab: implications for optimised dosing strategies and clinical efficacy in the treatment of allergic asthma. Curr Med Res Opin 19(6):491–8.

IFNb Multiple Sclerosis Study Group. (1993). Interferon beta-1b is effective in relapsing-remitting multiple sclerosis. I. Clinical results of a multicenter, randomized, double-blind, placebo-controlled trial. Neurology 43:655–61.

Jacobs LD, Cookfair DL, Rudick RA, et al. (1996). Intramuscular interferon beta-1a for disease progression in relapsing multiple sclerosis. Ann Neurol 39:285–94.

Johnson KP, Brooks BR, Cohen JA, et al. (1995). Copolymer 1 reduces relapse rate and improves disability in relapsing-remitting multiple sclerosis: results of a phase III multicenter, double-blind placebo-controlled trial. Neurology 45:1268–76.

Joshi A, Bauer R, Kuebler P, et al. (2006). An overview of the pharmacokinetics and pharmacodynamics of efalizumab: a monoclonal antibody approved for use in psoriasis. J Clin Pharm 46(1):10–20.

Kleinschmidt-DeMasters BK, Tyler KL. (2005). Progressive multifocal leukoencephalopathy complicating treatment with natalizumab and interferon beta-1a for multiple sclerosis. N Engl J Med 353(4):369–74.

Lublin FD, Reingold SC. (1996). Defining the clinical course of multiple sclerosis: results of an international survey. Neurology 46:907–11.

Martin F, Chan AC. (2006). B Cell Immunobiology in Disease: Evolving Concepts from the Clinic. Annu Rev Immunol 24:467–96.

Mortensen DL, Walicke PA, Wang X, et al. (2005). Pharmacokinetics and pharmacodynamics of multiple weekly subcutaneous efalizumab doses in patients with plaque psoriasis. J Clin Pharm 45(3):286–98.

Olsen NJ, Stein CM. (2004). New drugs for rheumatoid arthritis. N Engl J Med 350:2167–79.

Package insert for Enbrel (etanercept). (Accessed December 2006 at www.enbrel.com).

Package insert for Humira (adalimumab). (Accessed December 2006 at www.humira.com).

Package insert for Orencia (abatacept). (Accessed December 2006 at www.orencia.com).

Package insert for Raptiva (efalizumab). (Accessed December 2006 at www.raptiva.com).

Package insert for Remicade(infliximab). (Accessed December 2006 at www.remicade.com).

Package insert for Rituxan (rituximab). (Accessed December 2006 at www.rituxan.com).

Package insert for Tysabri® (natalizumab). (Accessed December 2006 www.tysabri.com).

Package insert for Xolair (omalizumab). (Accessed December 2006 at www.xolair.com).

Polman CH, O'Connor PW, Havrdova E, et al. (2006). A randomized, placebo-controlled trial of natalizumab for relapsing multiple sclerosis. N Eng J Med 354(9):899–910.

Presta, L, Shields, R, O'Connell, L, et al. (1994). The binding site on human immunoglobulin E for its high affinity receptor. J Biol Chem 269:26368–73.

PRISMS (Prevention of Relapses and Disability by Interferon beta-1a Subcutaneously in Multiple Sclerosis) Study Group. (1998). Randomised double-blind placebo-controlled study of interferon beta-1a in relapsing/remitting multiple sclerosis. Lancet 352:1498–504.

Rudick RA, Sandrock A. (2004). Natalizumab: 4-integrin antagonist selective adhesion molecule inhibitors for MS. Expert Rev Neurotherapeutics 4(4):571–80.

Rudick RA, Stuart WH, Calabresi PA, et al. (2006). A randomized, placebo-controlled trial of natalizumab plus interferon beta-1a for relapsing multiple sclerosis. N Engl J Med 354:911–23.

Sandborn WJ, Colombel JF, Enns R, et al. (2005). Natalizumab induction and maintenance therapy for Crohn's disease. N Engl J Med 353(18):1912–25.

Silverman GJ. (2006). Therapeutic B Cell Depletion and Regeneration in Rheumatoid Arthritis: Emerging Patterns and Paradigms. Arth Rheum 43(8):2356–67.

St. Clair EW, Wagner CL, Fasanmade AA, et al. (2002). The relationship of serum infliximab concentrations to clinical improvement in rheumatoid arthritis: results from ATTRACT, a multicenter, randomized, double-blind, placebo-controlled trial. Arthritis Rheum 46:1451—9.

Tchilian EZ, Owen JJ, Jenkinson EJ. (1997). Anti- 4 integrin antibody induces apoptosis in murine thymocytes and staphylococcal enterotoxin B-activated lymph node T cells. Immunology 92(3):321–7.

Van Assche G, Van Ranst M, Sciot R, et al. (2005). Progressive multifocal leukoencephalopathy after natalizumab therapy for Crohn's disease. N Engl J Med 353(4):362–8.

Vollmer TL, Phillips JT, Goodman AD, et al. (2004). An open-label safety and drug interaction study of natalizumab (Antegren™) in combination with interferon-beta (Avonex®) in patients with multiple sclerosis. Mult Scler 10:511–20.

Weinshenker BG, Bass B, Rice GPA, et al. (1989). The natural history of multiple sclerosis: a geographically based study. I. Clinical course and disability. Brain 112:133–46.

Yousry TA, Major EO, Ryschkewitsch C, et al. (2006). Evaluation of patients treated with natalizumab for progressive multifocal leukoencephalopathy. N Eng J Med 2006; 354(9):924–33.

# 19

# Recombinant Human Deoxyribonuclease I

*Robert A. Lazarus*
Genentech, Inc., South San Francisco, California, U.S.A.

*Jeffrey S. Wagener*
Department of Pediatrics, University of Colorado Medical School, Denver, Colorado, U.S.A.

## PHARMACOTHERAPY INFORMATION

Further information on the applied pharmacotherapy with recombinant human DNase I can be found in the following frequently used textbooks:

- *Applied Therapeutics: The Clinical Use of Drugs* (Koda-Kimble, MA, et al., Eds.), 8th edition, Lippincott Williams & Wilkins, Baltimore 2005: Chapter 98.
- *Pharmacotherapy: A Pathophysiologic Approach* (DiPiro, JT, et al., Eds.), 6th edition, McGraw-Hill, New York 2005: Chapter 30.
- *Textbook of Therapeutics: Drug and Disease Management* (Helms, RA, et al., Eds.), 8th edition, Lippincott Williams & Wilkins Baltimore 2006: Chapters 7, 36.

## INTRODUCTION

Human deoxyribonuclease I (DNase I) is an endonuclease that catalyzes the hydrolysis of extracellular DNA. It is the most extensively studied member of a family of DNase I-like nucleases (Lazarus, 2002; Baranovskii et al., 2004; Shiokawa and Tanuma, 2001); the homologous bovine DNase I has received even greater attention historically (Laskowski, 1971; Moore, 1981; Chen and Liao, 2006). Mammalian DNases have been broadly divided into several families initially based upon their products, pH optima and divalent metal ion requirements. These include the neutral DNase I family (EC 3.1.21.1), the acidic DNase II family (EC 3.1.22.1), as well as apoptotic nucleases such as DFF40/CAD and endonuclease G (Lazarus, 2002; Evans and Aguilera, 2003; Widlak and Garrard, 2005). The human DNase I gene resides on chromosome 16p13.3 and contains 10 exons and 9 introns, which span 15 kb of genomic DNA (Kominato et al. 2006). DNase I is synthesized as a precursor and contains a 22-residue signal sequence that is cleaved upon secretion, resulting in the 260-residue mature enzyme. It is secreted by the pancreas and parotid glands, consistent with its proposed primary role of digesting nucleic acids in the gastrointestinal tract. However it is also present in blood and urine as well as other tissues, suggesting additional functions.

Recombinant human DNase I (rhDNase I, rhDNase, Pulmozyme® dornase alfa) has been developed clinically where it is aerosolized into the airways for treatment of pulmonary disease in patients with cystic fibrosis (CF) (Suri, 2005). CF is an autosomal recessive disease caused by mutations in the cystic fibrosis transmembrane conductance regulator (CFTR) gene (Kerem et al., 1989; Riordan et al., 1989). Mutations of this gene result in both abnormal quantity and function of an apical membrane protein responsible for chloride ion transfer. The CFTR protein is a member of the ATP-binding cassette transporter superfamily (member ABCC7) and in addition to transporting chloride has many other functions including the regulation of epithelial sodium channels, ATP-release mechanisms, anion exchangers, sodium bicarbonate transporters, and aquaporin water channels found in airways, intestine, pancreas, sweat duct and other fluid-transporting tissues (Guggino and Stanton, 2006). Clinical manifestations of the disease include chronic obstructive airway disease, increased sweat electrolyte excretion, male infertility due to obstruction of the vas deferens, and exocrine pancreatic insufficiency. In the airways, abnormal CFTR is associated with formation of dehydrated, viscous mucus that results in obstructions. These obstructed airways become chronically infected with bacteria, which then leads to chronic, excessive neutrophilic airway inflammation. Necrosis of neutrophils results in airway damage and further obstruction from release of cell constituents precipitating a progressive downward spiral of lung damage and loss of lung function, ultimately resulting in premature death (Fig. 1).

The use of rhDNase I has been investigated in other diseases where exogenous DNA has been implicated pathologically, although it is only approved for use in CF. rhDNase I has been studied in

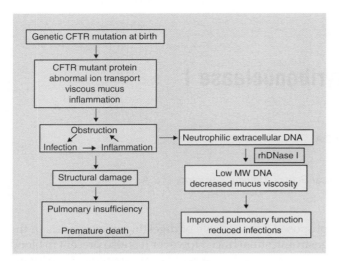

**Figure 1** ▨ Cystic fibrosis and rhDNase I. CFTR genetic mutation at birth leads to either reduced or improperly folded CFTR protein, which results in altered ion transport, viscous mucus and inflammation in the airways. Eventually this leads to obstruction of the airways, bacterial infection and further inflammation. After neutrophils arrive to fight the infection, they die and release cellular contents, one of which is DNA. Persistent obstruction, infection and inflammation leads to structural damage and eventually pulmonary insufficiency and premature death. rhDNase I is aerosolized into the airways where it degrades DNA to lower molecular weight fragments, thus reducing CF mucus viscosity and allowing expectoration, which improves lung function and reduces bacterial infections. *Abbreviations*: CF, cystic fibrosis; CFTR, cystic fibrosis transmembrane conductance regulator.

systemic lupus erythematosus (SLE), where degradation or prevention of immune complexes containing anti-DNA antigens may have therapeutic benefit (Davis et al., 1999). rhDNase I has also been studied in a variety of other diseases where extracellular DNA has been postulated to play a pathological role, including mechanical ventilation (Riethmueller et al., 2006), atelectasis (Hendriks et al., 2005), chronic sinusitis (Cimmino et al., 2005) and empyema (Simpson et al., 2003).

■ **Historical Perspective and Rationale**

Macromolecules that contribute to the physical properties of lung secretions include mucus glycoproteins, filamentous actin and DNA. Experiments in the 1950s and 1960s revealed that DNA is present in very high concentrations (3–14 mg/mL) only in infected lung secretions (Matthews et al., 1963). This implied that the DNA that contributes to the high viscoelastic nature of CF sputum is derived from neutrophils responding to chronic infections (Potter et al., 1969). These DNA-rich secretions also bind aminoglycoside antibiotics commonly used for treatment of pulmonary infections and thus may reduce their efficacy (Ramphal et al., 1988; Batallion et al., 1992).

Early in vitro studies in which lung secretions were incubated for several hours with partially purified bovine pancreatic DNase I showed a large reduction in viscosity (Armstrong and White, 1950; Chernick et al., 1961). Based on these observations, bovine pancreatic DNase I (Dornavac or Pancreatic Dornase) was approved in the United States for human use in 1958. Numerous uncontrolled clinical studies in patients with pneumonia and one study in patients with CF suggested that bovine pancreatic DNase I was effective in reducing the viscosity of lung secretions (Lieberman, 1968). However, severe adverse reactions occurred occasionally, perhaps due to allergic reactions to a foreign protein or from contaminating proteases, since up to 2% trypsin and chymotrypsin were present in the final product (Raskin, 1968; Lieberman, 1962). Both bovine DNase I products were eventually withdrawn from the market.

In the late 1980s human deoxyribonuclease I was cloned from a human pancreatic cDNA library, sequenced and expressed recombinantly using mammalian cell culture in Chinese hamster ovary (CHO) cells to re-evaluate the potential of DNase I as a therapeutic for CF (Shak et al., 1990). In vitro incubation of purulent sputum from CF patients with catalytic concentrations of rhDNase I reduced its viscoelasticity (Shak et al., 1990). The reduction in viscoelasticity was directly related to both rhDNase I concentration and to reduction in the size of the DNA in the samples. Therefore, reduction of high molecular weight DNA into smaller fragments by treatment with aerosolized rhDNase I was proposed as a mechanism to reduce the mucus viscosity and improve mucus clearability from obstructed airways in patients. It was hoped that improved clearance of the purulent mucus would enhance pulmonary function and reduce recurrent exacerbations of respiratory symptoms requiring parenteral antibiotics. This proved to be the case and rhDNase I was approved by the Food and Drug Administration in 1993.

## PROTEIN CHEMISTRY, ENZYMOLOGY, AND STRUCTURE

The protein chemistry of human DNases including DNase I, has been recently reviewed by Lazarus (2002) and Baranovskii et al. (2004). Recombinant human DNase I is a monomeric, 260-amino acid glycoprotein (Fig. 2) produced by mammalian CHO cells (Shak et al. 1990). The protein has four cysteines, which are oxidized into two disulfides between Cys101-Cys104 and Cys173-Cys209 as well as two potential N-linked glycosylation sites at Asn18 and Asn106 (Fig. 2). rhDNase I is glycosylated at both sites and migrates as a broad band on polyacrylamide gel

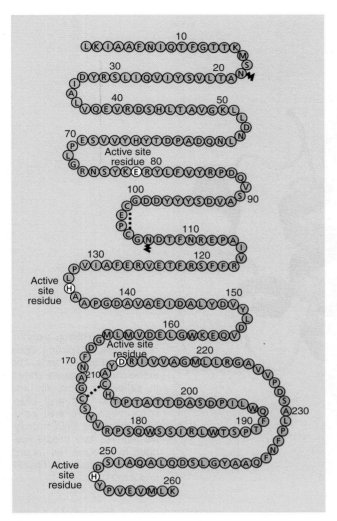

**Figure 2** ▪ Primary amino acid sequence of rhDNase I. Active site residues, disulfide bonds and N-linked glycosylation sites are highlighted.

electrophoresis gels with an approximate molecular weight of 37 kDa, which is significantly higher than the predicted molecular mass from the amino acid sequence of 29.3 kDa. rhDNase I is an acidic protein and has a calculated pI of 4.58. The primary amino acid sequence is identical to that of the native human enzyme purified from urine.

DNase I cleaves double-stranded DNA, and to a much lesser degree single-stranded DNA, non-specifically by nicking phosphodiester linkages in one of the strands between the 3′-oxygen atom and the phosphorus to yield 3′-hydroxyl and 5′-phosphoryl oligonucleotides with inversion of configuration at the phosphorus. rhDNase I enzymatic activity is dependent upon the presence of divalent metal ions for structure, as there are two tightly bound $Ca^{2+}$ atoms, and catalysis, which requires either $Mg^{2+}$ or $Mn^{2+}$ (Pan and Lazarus, 1999). The active site includes two histidine residues (His134 and His252) and two acidic

residues (Glu78 and Asp 212), all of which are critical for the general acid–base catalysis of phosphodiester bonds since alanine substitution of any of these results in a total loss of activity (Ulmer et al., 1996). The two $Ca^{2+}$ binding sites require acidic or polar residues for coordination of $Ca^{2+}$; for site 1 these include Asp201 and Thr203 and for site 2 these include Asp99, Asp107, and Glu112 (Pan and Lazarus, 1999). Other residues involved in the coordination of divalent metal ions at the active site and DNA contact residues have been identified by mutational analysis (Pan et al., 1998a). DNase I is a relatively stable enzyme and shows optimal activity at pH 5.5 to 7.5. It is inactivated by heat and is potently inhibited by EDTA and G-actin. Surprisingly, DNase I is also inhibited by NaCl and has only ca. 30% of the maximal activity in physiological saline.

The X-ray crystal structure of rhDNase I has been solved at 2.2 Å resolution and superimposes with the biochemically more widely studied bovine DNase I, which shares 78% sequence identity, with an rms deviation for main chain atoms of 0.56 Å (Wolf et al., 1995). DNase I is a compact α/β protein having a core of two tightly packed six-stranded β-sheets surrounded by eight α-helices and several loop regions (Fig. 3). Bovine DNase I has also been crystallized in complex with G-actin (Kabsch et al., 1990) as well as with several short oligonucleotides, revealing key features of DNA recognition in the minor groove and catalytic hydrolysis (Suck, 1994).

Several variants of rhDNase I with greatly improved enzymatic properties have been engineered by site-directed mutagenesis. The methods for production of the variants and the assays to characterize them have been reviewed recently (Pan and Lazarus, 1997; Sinicropi et al., 2001). The rationale for improving activity was to increase binding affinity to DNA by introducing positively charged residues (Arg or Lys) on rhDNase I loops at the DNA binding interface to form a salt bridge with phosphates on the DNA backbone. These so-called "hyperactive" rhDNase I variants are substantially more active than wildtype rhDNase I, and are no longer inhibited by physiological saline. The greater catalytic activity of the hyperactive variants is due to a change in the catalytic mechanism from a "single nicking" activity in the case of wildtype rhDNase I to a "processive nicking" activity in the hyperactive rhDNase I variants (Pan and Lazarus, 1997), where gaps rather than nicks result in a higher frequency of double strand cleavages.

It is interesting to note that significantly greater activity can result from just a few mutations on the surface that are not important for structural integrity. For whatever reason DNase I is not as efficient an enzyme as it could be for degrading DNA into small fragments. Furthermore the inhibition by G-actin can

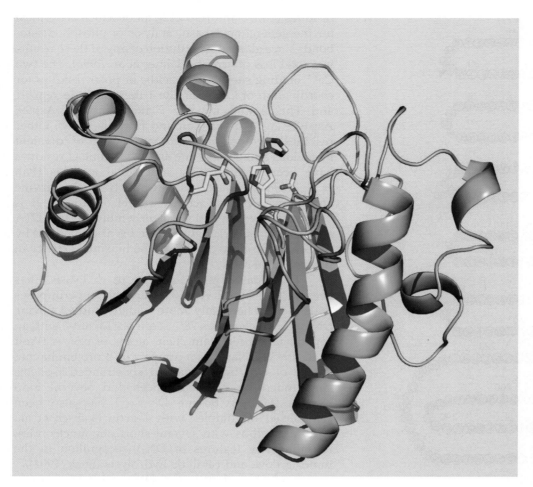

**Figure 3** ▨ Ribbon diagram of rhDNase I depicting alpha helices and beta strands. The active site residues are shown in yellow and oxygen and nitrogen in red and blue, respectively. General acid-base catalyzed DNA hydrolysis requires four critical residues: foreground, His134 and Glu78; background, His252 and Asp212.

be eliminated by a single amino acid substitution (see below). Thus DNase I is under some degree of regulation in vivo. One can only speculate that nature may have wanted to avoid an enzyme with too much DNA degrading activity that could result in undesired mutations in the genome.

## PHARMACOLOGY

### ■ In Vitro Activity in CF Sputum

In vitro, rhDNase I hydrolyzes the DNA in sputum of CF patients and reduces sputum viscoelasticity (Shak et al., 1990). Effects of rhDNase I were initially examined using a relatively crude "pourability" assay. Pourability was assessed qualitatively by inverting the tubes and observing the movement of sputum after a tap on the side of the tube. Catalytic amounts of rhDNase I (50 μg/mL) greatly reduced the viscosity of the sputum, rapidly transforming it from a viscous gel to a flowing liquid. More than 50% of the sputum moved down the tube within 15 minutes of incubation, and all the sputum moved freely down the tube within 30 minutes. The qualitative results of the pourability assay were confirmed by quantitative measurement of viscosity using a Brookfield Cone-Plate viscometer (Fig. 4). The reduction of viscosity by rhDNase I is rhDNase I concentration-dependent and is associated with reduction in size of sputum DNA as measured by agarose gel electrophoresis (Fig. 5).

Additional in vitro studies of CF mucus samples treated with rhDNase I demonstrated a dose-dependent improvement in cough transport and mucociliary transport of CF mucus using a frog palate model and a reduction in adhesiveness as measured by mucus contact angle (Zahm et al., 1995). The improvements in mucus transport properties and adhesiveness were associated with a decrease in mucus viscosity and mucus surface tension, suggesting rhDNase I treatment may improve the clearance of mucus from airways. The in vitro viscoelastic properties of rhDNase I have also been studied in combination with normal saline, 3% hypertonic saline or Nacystelyn, the L-lysine salt of N-acetyl cysteine (King et al., 1997; Dasgupta and King, 1996). The major impact of rhDNase I on CF sputum is to decrease spinnability, which is the thread forming ability of mucus under the influence of low amplitude stretching. CF sputum spinnability decreases 25%

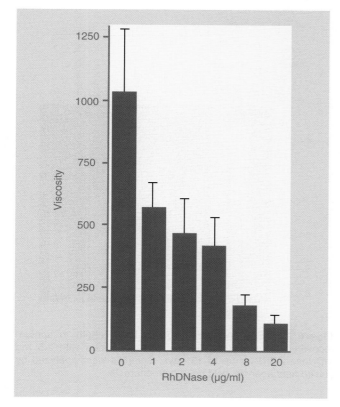

**Figure 4** ▨ In vitro reduction in viscosity (in centipoise) of cystic fibrosis sputum by cone-plate viscometry. Cystic fibrosis sputum was incubated with various concentrations of rhDNase I of 15 minutes at 37°C.

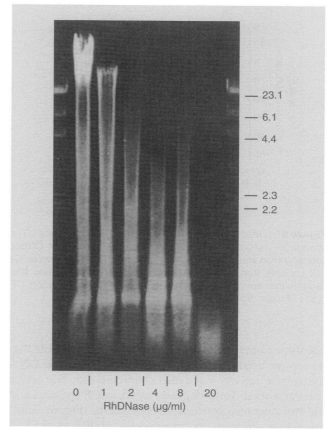

**Figure 5** ▨ In vitro reduction in sputum DNA size as measured by agarose gel electrophoresis. Cystic fibrosis sputum was incubated with increasing concentrations (0–20 μg/mL) of rhDNase I for 150 minutes at 37°C. Outside lanes are molecular weight standards for DNA in kDa.

after 30 minutes incubation with rhDNase I (King et al., 1997). rhDNase I in normal saline and saline alone both increased the cough clearability index. With the combination of rhDNase I and 3% hypertonic saline, there was minimal effect on spinnability, however, mucus rigidity and cough clearability improved greater than with either agent alone. The predicted mucociliary clearance did not significantly increase with 3% saline either alone or in combination with rhDNase I. Combining rhDNase I with Nacystelyn has an additive benefit on spinnability, but no effect on mucus rigidity or cough clearability (Dasgupta and King, 1996). These effects of rhDNase I can be variable in vivo and do not necessarily correlate with the level of DNA in sputum. For example, sputum from CF patients that clinically responded to rhDNase I contains significantly higher levels of magnesium ions compared with sputum from patients who do not have a clear response (Sanders et al., 2006). Although this response is consistent with the requirement for divalent cations and their mode of action on DNase I (Campbell and Jackson, 1980), the mechanism of increased rhDNase I activity by magnesium ions has been attributed to altering the polymerization state of actin such that

equilibrium favors increased F-actin and decreased G-actin (see below).

The mechanism of action of rhDNase I to reduce CF sputum viscosity has been ascribed to DNA hydrolysis (Shak et al., 1990). However, an alternative mechanism involving depolymerization of filamentous actin (F-actin) has been suggested since F-actin contributes to the viscoelastic properties of CF sputum and the actin-depolymerizing protein gelsolin also reduces sputum viscoelasticity (Vasconcellos et al., 1994). F-actin is in equilibrium with its monomeric form (G-actin), which binds to rhDNase I with high affinity and is also a potent inhibitor of DNase I activity (Lazarides and Lindberg, 1974). DNase I is known to depolymerize F-actin by binding to G-actin with high affinity, shifting the equilibrium in favor of rhDNase I/G-actin complexes (Hitchcock et al., 1976). To elucidate the mechanism of rhDNase I in CF sputum, the activity of two types of rhDNase I variants were compared in CF sputum (Ulmer et al., 1996). Active site variants were engineered that were unable to catalyze DNA hydrolysis but retained

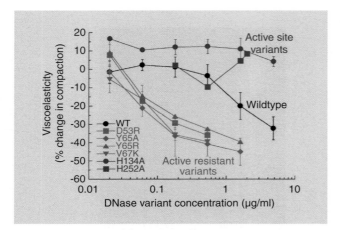

**Figure 6** ▪ Mechanism of action in CF mucus for rhDNase I. The change in viscoelasticity in CF mucus as a function of DNase concentration was determined for wildtype rhDNase I, two active site variants that no longer catalyze DNA hydrolysis and four variants that are no longer inhibited by G-actin. *Abbreviation*: CF, cystic fibrosis. *Source*: From Ulmer et al., 1996.

wildtype G-actin binding. Actin-resistant variants that no longer bound G-actin but retained wildtype DNA hydrolytic activity were also characterized. The active site variants did not degrade DNA in CF sputum and did not decrease sputum viscoelasticity (Fig. 6). Since the active site variants retained the ability to bind G-actin these results argue against depolymerization of F-actin as the mechanism of action. In contrast, the actin-resistant variants were more potent than wildtype DNase I in their ability to degrade DNA and reduce sputum viscoelasticity (Fig. 6). The increased potency of the actin-resistant variants indicated that G-actin was a significant inhibitor of wildtype DNase I in CF sputum and confirmed that hydrolysis of DNA was the mechanism by which rhDNase I decreases sputum viscoelasticity. The mechanism for reduction of sputum viscosity by gelsolin was subsequently determined to result from an unexpected second binding site on actin that competes with DNase I, thus relieving the inhibition by G-actin (Davoodian et al., 1997). Additional in vitro studies characterizing the relative potency of actin-resistant and hyperactive rhDNase I variants in serum and CF sputum have been reported (Pan et al., 1998b).

■ **In Vivo Activity in CF Sputum**

In vivo confirmation of the proposed mechanism of action for rhDNase I has been obtained from direct characterization of apparent DNA size (Fig. 7) and measurements of enzymatic and immunoreactive (ELISA) activity of rhDNase I (Fig. 8) in sputum from CF patients (Sinicropi et al., 1994a). Sputum samples were obtained one to six hours post-dose from adult CF patients after inhalation of 5 to 20 mg of rhDNase I.

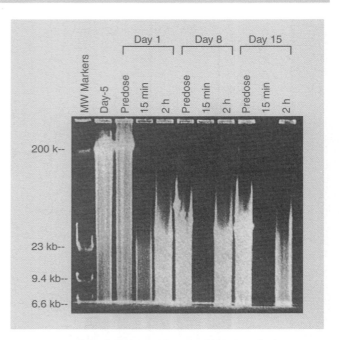

**Figure 7** ▪ Sustained reduction in DNA length in sputum recovered from a cystic fibrosis patient treated with 2.5 mg rhDNase I BID for up to 15 days. Samples were analyzed by pulsed field agarose field gel electrophoresis.

rhDNase I therapy produced a sustained reduction in DNA size in recovered sputum (Fig. 7), in good agreement with the in vitro data.

Inhalation of the therapeutic dose of rhDNase I produced sputum levels of rhDNase I which have been shown to be effective in vitro (Fig. 8) (Shak, 1995).

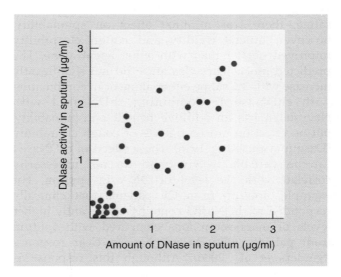

**Figure 8** ▪ Immunoreactive concentrations and enzymatic activity of rhDNase I in sputum following aerosol administration of either 10 mg (•) or 20 mg (•) rhDNase I to patients with cystic fibrosis. Each data point is a separate sample measured in duplicate.

The recovered rhDNase I was also enzymatically active. Enzymatic activity was directly correlated with rhDNase I concentrations in the sputum. Viscoelasticity was reduced in the recovered sputum, as well. Furthermore, results from scintigraphic studies in using twice daily 2.5 mg of rhDNase I in CF patients suggested possible reductions in pulmonary obstruction and increased rates of mucociliary sputum clearance from the inner zone of the lung compared to controls (Laube et al., 1996). This finding was not confirmed in a cross-over design study using once daily dosing, suggesting that improvement of mucociliary clearance may require higher doses (Robinson et al., 2000).

## ■ Pharmacokinetics and Metabolism

Non-clinical pharmacokinetic data in rats and monkeys suggest minimal systemic absorption of rhDNase I following aerosol inhalation of clinically-equivalent doses. rhDNase I is cleared from the systemic circulation without any accumulation in tissues following acute exposure (Green, 1994). Additionally, non-clinical metabolism studies suggest that the low rhDNase I concentrations present in serum following inhalation will be bound to binding proteins (Green, 1994; Mohler et al., 1993). The low concentrations of endogenous DNase I normally present in serum and the low concentrations of rhDNase I in serum following inhalation are inactive due to the ionic composition and presence of binding proteins in serum (Prince, 1998).

When 2.5 mg of rhDNase I was administered twice daily by inhalation to 18 CF patients, mean sputum concentrations of 2 µg/mL DNase I were measurable within 15 minutes after the first dose on Day 1 (Fig. 9). Mean sputum concentrations declined to an average of 0.6 µg/mL two hours following inhalation. The peak rhDNase I concentration

measured two hours after inhalation on Days 8 and 15 increased to 3.0 and 3.6 µg/mL, respectively. Sputum rhDNase I concentrations measured six hours after inhalation on Days 8 and 15 were similar to Day 1. Predose trough concentrations of 0.3 to 0.4 µg/mL rhDNase I measured on Days 8 and 15 (sample taken approximately 12 hours after the previous dose) were, however, higher than Day 1, suggesting possible modest accumulation of rhDNase I with repeated dosing. Inhalation of up to 10 mg three times daily of rhDNase I by four CF patients for six consecutive days did not result in significant elevation of serum concentrations of DNase above normal endogenous levels (Aitken et al., 1992; Hubbard et al., 1992). After administration of up to 2.5 mg of rhDNase I twice daily for six months to 321 CF patients, no accumulation of serum DNase was noted (assay limit of detection = approximately 0.5 ng DNase/mL serum).

## PROTEIN MANUFACTURING AND FORMULATION

rhDNase I is expressed in mammalian cell culture and purified to homogeneity using a variety of chromatographic steps. The development of the formulation of rhDNase I is especially important in that a suitable formulation is required to take into account protein stability, aerosolization properties, tonicity and the sealed container for storage (Shire, 1996). rhDNase I (Pulmozyme® dornase alpha) is manufactured by Genentech, Inc. and formulated as a sterile, clear, colorless aqueous solution containing 1.0 mg/mL dornase alpha, 0.15 mg/mL calcium chloride dihydrate and 8.77 mg/mL sodium chloride. The solution contains no preservative and has a nominal pH of 6.3. Pulmozyme® is administered by the inhalation of an aerosol mist produced by a compressed air-driven nebulizer system. Pulmozyme® is supplied as single-use ampoules, which deliver 2.5 mL of solution to the nebulizer.

The choice of formulation components was determined by a need to provide one to two years of stability and to meet additional requirements unique to aerosol delivery (Shire, 1996). A simple colorimetric assay for rhDNase I activity was used to evaluate the stability of rhDNase I in various formulations (Sinicropi et al., 1994b). In order to avoid adverse pulmonary reactions, such as cough or bronchoconstriction, aerosols for local pulmonary delivery should be formulated as isotonic solutions with minimal or no buffer components and should maintain pH > 5.0. rhDNase I has an additional requirement for calcium to be present for optimal enzymatic activity. Limiting formulation components raised concerns about pH control, since protein stability and solubility can be highly pH-dependent. Fortunately, the protein itself provided sufficient buffering capacity at 1 mg/mL to maintain pH stability over the storage life of the product.

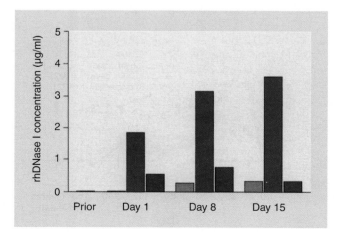

**Figure 9** ▪ rhDNase I concentration in sputum following administration of 2.5 mg of rhDNase I twice daily by inhalation to cystic fibrosis patients (mean ± SD N = 18).

## DRUG DELIVERY

The droplet or particle size of an aerosol is a critical factor in defining the site of deposition of the drug in the patient's airways (Gonda, 1990). A distribution of particle or droplet size of 1 to 6 μm was determined to be optimal for the uniform deposition of rhDNase I in the airways (Cipolla et al., 1994). Jet nebulizers have been used since they are the simplest method of producing aerosols in the desired respirable range. However, recirculation of protein solutions under high shear rates in the nebulizer bowl can present risks to the integrity of the protein molecule. rhDNase I survived recirculation and high shear rates during the nebulization process with no apparent degradation in protein quality or enzymatic activity (Cipolla et al., 1994).

Approved nebulizers produce aerosol droplets in the respirable range (1–6 μm) with a mass median aerodynamic diameter (MMAD) of 4 to 6 μm. The delivery of rhDNase I with a device that produces smaller droplets leads to more peripheral deposition in the smaller airways and thereby improves efficacy (Geller et al., 1998). Results obtained in 749 CF patients with mild disease confirmed that patients randomized to the Sidestream nebulizer powered by the Mobil Aire Compressor (MMAD = 2.1 μm) tended to have greater improvement in pulmonary function than patients using the Hudson T nebulizer with PulmoAide Compressor (MMAD = 4. μm). These results indicate that the efficacy of rhDNase I is dependent, in part, on the physical properties of the aerosol produced by the delivery system.

## CLINICAL USE

### ■ Indication and Clinical Dosage

rhDNase I (Pulmozyme® dornase alpha) is currently approved for use in CF patients, in conjunction with standard therapies, to reduce the frequency of respiratory infections requiring parenteral antibiotics and to improve pulmonary function (Fig. 1). The recommended dose for use in most CF patients is one 2.5 mg dose inhaled daily using a tested, recommended nebulizer.

### ■ Cystic Fibrosis

rhDNase I has been evaluated in a large, randomized, placebo-controlled trial of clinically stable CF patients, 5 years of age or older, with baseline forced vital capacity (FVC) greater than or equal to 40% of predicted (Fuchs et al., 1994). All patients received additional standard therapies for CF. Patients were treated with placebo or 2.5 mg of rhDNase I once or twice a day for six months. When compared to placebo, both once daily and twice daily doses of

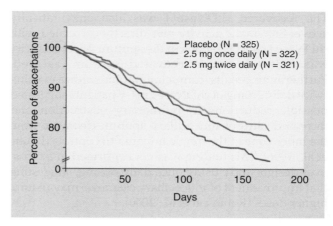

**Figure 10** ■ Proportion of patients free of exacerbations of respiratory symptoms requiring parenteral antibiotic therapy from a 24-week study.

rhDNase I resulted in a 28% to 37% reduction in respiratory tract infections requiring use of parenteral antibiotics (Fig. 10). Within eight days of the start of treatment with rhDNase I, mean forced expiratory volume in one second ($FEV_1$) increased 7.9% in patients treated once a day and 9.0% in those treated twice a day compared to the baseline values. The mean $FEV_1$ observed during long-term therapy increased 5.8% from baseline at the 2.5 mg daily dose level and 5.6% from baseline at the 2.5 mg twice daily dose level (Fig. 11). The risk of respiratory tract infection was reduced even in patients whose pulmonary function ($FEV_1$) was not improved. This finding is thought to result from improved clearance of mucus from the small airways in the lung, which may have little effect on $FEV_1$ or FVC, but may significantly reduce the risk of exacerbations of infection (Shak, 1995). The administration of rhDNase I also lessened shortness of breath, increased the general perception of well-being, and reduced the severity of other CF-related symptoms.

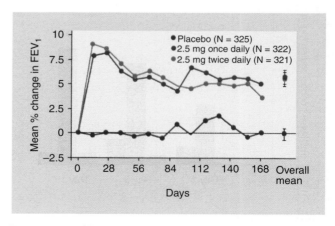

**Figure 11** ■ Mean percent change in $FEV_1$ from baseline through a 24-week study.

rhDNase I did not produce a pulmonary function benefit in short-term usage in the most severely ill CF patients (FVC less than 40% of predicted) (Shak, 1995; McCoy et al., 1996). These patients with end-stage lung disease represent approximately 7% of the CF population. Many are being prepared for lung transplantation but die while still awaiting an organ due to the shortage of donors. Studies are in progress to assess the impact of chronic usage on pulmonary function and infection risk in this population.

Since rhDNase I therapy may provide clinical benefit for young CF patients with mild disease by slowing progression of the disease, a study was done to investigate the safety and deposition of rhDNase I in the airways of CF patients <5 years old (3 months–5 years) compared with patients 5 to 10 years of age (Wagener et al., 1998). After two weeks of daily administration of 2.5 mg rhDNase I, comparable levels of rhDNase I were deposited in the lower airways of both age groups. Moreover, rhDNase I was well tolerated in the younger age group with an adverse event frequency similar to that in the older age group. Children with mild CF related lung disease were treated for 2 years in a randomized controlled trial to assess the effect of rhDNase I in early disease (Quan et al., 2001). Children with a mean age of 8.4 years and an FVC greater than 85% of predicted (Ramsey et al., 1999) were treated once daily with either placebo or 2.5 mg rhDNase I. After 96 weeks lung function was significantly better in the treated group compared with placebo, particularly for tests measuring function of smaller airways. Respiratory exacerbations were also reduced in the treated group.

Clinical trials have indicated that rhDNase I therapy can be continued or initiated during an acute respiratory exacerbation (Wilmott et al., 1996). Short-term dose ranging studies demonstrated that doses in excess of 2.5 mg twice daily did not provide further significant improvement in $FEV_1$ (Aitken et al., 1992; Hubbard et al., 1992; Ramsey et al., 1993). Patients who have received drug on a cyclical regimen (i.e., administration of rhDNase I 10 mg twice daily for 14 days, followed by a 14-day washout period) showed rapid improvement in $FEV_1$ with the initiation of each cycle and a return to baseline with each rhDNase I withdrawal (Eisenberg et al., 1997).

Concomitant therapy with rhDNase I and other standard CF therapies often show additive effects. The intermittent administration of aerosolized tobramycin was approved for use in CF patients with or without concomitant use of rhDNase I (Ramsey et al., 1999). Aerosolized tobramycin was well tolerated, enhanced pulmonary function and decreased the density of *Pseudomonas aeruginosa* in sputum. In combination with rhDNase I a larger treatment effect was noted but did not reach statistical significance. No differences in safety profile were observed following aerosolized tobramycin in patients that did or did not use rhDNase I. Chronic use of azithromycin has also been studied in CF patients chronically infected with *P. aeruginosa* (Saiman et al., 2005). Similar improvement in lung function and reduction in respiratory exacerbations was seen in patients receiving rhDNase I as those not, suggesting an additive, but not synergistic, benefit of the two therapies used together. The combination of hypertonic saline therapy with chronic use of rhDNase I has similar additive benefit (Elkins et al., 2006), in agreement with the previously mentioned in vitro studies. Additionally there was no evidence of a change in adverse events related to combination therapy in either of these studies.

### ■ Non-CF Respiratory Disease

Although originally considered beneficial for the treatment of non-CF related bronchiectasis (Wills et al., 1996), rhDNase I had no effect on pulmonary function or the frequency of respiratory exacerbations in a randomized controlled trial (O'Donnell et al., 1998). In another randomized controlled trial of rhDNase I, young children had shorter periods of ventilatory support following cardiac surgery when rhDNase I was instilled twice daily into the endotracheal tube (Riethmueller et al., 2006). Complicating atelectasis was less frequent in the treated group, consistent with numerous case reports suggesting that rhDNase I decreases, and can be used to treat, atelectasis when directly instilled into the airway (Hendriks et al., 2005). Finally, limited benefit has been described in children with asthma (Puterman and Weinberg, 1997) or with bronchiolitis due to respiratory syncytial virus infection (Nasr et al., 2001).

### ■ Systemic Lupus Erythematosus

The presence of antibodies to nuclear antigens including DNA is a hallmark of SLE, an autoimmune disease that affects multiple organ systems; antibodies directed against double-stranded DNA appear to play a prominent role in lupus nephritis and are generally present at elevated serum levels in clinically active disease. The observation that DNase I-deficient mice develop a lupus-like syndrome supports the hypothesis that a reduction in serum DNase may be a factor in the initiation of SLE (Napirei et al., 2000). Therefore, systemic administration of rhDNase I may be effective in the treatment of SLE (Lachmann, 2003). Degradation of extracellular DNA or the DNA component of DNA/anti-DNA immune complexes may be of clinical benefit in SLE by decreasing inflammation in tissues or by reducing the antigen load leading to a decrease in production of antibodies to DNA. A clinical study demonstrated that systemic administration of rhDNase I was well tolerated and did not induce the production of antibodies to rhDNase I (Davis et al., 1999). However, serum concentrations of rhDNase I were insufficient for catalytic activity of rhDNase I in serum (Prince et al., 1998). In a murine model of SLE, an actin/salt-resistant hyperactive DNase I variant showed significant protection from the development of anti-ssDNA and anti-histone antibodies, but not of renal disease (Manderson et al., 2006). Additional studies utilizing higher doses or more potent versions of rhDNase I variants are needed to determine whether systemic administration has any clinical benefit in SLE.

### ■ Other Medical Conditions

In principle rhDNase I may be useful for treating any condition where high levels of extracellular DNA and associated viscoelastic properties are pathological. A number of other clinical diseases with high potential for this have been investigated, although only to a limited extent. Pulmonary empyema involves the collection of purulent material in the pleural space and the use of rhDNase I instilled into the pleural space has been proposed (Simpson et al., 2003). rhDNase I has also been instilled into the nasal sinuses after surgery for chronic infections (Cimmino et al., 2005; Raynor et al., 2000).

### ■ Safety

The administration of rhDNase I has not been associated with an increase in major adverse events. Most adverse events were not more common with rhDNase I than with placebo treatment and probably reflect complications related to the underlying lung disease. Most events associated with dosing were mild, transient in nature, and did not require alterations in dosing. Observed symptoms included hoarseness, pharyngitis, laryngitis, rash, chest pain, and conjunctivitis. Within all the studies a small percentage (average 2–4%) of patients treated with rhDNase I developed serum antibodies to rhDNase I. None of these patients developed anaphylaxis, and the clinical significance of serum antibodies to rhDNase I is unknown.

## SUMMARY

DNase I, a secreted human enzyme whose normal function is thought to be for digestion of extracellular DNA, has been developed as a safe and effective adjunctive agent in the treatment of pulmonary disease in CF patients. rhDNase I reduces the viscoelasticity and improves the transport properties of viscous mucus both in vitro and in vivo. Inhalation of aerosolized rhDNase I reduces the risk of infections requiring antibiotics, improves pulmonary function and the well-being of CF patients with mild to moderate disease. Studies also suggest that rhDNase I has benefit in infants and young children with CF and in patients with early disease and "normal" lung function. Continuing studies will assess the usefulness of rhDNase I in early-stage CF pulmonary disease and other diseases where extracellular DNA may play a pathological role.

## ACKNOWLEDGMENTS

We would like to gratefully acknowledge Melinda Marion and Dominick Sinicropi for their encouragement to update their previous chapter in the second edition of this book.

## REFERENCES

Aitken ML, Burke W, McDonald G, et al. (1992). Recombinant human DNase inhalation in normal subjects and patients with cystic fibrosis. A phase 1 study. JAMA 267(14):1947–51.

Armstrong JB, White JC. (1950). Liquifaction of viscous purulent exudates by deoxyribonuclease. Lancet 2:739–42.

Baranovskii AG, Buneva VN, Nevinsky GA. (2004). Human deoxyribonucleases. Biochemistry (Mosc) 69 (6):587–601.

Bataillon V, Lhermitte M, Lafitte JJ, et al. (1992). The binding of amikacin to macromolecules from the sputum of patients suffering from respiratory diseases. J Antimicrob Chemother 29(5):499–508.

Campbell VW, Jackson DA. (1980). The effect of divalent cations on the mode of action of DNase I. The initial reaction products produced from covalently closed circular DNA. J Biol Chem, 255(8):3726–35.

Chen WJ, Liao TH. (2006). Structure and function of bovine pancreatic deoxyribonuclease I. Protein Pept Lett 2006, 13(5):447–53.

Chernick WS, Barbero GJ, Eichel HJ. (1961). In-vitro evaluation of effect of enzymes on tracheobronchial secretions from patients with cystic fibrosis. Pediatrics 27:589–96.

Cimmino M, Nardone M, Cavaliere M, et al. (2005). Dornase alfa as postoperative therapy in cystic fibrosis sinonasal disease. Arch Otolaryngol Head Neck Surg 2005, 131(12):1097–101.

Cipolla D, Gonda I, Shire SJ. (1994). Characterization of aerosols of human recombinant deoxyribonuclease I (rhDNase) generated by jet nebulizers. Pharm Res 11(4):491–8.

Dasgupta B, King M. (1996). Reduction in viscoelasticity in cystic fibrosis sputum *in vitro* using combined treatment with nacystelyn and rhDNase. Pediatr Pulmonol 22(3):161–6.

Davis JC, Jr., Manzi S, Yarboro C, et al. (1999). Recombinant human Dnase I (rhDNase) in patients with lupus nephritis. Lupus 8(1):68–76.

Davoodian K, Ritchings BW, Ramphal R, et al. (1997). Gelsolin activates DNase I *in vitro* and cystic fibrosis sputum. Biochemistry 36(32):9637–41.

Eisenberg JD, Aitken ML, Dorkin HL, et al. (1997). Safety of repeated intermittent courses of aerosolized recombinant human deoxyribonuclease in patients with cystic fibrosis. J Pediatr 131(1.1):118–24.

Elkins MR, Robinson M, Rose BR, et al. (2006). A controlled trial of long-term inhaled hypertonic saline in patients with cystic fibrosis. N Engl J Med 354(3):229–40.

Evans CJ, Aguilera RJ. (2003). DNase II: genes, enzymes and function. Gene 322:1–15.

Fuchs HJ, Borowitz DS, Christiansen DH, et al. (1994). Effect of aerosolized recombinant human DNase on exacerbations of respiratory symptoms and on pulmonary function in patients with cystic fibrosis. N Engl J Med 331(10):637–42.

Geller DE, Eigen H, Fiel SB, et al. (1998). Effect of smaller droplet size of dornase alfa on lung function in mild cystic fibrosis. Pediatr Pulmonol 25(2):83–7.

Gonda I. (1990). Aerosols for delivery of therapeutic and diagnostic agents to the respiratory tract. Crit Rev Ther Drug Carrier Syst 6(4):273–313.

Green JD. (1994). Pharmaco-toxicological expert report Pulmozyme rhDNase Genentech, Inc. Hum Exp Toxicol 13(Suppl 1):S1–42.

Guggino WB, Stanton BA. (2006). New insights into cystic fibrosis: molecular switches that regulate CFTR. Nat Rev Mol Cell Biol 7(6):426–36.

Hendriks T, de Hoog M, Lequin MH, et al. (2005). DNase and atelectasis in non-cystic fibrosis pediatric patients. Crit Care 9(4):R351–6.

Hitchcock SE, Carisson L, Lindberg U. (1976). Depolymerization of F-actin by deoxyribonuclease I. Cell 7(4):531–42.

Hubbard RC, McElvaney NG, Birrer P, et al. (1992). A preliminary study of aerosolized recombinant human deoxyribonuclease I in the treatment of cystic fibrosis. N Engl J Med 326(12):812–15.

Kabsch W, Mannherz HG, Suck D, et al. (1990). Atomic structure of the actin:DNase I complex. Nature 347(6288):37–44.

Kerem B, Rommens JM, Buchanan JA, et al. (1989). Identification of the cystic fibrosis gene: genetic analysis. Science 245(4922):1073–80.

King M, Dasgupta B, Tomkiewicz RP, et al. (1997). Rheology of cystic fibrosis sputum after *in vitro* treatment with hypertonic saline alone and in combination with recombinant human deoxyribonuclease I. Am J Respir Crit Care Med 156(1):173–7.

Kominato Y, Ueki M, Iida R, et al. (2006). Characterization of human deoxyribonuclease I gene (DNASE1) promoters reveals the utilization of two transcription-starting exons and the involvement of Sp1 in its transcriptional regulation. FEBS J 273(13):3094–105.

Lachmann PJ. (2003). Lupus and desoxyribonuclease. Lupus 12(3):202–6.

Laskowski Sr. M. Deoxyribonuclease I. (1971). In: Boyer PD, ed. The Enzymes. 3rd ed., Vol. 4. New York: Academic Press, 289–311.

Laube BL, Auci RM, Shields DE, et al. (1996). Effect of rhDNase on airflow obstruction and mucociliary clearance in cystic fibrosis. Am J Respir Crit Care Med 153(2):752–60.

Lazarides E, Lindberg U. (1974). Actin is the naturally occurring inhibitor of deoxyribonuclease I. Proc Natl Acad Sci USA 71(12):4742–6.

Lazarus RA. (2002). Human deoxyribonucleases. In: Creighton TE, ed. Wiley Encyclopedia of Molecular Medicine. New York: John Wiley and Sons, 1025–8.

Lieberman J. (1962). Enzymatic dissolution of pulmonary secretions. An in vitro study of sputum from patients with cystic fibrosis of pancreas. Am J Dis Child, 104:342–8.

Lieberman J. (1968). Dornase aerosol effect on sputum viscosity in cases of cystic fibrosis. JAMA 205(5):312–13.

Manderson AP, Carlucci F, Lachmann PJ, et al. (2006). The in vivo expression of actin/salt-resistant hyperactive DNase I inhibits the development of anti-ssDNA and anti-histone autoantibodies in a murine model of systemic lupus erythematosus. Arthritis Res Ther 8(3): R68.

Matthews LW, Specter S, Lemm J, et al. (1963). The over-all chemical composition of pulmonary secretions from patients with cystic fibrosis, bronchiectatis and laryngectomy. Am Rev Respir Dis 88:119–204.

McCoy K, Hamilton S, Johnson C. (1996). Effects of 12-week administration of dornase alfa in patients with advanced cystic fibrosis lung disease. Chest, 110(4):889–95.

Mohler M, Cook J, Lewis D, et al. (1993). Altered pharmacokinetics of recombinant human deoxyribonuclease in rats due to the presence of a binding protein. Drug Metab Dispos 21(1):71–5.

Moore S. (1981). Pancreatic DNase. In: Boyer PD, ed. The Enzymes, 3rd ed., Vol. 14. New York: Academic Press, 281–96.

Napirei M, Karsunky H, Zevnik B, et al. (2000). Features of systemic lupus erythematosus in Dnase1-deficient mice. Nat Genet 25(2):177–81.

Nasr SZ, Strouse PJ, Soskolne E, et al. (2001). Efficacy of recombinant human deoxyribonuclease I in the hospital management of respiratory syncytial virus bronchiolitis. Chest 120(1):203–8.

O'Donnell AE, Barker AF, Ilowite JS, et al. (1998). Treatment of idiopathic bronchiectasis with aerosolized recombinant human DNase I. rhDNase Study Group. Chest 113(5):1329–34.

Pan CQ, Lazarus RA. (1997). Engineering hyperactive variants of human deoxyribonuclease I by altering its functional mechanism. Biochemistry 36(22):6624–32.

Pan CQ, Ulmer JS, Herzka A, et al. (1998a). Mutational analysis of human DNase I at the DNA binding interface: implications for DNA recognition, catalysis, and metal ion dependence. Protein Sci 7(3):628–36.

Pan CQ, Dodge TH, Baker DL, et al. (1998b). Improved potency of hyperactive and actin-resistant human DNase I variants for treatment of cystic fibrosis and systemic lupus erythematosus. J Biol Chem 273(29):18374–81.

Pan CQ, Lazarus RA. (1999). $Ca^{2+}$-dependent activity of human DNase I and its hyperactive variants. Protein Sci 1999, 8(9):1780–8.

Pan CQ, Sinicropi DV, Lazarus RA. (2001). Engineered properties and assays for human DNase I mutants. Methods Mol Biol 160:309–21.

Potter JL, Specter S, Matthews LW, et al. (1969). Studies on pulmonary secretions. 3. The nucleic acids in whole pulmonary secretions from patients with cystic fibrosis bronchiectasis and laryngectomy. Am Rev Respir Dis 99:909–15.

Prince WS, Baker DL, Dodge AH, et al. (1998). Pharmacodynamics of recombinant human DNase I in serum. Clin Exp Immunol 113(2):289–96.

Puterman AS, Weinberg EG. (1997). rhDNase in acute asthma. Pediatr Pulmonol 23(4):316–17.

Quan JM, Tiddens HA, Sy JP, et al. (2001). A two-year randomized, placebo-controlled trial of dornase alfa in young patients with cystic fibrosis with mild lung function abnormalities. J Pediatr 139(6): 813–20.

Ramphal R, Lhermitte M, Filliat M, et al. (1988). The binding of anti-pseudomonal antibiotics to macromolecules from cystic fibrosis sputum. J Antimicrob Chemother 22(4):483–90.

Ramsey BW, Astley SJ, Aitken ML, et al. (1993). Efficacy and safety of short-term administration of aerosolized recombinant human deoxyribonuclease in patients with cystic fibrosis. Am Rev Respir Dis 148 (1):145–51.

Ramsey BW, Pepe MS, Quan JM, et al. (1999). Intermittent administration of inhaled tobramycin in patients with cystic fibrosis. N Engl J Med 340(1):23–30.

Raskin P. (1968). Bronchospasm after inhalation of pancreatic dornase. Am Rev Respir Dis 98(4):697–8.

Raynor EM, Butler A, Guill M, et al. (2000). Nasally inhaled dornase alfa in the postoperative management of chronic sinusitis due to cystic fibrosis. Arch Otolaryngol Head Neck Surg 126(5):581–3.

Riethmueller J, Borth-Bruhns T, Kumpf M, et al. (2006). Recombinant human deoxyribonuclease shortens ventilation time in young, mechanically ventilated children. Pediatr Pulmonol 41(1):61–6.

Riordan JR, Rommens JM, Kerem B, et al. (1989). Identification of the cystic fibrosis gene: cloning and characterization of complementary DNA. Science 245(4922):1066–73.

Robinson M, Hemming AL, Moriarty C, et al. (2000). Effect of a short course of rhDNase on cough and mucociliary clearance in patients with cystic fibrosis. Pediatr Pulmonol 30(1):16–24.

Saiman L, Mayer-Hamblett N, Campbell P, et al. (2005). Heterogeneity of treatment response to azithromycin in patients with cystic fibrosis. Am J Respir Crit Care Med 172(8):1008–12.

Sanders NN, Franckx H, De Boeck K, et al. (2006). Role of magnesium in the failure of rhDNase therapy in patients with cystic fibrosis. Thorax 61(11):962–8.

Shah PI, Bush A, Canny GJ, et al. (1995). Recombinant human DNase I in cystic fibrosis patients with severe pulmonary disease: a short-term, double-blind study followed by six months open-label treatment. Eur Respir J 8(6):954–8.

Shak S, Capon DJ, Hellmiss R, et al. (1990). Recombinant human DNase I reduces the viscosity of cystic fibrosis sputum. Proc Natl Acad Sci USA 87 (23):9188–92.

Shak S. (1995). Aerosolized recombinant human DNase I for the treatment of cystic fibrosis. Chest 107(2):65S–70S.

Shiokawa D, Tanuma S. (2001). Characterization of human DNase I family endonucleases and activation of DNase gamma during apoptosis. Biochemistry 40(1):143–52.

Shire SJ. (1996). Stability characterization and formulation development of recombinant human deoxyribonuclease I [Pulmozyme, (dornase alpha)]. In: Pearlman R, Wang YJ, eds. Pharmaceutical Biotechnology: Formulation, Characterization and Stability of Protein Drugs, Vol. 9. New York: Plenum Press, 393–426.

Simpson G, Roomes D, Reeves B. (2003). Successful treatment of empyema thoracis with human recombinant deoxyribonuclease. Thorax 58(4):365–6.

Sinicropi DV, Prince WS, Lofgren JA, et al. (1994a). Sputum pharmacodynamics and pharmacokinetics of recombinant human DNase I in cystic fibrosis. Am J Respir Crit Care Med 149(Suppl 1):A671.

Sinicropi DV, Baker DL, Prince WS, et al. (1994b). Colorimetric determination of DNase I activity with a DNA-methyl green substrate. Anal Biochem 222(2):351–8.

Sinicropi DV, Lazarus RA. (2001). Assays for human DNase I activity in biological matrices. Methods Mol Biol 160:325–33.

Suck D. (1994). DNA recognition by DNase I. J Mol Recognit 7(2):65–70.

Suri R. (2005). The use of human deoxyribonuclease (rhDNase) in the management of cystic fibrosis. BioDrugs 19(3):135–44.

Ulmer JS, Herzka A, Toy KJ, et al. (1996). Engineering actin-resistant human DNase I for treatment of cystic fibrosis. Proc Natl Acad Sci USA 93(16):8225–9.

Vasconcellos CA, Allen PG, Wohl ME, et al. (1994). Reduction in viscosity of cystic fibrosis sputum in vitro by gelsolin. Science 263(5149):969–71.

Wagener JS, Rock MJ, McCubbin MM, et al. (1998). Aerosol delivery and safety of recombinant human deoxyribonuclease in young children with cystic fibrosis: a bronchoscopic study. J Pediatr 133 (4):486–91.

Widlak P, Garrard WT. (2005). Discovery, regulation, and action of the major apoptotic nucleases DFF40/CAD and endonuclease G. J Cell Biochem 94(6):1078–87.

Wills PJ, Wodehouse T, Corkery K, et al. (1996). Short-term recombinant human DNase in bronchiectasis. Effect on clinical state and in vitro sputum transportability. Am J Respir Crit Care Med 154(2.1):413–17.

Wilmott RW, Amin RS, Colin AA, et al. (1996). Aerosolized recombinant human DNase in hospitalized cystic fibrosis patients with acute pulmonary exacerbations. Am J Respir Crit Care Med 153(6.1):1914–17.

Wolf E, Frenz J, Suck D. (1995). Structure of human pancreatic DNase I at 2.2 Å resolution. Protein Eng 8 (Suppl):79.

Zahm JM, Girod de Bentzmann S, Deneuville E, et al. (1995). Dose-dependent in vitro effect of recombinant human DNase on rheological and transport properties of cystic fibrosis respiratory mucus. Eur Respir J8(3):381–6.

# 20

# Follicle-Stimulating Hormone

*Tom Sam*
*Global Regulatory Affairs, N.V. Organon, Oss, The Netherlands*

## PHARMACOTHERAPY INFORMATION

Further information on the applied pharmacotherapy with follicle-stimulating hormone can be found in the following frequently used textbooks:

- **Applied Therapeutics: The Clinical Use of Drugs** (*Koda-Kimble, MA, et al., Eds.*), *8th edition, Lippincott Williams & Wilkins, Baltimore 2005*: Chapter 45.
- **Pharmacotherapy: A Pathophysiologic Approach** (*DiPiro, JT, et al., Eds.*), *6th edition, McGraw-Hill, New York 2005*: Chapters 75, 77, 78.
- **Textbook of Therapeutics: Drug and Disease Management** (*Helms, RA, et al., Eds.*), *8th edition, Lippincott Williams & Wilkins, Baltimore 2006*: Chapter 18.

## INTRODUCTION

About 15% of all couples experience infertility at some time during their reproductive lives. Increasingly, infertility can be treated by the use of assisted reproductive technologies, such as in vitro fertilization (IVF), gamete intra-fallopian transfer, and intracytoplasmic sperm injection. Gonadotropin treatment to increase the number of oocytes is a common element of these programs. A major cause for female infertility is chronic anovulation. Patients suffering from this condition are also treated with gonadotropins with the aim to achieve monofollicular development.

Gonadotropin preparations for infertility treatment are traditionally derived from postmenopausal urine. The urinary preparations contain follicle-stimulating hormone (FSH), but are typically less than 5% pure. The preparations also contain luteinizing hormone (LH) as a contaminant. Recombinant DNA technology allows the reproducible manufacturing of FSH preparations of high purity and specific activity, devoid of urinary contaminants. Recombinant FSH is produced using a Chinese hamster ovary (CHO) cell line, transfected with the genes encoding for the two human FSH subunits (van Wezenbeek, 1990; Howles, 1996). The isolation procedures render a product of high purity (at least 97%), devoid of LH activity and very similar to natural FSH.

Currently, there are two clinically approved recombinant FSH-containing drug products on the market. These are Gonal-F®, manufactured by Merck Serono S.A., and Puregon®, with the brand name of Follistim® in the United States, manufactured by NV Organon. Regulatory authorities have issued two distinct International Non-proprietary Names for the two corresponding recombinant FSH drug substances, i.e. follitropinα (Gonal-F®) and follitropinβ (Puregon®/Follistim®). Thus, the two products should be considered similar, but not identical preparations containing distinct active ingredients.

## BIOLOGICAL ROLE

The primary function of the glycoprotein hormone FSH in the female is the regulation of follicle growth. FSH is produced and secreted by the anterior lobe of the pituitary, a gland at the base of the brain. Its target is the FSH receptor at the surface of the granulosa cells that surround the oocyte. FSH acts synergistically with oestrogens and LH to stimulate proliferation of these granulosa cells, which leads to follicular growth. This process explains why deficient endogenous production of FSH may cause infertility.

## CHEMICAL DESCRIPTION

FSH belongs to a family of structurally related glycoproteins which includes LH, chorionic gonadotropin and thyroid-stimulating hormone. Each hormone is a dimeric protein consisting of two non-covalently associated glycoprotein subunits, denoted α and β. The α-subunit is identical for all these gonadotropins, and it is the β-subunit that provides each hormone with its specific biological function.

The glycoprotein subunits of FSH consist of two polypeptide backbones with carbohydrate side chains attached to the two asparagine (Asn) amino acid residues on each subunit. The oligosaccharides are attached to Asn-52 and Asn-78 on the α-subunit (92 amino acids), and to Asn-7 and Asn-24 on the β-subunit (111 amino acids). The glycoprotein FSH has a molecular mass of

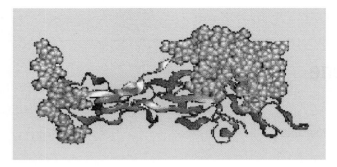

**Figure 1** ■ A three-dimensional model of FSH. The ribbons represent the polypeptide backbones of the α-subunit (*green ribbon*) and the β-subunit (*blue ribbon*). The carbohydrate side chains (*yellow and pink space filled globules*) cover large areas of the surface of the polypeptide subunits. The sialic acid carbohydrates are depicted in pink.

approximately 35 kDa. For the FSH preparation to be biologically active, the two subunits must be correctly assembled into their three-dimensional dimeric protein structure and post-translationally modified (Fig. 1).

Assembly and glycosylation are intracellular processes that take place in the endoplasmatic reticulum and in the Golgi apparatus. This glycosylation process leads to the formation of a population of hormone isoforms differing in their carbohydrate side-chain composition. The carbohydrate side-chains of FSH are essential for its biological activity since they (*i*) influence FSH receptor binding, (*ii*) play an important role in the signal transduction into the FSH target cell, and (*iii*) affect the plasma residence time of the hormone.

Recombinant FSH contains approximately 36% carbohydrate on a mass per mass basis. The carbohydrate side chains are composed of mannose, fucose, N-acetyl-glucosamine, galactose, and sialic acid. Structure analysis by $^1$H-NMR-spectroscopy on oligosaccharides enzymatically cleaved from follitropin β, reveals minor differences with natural FSH. For instance, the bisecting GlcNAc residues are lacking in the recombinant molecule, simply because the FSH-producing CHO1 cells do not possess the enzymes to incorporate these residues. Furthermore, the carbohydrate side-chains of recombinant FSH exclusively contain α 2-3 linked sialic acid, whereas in the natural hormone α 1-6 linked sialic acid occurs, as well. All carbohydrate side-chains identified in recombinant FSH are, however, moieties normally found in other natural human glycoproteins.

## PRODUCTION OF RECOMBINANT FSH

The genes coding for the human FSH α-subunit and β-subunit were inserted in cloning vectors (plasmids) to enable efficient transfer into recipient cells. These vectors also contained promoters that could direct transcription of foreign genes in recipient cells. CHO cells were selected as recipient cells since they were easily transfected with foreign DNA, and are capable of synthesizing glycoproteins. Furthermore they could be grown in cell cultures on a large scale. To construct a FSH-producing cell line NV Organon, the manufacturer of Puregon®/Follistim®, used one single vector containing the coding sequences for both subunit genes (Olijve, 1996). Merck Serono S.A., the manufacturer of Gonal-F®, used two separate vectors, one for each subunit gene (Howles, 1996). Following transfection, a genetically stable transformant producing biologically active recombinant FSH was isolated. For the CHO cell line used for manufacturing Puregon®/Follistim® it was shown that approximately 150 to 450 gene copies were present.

To establish a master cell bank (MCB) identical cell preparations of the selected clone are stored in individual vials and cryopreserved until needed. Subsequently a working cell bank (WCB) is established by the expansion of cells derived from a single vial of the MCB and aliquots are put in vials and cryopreserved, as well. Each time a production run is started cells from one or more vials of the WCB are cultured.

Both recombinant FSH products are isolated from cell culture supernatant. This supernatant is collected from a perfusion-type bioreactor containing recombinant FSH-producing CHO cells grown on microcarriers. This is because CHO cells are anchorage-dependent cells, which implies that a proper surface must be provided for cell growth. The reactor is perfused with growth-promoting medium during a period that may continue for up to three months (see Chapter 3). The down-stream purification processes for the isolation of the two recombinant FSH products are different. For Puregon®/Follistim® a series of chromatographic steps, including anion and cation exchange chromatography, hydrophobic chromatography and size-exclusion chromatography is used. Recombinant FSH in Gonal-F® is obtained by a similar process of five chromatographic steps, but also includes an immunoaffinity step using a murine FSH-specific monoclonal antibody. In both production processes, each purification step is rigorously controlled in order to ensure the batch-to-batch consistency of the purified product.

## ISOHORMONES

### ■ Structural Characteristics

As explained above, FSH exists in many distinct molecular forms (isohormones), with identical polypeptide backbones but diffences in oligosaccharide structure, in particular in the degree of terminal sialylation. These isohormones can be separated by chromatofocusing or isoelectric focusing on the basis of their different isoelectric points [pI, as has been demonstrated for follotropin β (de Leeuw et al., 1996)] (Fig. 2). The typical pattern for FSH indicates an

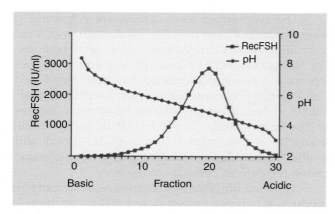

**Figure 2** ▪ Isohormone profile of recombinant FSH (follitropin) after preparative free flow focusing (De Leeuw et al., 1996). The FSH concentration was determined by a two-site immunoassay that is capable of quantifying the various isohormones equally well.

isohormone distribution between pI values of 6 and 4. To obtain structural information at the subunit level, the two subunits were separated by RP-HPLC and treated to release the N-linked carbohydrate side-chains. Fractions with low pI values (acidic fractions) displayed a high content of tri- and tetrasialo oligosaccharides and a low content of neutral and monosialo oligosaccharides. For fractions with a high pI (basic fractions) value the reverse was found. The β-subunit carbohydrate side chains appeared to be more heavily sialylated and branched than the α-subunit carbohydrate side chains. The low pI value isohormones of follitropin β have a high sialic acid/galactose ratio and are rich in tri- and tetra-antennary N-linked carbohydrate side chains, as compared with the side chains of the high pI value isohormones.

## ▪ Biological Properties of Recombinant FSH Isohormones

A FSH preparation can be characterized with four essentially different assays, each having its own specific merits: (*i*) The immunoassay determines FSH-specific structural features and provides a relative measure for the quantity of FSH. (*ii*) The receptor binding assay provides information on the proper conformation for interaction with the FSH receptor. Receptor binding studies with calf testis membranes have shown that FSH isoform activity in follitropin β decreases when going from high to low pI isoforms. (*iii*) The in vitro bioassay measures the capability of FSH to transduce signals into target cells (the intrinsic bioactivity). The in vitro bioactivity, assessed in the rat Sertoli cell bioassay, also decreases when going from high to low pI isoforms. (*iv*) The in vivo bioassay provides the overall bioactivity of a FSH preparation. It is determined by the number of molecules, the plasma residence time, the receptor

binding activity and the signal transduction. Surprisingly, in contrast to the receptor binding and in vitro bioassays, the in vivo biological activity determined in rats shows an approximate 20-fold increase between isoforms with a pI value of 5.49, as compared to those with a pI of 4.27. These results indicate that the basic isohormones exhibit the highest receptor binding and signal transduction activity, whereas the acidic isohormones are the more active forms under in vivo conditions.

## ▪ Pharmacokinetic Behavior of Recombinant FSH Isohormones

The pharmacokinetic behavior of follitropin β and its isohormones was investigated in Beagle dogs that were given an intramuscular bolus injection of a number of FSH isohormone fractions, each with a specific pI value. With a decrease in pI value from 5.49 (basic) to 4.27 (acidic), the AUC increased and the clearance decreased, each more than 10-fold (Fig. 3). A more than twofold difference in elimination half-life between the most acidic and the most basic FSH isohormone fraction was calculated. The absorption rate of the two most acidic isoforms was higher than the absorption rates of all other isoforms. The AUC and the clearance for the follitropin β preparation, being a mixture of all isohormone fractions, corresponded with the centre of the isohormone profile (Fig. 3). In contrast, the elimination of the follitropin β preparation occurred at a rate similar to that of the most acidic fractions, indicating that the elimination rate is largely determined by the removal of the most acidic isoforms from the plasma.

Thus, for follitropin β isohormone fractions, a clear correlation exists between pI value and pharmacokinetic behavior. Increasing acidity leads to an increase in the extent of absorption and elimination half-life and to a decrease in clearance.

## PHARMACEUTICAL FORMULATIONS

Recombinant FSH preparations distinguish themselves by their high purity (at least 97%) for example from urinary FSH preparations, which typically have a purity of less than 5%. Pure proteins are, however, relatively unstable and are generally lyophilized, unless some specific stabilizing measures can be taken. FSH preparations are available in different strengths and presentation forms, both as freeze-dried products (powder, cake, lyosphere) and as solution for injection (Table 1). Lyospheres are frozen drops of aqueous solution, which are freeze-dried in bulk and subsequently put in ampoules. Compared to the traditional freeze-dried cake formulation, lyospheres have the advantage of high dose uniformity, less adsorption to the glass walls of the

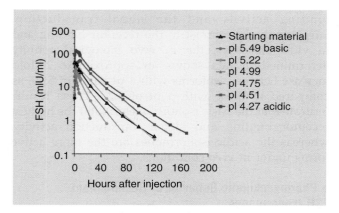

**Figure 3** ■ Kinetic behavior of FSH isoforms after a single intramuscular injection (20 IU/kg) in Beagle dogs.

ampoule, instantaneous dissolution, and in case of FSH, improved stability. Follitropin α was originally formulated with sucrose (bulking agent, lyoprotectant), sodium dihydrogen phosphate/disodium hydrogen phosphate, phosphoric acid and sodium hydroxide (for pH adjustment). In 2002, L-methionine (antioxidant) and polysorbate 20 (to prevent adsorption losses) were added to the single dose formulation. Follitropin β is formulated with sucrose, sodium citrate (stabilizer), polysorbate 20 (lyoprotectant and agent to prevent adsorption losses), and hydrochloride/sodium hydroxide (for pH adjustment). The lyophilized preparations are to be reconstituted before use to obtain a ready-for-use solution for injection. In addition to the freeze-dried presentation form, a solution for injection with several strengths of follitropin β could be developed. To stabilize the solutions 0.25 mg of L-methionine had to be added. Furthermore, the solution in the cartridge contains benzyl alcohol as preservative. For follitropin a multidose solution for injection in a pre-filled pen became available in 2004. This solution contains poloxamer 188 instead of polysorbate 20 and m-cresol has been added as preservative.

The lyophilized formulations are registered in strengths from 37.5 to 1050 IU. The dosage is not fixed, but is individually titrated based on ovarian response. For the convenience of both patient and healthcare worker a solution presentation has been developed. The Puregon/Follistim solution for injection is available in vials and is very suitable for titration because of the large range of 50 to 250 IU of available strengths. A pen injector has been developed with multidose cartridges containing solution for injection, giving the patient optimal convenience.

The shelf-life of the freeze-dried recombinant FSH products is two years when stored in the containers in which they are supplied, at temperatures below 30°C, not frozen and protected from light. The solutions for injection should be stored in the refrigerator for a maximum of three years with the container kept in the outer carton to protect the solution from light. The patient can keep the solutions at room temperature for a maximum of three months. The multidose solution of follitropin has a shelf-life of two years and can be stored for one month at room temperature.

## CLINICAL ASPECTS

Both recombinant FSH products on the market have been approved for two female indications. The first indication is anovulation (including polycystic ovarian disease) in women who are unresponsive to clomiphene citrate. The second indication is controlled ovarian hyperstimulation to induce the development of multiple follicles in medically assisted reproduction programs, such as IVF and embryo transfer. In addition, recombinant FSH may be used in men with congenital or required hypogonadotropic hypogonadism to stimulate spermatogenesis.

In anovulatory infertility in females, FSH treatment aims for the development of a single follicle, whereas IVF FSH treatment is aimed at multifollicular development. For the treatment of anovulatory patients it is recommended to start Puregon®/

| Market preparation | Presentation | Container | Strength |
|---|---|---|---|
| Gonal-F (follitropin α) (Merck Serono S.A.) | Powder | Ampule | 37.5, 75 and 150 IU |
| | Powder | Vial | 37.5 IU (2.8 μg), 75 IU (5.5 μg), 150 IU (11 μg) |
| | Powder | Multidose vial | 300 IU (22 μg), 450 IU (33 μg), 1050 IU (77 μg) |
| | Solution for injection | Cartridge | 300 IU (22 μg), 450 IU (33 μg), 900 IU (66 μg) |
| Puregon/Follistim (follitropin β) (NV Organon) | Lyosphere | Ampule | 50, 100 and 150 IU |
| | Cake | Vial | 75 and 150 IU |
| | Solution for injection | Vial | 50, 75, 100, 150, 200, 225, and 250 IU |
| | Solution for injection | Cartridge | 150, 300, 600, and 900 IU |

**Table 1** ■ The presentation forms of recombinant follicle-stimulating hormone products.

Follistim® treatment with 50 IU per day for 7 to 14 days and gradually increase dosing with steps of 50 IU if no sufficient response is seen. This gradual dose-increasing schedule is followed in order to prevent multifollicular development and the induction of ovarian hyperstimulation syndrome (a serious condition of unwanted hyperstimulation).

In the most commonly applied treatment regimens in IVF, endogenous gonadotropin levels are suppressed by a GnRH agonist or by the more recently approved GnRH antagonists (Cetrotide® and Orgalutran®/Antagon®). It is recommended to start Puregon® treatment with 100 to 200 IU of recombinant FSH followed by maintenance doses of 50 to 350 IU. The availability of a surplus of collected oocytes allows the replacement of two to three embryos. Similar treatment regimens are recommended for Gonal-F®.

Serum levels of FSH do not correlate with pharmacological responses, such as the production of estradiol, inhibin response or follicular development. Moreover, there is a large variability found in the individual pharmacological response to a fixed dose of recombinant FSH. This variability emphasizes the importance of a patient individualized dosing and treatment regimen when using recombinant FSH.

Follitropin β has an elimination half-life of approximately 40 hours. Steady-state levels of follitropin β are therefore reached after four daily doses. At that time, the concentrations of circulating immunoreactive FSH are about a factor of 1.5–2.5 higher than after a single dose. This increase is relevant in attaining therapeutically effective plasma concentrations of FSH. Follitropin β can be administered via the intramuscular, as well as via the subcutaneous route, because the absence of impurities results in an improved local tolerance. Bioavailability via both routes is approximately 77%. Injections of the highly pure follitropin preparations do not require medical personnel, but can be given by the patient herself or her partner. In a large number of patients treated with follitropin β, no formation of antibodies against recombinant FSH or CHO-cell derived proteins was observed.

### ■ Differences with Urinary FSH Preparations

In IVF, follitropin β treatment was found to be more effective and efficient than treatment with urinary FSH, since more follicles, oocytes, embryos and pregnancies are obtained with a lower total dose of recombinant FSH in a shorter treatment period. In a recent meta analysis the occurrence of higher pregnancy rates with recombinant FSH versus urinary FSH was confirmed (Daya, 2002). Treatment of patients with anovulatory infertility with either follitropin® or urinary FSH was equally effective, but follitropin® treatment was more efficient (a lower total dose was needed in a shorter duration of treatment).

## REFERENCES

Daya S. (2002). Updated meta-analysis of recombinant follicle stimulating hormone (FSH) versus urinary FSH for ovarian stimulation in assisted reproduction. Fertility Sterility 77:711–714.

De Boer W, Mannaerts B. (1990). Recombinant follicle stimulating hormone. II. Biochemical and biological characteristics. In: Crommelin DJA, Schellekens H, eds. From Clone to Clinic, Developments in Biotherapy, Vol. 1. Dordrecht: Kluwer Academic Publishers, 253–259.

De Leeuw R, Mulders J, Voortman G, Rombout F, Damm J, Kloosterboer L. (1996). Structure-function relationship of recombinant follicle stimulating hormone (Puregon®). Mol Human Reprod 2:361–369.

Dias JA. (2001). Is there any physiological role for gonadotrophin oligosaccharide heterogeneity in humans? II. A biochemical point of view. Human Reprod 16:825–830.

European Public Assessment Report Gonal-F (Follitropin alpha), CPMP/415/95, revision 8, 3 November 2004. European Agency for the Evaluation of Medicinal Products.

European Public Assessment Report Puregon (Follitropin beta), CPMP/003/96, revision 9, 19 May 2005. European Agency for the Evaluation of Medicinal Products.

Geurts TBP, Peters MJH, Bruggen JGC, van de Boer W, Out HJ. (1996). Puregon® (Org 32489)—Recombinant human follicle-stimulating hormone. Drugs Today 32:239–58.

Howles CM. (1996). Genetic engineering of human FSH (Gonal-F®) Human Reprod Update 2:172–191.

Olijve W, de Boer W, Mulders JWM, van Wezenbeek PMGF. (1996). Molecular biology and biochemistry of human recombinant follicle stimulating hormone (Puregon®). Mol Human Reprod 2:371–382.

Out HJ, Mannaerts BMJL, Driessen SGAJ, Coelingh Bennink HJT. (1996). Recombinant follicle stimulating hormone (rFSH; Puregon) in assisted reproduction: More oocytes, more pregnancies. Results from five comparative studies. Human Reprod Update 2:162–171.

Sansom C, Markman O. (2007). Glycobiology. Scion Publishing Ltd, p. 374.

Van Wezenbeek P, Draaijer J, Van Meel F, et al. (1990). Recombinant follicle stimulating hormone. I. Construction, selection and characterization of a cell line. In Crommelin DJA and Schellekens H. (eds), From Clone to Clinic, Developments in Biotherapy. Kluwer, Amsterdam, pp. 245–251.

Voortman G, van de Post J, Schoemaker RC, van Gerwen J. (1999). Bioequivalence of subcutaneous injections of recombinant human follicle stimulating hormone (Puregon®) by Pen-injector and syringe. Human Reprod 14:1698–1702.

Woodcock J. Griffin J. Behrman R, et al. (2007). The FDA's assessment of follow-on protein products: a historical perspective. Nature Reviews Drug Discovery 6:437–422.

# 21

# Vaccines

*Wim Jiskoot*
*Division of Drug Delivery Technology, Leiden/Amsterdam Center for Drug Research, Leiden University, Leiden, The Netherlands*

*Gideon F. A. Kersten*
*Netherlands Vaccine Institute (NVI), Bilthoven, The Netherlands*

*Enrico Mastrobattista*
*Department of Pharmaceutical Sciences, Utrecht University, Utrecht, The Netherlands*

## PHARMACOTHERAPY INFORMATION

Further information on the applied pharmacotherapy with vaccines can be found in the following frequently used textbooks:

- **Applied Therapeutics: The Clinical Use of Drugs** (Koda-Kimble, MA, et al., Eds.), 8th edition, Lippincott Williams & Wilkins, Baltimore 2005 : Chapters 60, 61, 65, 72, 73, 94, 95
- **Pharmacotherapy: A Pathophysiologic Approach** (DiPiro, JT, et al., Eds.), 6th edition, McGraw-Hill, New York 2005 : Chapter 122.
- **Textbook of Therapeutics: Drug and Disease Management** (Helms, RA, et al., Eds.), 8th edition, Lippincott Williams & Wilkins, Baltimore 2006 : Chapters 35, 49, 73.

## INTRODUCTION

Traditionally, vaccination aims to prevent infectious diseases. It can be considered as one of the most successful medical strategies. The conventional vaccines routinely applied in man are very effective in preventing a number of infectious diseases. This is illustrated by the fact that mass vaccination has resulted in the worldwide eradication of smallpox in the 1970s. Moreover, diphtheria, tetanus, poliomyelitis, measles, mumps, and rubella are under control in the developed countries as well as in an increasing number of developing countries, because of the application of childhood vaccines. Currently, vaccines are not only developed against infectious diseases. Vaccines in the pipeline include anti-drug abuse vaccines (nicotine, cocaine) and vaccines against allergies, cancer and Alzheimer's disease.

In the rapidly evolving field of new vaccine technologies one can discern the improvement of existing vaccines and the development of vaccines for diseases against which no vaccine is available yet. Modern biotechnology has an enormous impact on current vaccine development. The elucidation of the molecular structures of pathogens and the tremendous progress made in immunology during the past few decades have led to the identification of protective antigens and ways to deliver them. Together with technological advances, this has caused a move from empirical vaccine development to more rational approaches. A major goal of modern vaccine technology is to fulfill all requirements of the ideal vaccine as summarized in Figure 1, by expressing antigen epitopes (= the smallest molecular structures recognized by the immune system) and/or isolating those antigens that confer an effective immune response, and eliminating structures that cause deleterious effects. Thus, "cleaner," well-defined products can be obtained, resulting in improved safety. In addition, modern methodologies may provide simpler production processes for selected vaccine components.

In the following section immunological principles that are important for vaccine design are summarized. Subsequently, conventional vaccines, which are not a result of modern genetic or chemical engineering technologies will be addressed. Conventional and modern vaccines are listed in Table 1. Current strategies used in the development and manufacture of new vaccines are discussed in the section "Modern vaccine technologies". It is not our intent to provide a comprehensive review of all possible vaccine options for all possible diseases. Rather, we will explain modern approaches to vaccine development and illustrate these approaches with representative examples. In the last section pharmaceutical aspects of vaccines are dealt with.

The ideal vaccine

■ is 100% efficient in all individuals of any age
■ provides lifelong protection after single administration
■ does not evoke any adverse reaction
■ is stable under various conditions (temperature, light, transportation)
■ is easy to administer, preferably orally
■ is available in unlimited quantitites
■ is cheap

**Figure 1** ■ Characteristics of the (hypothetical) ideal vaccine.

## IMMUNOLOGICAL PRINCIPLES

After a natural infection the human immune system in most cases launches an immunological response to the particular pathogen. After recovery from the disease, the immunological response indeed protects the affected individual from that disease, in the ideal case forever. This phenomenon is called immunity and is due to the presence of circulating antibodies, activated cytotoxic cells and memory cells. Memory cells become active when the same type of antigenic material enters the body on a later occasion. Unlike the primary response after the first infection, the response after repeated infection is very fast and usually sufficiently strong to prevent reoccurrence of the disease.

The principle of vaccination is mimicking an infection in such a way that the natural specific defense mechanism of the host against the pathogen will be activated, but the host will remain free of the disease that normally results from a natural infection. This is effectuated by administration of antigenic components that (1) consist of, (2) are derived from, or (3) are related to the pathogen. The success of vaccination relies on the induction of a long-lasting immunological memory. Vaccination is also referred to as active immunization, because the host's immune system is activated to respond to the "infection" through humoral and cellular immune responses, resulting in adaptive immunity against the particular pathogen. The immune response is generally highly specific: it discriminates not only between pathogen species, but often also between different strains within one species (e.g., strains of meningococci, poliovirus, influenza virus). Albeit sometimes a hurdle for vaccine developers, this high specificity of the immune system allows an almost perfect balance between response to foreign antigens and tolerance with respect to self-antigens. Apart from active immunization, administration of specific antibodies can be utilized for short-lived immunological protection of the host. This is termed passive immunization (Fig. 2).

Traditionally, active immunization has mainly served to prevent infectious diseases, whereas passive immunization has been applied for both prevention and therapy of infectious diseases. Through recent developments new potential applications of vaccines for active immunization have emerged, such as the prevention of other diseases than infectious diseases (e.g., cancer) and for the treatment of substance abuse

| Category | Technology | Liver/non-living | Characteristics |
|---|---|---|---|
| Attenuated vaccines | Conventional | Live | Bacteria or viruses attenuated in culture; empirically developed |
| Inactivated vaccines | Conventional | Non-living | Heat-inactivated or chemically inactivated bacteria or viruses; empirically developed |
| Subunit vaccines | Conventional | Non-living | Extracts of pathogens; combination of purified proteins with killed suspension; purified single components (proteins, polysaccharides); combination of purified components with adjuvant; purified components in a suitable presentation form; polysaccharide-protein conjugates |
| Genetically improved live vaccines | Modern | Live | Genetically attenuated microorganisms; live viral or bacterial vectors |
| Genetically improved subunit vaccines | Modern | Non-living | Genetically detoxified proteins; proteins expressed in host cells; recombinant peptide vaccines |
| Recombinant subunit vaccines identified by reverse vaccinology | Modern | Non-living | Recombinant antigenic proteins obtained from the genomic sequence of the pathogen |
| Synthetic peptide-based vaccines | Modern | Non-living | Linear or cyclic peptides; multiple antigen peptides; peptide-protein conjugates |
| Nucleic acid-based vaccines | Modern | Non-living | DNA or mRNA coding for antigen |

**Table 1** ■ Categories of conventional vaccines and vaccines obtained by modern technologies.

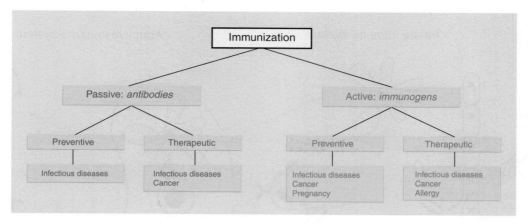

**Figure 2** ▦ Scheme of active immunization (= vaccination) and passive immunization and examples of their fields of application.

(e.g., nicotine addiction). Such vaccines are referred to as therapeutic vaccines. The difference between passive and active immunization for preventive and therapeutic applications is outlined in Figure 2. Since antibody preparations for passive immunization do not fall under the strict definition of a vaccine, they are not discussed here.

### ■ Active Immunization: Generation of an Immune Response

The generation of an immune reaction against a pathogen by vaccination follows several distinct steps that should ultimately lead to long-lasting protection against the pathogen through memory cells. These steps are uptake of the vaccine (consisting of either the entire pathogen or antigenic components thereof) by phagocytic cells, activation and migration of professional antigen-presenting cells (APCs) from infected tissue to peripheral lymphoid organs, antigen presentation to T-lymphocytes and finally activation (or inhibition) of T- and B-lymphocytes. The entire process is illustrated in Figure 3. Below we will describe the successive steps leading to an immune response to a pathogen, which are important for the design and fate of vaccines against the pathogen.

### ■ Uptake

Every immune reaction against a pathogen starts with its uptake by specialized phagocytic cells in the infected tissue. These cells carry receptors on their surface; pattern-recognition receptors (PRRs) that recognize common features of pathogens called pathogen associated molecular patterns (PAMPs). Binding of PAMPs to these PRRs results in phagocytosis of the pathogens. Examples of PRRs are toll-like receptors (TLRs), scavenger receptors and C-type lectins (Table 2). TLRs consist of a family of receptors, with each member recognizing different patterns on the surface of pathogens ( Akira et al., 2006). TLRs can

be found on many cells including macrophages and dendritic cells (DCs). DCs can also engulf materials from their extracellular environment by a receptor independent process called micropinocytosis.

### ■ Activation and Migration

Besides mediating uptake of antigenic material from the surrounding tissue, the PRRs also play an important role in triggering the cytokine network that will eventually influence the type of adaptive immune response that will be evoked against the pathogen. The phagocytic cells that have taken up pathogens from the infected tissue become activated and start to produce pro-inflammatory cytokines such as interleukin-1$\beta$, interleukin-6 and tumor necrosis factor-$\alpha$ as well as chemokines. The chemokines recruit more phagocytic cells such as neutrophils and monocytes to the infection site, whereas the pro-inflammatory cytokines induce fever and the production of acute-phase response proteins that can opsonize pathogens.

Most phagocytic cells, including DCs and macrophages, but also B-cells can serve as professional APCs to present processed antigenic determinants to lymphocytes in the peripheral lymphoid organs. For instance, DCs that have taken up antigens from infected tissue become activated and migrate via the afferent lymphatic vessels towards nearby lymph nodes where the encounter with pathogen-specific lymphocytes can take place.

### ■ Antigen Presentation and Lymphocyte Activation

The peripheral lymphoid organs are the primary meeting place between cells of the innate immune system (APCs) and cells of the adaptive immune system (T-cells and B-cells). Upon interaction with APCs, pathogen-specific T-cells and B-cells will be activated, provided that they acquire the appropriate signals from the APCs. Besides antigen-specific binding via their antigen receptors, lymphocytes

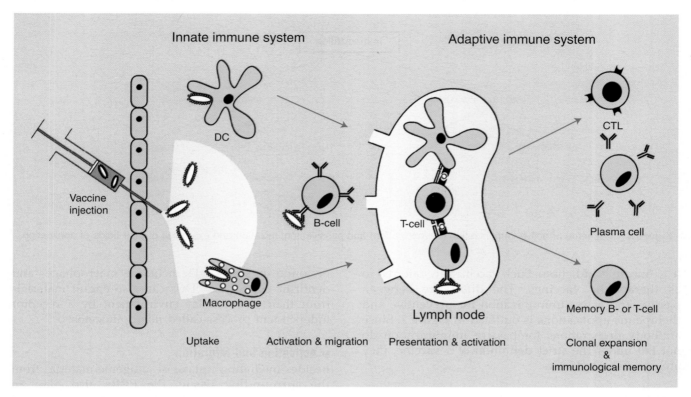

**Figure 3** ■ Overview of the steps leading to immunization after administration of a vaccine. Upon subcutaneous or intramuscular administration the vaccine components are taken up by phagocytic cells such as macrophages and dendritic cells (DCs) that reside in the peripheral tissue and express PRRs that recognize PAMPs. Professional APCs that have taken up antigens become activated and start migrating towards nearby lymph nodes. Inside the lymph nodes, the antigen processed by the APCs is presented to lymphocytes, which, when recognizing the antigen and receiving the appropriate co-stimulatory signals, become activated. These antigen-specific B- and T-lymphocytes clonally expand to produce multiple progenitors recognizing the same antigen. In addition, memory B- and T-cells are formed that provide long-term (sometimes lifelong) protection against infection with the pathogen. *Abbreviations*: APC, antigen presenting cell; CTL, cytotoxic T-lymphocyte; PAMP, pathogen-associated molecular pattern; PRR, pattern recognition receptor.

require co-stimulatory signals via interaction of accessory and co-stimulatory molecules between lymphocytes and APCs. This cell-cell interaction is essential for proper stimulation of lymphocytes and without those accessory signals, antigen-specific T-cells may become anergic. Lymphocytes receiving the appropriate signals for activation will clonally expand and generate multiple progenitors all recognizing the same antigen. Clonal expansion is a typical feature of the adaptive immune system, which will be discussed in more detail below.

### ■ The Adaptive Immune System

The adaptive immune system is involved in elimination of pathogens in the late phase of infection and in the generation of immunological memory. It consists of B- and T-lymphocytes both bearing antigen-specific receptors. The adaptive immune system can be divided into humoral and cell-mediated immunity (CMI) (Fig. 4 and Table 3). The humoral response results in antibody formation (but contains cell-mediated events, Fig. 4A,B); CMI results in the generation of cytotoxic cells (Fig. 4A,B). The action

of antibodies and T-cells is dependent on accessory factors, some of which are mentioned in Table 3. In general, after infection with a pathogen or a protective vaccine, both humoral and cellular responses are generated. This indicates that both are needed for efficient protection. The balance between humoral and cellular responses, however, can differ widely between pathogens and is dependent on how the pathogen is presented to the adaptive immune system by APCs. This may have consequences for the design of a particular vaccine (see section "Vaccine design in relation to the immune response").

Antibodies are the typical representatives of humoral immunity. An antibody belongs to one of four different immunoglobulin classes (IgM, IgG, IgA, or IgE). Upon immunization, the B-cells expressing specific antibodies on their cell surface (representing a fifth immunoglobulin class, IgD) are activated. The surface-bound antibodies bind specific epitopes of the pathogen, and in close cooperation with T-helper cells ($T_h$-cells), the B-cell becomes activated eventually resulting in massive clonal proliferation. The proliferated B-cells are called plasma cells and excrete large

| PRR | PAMP |
|---|---|
| TLR-1 | Triacyl lipoproteins |
| TLR-2 | Peptidoglycans |
| | Lipoproteins |
| | Lipoarabinomannan |
| | Zymosan |
| TLR-3 | Viral dsRNA |
| TLR-4 | Lipopolysaccharide, lipid A, taxol |
| TLR-5 | Flagellin |
| TLR-6 | Diacyl lipoproteins |
| TLR-7 | Small, synthetic compounds, ssRNA |
| TLR-8 | Small, synthetic compounds |
| TLR-9 | Unmethylated CpG DNA |
| TLR-10 | Unknown |
| TLR-11 | Components from uropathogenic bacteria |
| Scavenger receptors | Polyanionic ligands |
| C-type lectin receptors | Sulfated sugars, mannose-, fucose- and galactose-modified polysaccharides and proteins |
| NOD-1, NOD-2 | Peptidoglycans |
| Type 3 complement receptors | Zymosan particles, β-glucan |

*Abbreviations*: PRR, pattern-recognition receptor; PAMP, pathogen associated molecular pattern; TRR, toll-like receptor.
*Source*: Adapted from Pashine et al. (2005).

**Table 2** ■ Pattern-recognition receptors (PRRs) and their ligands (PAMPs).

amounts of soluble antibodies (Fig. 4B). Antibodies are able to prevent infection or disease by several mechanisms:

1. Binding of antibody covers the antigen with Fc (constant fragment), the "rear-end" of immunoglobulins. Phagocytic cells, like macrophages express surface receptors for Fc. This allows targeting of the opsonized (antibody-coated) antigen to these cells, followed by enhanced phagocytosis.
2. Immune complexes (i.e., antibodies bound to target antigens) can activate complement, a system of proteins which then becomes cytolytic to bacteria, enveloped viruses or infected cells.
3. Phagocytic cells may express receptors for complement factors associated with immune complexes. Binding of these activated complement factors enhances phagocytosis.

4. Viruses can be neutralized by antibodies through binding at or near receptor binding sites on the virus surface. This may prevent binding to and entry into the host cell.

Antibodies are effective against certain but not all infectious microorganisms; they may have limited value when CMI is the major protective mechanism. Of the cell types that are known to exhibit cytotoxicity, two are antigen-sensitized. Because of their specificity, they are of special importance with respect to vaccine design:

1. Cytotoxic T-lymphocytes (CTLs) react with target cells and kill them by release of cytolytic proteins like perforin. Target cells express non-self antigens like viral proteins or tumor antigens, by which they are identified. CTL responses, as antibody responses, are highly specific.
2. T-cells involved in delayed type hypersensitivity ($T_{DTH}$) are able to kill target cells as CTLs do, but also have helper ($T_{h1}$-type, see below) functions that enable them to activate macrophages.

Other, less specific cells involved in cytotoxic immune responses are natural killer cells (NK-cells). They play a role in antibody-dependent cellular cytotoxicity. NK-cells recognize opsonized (antibody coated) cells with their Fc-receptors.

Besides plasma cells and cytotoxic cells, in many cases memory B- and T-cells develop. Memory B-cells do not produce soluble antibody, but on repeated antigen contact their response time to develop into antibody-excreting plasma cells is shorter compared to naïve B-cells.

The occurrence of different types of immune response to vaccines is the result of differences in antigen processing of the vaccine by APCs and, as a result, in the activation of $T_h$-cells (Figs. 3 and 4). Major histocompatibility complex (MHC) molecules play an important role in the presentation of processed antigens to T-cells. Cells expose either MHC class I or II molecules on their surface.

APCs carrying class II molecules process soluble, exogenous (extracellular) proteins or more complicated structures such as microorganisms (Fig. 4A). After their endocytosis, the proteins are subject to limited proteolysis before they return as peptides to the surface of the APC in combination with the class II molecules for presentation to a T-cell receptor (TCR) of CD4 positive $T_h$-cells. The $T_h$-cells provide type 2 help necessary for the effector function of B-cells. This type 2 help is characterized by the lymphokine pattern produced: interleukin-4 (IL-4), IL-5, IL-6, IL-10, and IL-13. These lymphokines trigger B-cells, which eventually results in the production of IgM and IgG antibodies.

410

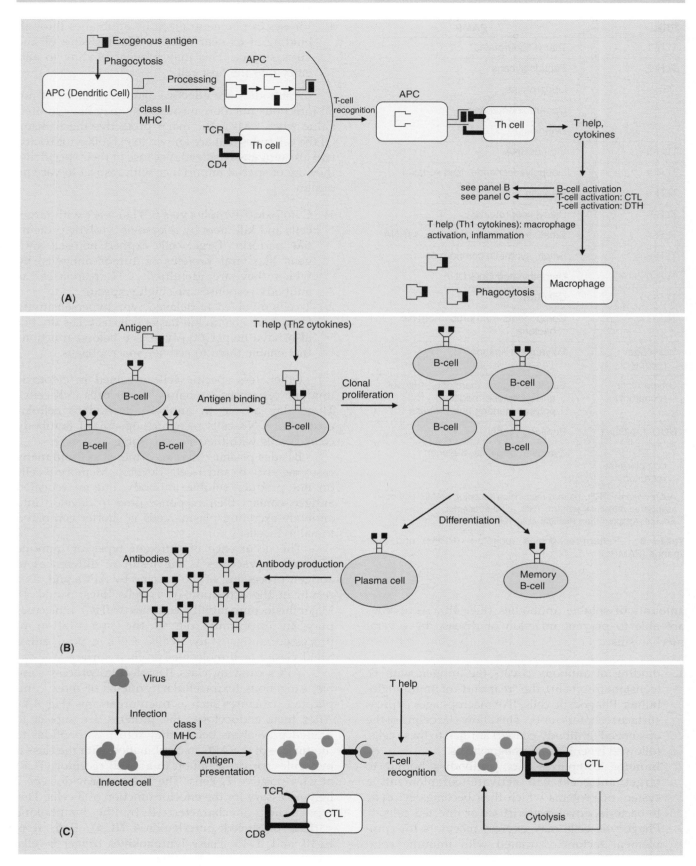

**Figure 4** ▪ Schematic representation of antigen-dependent immune responses.

| Immune response | Immune product | Accessory factors | Infectious agents |
|---|---|---|---|
| Humoral | IgG | Complement, neutrophils | Bacteria and viruses |
| | IgA | Alternative complement pathway | Micro-organisms causing respiratory and enteric infections |
| | IgM | Complement, macrophages | (Encapsulated) bacteria |
| | IgE | Mast cells | Parasites |
| Cell-mediated | CTL | Cytolytic proteins | Viruses and mycobacteria |
| | $T_{DTH}$ | Macrophages | Viruses, mycobacteria, treponema (syphilis), fungi |

*Source*: Adapted from Sell and Hsu,1993.

**Table 3** ▪ Immune products protecting against infectious diseases.

Cells carrying MHC class I molecules process endogenous (intracellularly produced) antigens like viral and tumor antigens, and present them in combination with class I molecules on the cell surface (Fig. 4C). The class I-antigen combination on the APC is recognized by the TCR of CD8 positive CTLs. $T_h$-cells provide help for the CTLs. For the induction of CMI (Fig. 4A, C), type 1 help is needed (production of IL-2 and IL-12, interferon-γ, and tumor necrosis factor). $T_h$-cells are CD4 positive, regardless whether they have $T_{h1}$or $T_{h2}$ functions. There is increasing evidence that the $T_{h1}/T_{h2}$ balance is an important immunological parameter since some diseases coincide with $T_{h1}$ (autoimmunity) or $T_{h2}$ (allergy) type responses.

### ■ Vaccine Design in Relation with the Immune Response

For the rational design of a new vaccine, understanding of the mechanisms of the protective immunity to the pathogen against which the vaccine is developed is crucial. For instance, to prevent tetanus a high blood titer of antibody against tetanus toxin is required; in mycobacterial diseases such as tuberculosis a macrophage-activating CMI is most effective; in case of an influenza virus infection CTLs probably play a significant role. Importantly, the immune effector mechanisms triggered by a vaccine and, hence, the success of immunization not only depend on the nature of the protective components but also on their presentation form, the presence of adjuvants, and the route of administration.

The presentation form of the vaccine is one of the determinants that influence the extent and type of immune response that will be evoked (Pashine et al., 2005; Pulendran and Ahmed, 2006). DCs and other APCs play a pivotal role in how the antigenic determinants of a vaccine will be processed and presented to T-cells in the peripheral lymphoid organs. Through various PRRs, DCs are more or less able to "sense" the type of pathogen that is encountered. This determines the set of co-stimulatory signals and pro-inflammatory cytokines that will be generated by APCs when presenting the antigen to Th-cells in the peripheral lymphoid organs. For instance, pathogens or vaccines containing lipoproteins or peptidoglycans will trigger DCs via TLR-2, which predominantly generates a $T_{h2}$ response, whereas stimulation of DCs through TLR-3, -4, -5 or -8 is known to yield robust $T_{h1}$ responses. Therefore, vaccines should be formulated in such a way that the appropriate $T_h$ response will be triggered. This can be done by presenting the antigen in its native format, as is the case for the conventional vaccines, or by adding adjuvants that stimulate the desired response (see below).

The response by B-cells is dependent upon the nature of the antigen and two types of antigens can be distinguished:

1. Thymus-independent antigens include certain linear antigens that are not readily degraded in the body and have a repeating determinant, such as bacterial polysaccharides. They are able to stimulate B-cells without the $T_h$-cell involvement. Thymus-independent antigens do not induce immunological memory.

2. Thymus-dependent antigens provoke little or no antibody response in animals with few T-cells. Proteins are the typical representatives of thymus-dependent antigens. A prerequisite for thymus-dependency is that a physical linkage exists between the sites recognized by B-cells and those by $T_h$-cells. When a thymus-independent antigen is coupled to a carrier protein containing $T_h$-epitopes, it becomes thymus-dependent. As a result, these conjugates are able to induce memory.

When the antigen is a protein, the epitopes can be continuous or discontinuous. Continuous epitopes involve linear peptide sequences (usually consisting of up to ten amino acid residues) of the protein (Fig. 7A). Discontinuous epitopes comprise amino acid residues sometimes far apart in the primary sequence, which are brought together through the unique folding of the protein (Fig. 7B). Antibody recognition of B-cell epitopes, whether continuous or discontinuous, is usually dependent on the conformation (= three-dimensional structure). T-cell epitopes, on the other hand, are continuous peptide sequences, the conformation of which does not seem to play a role in T-cell recognition.

### ■ Route of Administration

The immunological response to a vaccine is dependent on the route of administration. Most current vaccines are administered intramuscularly or subcutaneously, with some exceptions such as live polio vaccine and live typhoid vaccine, which are administered orally. Parenteral immunization usually induces systemic immunity. However, mucosal (e.g., oral, intranasal, or intravaginal) immunization may be preferred, because mucosal surfaces are the common entrance of many pathogens. The induction of a mucosal secretory IgA response may prevent the attachment and entry of pathogens into the host. For example, antibodies against cholera need to be in the gut lumen to inhibit adherence to and colonization of the intestinal wall. Moreover, mucosal immunization is attractive because it may induce both mucosal and systemic immunity. For example, orally administered *Salmonella typhi* not only invades the mucosal lining of the gut, but also infects cells of the phagocytic system throughout the body, thereby stimulating the production of both secretory and systemic antibodies, as well as CMI. Additional advantages of mucosal immunization are the ease of administration and the avoidance of systemic side effects (Shalaby, 1995; Bouvet et al., 2002; Walker, 2005). Up to now, however, successful local immunization has only been achieved with a limited number of oral vaccines. The formulation of the antigens is probably crucial for the success of mucosal immunization.

Apart from mucosal routes research groups are working on needle free jet injection of powders and fluids and dermal delivery with micro needles (Kersten and Hirschberg, 2004). A prerequisite of these approaches is that they must be painless. In that case several immunizations can be given with monovalent vaccines, replacing one multivalent vaccine. Up to now these products have not yet been registered.

## CONVENTIONAL VACCINES

### ■ Classification

Conventional vaccines originate from viruses or bacteria and can be divided in live attenuated vaccines and non-living vaccines. In addition, three vaccine generations can be distinguished for non-living vaccines. *First generation* vaccines consist of an inactivated suspension of the pathogenic microorganism. Little or no purification is applied. For *second generation* vaccines purification steps are applied, varying from the purification of a pathogenic microorganism (e.g., improved non-living polio vaccine) to the complete purification of the protective component (e.g., polysaccharide vaccines). *Third generation* vaccine are either a well-defined combination of protective components (e.g., acellular pertussis vaccine) or the protective component with the desired immunological properties (e.g., polysaccharides conjugated with carrier proteins). An overview of the various groups of conventional vaccines and their generations is given in Table 4.

### ■ Live Attenuated Vaccines

Before the introduction of recombinant-DNA (rDNA) technology, a first step to improved live vaccines was the attenuation of virulent microorganisms by serial passage and selection of mutant strains with reduced virulence or toxicity. Examples are vaccine strains for oral polio vaccine, measles-rubella-mumps (MMR) combination vaccine, and tuberculosis vaccine consisting of bacille Calmette-Guérin (BCG). An alternative approach is chemical mutagenesis. For instance, by treating *Salmonella typhi* with nitrosoguanidine, a mutant strain lacking some enzymes that are responsible for the virulence was isolated (Germanier and Fuer, 1975).

Live attenuated organisms have a number of advantages as vaccines over non-living vaccines. After administration, live vaccines may replicate in the host similar to their pathogenic counterparts. This confronts the host with a larger and more sustained dose of antigen, which means that few and low doses are required. In general, the vaccines give long-lasting humoral and cell-mediated immunity.

Live vaccines also have drawbacks. Live viral vaccines bear the risk that the nucleic acid is incorporated into the host's genome. Moreover, reversion to a virulent form may occur, although this is unlikely when the attenuated seed strain contains several mutations. Nevertheless, for diseases such as viral hepatitis, AIDS and cancer, this drawback makes the use of conventional live vaccines virtually unthinkable. Furthermore, it is important to recognize that immunization of immunodeficient children with live organisms can lead to serious complications. For instance, a child with T-cell deficiency may become overwhelmed with BCG and die.

### ■ Non-Living Vaccines: Whole Organisms

An early approach for preparing vaccines is the inactivation of whole bacteria or viruses. A number of reagents (e.g., formaldehyde, glutaraldehyde) and heat are commonly used for inactivation. Examples of

| Type | | Example | Marketed | Characteristics[a] |
|---|---|---|---|---|
| **Live** | | | | |
| Viral | | Adenovirus | Yes | Oral vaccine, USA military services only, whole |
| | | Poliovirus (Sabin) | Yes | Whole |
| | | Hepatitis A virus | No | |
| | | Measles virus | Yes | |
| | | Mumps virus | Yes | |
| | | Rubella virus | Yes | |
| | | Varicella zoster virus | Yes | |
| | | Vaccinia virus | Yes | |
| | | Yellow fever virus | Yes | |
| | | Rotavirus | No | |
| | | Influenza virus | No | |
| Bacterial | | Bacille Calmette–Guérin | Yes | Inactivated whole organism, oral vaccine |
| | | *Salmonella typhi* | Yes | Inactivated whole |
| **Non-living (first generation products)** | | | | |
| Viral | | Poliovirus (Salk) | Yes | Purified inactivated whole |
| | | Influenza virus | Yes | |
| | | Japanese B encephalitis virus | Yes | |
| Bacterial | | Bordetella pertussis | Yes | |
| | | *Vibrio cholerae* | Yes | |
| | | *Salmonella typhi* | Yes | |
| **Non-living (second generation products)** | | | | |
| Viral | | Poliovirus | Yes | |
| | | Rabies virus | Yes | |
| | | Hepatitis A virus | Yes | |
| | | Influenza virus | Yes | Subunit vaccine |
| | | Hepatitis B virus | Yes | Plasma-derived hepatitis B surface antigen |
| Bacterial | | Bordetella pertussis | Yes | Bacterial protein extract |
| | | *Haemophilus influenzae* type b | Yes | Capsular polysaccharides |
| | | Neisseria meningitidis | Yes | Capsular polysaccharides |
| | | Streptococcus pneumoniae | Yes | Capsular polysaccharides |
| | | *Vibrio cholerae* | Yes | Bacterial suspension + B subunit of cholera toxin |
| | | *Corynebacterium diphtheriae* | Yes | Diphtheria toxoid |
| | | *Clostridium tetani* | Yes | Tetanus toxoid |
| **Non-living (third generation products)** | | | | |
| Viral | | Measles virus | No | Subunit vaccine, ISCOM formulation |
| Bacterial | | Bordetella pertussis | Yes | Mixture of purified protein antigens |
| | | *Haemophilus influenzae* type B | Yes | Polysaccharide-protein conjugates |
| | | Neisseria meningitidis | No | Polysaccharide-protein conjugates |
| | | Streptococcus pneumoniae | No | Polysaccharide-protein conjugates |

[a] Unless mentioned otherwise, the vaccine is administered parenterally.
*Source*: From Plotkin and Orenstein, 2004.

**Table 4** ▪ Conventional vaccines.

this first generation approach are pertussis, cholera, typhoid fever, and inactivated polio vaccines. These non-living vaccines have the disadvantage that little or no CMI is induced. Moreover, they more frequently cause adverse effects as compared to live attenuated vaccines and second and third generation non-living vaccines.

## ■ Non-Living Vaccines: Subunit Vaccines

### Diphtheria and Tetanus Toxoids

Some bacteria such as *Corynebacterium diphtheriae* and *Clostridium tetani* form toxins. Antibody-mediated immunity to the toxins is the main protection mechanism against infections with these bacteria. Both toxins are proteins. Around the beginning of the twentieth century, a combination of diphtheria toxin and antibodies to diphtheria toxin was used as diphtheria vaccine. This vaccine was far from ideal and was replaced in the 1920s with formaldehyde-treated toxin. The chemically treated toxin is devoid of toxic properties and is called toxoid. The immunogenicity of this preparation was relatively low and was improved after adsorption of the toxoid to a suspension of aluminum salts. This combination of an antigen and an adjuvant is still used in existing combination vaccines. Similarly, tetanus toxoid vaccines have been developed.

Diphtheria toxin has also been detoxified by chemical mutagenesis of *Corynebacterium diphtheriae* with nitrosoguanidine. These diphtheria toxoids are referred to as cross-reactive materials (e.g., $CRM_{197}$).

### Acellular Pertussis Vaccines

The relatively frequent occurrence of side effects of whole-cell pertussis vaccine was the main reason to develop subunit vaccines in the 1970s, which are referred to as acellular pertussis vaccines. These vaccines were prepared by either extraction of the bacterial suspension followed by purification steps, or purification of the cell-free culture supernatant. These second generation vaccines showed relatively large lot-to-lot variations, as a result of their poorly controlled production processes.

The development of third generation acellular pertussis vaccines in the 1980s exemplifies how a better insight into factors that are important for pathogenesis and immunogenicity can lead to an improved vaccine. It was conceived that a subunit vaccine consisting of a limited number of purified immunogenic components and devoid of (toxic) lipopolysaccharide would significantly reduce undesired effects. Four protein antigens important for protection have been identified. However, as yet there exists no consensus about the optimal composition of an acellular pertussis vaccine. Current vaccines contain different amounts of two to four of these proteins.

### Polysaccharide Vaccines

Bacterial capsular polysaccharides consist of pathogen-specific multiple repeating carbohydrate epitopes, which are isolated from cultures of the pathogenic species. Plain capsular polysaccharides (second generation vaccines) are thymus-independent antigens that are poorly immunogenic in infants and show poor immunological memory when applied in older children and adults. The immunogenicity of polysaccharides is highly increased when they are chemically coupled to carrier proteins containing $T_h$-epitopes. This coupling makes them T-cell dependent, which is due to the participation of $T_h$-cells that are activated during the response to the carrier. Examples of such third generation polysaccharide conjugate vaccines include meningococcal type C, pneumococcal and *Haemophilus influenzae* type b (Hib) polysaccharide vaccines that have recently been introduced in many national immunization programs. Four different conjugated Hib polysaccharide structures are presently available, i.e., chemically linked to either tetanus toxoid, diphtheria toxoid, $CRM_{197}$ (mutagenically detoxified diphtheria toxin, see above) or meningococcal outer membrane complexes. Apart from the carrier, the four structures vary in the size of the polysaccharide moiety, the nature of the spacer group, the polysaccharide-to-protein ratio, and the molecular size and aggregation state of the conjugates. As a result, they induce different immunological responses. This illustrates that not only the antigen, but also its presentation form determines the immunogenicity of a vaccine. Therefore, the determination of optimal conjugation procedures, the standardization of conjugation, as well as the separation of conjugates from free proteins and polysaccharides are of utmost importance.

## MODERN VACCINE TECHNOLOGIES

### ■ Genetically Improved Live Vaccines

#### Genetically Attenuated Microorganisms

Emerging insights in molecular pathogenesis of many infectious diseases make it possible to attenuate microorganisms very efficiently nowadays. By making multiple deletions the risk of reversion to a virulent state during production or after administration can be virtually eliminated. A prerequisite for attenuation by genetic engineering is that the factors responsible for virulence and the life cycle of the pathogen are known in detail. It is also obvious that the protective antigens must be known: attenuation must not result in reduced immunogenicity.

An example of an improved live vaccine obtained by homologous genetic engineering is an experimental, oral cholera vaccine. An effective cholera vaccine should induce a local, humoral response in order to prevent colonization of the small intestine. Initial trials with *Vibrio cholerae* cholera toxin (CT) mutants caused mild diarrhea, which was thought to be caused by the expression of accessory toxins. A natural mutant was isolated that was negative for these toxins. Next, CT was detoxified by rDNA technology. The resulting vaccine strain, called CVD 103, is well tolerated by volunteers (Suharyono et al., 1992; Tacket et al., 1999) and challenge experiments with adult volunteers showed protection (Garcia et al., 2005).

Genetically attenuated live vaccines have the general drawbacks mentioned in the section "Live Attenuated Vaccines." For these reasons, it is not surprising that homologous engineering is mainly restricted to pathogens that are used as starting materials for the production of subunit vaccines (see section "Genetically Improved Subunit Vaccines," below).

## Live Vectored Vaccines

A way to improve the safety or efficacy of vaccines is to use live, avirulent or attenuated organisms as a carrier to express protective antigens from a pathogen. Both bacteria and viruses can be used for this purpose; some of them are listed in Table 5. Live vectored vaccines are created by recombinant technology, wherein one or more genes of the vector organism are replaced by one or more protective genes from the pathogen. Administration of such live vectored vaccines results in efficient and prolonged expression of the antigenic genes either by the vaccinated individual's own cells or by the vector organism itself (e.g., in case of bacteria as carriers).

Most experience has been acquired with vaccinia virus by using the principle that is schematically shown in Figure 5. Advantages of vaccinia virus as vector include (*i*) its proven safety in humans as a smallpox vaccine, (*ii*) the possibility for multiple immunogen expression, (*iii*) the ease of production, (*iv*) its relative heat-resistance, and (*v*) its various possible administration routes. A multitude of live recombinant vaccinia vaccines with viral and tumor antigens have been constructed (Sutter and Staib, 2003), several of which have been tested in the clinic. It has been demonstrated that the products of genes coding for viral envelope proteins can be correctly processed and inserted into the plasma membrane of infected cells. Problems related with the side effects or immunogenicity of

| Vector | Antigens from | Advantages of vector | Disadvantages of vector |
|---|---|---|---|
| **Viral** | | | |
| Vaccinia | RSV, HIV, VSV, rabies virus, HSV, influenza virus, EBV, *Plasmodium* spp. (malaria) | Widely used in man (safe) Large insertions possible (up to 41 kB) | Sometimes causing side effects Very immunogenic: repeated use difficult |
| Avipoxviruses (canarypox, fowlpox) | Rabies virus, measles virus | Abortive replication in man Low immunogenicity | |
| Poliovirus | *Vibrio cholerae*, influenza virus, HIV, *Chlamydia* | Widely used in man (safe) Live/oral and inactivated/ parenteral forms possible | Small genome |
| Adenoviruses | RSV, HBV, EBV, HIV, CMV | Oral route applicable | Small genome |
| Herpesviruses (HSV, CMV, varicella virus) | EBV, HBV | Large genome | |
| **Bacterial** | | | |
| *Salmonella* spp. | *B. pertussis*, HBV, *Plasmodium* spp., *E. coli*, influenza virus, Streptococci, *Vibrio cholerae*, *Shigella* spp. | Strong mucosal responses | |
| Mycobacteria (BCG) | *Borrelia burgdorferi* (Lyme disease) | Widely used in man (safe) Large insertions possible | |
| *E. coli* | Bordetella pertussis; *Shigella flexneri* | | |

*Abbreviations*: BCG, Bacille Calmette-Guérin; CMV, cytomegalovirus; EBV, Epstein-Barr virus; HBV, Hepatitis B virus; HIV, Human immunodeficiency virus; HSV, herpes simplex virus; RSV, respiratory syncytial virus; VSV, vesicular stomatitis virus.

**Table 5** Recombinant live vaccines.

vaccinia virus may be circumvented by the use of attenuated strains or poxviruses with a non-human natural host.

Adenoviruses can also be used as vaccine vectors (see also Chapter 8). Adenoviruses have several characteristics that make them suitable as vaccine vectors: (i) They can infect a broad range of both dividing and non-dividing mammalian cells; (ii) transgene expression is generally high and can be further increased by using heterologous promoter sequences; (iii) adenovirus vectors are mostly replication deficient and do not integrate their genomes into the chromosomes of host cells, making these vectors very safe to use; (iv) upon parenteral administration, adenovirus vectors induce strong immunity and evoke both humoral and cellular responses against the expressed antigen. A number of clinical trials with human adenovirus vectors (HAd5) expressing antigens of Ebola virus, human immunodeficiency virus (HIV) and severe acute respiratory syndrome as vaccines against these diseases are currently in progress (Bangari and Mittal, 2006).

A major limitation of the use of live vectored vaccines is the prevalence of preexisting immunity against the vector itself, which could neutralize the vaccine before the immune system can be primed. Such preexisting immunity has been described for adenoviral vectors, for which the prevalence of neutralizing antibodies can be as high as 90% of the total population. The use of strains with no or low prevalence of preexisting immunity as live vectors is therefore recommended (Holterman et al., 2004; Bangari and Mittal, 2006).

## ■ Genetically Improved Subunit Vaccines

### Genetically Detoxified Proteins

A biotechnological improvement of the acellular pertussis vaccine has been the switch from chemically to genetically inactivated pertussis toxin. The principle of both chemical and genetic inactivation is schematically illustrated in Figure 6. Chemical treatment with formaldehyde results in a cripple protein molecule with partial loss of conformational and antigenic properties (Fig. 6B). This reduces its immunogenicity, whereas potential reversal to a biologically active toxin is a major concern. Variations in the extent of detoxification can affect both the immunogenicity and the toxicity of the product. In contrast, genetic detoxification by site-directed mutagenesis warrants the reproducible production of a non-toxic mutant protein that is highly immunogenic because the integrity of immunogenic sites is fully retained (Fig. 6C). In the pertussis toxin example, codons for two amino acids were mutated in the cloned pertussis gene, which abolished the

toxicity of the protein without changing its immunological properties. The altered gene was then substituted in *Bordetella pertussis* for the native gene (Nencioni et al., 1990). Other candidates for genetic detoxification are diphtheria toxin, tetanus toxin, and cholera toxin.

### Proteins Expressed in Host Cells

To improve the yield, facilitate the production, and/or improve the safety of protein-based vaccines, protein antigens are sometimes expressed by host cells of the same (homologous) species or of different (heterologous) species that are safe to handle and/or allow high expression levels.

Heterologous hosts used for the expression of immunogenic proteins include yeasts, bacteria, and mammalian cell lines. Hepatitis B surface antigen (HBsAg), which previously was obtained from plasma of infected individuals, has been expressed in bakers' yeast (*Saccharomyces cerevisae*); (Valenzuela et al., 1982; Vanlandschoot et al., 2002) and in mammalian cells (Chinese hamster ovary cells) (Burnette et al., 1985; Raz et al., 2001) by transforming the host cell with a plasmid containing the HBsAg-encoding gene. Both expression systems yield 22-nm HBsAg particles (also called virus like particles or VLPs) that are structurally identical to the native virus. Advantages are safety, consistent quality, and high yields. The yeast-derived vaccine has become available worldwide and appears to be as safe and efficacious as the classical plasma-derived vaccine.

The experimental multivalent meningococcal vesicle vaccine is an example of the expression of multiple antigens in homologous host cells (van der Ley et al., 1995). The vaccine is prepared by extraction of vesicles from the meningococcal outer membrane. These vesicles serve as a natural carrier for immunogenic outer membrane proteins (OMPs), which are incorporated into the vesicle membrane. Each wild-type meningococcus strain expresses strain-specific OMPs. Taking a wild-type strain as starting point, mutant strains expressing OMPs specific for three strains have been made through transformation with plasmid constructs in *Escherichia coli* and their recombination into the meningococcal chromosome. Outer membrane vesicles of two trivalent strains have been prepared and combined to a hexavalent vaccine, which has been shown to be immunogenic in infants (Cartwright et al., 1999).

An interesting development is the exploration of transgenic plants for their potential as heterologous expression system for antigenic components (Sala et al., 2003). The aim of this approach is to express antigenic components in edible (parts of) plants, such as bananas. Advantages of edible vaccines include: (*i*)

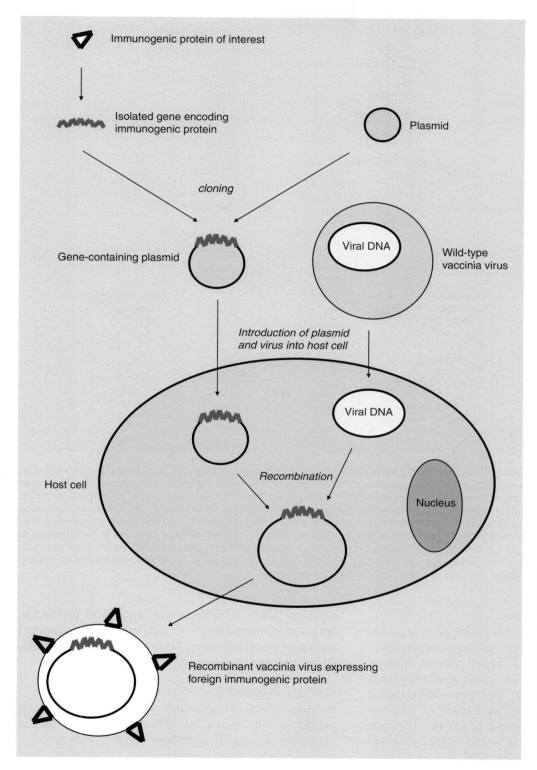

Immunogenic protein of interest

Isolated gene encoding
immunogenic protein

Plasmid

*cloning*

Gene-containing plasmid

Viral DNA

Wild-type
vaccinia virus

*Introduction of plasmid
and virus into host cell*

Viral DNA

Host cell

*Recombination*

Nucleus

Recombinant vaccinia virus expressing
foreign immunogenic protein

**Figure 5** ■ Construction of recombinant vaccinia virus as a vector of foreign protein antigens. The gene of interest encoding an immunogenic protein is inserted into a plasmid. The plasmid containing the protein gene and wild-type vaccinia virus are then simultaneously introduced into a host cell line to undergo recombination of viral and plasmid DNA, after which the foreign protein is expressed by the recombinant virus.

no need for purification, (*ii*) ease of immunization, (*iii*) built-in protection of antigens by cell walls and cellular membranes, and (*iv*) possibility of local production in developing countries. Problems related with the production of edible vaccines are the low expression levels and the control of the level and quality of the antigen. Examples of candidate vaccine components are VLPs, such as HBsAg and Norwalk virus capsid protein, which have entered into clinical trials.

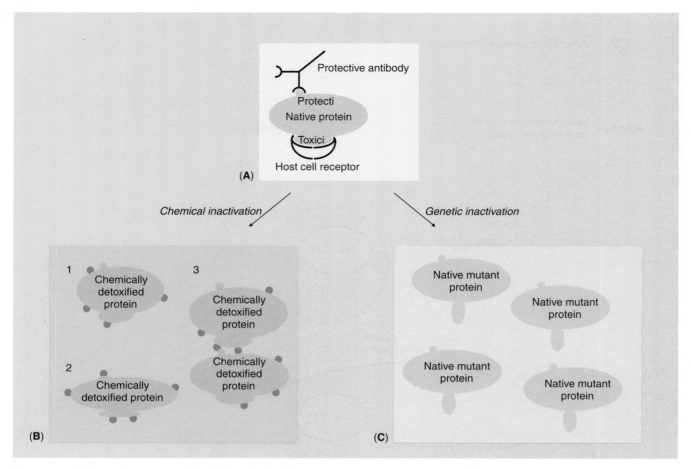

**Figure 6** ■ Schematic representation of chemical and genetic detoxification of immunogenic toxins. A hypothetical toxin contains an epitope recognized by protective antibodies and a site responsible for toxicity through interaction with a host cell receptor (**A**). Toxins can be chemically inactivated by treatment with (usually) formaldehyde, resulting in a heterogeneous population of chemically detoxified proteins that carry covalently bound formaldehyde residues on their surface (represented by black spheres in (**B**). Chemically detoxified proteins preferably retain protective epitopes while the toxicity-related site is blocked (B1). However, part of the protein population may contain epitopes that are no longer recognized by protective antibodies (B2). Formaldehyde treatment may also lead to the formation of covalent multimers (B3) and slight perturbations of the three-dimensional protein structure (B2, B3). (**C**) Apart from chemical inactivation, toxins can be genetically detoxified by selectively changing the amino acid sequence in the site responsible for toxicity without affecting the protective epitope, resulting in a homogeneous toxoid population.

## Recombinant Peptide Vaccines

After identification of a protective epitope, it is possible to incorporate the corresponding peptide sequence through genetic fusion into a carrier protein, such as HBsAg, hepatitis B core antigen, and β-galactosidase (Francis and Larche, 2005). The peptide-encoding DNA sequence is synthesized and inserted into the carrier protein gene. An example of the recombinant peptide approach is a malaria vaccine based on a 16-fold repeat of the Asn-Ala-Asn-Pro sequence of a *Plasmodium falciparum* surface antigen. The gene encoding this peptide was fused with the HBsAg gene and the fusion product was expressed by yeast cells (Vreden et al., 1991). Genetic fusion of peptides with proteins offers the possibility to produce protective epitopes of toxic antigens derived from pathogenic species as part of non-toxic proteins expressed by

harmless species. Furthermore, a uniform product is obtained in comparison with the variability of chemical conjugates (see following section "Synthetic Peptide-Based Vaccines").

## Synthetic Peptide-Based Vaccines

Another form of molecular mimicry are synthetic peptides, which can be obtained by solid phase synthesis. Primarily, peptide-based vaccines have been designed based on antibody recognition. Two approaches can be discerned, as outlined in Figure 7, depending on whether the epitope is continuous or discontinuous.

In the first approach (Fig. 7A) immunogenic epitopes are determined by DNA cloning and nucleotide sequencing of protein antigens, and serology studies. The small linear peptide sequence is

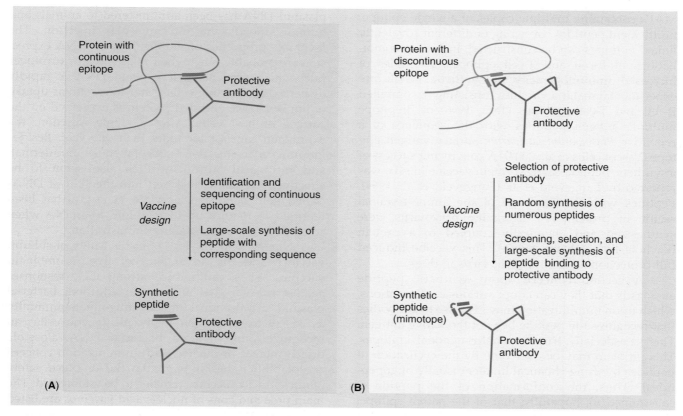

**Figure 7** ▪ Two approaches for the design of synthetic peptide vaccines. (**A**): identification and sequencing of a continuous epitope on an immunogenic protein is followed by the synthesis of peptides with the amino acid sequence corresponding to that of the epitope. (**B**) synthesis of peptides mimicking discontinuous epitopes that are determined by the three-dimensional structure of the immunogenic protein; a peptide that strongly binds to a protective antibody recognizing the discontinuous epitope is selected. The peptide (mimotope) does not necessarily contain the exact amino acid sequence of the constituent fragments that form the epitope.

chemically synthesized and can be used as a vaccine component. A limitation of this concept is that it is only applicable to continuous epitopes that are solely determined by the primary amino acid sequence and not by the conformation of the epitope. Many B-cell epitopes, however, are conformationally determined and/or discontinuous. For continuous conformational epitopes, synthetic peptides can be forced to adopt the proper conformation by cyclization (see below).

The second approach (Fig. 7B) is particularly useful for discontinuous epitopes. In this case, the optimal sequence of a synthetic peptide is not easy to determine a priori. With current technology, however, thousands of peptides can be rapidly synthesized at random and screened for optimal binding to protective antibodies. The sequence of a selected peptide can, if necessary, be optimized for antibody binding by selectively substituting one or more amino acid residues. Such peptides approximating the native epitope—but not necessarily containing the exact (linear or non-linear) sequence of the epitope—are referred to as mimotopes. In theory, analogous with anti-idiotype antibodies, mimotopes may be useful as

internal image not only of peptide epitopes but also of non-protein structures.

Similar to B-cell epitope peptides, T-cell epitope peptide vaccines can also be designed. T-cell epitopes usually have a continuous, non-conformational nature and are therefore relatively easy to mimic after their sequence has been identified, in analogy with the approach for continuous B-cell epitopes.

Synthetic peptide vaccines have the following advantages:

1. They can be prepared in unlimited quantities using solid-phase technology.
2. They are easily purified by HPLC methods.
3. They do not contain infectious or toxic material.

The use of synthetic peptides as vaccine has two main complications regarding their immunogenicity. First, plain short peptide antigens are usually poorly immunogenic. This can be alleviated by (*a*) synthesizing them as multiple antigen peptides (MAPs; (Tam, 1996)) or (*b*) by coupling them to a carrier protein (Francis, 1991). MAPs consist of branched multimers with a small oligolysine core at the center. Apart from

MAPs containing multiple copies of a single epitope, multivalent peptides consisting of different covalently linked epitopes can be constructed, including combinations of B-cell and T-cell epitopes. Examples of increased immunogenicity of synthetic MAPs are experimental malaria vaccines consisting of combined B-cell and T-cell epitopes (Tam, 1996) or diepitope multiple antigen peptides with the sequence of a repetitive *Plasmodium falciparum* surface antigen epitope (Vasconcelos et al., 2004). A convincing success of a synthetic peptide-carrier protein vaccine in vivo was reported by Langeveld et al. (Langeveld et al., 1994). Peptides with the sequence of the amino-terminal region of protein VP2 of canine parvovirus were synthesized and chemically coupled to a protein (keyhole limpet hemocyanin). This vaccine induced full protection against virulent virus in dogs.

A second concern about synthetic peptide analogs is that they can adopt various conformations, which upon immunization may give rise to antibodies that recognize the peptide but not the native antigen. This is especially true for conformational epitopes. This problem may be overcome by the cyclization of peptides by using chemical linkers (usually oligopeptides). Thus, the conformation of the peptide is constrained to, hopefully, that of the native epitope. The nature of the peptide as well as the length and conformation of the cyclic construct determine the success of cyclization, as illustrated in Figure 8. One of the first examples of the successful induction of the proper conformation through cyclization has been reported by Muller et al. (1990). Antibodies raised to ovalbumin conjugates of cyclic peptide analogs of influenza virus hemagglutinin reacted with native hemagglutinin. The immunogenicity of the peptides was strongly dependent on the loop conformation and on the orientation of the peptide on the carrier protein. Hoogerhout et al. (1995) showed that the ring size and the cyclization chemistry are of crucial importance for the immunogenicity of cyclic peptide analogs (coupled to tetanus toxoid) of a meningococcal OMP epitope.

### Nucleic Acid Vaccines

A revolutionary application of rDNA technology in vaccinology has been the introduction of nucleic acid vaccines (Davis and Whalen, 1995; Donnelly et al., 2005). In this approach plasmid DNA or messenger RNA encoding the desired antigen is directly administered into the vaccinee. The foreign protein is then expressed by the host cells and generates an immune response.

Plasmid DNA is produced by replication in *E. coli* or other bacterial cells and purification by established methods (e.g., density gradient centrifugation, ion-exchange chromatography). Up until now plasmid DNA has been administered to animals and humans mostly via intramuscular injection. The favorable properties of muscle cells for DNA expression are probably due to their relatively low turn-over rate, which prevents that plasmid DNA is rapidly dispersed in dividing cells. After intracellular uptake of the DNA, the encoded protein is expressed on the surface of host cells. After a single injection, the expression can last for more than one year. Besides intramuscular injection, subcutaneous, intradermal, and intranasal administrations also seem to be effective. Needleless injection into the skin of DNA-coated gold nanoparticles via a gene gun has been reported to require up to 1000-fold less DNA when compared to intramuscular administration.

Nucleic acid vaccines offer the safety of subunit vaccines and the advantages of live recombinant vaccines. They can induce strong CTL responses against the encoded antigen. In addition, bacterial plasmids are also ideal for activating innate immunity as TLR-9 expressed on many phagocytic cells can recognize unmethylated bacterial DNA. Possible disadvantages of nucleic acid immunization concern acceptability issues. In particular, the long-term safety of nucleic acid vaccines remains to be established. The main pros and cons of nucleic acid vaccines are listed in Table 6. An advantage of RNA over DNA is that it is not able to incorporate into host DNA. A drawback of RNA, however, is that it is less stable than DNA. Nucleic acids coding for a variety of antigens have shown to induce protective, long-lived humoral and cellular immune responses in various species including man. Examples of DNA vaccines that have been tested in clinical trials comprise plasmids encoding HIV-1 antigens and malaria antigens.

### ■ Reverse Vaccinology

Nowadays vaccines can be designed based on the information encoded by the genome of a particular pathogen (Masignani et al., 2002; Rappuoli and Covacci, 2003). From many pathogens the entire genomes have been sequenced and this number is increasingly growing (http://www.sanger.ac.uk/Projects/Pathogens). The genome sequence of a pathogen provides a complete picture of all proteins that can be produced by the pathogens at any given time. Using computer algorithms, proteins that are either excreted or expressed on the surface of the pathogen, and thus most likely available for recognition by the host's immune system, can be identified. After recombinant production and purification, these vaccine candidates can be screened for immunogenicity in mice. From these, the best candidates can be selected and used as subunit vaccines (Fig. 9).

A big advantage of reverse vaccinology is the ease at which novel candidate antigens can be selected

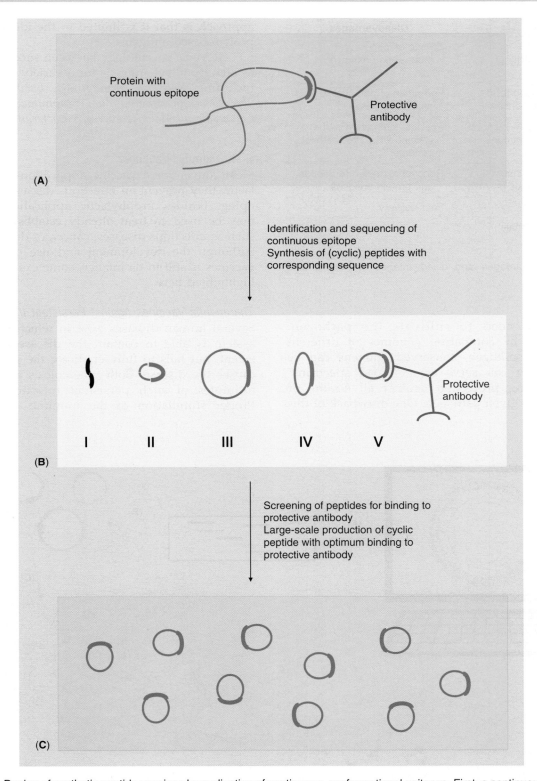

**Figure 8** ☐ Design of synthetic peptide vaccines by cyclization of continuous, conformational epitopes. First, a continuous epitope that evokes protective antibodies is identified and sequenced (**A**). Next, peptides with the amino acid sequence corresponding to that of the epitope are synthesized whether or not with a linker to form a loop structure—and are screened for binding to protective antibody (**B**). In this example, immunization with peptides I to IV would induce non-protective antibodies to the misfolded epitope. Linear peptide I does not have the proper conformation corresponding to that on the native protein. Loops for cyclization in peptides II-IV are too short (II), too long (III) or improperly folded (IV), thereby inducing incorrect peptide conformations. (**C**) Cyclic peptide V has the correct native conformation and is likely to induce protective antibody formation upon immunization. Therefore, cyclic peptide V is produced for vaccine purposes.

| Advantages | Disadvantages |
|---|---|
| Low intrinsic immunogenicity of nucleic acids | Effects of long-term expression unknown |
| Induction of long-term immune responses | Formation of anti-nucleic acid antibodies possible |
| Induction of both humoral and cellular immune responses | Possible integration of the vaccine DNA into the host genome |
| Possibility of constructing multiple epitope plasmids | Concept restricted to peptide and protein antigens |
| Heat-stability | Poor delivery |
| Ease of large-scale production | |

**Table 6** ▪ Advantages and disadvantages of nucleic acid vaccines.

without the need to cultivate the pathogen. Furthermore, by comparing genomes of different strains of a pathogen, conserved antigens can be identified that can serve as a "broad spectrum" vaccine, giving protection against all strains or serotypes of a given pathogen. One drawback of this

approach is that it is limited to the identification of protein-based antigens.

Reverse vaccinology has been successfully used to identify novel antigens for a variety of pathogens, including *Neisseria meningitidis*, *Bacillus anthracis*, *Streptococcus pneumoniae*, *Staphylococcus aureus*, *Chlamydia pneumoniae* and *Mycobacterium tuberculosis*.

## ▪ Therapeutic Vaccines

Most conventional vaccine applications are prophylactic: they prevent an infectious disease from developing. Besides prophylactic applications, vaccines may be used to treat already established diseases, such as infectious diseases, cancer, or drug addiction. Although the development and use of therapeutic vaccines is still in its infancy, some examples will be highlighted here.

### Therapeutic Vaccines Against Persistent Infections

Several human diseases exist in which the immune system is able to contain the disease to a certain extent, but fails to fully eradicate the pathogen that causes the disease. Both tuberculosis and AIDS are examples of such persistent infectious diseases. Proper stimulation of the immune system using

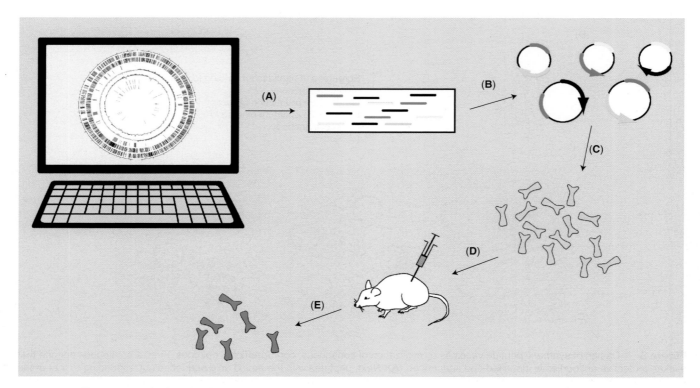

**Figure 9** ▪ Reverse vaccinology involves the analysis of genome sequences of pathogens in silico with the aim to identify potential antigens (**A**). These potential antigens can then be cloned (**B**), produced recombinantly (**C**) and subsequently used for immunological screening (**D**). The entire process leads to a quick identification of a limited number of vaccine candidates that can give protection against infection with the pathogen without the need to test all proteins produced by this pathogen (**E**). *Source*: Adapted from Scarselli et al., 2005.

therapeutic vaccines may break the status quo and shift the equilibrium towards full eradication of the disease-causing pathogen.

Tuberculosis is caused by infection with *M. tuberculosis* via the lungs. The mycobacteria are taken up by alveolar macrophages and DCs, but these cells somehow fail to destroy the pathogens. As a result, a local inflammation occurs causing influx of monocytes and the formation of granulomas, which can persist for years. Although a vaccine against tuberculosis based on an attenuated strain of *Mycobacterium bovis* (bacille Calmette-Guérin, or BCG) already exists, this vaccine is only effective in severe forms of childhood tuberculosis and not for treating latent infections with *M. tuberculosis*. Currently, therapeutic vaccines are under development containing the antigen HspX that is expressed during the dormant stage of the mycobacterium. Vaccines based on this antigen have proven to be effective in mice, and are currently tested in phase I clinical trials (Haile and Kallenius, 2005).

Acquired immunodeficiency syndrome (AIDS) is caused by infection with the HIV. HIV predominantly resides in CD4 positive T-cells, monocytes and macrophages. The virus is cytopathic in activated T-cells, but less in macrophages and not at all in latently infected cells with integrated provirus. Although HIV infection does not immediately cause AIDS, and some seropositive patients never develop AIDS, most infected patients progress to AIDS over a period of years and eventually die if not adequately treated.

Vaccines against HIV should ideally elicit both humoral and cellular immunity. The humoral response should give protection against non-infected individuals (prophylactic) or against spread or re-infection of already infected individuals, whereas the cellular immunity should reduce the intracellular virus pool by killing infected cell populations. A humoral response against HIV has proven difficult to obtain: vaccination against the viral glycoprotein gp120 has resulted in protection against the culture-adapted HIV strains, but not against a challenge with native virus (Gilliam and Redfield, 2003; Kaufmann and McMichael, 2005). Also protective cellular responses are difficult to obtain as $T_h$-cells are the prime target of the virus.

To date, the best results with therapeutic vaccines against HIV were achieved with a replication-defective recombinant adenovirus-5 (rAd5) vector (Shiver et al., 2002; Shiver and Emini, 2004). Vaccination of rhesus monkeys with rAd5 vectors resulted in partial protection against reinfection with fresh isolates of infectious virus. In humans rAd5 vectors have been tested in a phase I study, showing that these vectors could induce strong cellular immune responses in humans. A recently started phase IIb clinical study should demonstrate whether these vectors can convey protection in HIV-infected patients.

## Cancer Vaccines

Cancer is caused by the malignant outgrowth of a single transformed cell. Multiple mutations in genes may give them a growth advantage, but may also lead to different antigens or a different pattern of antigen expression, as has been demonstrated in several types of tumors. In principle specific T-cell responses can be mounted against such tumor-specific or tumor-associated antigens. However, despite the presence of tumor infiltrating lymphocytes in certain sets of tumors, the immune system somehow fails to mount an effective response that can eradicate the tumor. It is the hope that active vaccination may be able to augment the already-existing immune reaction against tumors in such a way that this will lead to eradication of the tumor (Finn, 2003). However, this is not an easy task. Patients with cancer are often of advanced age and therefore have a smaller repertoire of circulating T-cells that can mount a tumor-specific response. Anti-cancer treatments received by the patient may further suppress antitumor immune responses. Furthermore, tumor cells can evade immune suppression in various ways. Tumors tend to be genetically unstable and can lose their antigens by mutation. Moreover, CTL-based responses sometimes result in selection of tumor cells lacking MHC class I molecules that cannot be recognized and killed by cytotoxic T-cells. Some tumors excrete immunosuppressive cytokines (e.g., TGF-β) to prevent or reduce immune attack.

Immunotherapy against cancer requires the activation of tumor specific T-cells, although humoral responses may in some cases (e.g., non-Hodgkin lymphoma) also be effective. There are several strategies to boost such a tumor-specific CTL response. Vaccines can be prepared from the patient's tumor itself by mixing irradiated tumor cells or cell extracts with bacterial adjuvants such as BCG to enhance their immunogenicity. Alternatively, heat shock proteins isolated from the patient's tumor that contain associated tumor antigens can be used as a tumor-specific vaccine. In combination with adjuvants, these heat-shock proteins can be very potent in stimulating CTL responses against tumor cells as has been demonstrated in several clinical trials (Liu et al., 2002). Another approach is to genetically alter tumor cells in order to make them more immunogenic. Transfection of tumor cells with the gene encoding the co-stimulatory molecule B7 has resulted in direct activation of tumor-specific CTLs by the transformed tumor cells (Garnett et al., 2006). Similar results can be achieved by transforming tumor cells with genes encoding cytokines (e.g., GM-CSF, IL-2, IL-4, and IL-12).

### Vaccines Against Drug Abuse

Therapeutic vaccines are also being developed for the treatment of drug abuse, such as addiction to nicotine, cocaine or metamphetamine (Haney and Kosten, 2004). The idea is to evoke a humoral immune reaction against the drug molecules. As most of these drugs have their addictive action within the central nervous system, antibodies raised against the drug molecules can prevent the passage of these molecules over the blood brain barrier and thus prevent the addictive effects. Most abused drugs are small non-protein substances, which generally do not elicit an immune response. In order to activate the host immune system against these substances they need to be conjugated to proteins, such as ovalbumin or diphtheria toxin. This approach has been effective in animal models. Several clinical trials to test vaccines against nicotine are ongoing. The first outcomes show large variations between neutralizing antibody levels among patients, but those with high levels can successfully remain abstinent.

## PHARMACEUTICAL ASPECTS

### ■ Production

Except for synthetic peptides, vaccines are derived from microorganisms or from animal cells. For optimal expression of the required vaccine component(s), these microorganisms or animal cells can be genetically modified. Animal cells are used for the cultivation of viruses and for the production of some subunit vaccine components, and have the advantage that the vaccine components are released into the culture medium.

Three stages can be discerned in the manufacture of cell-derived vaccines: (1) cultivation or upstream processing, (2) purification or downstream processing, and (3) formulation. For the first two stages the reader is referred to Chapter 3, whereas the formulation is addressed in the following section.

### ■ Formulation

### Adjuvants and Delivery Systems

The success of immunization is not only dependent on the nature of the immunogenic components, but also on their presentation form. Therefore, the search for effective and acceptable adjuvants (Schijns, 2000) and delivery systems (Kersten and Hirschberg, 2004) is an important issue in modern vaccine development. Adjuvants are defined as any material that can increase the humoral and cellular response against an antigen. Colloidal aluminum salts (hydroxide,

phosphate) are widely used in many classical vaccine formulations. Other adjuvants are in experimental testing or are used in veterinary vaccines. Delivery systems are injectable devices that allow multimeric presentation of antigens. They can also contain adjuvants. Table 7 shows a list of some well-known adjuvants and delivery systems.

Adjuvants and delivery systems stimulate the immune system by several mechanisms of action (Schijns, 2000):

1. A depot effect leading to slow antigen release and prolonged antigen presentation.
2. Attraction and stimulation of APCs by some local tissue damage and binding to PRRs present on APCs.
3. Delivery of the antigen to regional lymph nodes by improved antigen uptake, transport and presentation by APCs.

A particular adjuvant may act by one or more of these mechanisms.

| Adjuvant | Characteristics |
|---|---|
| Aluminum salts | Antigen adsorption is crucial |
| Lipid A and derivatives | Fragment of lipopolysaccharide, a bacterial endotoxin |
| Muramyl peptides | Active fragments of bacterial cell walls |
| Saponins | Plant triterpene glycosides |
| NBP | Synthetic amphiphiles |
| DDA | Synthetic amphiphile |
| CpG | Non-methylated DNA-sequences containing CpG-oligodinucleotides |
| Cytokines | Interleukins (1, 2, 3, 6, 12), interferon, tumor necrosis factor |
| Cholera toxin, B subunit | Mucosal adjuvant |
| **Delivery system** | **Characteristics** |
| Emulsions | Both water-in-oil and oil-in-water emulsions are used; often contain amphiphilic adjuvants |
| Liposomes | Phospholipid membrane vesicles; aqueous interior as well as lipid bilayer may contain antigens and/or adjuvants |
| ISCOMs | Micellar lipid-saponin complex; not suitable for soluble antigens |
| Microspheres | Biodegradable polymeric spheres, often poly(lactide-co-glycolide) |

*Abbreviations*: DDA, dioctadecyldimethylammonium bromide; ISCOM, immune stimulating complex; NBP, non-ionic block copolymers.

**Table 7** ▪ Adjuvants and antigen delivery systems.

## Combination Vaccines

Since oral immunization is not possible for most available vaccines (see section "Route of Administration," above), the strategy to mix individual vaccines in order to limit the number of injections has been common practice since many years. Currently, vaccines are available containing up to six non-related antigens: diphtheria-tetanus-pertussis-hepatitis B-polio-*Haemophilus influenzae* type b vaccine. Another example is MMR vaccine, alone or in combination with varicella vaccine. Sometimes a vaccine contains antigens from several subtypes of a particular pathogen. Heptavalent pneumococcal vaccine is an example. This vaccine contains polysaccharides from seven pneumococcal strains, conjugated to a carrier protein to improve immunogenicity.

Combining vaccine components sometimes results in pharmaceutical as well as immunological problems. For instance, formaldehyde-containing components may chemically react with other components; an unstable antigen may need freeze drying whereas other antigens cannot be frozen. Components that are not compatible can be mixed prior to injection, if there is no short-term incompatibility. To this end, dual-chamber syringes have been developed.

From an immunological point of view, the immunization schedules of the individual components of combination vaccines should match. Even when this condition is fulfilled and the components are pharmaceutically compatible, the success of a combination vaccine is not warranted. Vaccine components in combination vaccines may exhibit a different behavior in vivo compared to separate administration of the components. For instance, enhancement (Paradiso et al., 1993) as well as suppression (Gold et al., 1994) of humoral immune responses has been reported.

## ■ Characterization

Second and third generation conventional vaccines and modern vaccines are well-defined products in terms of immunogenicity, structure, and purity. This means that the products can be characterized with a combination of appropriate biochemical, physico-chemical, and immunochemical techniques (see Chapter 2). Vaccines have to meet the same standards as other biotechnological pharmaceuticals. The use of modern analytical techniques for the design and release of new vaccines is gaining importance. Currently, animal experiments are needed for quality control of many vaccines but in vitro analytical techniques may eventually partly substitute preclinical tests in vivo. During the development of the production process of a vaccine component, a combination of suitable assays can be defined. These assays can subsequently be applied during its routine production.

Column chromatographic (HPLC) and electrophoretic techniques like gel electrophoresis and capillary electrophoresis provide information about the purity, molecular weight, and electric charge of the vaccine component. Physico-chemical assays comprise mass spectrometry, nuclear magnetic resonance spectroscopy, and light spectroscopy, including circular dichroism and fluorescence spectroscopy. Information is obtained mainly about the molecular weight and the conformation of the vaccine component. Immunochemical assays, such as enzyme-linked immunoassays and radioimmunoassays, are powerful methods for the quantification of the vaccine component. By using well-defined monoclonal antibodies (preferably with the same specificity as those of protective human antibodies) information can be obtained about the conformation and accessibility of the epitope to which the antibodies are directed. Moreover, the use of biosensors makes it possible to measure antigen-antibody interactions momentarily, allowing accurate determination of binding kinetics and affinity constants.

## ■ Storage

Depending on their specific characteristics, vaccines are stored as solution or as a freeze-dried formulation, usually at 2°C to 8°C. Their shelf-life depends on the composition and physico-chemical characteristics of the vaccine formulation and on the storage conditions, and typically is in the order of several years. The quality of the container can influence the long-term stability of vaccines, e.g., through adsorption or pH changes resulting from contact with the vial wall. The use of pH indicators or temperature or time sensitive labels ("vial vaccine monitors," which change color when exposed to extreme temperatures or after the expiration date) can avoid unintentional administration of inappropriately stored or expired vaccine.

## CONCLUDING REMARKS

Despite the tremendous success of conventional vaccines, there are still many infectious diseases and other chronic diseases (e.g., cancer, drug abuse) against which no effective vaccine exists. Although vaccines, like other biopharmaceuticals, are expensive, calculations may indicate cost effectiveness for vaccination against many of these diseases. In addition, the growing resistance to the existing arsenal of antibiotics increases the need to develop vaccines against common bacterial infections. It is expected that novel vaccines against several of these diseases will become available, and in these cases several technologies described in this chapter have great promise.

## REFERENCES

Akira S, Uematsu S, Takeuchi O. (2006). Pathogen recognition and innate immunity. Cell 124:783–801.

Bangari DS, and Mittal SK. (2006). Development of non-human adenoviruses as vaccine vectors. Vaccine 24:849–62.

Bouvet JP, Decroix N, Pamonsinlapatham P. (2002). Stimulation of local antibody production: parenteral or mucosal vaccination? Trends Immunol 23:209–13.

Burnette WN, Samal B, Browne J, Ritter GA. (1985) Properties and relative immunogenicity of various preparations of recombinant DNA-derived hepatitis B surface antigen. Dev Biol Stand 59:113–20.

Cartwright K, Morris R, Rumke H, et al. (1999). Immunogenicity and reactogenicity in UK infants of a novel meningococcal vesicle vaccine containing multiple class 1 (PorA) outer membrane proteins. Vaccine 17:2612–9.

Davis HL, Whalen RG. (1995). DNA-based immunization. Mol Cell Biol Hum Dis Ser 5:368–87.

Donnelly JJ, Wahren B, Liu MA. (2005). DNA vaccines: progress and challenges. J Immunol 175:633–9.

Finn OJ. (2003). Cancer vaccines: between the idea and the reality. Nat Rev Immunol 3:630–41.

Francis JN, Larche M. (2005). Peptide-based vaccination: where do we stand? Curr Opin Allergy Clin Immunol 5:537–43.

Francis MJ. (1991). Enhanced immunogenicity of recombinant and synthetic peptide vaccines. In: Gregoriadis GA, Allison AC, Poste G, eds. Vaccines: Recent Trends and Progress. New York: Plenum Press, 13–23.

Garcia L, Jidy MD, Garcia H, et al. (2005) The vaccine candidate Vibrio cholerae 638 is protective against cholera in healthy volunteers. Infect Immun 73:3018–24.

Garnett CT, Greiner JW, Tsang KY, et al. (2006) TRICOM vec-tor based cancer vaccines. Curr Pharm Des 12:351–61.

Germanier R, Fuer E. (1975) Isolation and characterization of Gal E mutant Ty 21a of Salmonella typhi: a candidate strain for a live, oral typhoid vaccine. J Infect Dis 131:553–8.

Gilliam BL, Redfield RR. (2003) Therapeutic HIV vaccines. Curr Top Med Chem 3:1536–53.

Gold R, Scheifele D, Barreto L, et al. (1994) Safety and immunogenicity of Haemophilus influenzae vaccine (tetanus toxoid conjugate) administered concurrently or combined with diphtheria and tetanus toxoids, pertussis vaccine and inactivated poliomyelitis vaccine to healthy infants at two, four and six months of age. Pediatr Infect Dis J 13:348–55.

Haile M, Kallenius G. (2005). Recent developments in tuberculosis vaccines. Curr Opin Infect Dis 18:211–15.

Haney M, Kosten TR. (2004). Therapeutic vaccines for substance dependence. Expert Rev Vaccines 3:11–18.

Holterman L, Vogels R, van der Vlugt R, et al. (2004). Novel replication-incompetent vector derived from adenovirus type 11 (Ad11) for vaccination and gene therapy: low seroprevalence and non-cross-reactivity with Ad5. J Virol 78:13207–15.

Hoogerhout P, Donders EM, van Gaans-van den Brink JA, et al. (1995). Conjugates of synthetic cyclic peptides elicit bactericidal antibodies against a conformational epitope on a class 1 outer membrane protein of Neisseria meningitidis. Infect Immun 63:3473–8.

Kaufmann SH, McMichael AJ. (2005). Annulling a dangerous liaison: vaccination strategies against AIDS and tuberculosis. Nat Med 11:S33–44.

Kersten G, Hirschberg H. (2004). Antigen delivery systems. Expert Rev Vaccines 3:453–62.

Langeveld JP, Casal JI, Osterhaus AD, et al. (1994). First peptide vaccine providing protection against viral infection in the target animal: studies of canine parvovirus in dogs. J Virol 68:4506–13.

Liu B, DeFilippo AM, Li Z. (2002). Overcoming immune tolerance to cancer by heat shock protein vaccines. Mol Cancer Ther 1:1147–51.

Masignani V, Rappuoli R, Pizza M. (2002). Reverse vaccinology: a genome-based approach for vaccine development. Expert Opin Biol Ther 2:895–905.

Muller S, Plaue S, Samama JP, Valette M, Briand JP, Van Regenmortel MH. (1990). Antigenic properties and protective capacity of a cyclic peptide corresponding to site A of influenza virus haemagglutinin. Vaccine 8:308–14.

Nencioni L, Pizza M, Bugnoli M, et al. (1990). Characterization of genetically inactivated pertussis toxin mutants: candidates for a new vaccine against whooping cough. Infect Immun 58:1308–15.

Paradiso PR, Hogerman DA, Madore DV, et al. (1993). Safety and immunogenicity of a combined diphtheria, tetanus, pertussis and Haemophilus influenzae type b vaccine in young infants. Pediatrics 92:827–32.

Pashine A, Valiante NM, Ulmer JB. (2005). Targeting the innate immune response with improved vaccine adjuvants. Nat Med 11:S63–8.

Plotkin SA, Orenstein, WA. (2004). Vaccines. 4th Ed. Philadelphia, PA: WB Saunders Company.

Pulendran B, Ahmed R. (2006). Translating innate immunity into immunological memory: implications for vaccine development. Cell 124:849–63.

Rappuoli R, Covacci A. (2003). Reverse vaccinology and genomics. Science 302:602.

Raz R, Koren R, Bass D. (2001). Safety and immunogenicity of a new mammalian cell-derived recombinant hepatitis B vaccine containing Pre-S1 and Pre-S2 antigens in adults. Isr Med Assoc J 3:328–32.

Sala F, Manuela Rigano M, Barbante A, Basso B, Walmsley AM, Castiglione S. (2003). Vaccine antigen production in transgenic plants: strategies, gene constructs and perspectives. Vaccine 21:803–8.

Scarselli M, Giuliani MM, Adu-Bobie J, Pizza M, Rappuoli R. (2005). The impact of genomics on vaccine design. Trends Biotechnol 23:84–91.

Schijns VE. (2000). Immunological concepts of vaccine adjuvant activity. Curr Opin Immunol 12:456–63.

Sell S, Hsu PL. (1993). Delayed hypersensitivity, immune deviation, antigen processing and T-cell subset selection in syphilis pathogenesis and vaccine design. Immunol Today 14:576–82.

Shalaby WS. (1995). Development of oral vaccines to stimulate mucosal and systemic immunity: barriers and novel strategies. Clin Immunol Immunopathol 74:127–34.

Shiver JW, Emini EA. (2004). Recent advances in the development of HIV-1 vaccines using replication-incompetent adenovirus vectors. Annu Rev Med 55:355–72.

Shiver JW, Fu TM, Chen L, et al. (2002). Replication-incompetent adenoviral vaccine vector elicits effective anti-immunodeficiency-virus immunity. Nature 415:331–5.

Suharyono, Simanjuntak C, Witham N, et al. (1992). Safety and immunogenicity of single-dose live oral cholera vaccine CVD 103-HgR in 5-9-year-old Indonesian children. Lancet 340:689–94.

Sutter G, Staib C. (2003). Vaccinia vectors as candidate vaccines: the development of modified vaccinia virus Ankara for antigen delivery. Curr Drug Targets Infect Disord 3:263–71.

Tacket CO, Cohen MB, Wasserman SS, et al. (1999). Randomized, double-blind, placebo-controlled, multi-centered trial of the efficacy of a single dose of live oral cholera vaccine CVD 103-HgR in preventing cholera following challenge with Vibrio cholerae O1 El tor inaba three months after vaccination. Infect Immun 67:6341–5.

Tam JP. (1996). Recent advances in multiple antigen peptides. J Immunol Methods 196:17–32.

Valenzuela P, Medina A, Rutter WJ, Ammerer G, Hall BD. (1982). Synthesis and assembly of hepatitis B virus surface antigen particles in yeast. Nature 298:347–50.

van der Ley P, van der Biezen J, Poolman JT. (1995). Construction of Neisseria meningitidis strains carrying multiple chromosomal copies of the porA gene for use in the production of a multivalent outer membrane vesicle vaccine. Vaccine 13:401–7.

Vanlandschoot P, Roobrouck A, Van Houtte F, Leroux-Roels G. (2002). Recombinant HBsAg, an apoptotic-like lipoprotein, interferes with the LPS-induced activation of ERK-1/2 and JNK-1/2 in monocytes. Biochem Biophys Res Commun 297:486–91.

Vasconcelos NM, Siddique AB, Ahlborg N, Berzins K. (2004). Differential antibody responses to plasmodium falciparum-derived B-cell epitopes induced by diepitope multiple antigen peptides (MAP) containing different T-cell epitopes. Vaccine 23:343–52.

Vreden SG, Verhave JP, Oettinger T, Sauerwein RW, Meuwissen JH. (1991). Phase I clinical trial of a recombinant malaria vaccine consisting of the circumsporozoite repeat region of Plasmodium falciparum coupled to hepatitis B surface antigen. Am J Trop Med Hyg 45:533–8.

Walker RI. (2005). Considerations for development of whole cell bacterial vaccines to prevent diarrheal diseases in children in developing countries. Vaccine 23: 3369–85.

## FURTHER READING

Alpar HO, Papanicolaou I, Bramwell VW. (2005). Strategies for DNA vaccine delivery. Expert Opin Drug Deliv, 2, 829–42.

Janeway CA, Travers P, Walport M, Shlomchik MJ. (2005). Immunobiology, the Immune System in Health and Disease. 5th Ed. London: Garland Science Publishing.

Levine MM, Kaper JB, Rappuoli R, Liu MA, Good MF. (2004). New Generation Vaccines. 3rd edn. New York, NY: Marcel Dekker.

Liljeqvist S, Ståhl S. (1999). Production of recombinant subunit vaccines: protein immunogens, live delivery systems and nucleic acid vaccines. J Biotechnol 73:1–33.

Plotkin SA, Orenstein WA. (2004). Vaccines. 4th Ed. Philadelphia, PA: WB Saunders Company.

Roitt I. (2001). Essential Immunology. 10th Edn. London: Blackwell Scientific Publications.

Roitt I, Brostoff J, Male D. (2001). Immunology, 6th edn. St. Louis, MO: Mosby.

O'Hagan DT, Rappuoli R. (2004). Novel approaches to vaccine delivery. Pharm Res 21:1519–30.

# Dispensing Biotechnology Products: Handling, Professional Education, and Product Information

*Peggy Piascik*
University of Kentucky College of Pharmacy, Lexington, Kentucky, U.S.A.

## INTRODUCTION

Preparation and/or dispensing of pharmaceuticals are primarily the responsibility of the pharmacist. Traditionally, parenteral products have been available in ready-to-use containers or required dilution with water or saline prior to use with no other special handling requirements. Hospital pharmacists, in particular, have prepared and dispensed parenteral products for individual patients for many years. While many pharmacists are skilled in handling parenteral products, biotechnology products may present additional challenges since they are proteins subject to denaturation and thus require special handling techniques. These challenges will be explained in greater detail in this chapter.

## PHARMACIST RELUCTANCE

Pharmacists may be reluctant to provide pharmaceutical care services to patients who require therapy with biotechnology drugs for a variety of reasons including (*i*) lack of knowledge about the tools of biotechnology; (*ii*) lack of understanding of the therapeutic aspects of recombinant protein products; (*iii*) lack of familiarity with the side effects and patient counseling information; (*iv*) lack of familiarity with the storage, handling and reconstitution of proteins; and (*v*) difficulty of handling reimbursement issues.

Pharmacists may view biotechnology drugs as quite different from traditional parenteral products like insulin and familiar oral dosage forms. However, in most respects, the services offered by pharmacists when dispensing biotechnology products are the same as those provided for traditional tablets or injectable products. It is important, regardless of the product being dispensed, to ensure that the patient understands the use, dosage regimen, potential adverse effects, proper storage and handling instructions as well as specific training on the administration of the drug and proper disposal of unused medication. When patients do not understand the administration and monitoring requirements of biotechnology products, scheduling training sessions for patients or including a caregiver during the counseling session should be considered to ensure appropriate patient care.

As more novel protein products have come to market and the indications for existing agents have expanded for ambulatory patients, pharmacists are increasingly required to deal with these protein pharmaceuticals. While the first protein/peptide recombinant products were used primarily in hospital settings, many of these agents are now commonplace in ambulatory settings. The traditional community pharmacy may now dispense products like colony stimulating factors, growth hormone, and interferons to name a few.

Traditional routes of delivery for pharmaceuticals have been challenged by the unique characteristics of biotech product delivery. Community pharmacies struggle with maintaining sufficient inventory of high cost products, with in-depth knowledge of the products and its characteristics and with product administration. Physicians also have difficulty with inventory and with slow reimbursement. Managed care organizations may have difficulty tracking claims for these products.

As a result, the majority of patients receiving biotech drugs are managed by home health, home infusion or specialty pharmacy services. Specialty pharmacies have evolved to manage out-patient biotechnology therapies for patients. The services offered by these pharmacies go far beyond dispensing biotech products (Suchanek, 2005). These pharmacies have expertise in the following areas:

- Insurance coverage and drug costs
- Pipeline monitoring and management
- Utilization management
- Promoting adherence to drug regimen
- Disease state management

Payers, in particular managed care organizations, now contract with specialty pharmacies to provide biotech and other expensive agents to solve many of the problems these products pose for the payer. The specialty pharmacy market is growing at a rate of 20% per year and is estimated by some experts to reach annual sales of $40 billion in the United States by the end of 2006 (Casemark, 2006).

## ■ Types of Information Needed by Pharmacists

What types of information do pharmacists require to be confident providers of biotech drugs and services? For pharmacists who have been out of school for more than ten years, a contemporary understanding of the immune system, autoimmune diseases and mechanisms by which drugs modify the immune system is essential. Several appropriate books that can provide a basic background in immunology are listed in Table 1. Additionally, practitioners may enroll in organized courses or continuing education programs that can provide up-to-date information in the discipline of immunology. Current pharmacy students and recent graduates should be sufficiently trained in basic immunology as part of their professional curriculum.

Many pharmacists, upon hearing the word biotechnology, imagine a discipline too technical or complicated to be understood by the typical practitioner. Pharmacists must recognize that biotechnology primarily refers to a set of tools that has allowed great strides to be made in basic research, the understanding of disease and development of new therapeutic agents. It is essential for pharmacists to have a basic understanding of recombinant DNA technology and monoclonal antibody technology. However, it is not necessary that pharmacy practitioners know how to use these tools in the laboratory but rather how the use of these tools provides new therapeutic agents and a greater understanding of disease processes.

Pharmacists may need to review or learn anew about protein chemistry and those characteristics that affect therapeutic activity, product storage and routes of administration of these drugs. Apart from this textbook, several publications, videotapes and continuing professional education programs from industry and academic institutions are available to pharmacists for learning about the technical aspects of product storage and handling. Pharmacists also need to become familiar with the drug delivery systems currently in use for biotech drugs as well as those that are in development (see Chapter 4).

## ■ Sources of Information for Pharmacists

Many pharmacists do not know where to obtain the information that will allow them to be good providers of products of biotechnology. This textbook provides much of the essential background information in one source.

An excellent source of information on biotechnology in general, and specific products in particular, is the biotech drug industry. Many manufacturer-sponsored programs are available describing approved biotech products and those likely to come to market in the near future. Manufacturer programs provide extensive information about the disease states for which their products are indicated as well as product-specific information. Manufacturers are prepared to help pharmacists in the most effective provision of products and services to hospital-based and ambulatory patients. However, many pharmacists are unaware of these services and how to obtain them. A web search of specific products will lead to the product and manufacturer's websites where this information can be accessed.

The information provided by manufacturers can help pharmacists confidently provide biotechnology products to their patients. The services provided generally fall into three categories: customer/medical services and support, educational materials, and reimbursement information. Manufacturers may have a separate number for reimbursement questions. Table 2 lists the manufacturer's toll-free assistance numbers and web addresses for obtaining product

---

■ **Cellular and Molecular Immunology**, 5th ed.
Abbas AK, Lichtman AH. Philadelphia: W.B. Saunders Company, 2005; 562 pages. *Provides basic immunology concepts and clinical issues;includes access to online edition.*

■ **Immunology: A Short Course**, 5th ed.
Coico R, Sunshine G, Benjamini E. New York: Wiley-Liss, 2003; 329 pages. *Elementary text with review questions for each chapter.*

■ **Concepts in Immunology and Immunotherapeutics**, 4th ed.
Koeller J, Tami J, eds. Bethesda, MD: American Society of Hospital Pharmacists, 2006; 360 pages. *Provides a review of basic immunology including therapeutic applications.*

■ **Medical Immunology Made Memorable**.
Playfair JHL, Lydyard PM. New York: Churchill Livingstone, 2000; 108 pages. *Gives a simple overview of basic immunology, immunopathology and clinical immunology.*

■ **Roitt's Essential Immunology**, 11th ed.
Burton D, Delves PJ, Martin S, Roitt I. Oxford; Boston: Blackwell Publishing 2006; 496 pages; *A basic immunology textbook.*

■ **Immunobiology**, 6th ed.
Janeway C, Travers P, Walport M, and Shlomchik M. Garland Science 2004; 756 pages. *Includes a CD-ROM that provides animations.*

**Table 1** ■ Selected texts to enhance immunology knowledge.

and reimbursement information in North America. Vaccines and insulin products are not included in this table since these products were previously available in a non-recombinant form which was used in a similar manner. Moreover, the recombinant form is not significantly higher in price than the non-recombinant product.

## ■ The Pharmacist and Handling of Biotech Drugs

The pharmacist is responsible for the storage, preparation and dispensing of biotechnology drugs as well as patient education regarding the use of these products. In many cases, pharmacists must have additional training in order to be prepared for this role. This is especially true for pharmacists who practice in the ambulatory care setting since these products are increasingly available for administration by the patient in the home. Pharmacies of the future may stock pumps, patches, timed-release tablets, liposomes, implants, and vials of tailored monoclonal antibodies. With gene therapy and gene splicing on the horizon, it is possible that the pharmacist may eventually prepare and dispense gene therapy products tailored for specific patients.

This chapter will discuss the general principles that pharmacists need to understand about storage, handling, preparation, administration of biotech products and issues related to outpatient/home care. Specific examples will be discussed for illustrative purposes. Table 3 lists selected products along with specific handling requirements for each. For specific products or recent updates, contact the manufacturer. For additional information regarding drug handling and preparation, pharmacist may consult the following publications: American Hospital Formulary Drug Information and the King Guide to Parenteral Admixture (Catania, 2006). In addition to hardcover publications with frequent updates, both of these references are available on-line at www.ashp.org/ahfs/ and www.kingguide.com. Pharmacy benefits management companies usually own specialty pharmacy companies and provide valuable information via their websites. Two well-known companies are RxSolutions and Caremark.

## STORAGE

Biotech products have unique storage requirements when compared to the majority of products that pharmacists normally dispense. The shelf life of these products is often considerably shorter than for traditional compounds. For example, interferon-α2a (Roche, 2005) is only stable in a refrigerator in the ready-to-use solution for 2 years. After the first dose, cartridges may be stored at less than 25°C for up to

28 days although refrigeration is recommended. Since most of these products need to be kept at refrigerated temperatures (as discussed below), some pharmacies may need to increase cold storage space in order to accommodate the storage needs.

## ■ Temperature Requirements

Since biotech products are primarily proteins, they are subject to denaturation when exposed to extreme temperatures. In general, most biotech products are shipped by the manufacturer in gel ice containers and need to be stored at 2°C to 8°C (Banga and Reddy, 1994). Once reconstituted, they should be stored under refrigeration until just prior to use. There are a few exceptions to this rule. For example, alteplase (tissue plasminogen activator) lyophilized powder is stable at room temperature for several years at temperatures not to exceed 30°C (86°F). However, after reconstitution, the product should be used within 8 hours (Genentech, 2005). For individual product temperature requirements, the product insert, product website or the manufacturer should be contacted. Table 3 lists temperature requirements for selected frequently prescribed products.

The variability between products with respect to temperature is exemplified by granulocyte-colony stimulating factor (G-CSF, filgrastim; Amgen, 2004) and erythropoietin (Amgen, 2006), which are stable in ready-to-use form at room temperature for 24 hours and 14 days, respectively. Granulocyte macrophage-colony stimulating factor (GM-CSF, sargramostim; Berlex, 2004) is packaged as a lyophilized powder, but still requires refrigeration and once reconstituted is stable at room temperature for 30 days or in the refrigerator for 2 years. Aldesleukin (interleukin-2) is stable for 48 hours at room temperature or under refrigeration (Chiron, 2000). Betaseron (interferon-β1b) must be stored in a refrigerator and should be used within three hours after reconstitution (Berlex, 2003). While most products require refrigeration to maintain stability due to denaturation by elevated temperatures, extreme cold such as freezing may be just as harmful to most products. The key is to avoid extremes in temperature whether it is heat or cold (Banga and Reddy, 1994).

## ■ Storage in Dosing and Administration Devices

Most biotech products may adhere to either plastic or glass containers such as syringes, polyvinyl chloride (PVC) intravenous bags, infusion equipment, and glass intravenous bottles. The effectiveness of the product may be reduced by three- or four-fold due to adherence. In order to decrease the amount of adherence, human serum albumin (HSA) is usually added to the solutions (see Chapter 4). The relative loss through adherence is concentration dependent,

| Manufacturer | Professional services | Reimbursement hotline/indigent patient programs | Manufacturer website |
|---|---|---|---|
| Amgen | 1-800-772-6436 | 1-800-272-9376 | www.amgen.com<br>www.imminex.com |
| Baxter Healthcare | 1-800-422-9837 | 1-800-548-4448 | www.baxter.com |
| Bayer Healthcare | 1-888-606-3780 | 1-800-288-8374 | www.bayerhealthcare.com |
| Bedford Laboratories | 1-800-521-5169 | 1-800-562-4797 | www.bedfordlabs.com |
| Berlex | 1-888-237-5394 | 1-800-237-5394 | www.berlex.com |
| Biogen Idec | 1-800-456-2255 | 1-800-386-9997 | www.biogenidec.com |
| BioMarin | 1-866-906-6100 | | www.biomarinpharm.com |
| Bristol-Myers Squibb | 1-800-673-6242 | 1-800-736-0003 | www.bms.com |
| Centocor | 1-800-457-6399 | 1-800-331-5773 | www.centocor.com |
| ChiRhoClin | 1-877-272-4888 | | www.chirhoclin.com |
| Chiron | 1-800-244-7668 | 1-866-385-4729 | www.chiron.com |
| Genentech | 1-866-582-3684<br>1-800-821-8590 | 1-800-232-0592<br>1-800-530-3083 | www.spoconline.com<br>www.gene.com<br>www.spoconline.com[2] |
| Genzyme | 1-800-745-4447 | 1-800-745-4447 | www.genzyme.com |
| GlaxoSmithKline | 1-888-825-5249 | 1-866-728-4368 | www.gsk.com |
| Hoffmann-La Roche | 1-800-526-6367 | 1-877-757-6243 | www.rocheusa.com |
| ImClone | 1-866-730-9324 | 1-800-736-0003 | www.imclone.com<br>www.bmspaf.org |
| Insmed | 1-866-464-7539 | 1-866-464-7539 | www.insmed.com |
| Intermune | 1-415-466-2200 | 1-877-305-7704 | www.intermune.com |
| Ligand | 1-800-964-5836 | 1-877-454-4263 | www.ligand.com |
| Lilly | 1-800-545-5979 | 1-800-545-6962 | www.lilly.com |
| Merck | 1-866-342-5683 | 1-800-994-2111 | www.merck.com |
| Novo Nordisk | 1-800-727-6500 | 1-866-310-7549 | www.novomedlink.com<br>www.novonordisk-us.com |
| Organon | 1-866-836-5633 | | www.organon-usa.com |
| Ortho Biotech | 1-800-325-7504 | 1-800-553-3851 | www.othobiotech.com |
| Ortho-McNeil | 1-800-526-7736 | 1-800-652-6227 | www.ortho-mcneil.com |
| OSI | 1-877-827-2382 | 1-800-530-3083 | www.spoconline.com |
| Pfizer | 1-800-398-2372 | 1-866-706-2400 | www.pfizerhelpfulanswers.com |
| Roche | 1-800-526-6367 | 1-877-757-6243 | www.roche.com |
| Sanofi-Aventis | 1-800-633-1610 | 1-800-221-4025 | www.sanofi-aventis.us |
| Schering-Plough | 1-800-222-7579 | 1-800-521-7157 | www.schering-plough.com |
| Serono | 1-888-275-7376 | 1-866-538-7879 | www.seronousa.com |
| Tercica | 1-866-837-2422 | 1-866-837-2422 | www.tercica.com |
| Unigene | 1-800-654-2299 | | www.unigene.com |
| Wyeth | 1-800-934-5556 | 1-800-568-9938 | www.wyeth.com |
| ZLB Behring | 1-610-878-4000 | | www.zlbbehring.com |

**Table 2** ▪ Toll-free assistance numbers and websites for selected biopharmaceutical manufacturers in the United States and Canada.

| Generic name | Brand name | Storage temperature | Stability | | Reconstitution solution | Stability after reconstitution | |
|---|---|---|---|---|---|---|---|
| | | | RT | Ref | | RT | Ref |
| Adalimumab | Humira® | 2–8°C | NA | ex da | RTU | NA | NA |
| Darbepoetin alfa | Aransep® | 2–8°C | NA | ex da | RTU | NA | NA |
| Epoetin alfa | Epogen®, Procrit® | 2–8°C | 14 d | 21 d aie, mdv | RTU | NA | NA |
| Etanercept | Enbrel® | 2–8°C | NA | ex da | dil (SBWFI) | NA | 14 d |
| Glatiramer acetate | Copaxone® | 2–8°C | 7 d | ex da | RTU | NA | NA |
| Interferon-β1a prefilled syringe | Avonex®, Rebif® | 2–8°C | 12 h | ex da | RTU | NA | NA |
| Interferon-β1a reconstitutable vial | Avonex®, Rebif® | 2–8°C | 30 d | ex da | dil (SWFI) | NA | 6 h |
| Interferon-β1b | Betaseron® | 25°C | ex da | NA | dil (NaCl 0.54%) | NA | 3 h |
| Pegfilgrastim | Neulasta® | 2–8°C | 48 h | ex da | RTU | NA | NA |
| Trastuzumab | Herceptin® | 2–8°C | NA | ex da | dil (SBWFI) | NA | 28 d |

*Abbreviations*: aie, after initial entry into vial; d, days; dil, supplied diluent; dil sol, once in diluted solution; ex da, see expiration date on package; h, hours; mdv, applies only to multi-dose vials; NA, not applicable/not available; Ref, under refrigeration; RT, room temperature; RTU, ready to use; SBWFI, sterile bacterial water for injection; SWFI, sterile water for injection.

**Table 3** ■ Storage, stability, and reconstitution of selected biotechnology products.

i.e., the more concentrated the final solution the less significant the adherence becomes. The amount of HSA added varies with the product (Banga and Reddy, 1994; Koeller and Fields, 1991). Some products that require the addition of HSA include filgrastim, sargramostim, aldesleukin, erythropoietin and interferon-α. In the case of filgrastim, the addition of 2 mg/mL of HSA to the final solution is required for concentrations of 5 to 15 µg/mL (Amgen, 2004). One mg of HSA per 1 mL 0.9% Sodium Chloride injection is added to achieve a final concentration of 0.1% HSA for sargramostim concentrations of <10 µg/mL. (Berlex, 2004). For aldesleukin 0.1%, HSA is required for all concentrations (Chiron, 2000). For erythropoietin, 2.5 mg HSA is present per mL in each single-dose and multi-dose vial (Amgen, 2006). One mg/mL of HSA is added to interferon-α in single dose and multi-dose vials and pens (Schering, 2004).

For additional information or to find information for other products, check the current product information or contact the manufacturer.

## ■ Storage in IV Solutions

Biotech product stability may vary when stored in different types of containers and syringes. Some products are only stable in plastic syringes, e.g., somatropin and erythropoietin, while others are stable in glass, polyvinyl chloride and polypropylene, e.g., aldesleukin. Batch prefilling of syringes is possible. However, it is important to make sure that the product you wish to provide in pre-filled syringes is stable in the type of syringe you wish to use. This may present a challenge to specialty pharmacy programs. Determining how far in advance doses may be prepared is also an important consideration. G-CSF is stable in Becton Dickinson (B-D) disposable plastic syringes for up to 7 days (Amgen, 2004) while erythropoietin is stable for up to 14 days (Amgen, 2006). Aldesleukin is recommended to be administered in PVC although glass has been used in clinical trials with comparable results (Chiron, 2000). Solutions are stable for 48 hours when refrigerated. GM-CSF and G-CSF can be administered in either PVC or polypropylene (Berlex, 2004).

## ■ Light Protection

Many biotech products are sensitive to light. Manufacturer's information usually suggests that products be protected from strong light until the product is used. Dornase-α is packaged in protective foil pouches by the manufacturer to protect it from light degradation and should be stored in these original light protective containers until use. For patients who travel, the manufacturer will provide special travel pouches on request (Genentech, 1994). Alteplase in the lyophilized form also needs to be protected from light but is not light sensitive when in solution (Genentech, 2005). Pharmacists must be aware of the specific storage requirements with respect to light for each of the products stocked in the pharmacy.

# HANDLING

## ■ Mixing and Shaking

Improper handling of protein products can lead to denaturation. Shaking and severe agitation of most of these products will result in degradation. Therefore special techniques must be observed in preparing biotech products for use. Biotech products should not be shaken when adding any diluent as this may cause the product to break down. Once the diluent is added to the container, the vial should be swirled rather than vigorously shaken. Some shaking during transport may be unavoidable and proper inspection of products should occur to make sure the products have not been damaged during transit. When a product is affected by excessive shaking, physical separation or frothing within the vial of liquid products can usually be observed. For lyophilized products, agitation is not harmful until the product has been reconstituted. In distributing individual products to patient or ward areas, pneumatic tubes should be avoided.

## ■ Travel Requirements

When patients travel with these products, certain precautions should be observed. The drugs should be stored in insulated, cool containers. This can be accomplished by using ice packs to keep the biotech drug at the proper temperature in warmer climates, whereas the insulated container in colder climates may be all that is required. When traveling in sub-freezing weather, the products should be protected from freezing (temperatures below 2°C). Keeping biotech drugs at proper temperature during automobile travel may present a problem with temperatures inside a parked car often exceeding 37°C (100°F) on a warm day. Patients and delivery personnel must take care not to leave products that are not in insulated containers inside the car, trunk or glove compartment while shopping or making deliveries. When ice is used, care should be taken not to place the product directly on the ice. Dry ice should be avoided since it has the potential for freezing the product. When traveling by air, biotech products should be taken onto the plane in insulated packages and not placed in a cargo container. Airplane cargo containers may be cold enough to cause freezing (Banga and Reddy, 1994; Koeller and Fields, 1991).

# PREPARATION

When preparing biotech products, aseptic technique must be employed as it is with traditional parenteral products. The product should be prepared in a clean room designed for this purpose with laminar air flow hoods, etc. Most of the products require reconstitution with sterile water or bacteriostatic water for injection depending on stability data. The compatibility of individual products varies and limited data are available. As mentioned previously, when adding diluent to these products, care should be taken not to shake them, but to swirl the container or roll it between the palms of the hands. In the case of lyophilized products, introduction of the diluent should be directed down the side of the vial and not directly on the powder to avoid denaturing the protein. It is important to mention that stability does not mean sterility. Biotech products require the same precautions as any other parenteral product. Sterility is particularly important when pre-filling and pre-mixing various doses for administration at home. Once the manufacturer's sterile packaging is entered, sterility can no longer be assured nor will the manufacturer be responsible for any subsequent related problems. Many biotech drugs are not compatible with preservative agents and single use vials do not contain a preservative. Individual manufacturers have not addressed the issue of sterility and each institution or organization must determine its own policy on this issue. Many of the currently available biotechnology-produced products are provided as single-dose vials and should not be reused. This does not, however, prevent preparing batches ("batching") of unit-of-use doses in order to be efficient. Many of the patients receiving these agents are likely to have suppressed immune systems and are vulnerable to infection. Therefore, a policy involving the maintenance of sterility of biotech products should be developed by each healthcare organization, especially hospitals, and specialty pharmacies. When products are made in a sterile environment under aseptic procedures they should remain sterile until used and thus could be stored for as long as physical compatibility data dictate. However, most institutions have shorter expiration dates, which are generally 72 hours or less, on reconstituted products. These expiration dates have been arbitrarily set due to lack of good sterility data to the contrary. Sterility studies should be performed in order to determine if reconstituted products could be stored for a longer period of time and still maintain sterility. For products reconstituted for home use in the pharmacy sterile products area, a seven day expiration date is used provided the product is stable and can be stored in the refrigerator. The American Society of Health-System Pharmacists has published a technical assistance bulletin on sterile products, which should be consulted for developing policies on storage of reconstituted parenteral products (American Society of Hospital Pharmacy, 2000). Patients need to be informed about specific storage requirements and expiration dates to assure sterility and stability.

## ADMINISTRATION

Prior to administering these products, pharmacists will need to use caution in reviewing dosage regimens. A potential source of medication error is the variation in units of measure for the various products. Some products are dosed in micrograms/kilogram (μg/kg) rather than milligrams/kilogram (mg/kg). Also, some units of measure may be unique to the product, e.g., Chiron or Roche units. Dosage calculations need to be carefully checked to avoid potential errors.

### ■ Routes of Administration

Biotech products are primarily administered parenterally although many other routes of administration are in development. Some products may be given by either the intravenous or subcutaneous route while others are restricted to the subcutaneous or intramuscular routes. In some cases, manufacturers have information on unapproved routes of administration or other new information that may be available by contacting the individual manufacturer. In any case, the manufacturer should always be consulted in order to obtain supporting evidence for a particular route that is not approved, but may be more convenient for the patient. For example, G-CSF should be administered by the subcutaneous or intravenous route only, while GM-CSF is given by intravenous infusion, over a two-hour period (McEvoy, 2005). Aldesleukin is approved for intravenous administration only. However, subcutaneous administration, while not approved, has been used by some (Chiron, 1992). Erythropoietin should only be administered by the intravenous or subcutaneous routes (Amgen, 2006), while alteplase is only approved for the intravenous route (Genentech, 2005; McEvoy, 2005). Alteplase has also been administered by the intracoronary, intra-arterial, and intraorbital routes as well (McEvoy, 2005).

### ■ Filtration

Filtering biotech products is not generally recommended since most of these proteins will adhere to the filter. Some hospitals and home infusion companies routinely use in-line filters for all intravenous solutions to minimize the introduction of particulate matter into the patient. In the case of biotech products, they should be infused below the filter to avoid a potential decrease in the amount of drug delivered to the patient (Banga and Reddy, 1994; Koeller et al., 1991).

### ■ Flushing Solutions

Pharmaceutical biotechnology products are usually flushed with either saline or dextrose 5% in water. The product literature should be consulted and care should be taken to assure that the proper solution is used with each agent. In general, biotech drugs should not be administered with other drugs since, in most cases, data do not exist that demonstrate whether biotech products are compatible with other drugs or fluids.

## BIOGENERICS—A FUTURE CONSIDERATION?

A huge potential exists for the development of biogeneric products or generic versions of existing biotech drugs. Another term, follow-on protein, is sometimes used to describe the same concept. It is estimated that biogenerics could be available in the United States as early as 2009. Factors driving the development of biogenerics include the growing number of products, size of the biotech drug market, and the high cost of existing patent-protected products.

The Food and Drug Administration (FDA) has said that creating generic versions of these drugs will be difficult due to the complexity of these products. It will be difficult, if not impossible, to demonstrate an equivalent chemical structure for biogenerics. However, legislation may be introduced to develop a regulatory process (none currently exists in the United States) for approval of this type of product (see Chapter 24).

The biotech market already contains several types of insulins, growth hormones, and second generation products such as Aranesp and Neulasta. Pharmacists and formulary committees in the future may need to choose between a variety of biotech drugs produced in different cell lines with differences in physical properties but producing essentially the same therapeutic effect.

## OUTPATIENT/HOME CARE ISSUES

As mentioned previously, the management of patients in the outpatient and home settings is now an accepted aspect of health care delivery. The use of biotech products outside the hospital is no exception to this trend. Home infusion and specialty pharmacy services dispense all forms of parenteral and enteral products including biotech drugs. These pharmacies have grown exponentially in the last twenty years due to cost savings for third party payers, technological advances that allow these services to occur in the home, and patient preference to be treated at home rather than an in-patient setting.

### ■ Patient Assessment and Education

Before a patient can be a candidate for home therapy, an assessment of the patient's capabilities must occur. The patient, family member, or caregiver will need to be able to administer the medication and comply with all of the storage, handling, and preparation requirements. If the patient is incapable, then a caregiver (usually a relative, spouse, or friend) needs to be recruited to assist the patient. The pharmacy staff or other health professional may also make home visits to assist the patient in these tasks. The use of aseptic technique is usually new to the patients and in some cases may be overwhelming. The healthcare provider must be sure that the patient or caregiver is competent and willing to follow these procedures. Self-instructional guides on specific products may be available from the manufacturer, and if so, should be provided to the patient providing they have the proper equipment for viewing.

Proper storage facilities will need to be available in the patient's home as well as a clean area for preparation and administration. Ideally, the patient will be able to prepare each dose immediately prior to the time of administration. If this is not possible, the pharmacy will have to prepare pre-filled syringes and provide appropriate storage and handling requirements to the patient. The patient will also need to be educated regarding the proper handling of the syringes as well as other required supplies and materials such as needles, syringes, alcohol wipes, etc. Proper disposal of these hazardous wastes must also be reviewed. Specific issues related to patient teaching include rotating injection sites, product handling, drug storage including transporting and traveling with biotech drugs, expiration dates, refrigeration, cleansing the injection site with alcohol, disposal of needles and syringes, potential adverse effects, and expected therapeutic outcomes.

### ■ Monitoring

For patients who receive biotech drug therapy in the home, it is particularly important that close patient monitoring occurs. This will require frequent phone calls to the patient and periodic home visits. Monitoring parameters should include adverse events, progress to expected outcomes, assessment of administration technique, review of storage and handling procedures, and adherence to aseptic technique.

### ■ Reimbursement

Reimbursement issues include third party billing information and availability of forms, cost sharing programs that limit the annual cost of therapy, financial assistance programs for patients who would otherwise have difficulty paying for therapy, and reimbursement assurance programs that are designed to remove reimbursement barriers when reimbursement has been denied. Any detailed discussion of reimbursement issues is beyond the scope of this book

and is subject to practice location. This discussion will deal only with the availability of information to pharmacists to appropriately handle reimbursement for products and services in the United States.

Pharmacists need to know current third party payment policies including those conditions under which insurance companies will disallow claims. Some examples include off-label prescribing or administration of the product in the home rather than administration in a hospital or physician's office. Prior authorization is usually required particularly with managed care or prepaid plans. Manufacturers will often assist the patient by contacting the carrier to verify coverage, providing sample prior-approval letters, and following up on claims to determine the claim's status and continuing to follow the case until it is resolved.

Manufacturers can also provide information that may convince the third-party payer to reconsider a denied claim. Some companies will intervene with the third party payer to evaluate the case for denial, provide additional clinical documentation or coding information, and will follow the appeal to conclusion. Pharmacists can act as facilitators to get qualified patients enrolled in programs to provide free medication to those who have insufficient insurance coverage or are otherwise unable to purchase the therapy. Manufacturers' websites and toll-free numbers for reimbursement issues are provided in Table 2. Websites and toll-free numbers for some of the patient assistance programs are provided in Table 4. The Partnership for Patient Assistance website provides information on a variety of patient assistance programs as well as the requirements to qualify for various programs.

## EDUCATIONAL MATERIALS

Therapy with biotech drugs is a rapidly growing, ever changing area of therapeutics. Pharmacists need to keep informed of current information about existing agents such as new indications, management of adverse effects, results of studies describing drug interactions or changes in information regarding

| Partnership for Patient Assistance | 1-888-477-2669 www.pparx.org |
|---|---|
| Rx Assist | 1-401-729-3284 www.rxassist.org |
| Together Rx Access | 1-800-444-4106 www.togetherrxaccess.org |

**Table 4** ■ Toll-free assistance numbers and websites for patient assistance programs.

■ **Biotechnology Medicines in Development**
Communications Division, Pharmaceutical Manufacturers Association, Washington, D.C., *202-835-3400, updated approximately every 18 months.* www.newmeds.pharma. org

■ **FDC Reports, "The Pink Sheet"**
Chevy Chase, MD, *published weekly.* www.thepinksheet. com/FDC/Weekly/pink/TOC.htm

■ **BioWorld Today**
Bioworld Publishing Group, Atlanta; *newspaper, 5 issues per week; also available on Netscape; Tel. (404)-262-7436; Fax (404)-814-0759.* www.bioworld.com

■ **Bio/Technology**
Nature Publishing Co., New York, *a monthly journal dealing with all aspects of biotechnology.* www.nature.com/nbt

■ **Genetic Engineering News**
GEN Publishing, New York, *bimonthly publication Tel. (914)-834-3100; Fax (914)-834-3771* www.genengnews. com

**Table 5** ■ Information sources for current trends in biotechnology

| Apidra | www.apidra.com |
|---|---|
| Avastin | www.avastin.com |
| Copegus, Pegasys | www.pegasys.com |
| Erbitux | www.erbitux.com |
| Follistim AQ | www.follistim.com |
| Fortical | www.fortical.com |
| Increlex | www.increlex.com |
| Iplex | www.go-iplex.com |
| Kepivance | www.kepivance.com |
| Levemir | www.levemir-us.com |
| Lucentis | www.lucentis.com |
| Macugen | www.macugen.com |
| Myozyme | www.myozyme.com |
| Naglazyme | www.naglazyme.com |
| Orencia | www.orencia.com |
| Tarceva | www.tarceva.com |
| Tysabri | www.tysabri.com |

**Table 6** ■ Examples of individual product websites.

product stability and reconstitution. Pharmacists will also be interested in the status of new agents as they move through the FDA approval process. Some good periodical sources of practical information about products of biotechnology are listed in Table 5.

■ **Educational Materials for Health Professionals**

Manufacturer and specific product websites (Table 6) provide a variety of educational materials including continuing education programs for physicians, pharmacists and nurses. These programs often focus on specific disease states as well as drug therapy. The programs sometimes include slides, videos and brochures. Since most biotechnology products are parenteral products, several manufacturers have produced videotapes, which show the proper procedure for product administration, storage and handling. These instructional tapes are beneficial not just for patients but also for health professionals who may not be skilled in injection techniques.

■ **Educational Materials for Patients**

Detailed patient information booklets exist for many of the products both in print and by downloading from the Internet. Patient education materials can assist the patient and family members in learning more about his or her disease and how it will be treated. Education allows the patient to participate more actively in the therapy and to feel a greater level of control over the process. By contacting the manufacturer and acquiring patient educational materials, pharmacists can offer support to the patient in learning to use a new product. Many patients are already overwhelmed by dealing with a diagnosis of serious or chronic disease. Learning about a new therapy, especially if it involves the necessity of self-injection, can cause additional stress for the patient and family.

Most commercially available biotech drugs now have individual websites to provide updated information to patients. These sites usually contain the following types of information: disease background, reimbursement information, dosing information, references, frequently asked questions, administration and storage information, and information specifically for health professionals. These websites also offer tools such as journals for patients to record administration of doses and monitoring information to assist health professionals in following the patient's progress. The websites also refer patients to disease-related associations and organizations whose services include a link to local chapters, meetings and support groups. These groups may provide support to the patient while he or she adjusts to the diagnosis and treatment of a potentially serious disease. A partial list of websites for current products is provided in Table 6.

■ **The Internet and Biotech Information**

The Internet has become a valuable site rich in up-to-date information concerning all aspects of pharmaceutical biotechnology. Sites including virtual libraries/catalogs, online journals (usually requiring a

| Internet site | Type of site | Web address |
|---|---|---|
| A Doctor's Guide to the Internet | Biomedical news | www.docguide.com |
| BioOnline | Information library/catalog | www.bio.com |
| BioCentury | Biotechnology industry new | www.biocentury.com/ |
| BioPharma | Database | www.biopharma.com |
| Genetic Engineering News | On-line journal | www.genengnews.com |
| Nature Biotechnology | On-line journal | www.nature.com/nbt |
| Pharmaceutical Research and Manufacturers of America | Professional organization | www.phrma.org |
| Physicians Guide to the Internet | Biomedical news | www.physiciansguide.com |
| Reuter's Health Information Services, Inc. | Biomedical news | www.reutershealth.com |
| The World Wide Web Virtual Library: Biotechnology | Information library/catalog | www.cato.com/biotech |

**Table 7** ▪ Examples of biotech-related internet sites.

subscription), biomedical newsletters and biotechnology specific homepages abound on the Internet. Since the number of biotech-related sites is constantly increasing, only a small sampling of sites of interest could be provided in Table 7.

## CONCLUDING REMARKS

The handling of biotechnology products requires similar skills and techniques as required for the preparation of other parenteral drugs, but there are often different nuances to the handling, preparation and administration of biotechnology-produced pharmaceuticals. The pharmacist can become an educator regarding the pharmaceutical aspects of biotechnology products and can serve as a valuable resource to other health care professionals. In addition, biotech products give the pharmacist the opportunity to provide enhanced patient care services since patient education and monitoring is required. To carry out this role successfully, the pharmacist will need to keep abreast of new developments as new literature and products become available.

## REFERENCES

American Society of Health-System Pharmacists. (2000). ASHP guidelines on quality assurance for pharmacy-prepared sterile products. Am J Health Syst Pharm 57 (12):1150–69.

Amgen Inc. (2006). Epogen® package insert. CA: Thousand Oaks.

Amgen Inc. (2004). Neupogen® package insert. CA: Thousand Oaks.

Banga AK, Reddy IK. (1994). Biotechnology drugs: pharmaceutical issues. Pharmacy Times 60(3):68–76.

Berlex Laboratories. (2003). Betaseron®: package insert. CA: Richmond.

Berlex Laboratories. (2004). Leukine® package insert. CA: Richmond.

Caremark. (2006). Focus on Specialty Pharmacy Trends Rx. IL: Northbrook.

Catania P. (2006). King Guide to Parenteral Admixture. MO: St Louis, MO.

Chiron Therapeutics. (2000). Proleukin® package insert. CA: Emeryville.

Genentech, Inc. (1994). Pulmozyme® package insert. CA: South San Francisco.

Genentech, Inc. (1995). Written information on storage, reconstitution, compatibility, stability, and administration on file. CA: South San Francisco.

Koeller J, Fields S. (1991).The pharmacist's role with biotechnology products. Kalamazoo, MI: The Upjohn Company.

McEvoy GK. (2005). American Hospital Formulary Service Drug Information. Bethesda, MD: American Society of Health-System Pharmacists.

Roche Laboratories. (2005). Summary of Product Characteristics. (Accessed at http://www.rocheuk.com/ProductDB/Documents/rx/spc/Roferon-A_Cartridge_SPC.pdf, 10/31/06.)

Schering Laboratories. (2004). Intron® package insert. NJ: Kennilworth.

Suchanek D. (2005). The rise and role of specialty pharmacy. Biotechnology Healthcare, 31–5.

## FURTHER READING

See Tables 1, 5, and 7 for suggested readings.

# 23

# Economic Considerations in Medical Biotechnology

*Eugene M. Kolassa*
*Medical Marketing Economics, LLC, and Department of Pharmacy, University of Mississippi,*
*Oxford, Mississippi, and University of the Sciences, Philadelphia, Pennsylvania, U.S.A.*

## INTRODUCTION

The biotechnology revolution has coincided with another revolution in health care: the emergence of finance and economics as major issues in the use and success of new medical technologies. Health care finance has become a major social issue in nearly every nation, and the evaluation and scrutiny of the pricing and value of new treatments has become an industry unto itself. The most tangible effect of this change is the establishment of the so-called "third hurdle" for new agents in many nations. Beyond the traditional requirements for demonstrating the efficacy and safety of new agents, some nations, and many private health care systems, now demand data on the economic costs and benefits of new medicines. Although currently required only in Canada (Blaker et al., 1994) and Australia (Drummond, 1992), methods to extend similar prerequisites are being examined by the governments of most developed nations. Many managed care organizations in the United States now prefer that an economic dossier be submitted along with the clinical dossier to make coverage decisions.

The licensing of new agents in most non-US nations has traditionally been accompanied by a parallel process of price and reimbursement approval, and the development of an economic dossier has emerged as a means of securing the highest possible rates of reimbursement. In recent years, sets of economic guidelines have been developed and adopted by the regulatory authorities of several nations to assist them in their decisions to reimburse new products. As many of the products of biotechnology are used to treat costly disorders and the products themselves are often costly to discover and produce, these new agents have presented new problems to those charged with the financing of medical care delivery. The movement to require an economic rationale for the pricing of new agents brings new challenges to those developing such agents. These requirements also provide firms with new tools to help determine which new technologies will provide the most value to society, as well as contribute the greatest financial returns to those developing and marketing the products.

## THE VALUE OF A NEW MEDICAL TECHNOLOGY

The task of determining the value of a new agent should fall somewhere within the purview of the marketing function of a firm. Although some companies have established health care economic capabilities within the clinical research structure of their organizations, it is essential that the group that addresses the value of a new product does so from the perspective of the market and not of the company or the research team. This is important for two reasons. First, evaluating the product candidate from the perspective of the user, and not from the team that is developing it, can minimize the bias that is inherent in evaluating one's own creations. Second, and most importantly, a market focus will move the evaluation away from the technical and scientifically interesting aspects of the product under evaluation and toward the real utility the product might bring to the medical care marketplace. Although the scientific, or purely clinical, aspects of a new product should not be discounted, when the time comes to measure the economic contribution of a new agent, those developing the new agent must move past these considerations. It is the tangible effects that a new treatment will have on the patient and the health care system that determine its value, not the technology supporting it. The phrase to keep in mind is "value in use."

The importance of a marketing focus when evaluating the economic effects of a new agent, or product candidate, cannot be overstated. Failing to consider the product's value in use can result in overly optimistic expectations of sales performance and market acceptance. Marketing is often defined as the process of identifying and filling the needs of the market. If this is the case, then the developers of new pharmaceutical technologies must ask two questions: "What does the market need?" and "What does the market want?" Analysis of the pharmaceutical market in the first decade of the twenty first century will show that the market needs and wants:

- Lower costs
- Controllable costs
- Predictable cost
- Improved outcomes

Note that this list does not include new therapeutic agents. From the perspective of many payers, authorities, clinicians, and buyers, a new agent, in and of itself, is a problem. The effort required to evaluate a new agent and prepare recommendations to adopt or reject it takes time away from other efforts. For many in the health care delivery system a new drug means more work—not that they are opposed to innovation, but newness in and of itself, regardless of the technology behind it, has no intrinsic value. The value of new technologies is in their efficiency, their ability to render results that are not available through other methods or at costs significantly lower than other interventions. Documenting and understanding the economic effects of new technologies on the various health care systems helps the firm to allocate its resources more appropriately, accelerate the adoption of new technologies into the health care system, and reap the financial rewards of its innovation.

There are many different aspects of the term "value," depending upon the perspective of the individual or group evaluating a new product and the needs that are met by the product itself. When developing new medical technologies, it is useful to look to the market to determine the aspects of a product that could create and capture the greatest amount of value. Two products that have entered the market in recent years provide good examples of the different ways in which value is assessed.

Activase® [tissue plasminogen activator (tPA)] from Genentech, one of the first biotechnology entrants in health care, entered the market priced at nearly ten times the price level of streptokinase, its nearest competitor. This product, which is used solely in the hospital setting, significantly increased the cost of medical treatment of patients suffering myocardial infarctions. But the problems associated with streptokinase and the great urgency of need for treatments for acute infarctions were such that many cardiologists believed that any product that proved useful in this area would be worth the added cost. The hospitals, which in the United States are reimbursed on a capitated basis for the bulk of such procedures, were essentially forced to subsidize the use of the agent, as they were unable to pass the added cost of tPA to many of their patients' insurers. The pricing of the product created a significant controversy, but the sales of Activase and its successors have been growing consistently since its launch. The key driver of value for tPA has been, and continues to be, the urgency of the underlying condition. The ability of the product to reduce the rate of immediate mortality is what drives its value. Once the product became a standard of care, incidentally, reimbursement rates were increased to accommodate it, making its economic value positive to hospitals.

A product that delivered a different type of value is the colony-stimulating factor from Amgen (G-CSF, Neupogen®). Neupogen was priced well below its economic value. The product's primary benefit is in the reduction of serious infections in cancer patients, who often suffer significant decreases in white blood cells due to chemotherapy. By bolstering the white count, Neupogen allows oncologists to use more efficacious doses of cytotoxic oncology agents while decreasing the rate of infection and subsequent hospitalization for cancer patients. It has been estimated that the use of Neupogen reduces the expected cost of treating infections by roughly $6,000 per cancer patient per course of therapy. At a price of roughly $1400 per course of therapy, Neupogen not only provides better clinical care but also offers savings of approximately $4600 per patient. The economic benefits of the product have helped it to gain use rapidly with significantly fewer restrictions than products such as tPA, whose economic value is not as readily apparent.

These two very successful products provide clear clinical benefits, but their sources of value are quite different. The value of a new product may come from several sources, depending on the needs of clinicians and their perceptions of the situations in which they treat patients. Some current treatments bring risk, either because of the uncertainty of their effects on the patient (positive or negative) or because of the effort or cost required to use or understand the treatments. A new product that reduces this risk will be perceived as bringing new value to the market. In such cases, the new product removes or reduces some negative aspects of treatment. Neupogen, by reducing the chance of infection and reducing the average cost of treatment, brought new value to the marketplace in this manner.

Value can come from the enhancement of the positive aspects of treatment as well. A product that has a higher rate of efficacy than current therapies is the most obvious example of such a case. But any product that provides benefits in an area of critical need, where few or no current treatments are available, will be seen as providing immediate value. This was, and remains, the case for tPA.

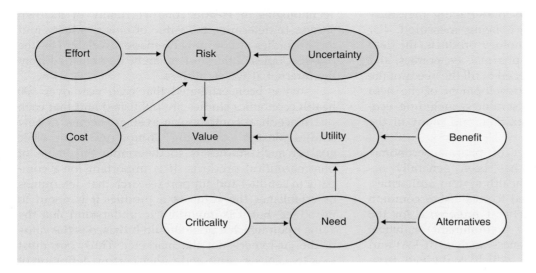

**Figure 1** ■ Generalized model of value. *Source*: Copyright © 2003, Medical Marketing Economics, LLC, Oxford, MS.

Any new product under development should be evaluated with these aspects of value in mind. A generalized model of value, presented in Figure 1, can be used to determine the areas of greatest need in the marketplace for a new agent and to provide guidance in product development. By talking with clinicians, patients, and others involved in current treatments and keeping this model in mind, the shortcomings of those current approaches can be evaluated and the sources of new incremental value can be determined.

Understanding the source of the value brought to the market by a new product is crucial to the development of the eventual marketing strategy. Using Figure 1 as a guide, the potential sources of value can be determined for a product candidate and appropriate studies, both clinical and economic, can be designed to measure and demonstrate that value.

## AN OVERVIEW OF ECONOMIC ANALYSIS FOR NEW TECHNOLOGIES

A thorough economic analysis should be used to guide the clinical research protocol to ensure that the end points measured are commercially relevant and useful. The analysis should describe important elements of the market to the firm, helping decision makers to understand the way decisions are made and providing guidance in affecting those decisions. Later, the results of economic analyses should inform and guide marketing and pricing decisions as the product is prepared for launch, as well as help customers to use the product efficiently and effectively.

To prepare a thorough economic analysis, the researchers must first have a comprehensive understanding of the flow of patients, services, goods, and money through the various health care systems. This process should begin as soon as the likely indications for a new product have been identified and continue throughout the product's development. The first step is to create basic economic models of the current treatment for the disorder(s) for which the product is likely to be indicated. This step will be used to provide better information to fine-tune financial assumptions and to provide critical input into the clinical development process to assure that the clinical protocols are designed to extract the greatest commercial potential from the product. If the product is likely to be used for more than one indication and/or if there is the potential that several different levels of the same indication (e.g., mild, moderate, and severe) would be treated by the same product, separate models should be prepared for each indication and level.

The purpose of the basic model is to provide a greater understanding of the costs associated with the disorder and to identify areas and types of cost that provide the greatest potential for the product to generate cost savings. For example, the cost of a disorder that currently requires a significant amount of laboratory testing offers the potential for savings, and thus better pricing, if the new product can reduce or eliminate the need for tests. Similarly, some indications are well treated, but the incidence of side effects is sufficiently high to warrant special attention. When developing a new agent, it is as important to understand the source of the value to be provided as it is to understand the clinical effects of the agent.

## PARMACOECONOMICS

The field of economic evaluation of medical technologies goes by several names, depending on the discipline of the researchers undertaking the study and the type of technology being measured. For pharmaceutical and biotechnology products, the field has settled on the name of pharmacoeconomics, and an entire discipline has emerged to fill the needs of the area. Contributions to the development of the field have come from several disciplines, including economics, pharmacy administration, and many of the behavioral sciences.

In recent years, a set of pharmacoeconomic standards, or guidelines, has been generally accepted by researchers and health system authorities. These standards have helped to establish a common set of techniques and a general preference for the type of analysis used. The predominant analytical techniques are cost-effectiveness analysis (CEA) and cost-utility analysis (CUA), which is derived from CEA and is often much more useful and meaningful than CEA. In a CEA of a product such as tPA for use in myocardial infarction, a typical measure used for the analysis would be the cost of saving an additional life (or preventing a death). This measure would be extended using life expectancy tables to determine the cost of providing a patient with an additional year of life. This measure is called the "cost per life year saved."

As patients are often left with less than ideal functional status and quality of life after a serious medical event, it is desirable to consider the outcome from the perspective of the patient and to factor in any reductions in quality of life. CUA allows researchers to factor in such differences, called patient preferences, by applying different weights to the value of additional years of life gained, depending on the functional status of the patient. In the case of myocardial infarction, a significant proportion of patients who survive will find their abilities to participate in strenuous recreational activities impaired, which would reduce the quality of life for many patients compared to those in a more ideal health state. CUA reduces the value of the additional years of life gained through the specific treatment under evaluation. The resultant revised figure is called a quality-adjusted life year, or QALY. The cost of achieving a QALY has become such a common measure in pharmacoeconomic evaluations that the Canadian government uses this figure to determine the appropriateness of the reimbursement of new agents.

Under the Canadian system, a product that renders a cost per QALY gained of $50,000 (Canadian) or less will be generally accepted into the system and reimbursed without difficulty. Products delivering an additional QALY for $100,000 or more will not be reimbursed, while those with costs between $50,000 and $100,000 will be subjected to more study, scrutiny, and negotiation. The Canadian Agency for Drugs and Technologies in Health conducts many of its own studies to determine the value of new products, and these studies are routinely made available to the public. Copies of the studies can be downloaded from the Internet at www.cadth.ca.

It has been estimated that each year over 600 health economics studies are published and that each pharmaceutical company, on average, begins 23 new studies (Boston Consulting Group, 1993). The basic goal of such studies is to determine the value of pharmaceutical products. It is important for a company to conduct and support research that determines or establishes the value of a product it is about to introduce, but it is important to understand that the value upon which a price should be based is the value to the customer—not the marketer. Thus, one must look to a conservative and rather narrow definition of value as a starting point.

The first, and perhaps most important, measure of value to determine after the economic studies have been completed is the break-even or "zero-based" value. This value is derived by modeling the new product in the treatment process, as determined through a burden of illness study, and measuring the difference with and without the new product, which has been assigned a cost of $0. The "economic value" of the new product is the difference between the two treatment approaches: the cost of the original treatment minus the cost of treatment with the new product. Ideally, the treatment with the new product results in lower costs than treatment without it. The alternative, that treatment with the new product is more costly than treatment without, requires serious decisions as to the launch of the product.

The economic value of the product may have elements besides the basic economic efficiency implied by the break-even level just discussed. Quality differences, in terms of reduced side effects, greater efficacy, or other substantive factors can result in increases in value beyond the break-even point calculated in a simple cost comparison. Should these factors be present, it is crucial to capture their value in the price of the product, but how much value should be captured?

It is important to recognize that a product can provide a significant economic benefit in one indication but none in another; therefore, it is prudent to perform these studies on all indications considered for a new product. A case in point is that of epoetin alfa (EPO). EPO was initially developed and approved for use in dialysis patients, where its principle benefit is to reduce, or even eliminate, the need for transfusion. Studies have shown that EPO doses that drive hematocrit levels to between 33% and 36% result in significantly lower total patient care costs than lower doses of EPO or none at all (Collins et al., 2000). The same product, when used to reduce the need for transfusion in elective surgery, however, has been shown not to be cost-effective (Coyle et al., 1999). Although EPO was shown to reduce the need for transfusion in this study, the cost of the drug far outweighed the savings from reduced transfusions as well as reductions in the transmission and treatment of blood-born pathogens. Economic efficiency is not automatically transferred from one indication to another.

The lack of economic savings in the surgical indication does not necessarily mean that the product should not be used, only that users must recognize that in this indication use results in substantially higher costs while in dialysis it actually reduces the total cost of care.

Similarly, the interferons and other agents used in multiple sclerosis and the disease-modifying agents for rheumatoid arthritis have added substantially to the cost of care for those disorders, but they have improved the lives of many patients. In these cases, the added cost has been accepted and the products appreciated. But when these same agents have been used in other indications, such as psoriasis, some payers have come to doubt their value, despite their efficacy. This brings a new set of considerations to the table: the value of the intervention itself.

The first biomedical agents to enter the market were for very serious disorders, most of them life-threatening. Activase could prevent death, as could Neupogen. EPO changed the way in which dialysis patients were treated and improved their outcomes. But when new, high-cost agents began to be used in disorders that were less life-threatening, first rheumatoid arthritis and multiple sclerosis and then other disorders, payers began to take steps to ensure appropriate use. Some question the need to spend thousands of dollars each month for arthritis treatments, and many, to date, have refused to pay these prices for the treatment of psoriasis, which some have deemed "cosmetic."

As new biomedical products are developed, society begins to ask, "Do we need a $1000 solution to a $100 problem?" The fact that a new agent *can* treat a disease does not address the societal question of whether or not it should be used. A recent evaluation of infliximab and etanercept in patients with rheumatoid arthritis, undertaken by the Canadian Coordinating Office for Health Technology Assessment (CCOHTA) (now CADTH), provides a clear example of how these technologies are being evaluated and why, in some cases, health authorities have decided not to cover their use (Coyle et al., 2006). To determine the economic value of these two agents, which are anti-TNF (tumor necrosing factor) agents for the treatment of rheumatoid arthritis, the CCOHTA undertook a comprehensive review of the

clinical and economic literature for the products. The researchers compiled the results of these studies and determined that these agents do, indeed, offer clinical advantages, in terms of improved efficacy and health outcomes, over standard therapies. The question they addressed, however, was not "Do they work?" but "Are they worth the prices charged?" The conclusion was that they are not.

The researchers first looked at the costs of treatment with gold therapy, the standard of care, and the two new agents. They compiled the costs of the agents, of managing adverse reactions, and of the monitoring that is needed for each intervention. The results of this phase are presented in Table 1. Although the monitoring costs for gold therapy were higher than those for the new agents, the costs of the anti-TNF agents were 14 to 16 times higher than the

| | Cost[a] | Probability distribution |
|---|---|---|
| **Costs for managing AEs** | | |
| Gold therapy | 62.88 | Normal (62.88, 15.72) |
| Infliximab and methotrexate | 62.88 | Normal (62.88, 15.72) |
| Etanercept | 62.88 | Normal (62.88, 15.72) |
| **Monitoring costs** | | |
| *First cycle* | | |
| Gold therapy | 488.90 | Normal (488.90, 122.23) |
| Infliximab plus methotrexate | 215.57 | Normal (215.57, 53.89) |
| Etanercept | 229.13 | Normal (229.13, 57.28) |
| *Subsequent cycles* | | |
| Gold therapy | 143.8 | Normal (143.80, 35.95) |
| Infliximab plus methotrexate | 87.58 | Normal (87.58, 21.89) |
| Etanercept | 120.19 | Normal (120.19, 30.05) |
| Costs of palliative care | 1,000.00 | Normal (1000, 500) |
| **Drug costs per cycle** | | |
| Gold therapy | 582.70 | Fixed |
| Infliximab plus methotrexate | 7,056.81 | Fixed |
| Etanercept | 8,580.00 | Fixed |

[a] In Canadian dollars.
*Abbreviation*: AEs, adverse events.

**Table 1** ◼ Unit costs for six-month cycle.

|  | Baseline strategy | Infliximab plus methotrexate before gold | Infliximab plus methotrexate after gold |
|---|---|---|---|
| Total costs | **$9200** | **$37,900** | **$30,900** |
| Years with ACR 20 response | 0.73 | 2.46 | 1.62 |
| Years with ACR 50 response | 0.13 | 1.08 | 0.59 |
| Years with ACR 70 response | 0.03 | 0.35 | 0.26 |
| Years on DMARDs | 1.78 | 3.54 | 3.63 |
| QALYs gained | 0.09 | 0.34 | 0.31 |
| **Incremental cost-effectiveness ratio in comparison with baseline strategy:** | | | |
| Per year with ACR 20 response |  | $16,700 | $24,500 |
| Per year with ACR 50 response |  | $30,400 | $47,900 |
| Per year with ACR 70 response |  | $89,800 | $95,700 |
| Per year on DMARDs |  | $16,300 | $11,700 |
| Incremental cost per QALY |  | $113,000 | $97,800 |

*Abbreviations*: ACR, American College of Rheumatology; DMARDs, disease-modifying antirheumatic drugs; QALYs, quality-adjusted life years.

**Table 2** ▪ Base economic results for infliximab plus methotrexate strategies.

older intervention. This fact alone warrants the review that was undertaken.

These health economics researchers then moved on to evaluating the clinical and humanistic outcomes (Table 2). From this study, it is evident that patients receive three times more benefit from the newer agents (see the improvement in QALYs for the anti-TNF agents in Table 2).

The conclusion of the study was that the cost for the improvements provided by these agents was roughly $100,000 (Canadian) per QALYs gained. This figure is well above the $50,000 upper limit agreed upon within the Canadian system and resulted in the recommendation not to cover these agents. Although anti-TNF agents are widely used in the United States, Canada's health system has determined that they do not provide sufficient value to support their current prices.

Payers within the U.S. healthcare system have begun to use similar methods of evaluation. Although it cannot be stated with certainty that the U.S. system will adopt this approach to coverage wholeheartedly, the consistent news reports of new drugs costing tens, and hundreds, of thousands of dollars would indicate that the importance of delivering demonstrable value will increase in that market as well.

## CONCLUSIONS

In the pharmaceutical marketing environment of the foreseeable future, it is wise, when possible, to first consider determining the true medical need for the intervention, then, if the need is real, to consider surrendering some value to the market—pricing the product at some point below its full economic value. This is appealing for several reasons:

- The measurement of economics is imprecise, and the margin for error can be large.
- If the market is looking for lower costs, filling that need enhances the market potential of the product.
- From a public relations and public policy perspective, launching a new product with the message that it provides savings to the system can also provide positive press and greater awareness.

As societies continue to focus on the cost of health care interventions, we must all be concerned about the economic and clinical implications of the products we bring into the system. Delivering value, in the form of improved outcomes, economic savings, or both, is an important part of pharmaceutical science. Understanding the value that is delivered should be the responsibility of everyone involved with new product development.

## REFERENCES

Blaker D, Detsky A, Hubbard E, et al., (1994). Guidelines for Economic Evaluation of Pharmaceuticals: Canada, Draft of Report of the Steering Committee, February 1.

Boston Consulting Group. (1993). The changing environment for U.S. pharmaceuticals. Boston: Boston Consulting Group, April.

Collins AJ, Li S, Ebben J, Ma JZ, Manning W. (2000). Hematocrit levels and associated medicare expenditures. Am J Kidney Dis 36(2):282–93.

Coyle D, Lee K, Laupacis A, Fergusson D. (1999). Economic analysis of erythropoietin in surgery, Canadian Coordinating Office for Health Technology Assessment, March 9.

Coyle D, Judd M, Blumenauer B, Cranney A, Maetzel A, Tugwell P, Wells GA. (2006). Infliximab and etanercept in patients with rheumatoid arthritis: a systematic review and economic evaluation, Canadian Coordinating Office for Health Technology Assessment, Technology Report No. 64. (Accessed at http://www.cadth.ca/media/pdf/123_infliximab_tr_e_no-appendices.pdf.)

Drummond M. (1992). Australian guidelines for cost-effectiveness studies of pharmaceuticals: the thin edge of the boomerang?, PharmacoEconomics 1 (Suppl. 1):61–9.

## FURTHER READING

### ■ Pharmacoeconomic Methods and Pricing Issues

Bootman JL, Townsend JT, McGhan WF. (1991). Principles of Pharmacoeconomics. Cincinnati: Harvey Whitney Books.

Bonk RJ. (1999). Pharmacoeconomics in Perspective. New York: Pharmaceutical Products Press.

Drummond MF, O'Brien BJ, Stoddart GL, Torrance GW. (1997). Methods for the Economic Evaluation of Health Care Programmes. 2nd Ed. Oxford: Oxford University Press.

Kolassa EM. (1997). Elements of Pharmaceutical Pricing. New York: Pharmaceutical Products Press.

### ■ Pharmacoeconomics of Biotechnology Drugs

Dana WJ, Farthing K. (1998). The pharmacoeconomics of high-cost biotechnology products. Pharm Practice Manage Q 18(2):23–31.

Hui JW, Yee GC. (1998). Pharmacoeconomics of biotechnology drugs (Part 1 of 2). J Am Pharma Assoc 38 (1):97–3.

Hui JW, Yee GC. (1998). Pharmacoeconomics of biotechnology drugs (Part 2 of 2). J Am Pharm Assoc 38 (2):231–3.

Reeder CE. (1995). Pharmacoeconomics and health care outcomes management: Focus on biotechnology (special supplement). Am J Health-Syst Pharm 52(19,S4): S1–28.

# Regulatory Issues and Drug Product Approval for Biopharmaceuticals

*Vinod P. Shah*
Pharmaceutical Consultant, North Potomac, Maryland, U.S.A.

*Daan J. A. Crommelin*
Utrecht University, Utrecht and Dutch Top Institute Pharma, Leiden, The Netherlands

## INTRODUCTION

The term "biopharmaceuticals" is used to describe biotechnologically derived drug products. Biopharmaceuticals are protein-based macromolecules and include, insulin, human growth hormone, the families of the cytokines and of the monoclonal antibodies, antibody fragments, and nucleotide based systems such as antisense oligonucleotides, siRNA and DNA preparations for gene delivery. These are large complex molecules and are often heterogeneous mixtures compared to synthetically manufactured, pure small molecules. This chapter focuses only on protein molecules.

In the first years of the new millennium the regulatory landscape for biopharmaceuticals changed. Before that time only original biopharmaceuticals were approved by FDA and EMEA (Table 1) following the normal pathway of approval including full scale clinical trials to ensure efficacy and safety and this pathway still stands for original biopharmaceuticals. Then, a number of biopharmaceutical drugs ran out of patent and the introduction of generic versions of biopharmaceuticals became the center of lively debates: the new products were called biosimilars (EMEA) or follow-on biologics (FDA) and issues of debate were, for instance, structuring of the clinical trial programs. The regulatory process for biosimilars/follow-on biologics is an evolutionary process. Up until recently we have considered biopharmaceuticals as one homogeneous class of compounds. But, that is an oversimplification. The requirements for approval of biosimilar products should be based on the structural complexity and clinical knowledge of and experience with the reference biopharmaceutical product. The information provided here reflects the status at December 2006.

## BACKGROUND

The aim of this chapter is to provide a comprehensive view on the regulatory issues for the approval of a biosimilar product. In order to have a better understanding of the regulatory process involved, it is essential to appreciate the basic difference between small drug molecules and macromolecules and their approval process. Table 1 provides the definitions of different classes of medicinal drug products. Table 2 provides the steps involved in the drug approval process of small molecules. For the approval of a (small molecule) generic product, it must be pharmaceutically equivalent and bioequivalent (Table 3). Biopharmaceuticals have a number of characteristics (Table 4) that set them aside from small molecule drugs (Crommelin et al., 2003). The efficacy and safety of biotech products depend on their complicated, rather labile shape built up of secondary, tertiary and sometimes quaternary structures.

The mission of a regulatory authority is to "Assure that safe, effective and high quality drugs are marketed in the country and are available to the people". Safety of an innovator's drug product, be it a small molecule or biopharmaceutical, is established through preclinical studies in animals and controlled clinical studies in humans. Efficacy is established through clinical studies in patients. A complete set of information on Chemistry, Manufacturing and Controls (CMC-section) is needed in the dossier submitted for approval to ensure that the drug substance and the drug product are, pure, potent and of high quality. The CMC section should include full analytical characterization, a description of the manufacturing process and test methods, and stability data. In addition to the establishment of safety and efficacy of the drug product, the approval process requires manufacturing of the drug product under controlled current good manufacturing practice (cGMP) conditions. The cGMP requirement ensures identity, potency, purity, quality and safety of the final product. These features include process robustness and reproducibility, validation, controls and testing. Batch release criteria are established to assure

| | |
|---|---|
| Biopharmaceutical drug | An original biotechnology-derived pharmaceutical and/or a medicinal product containing a biotechnology derived protein as an active product |
| Biosimilar product | A generic version of a biopharmaceutical product already approved and marketed (EMEA) |
| FDA | U.S. Food and Drug Administration |
| Follow-on biologics | A generic version of a biopharmaceutical product already approved and marketed (Food and Drug Administration, United States) |
| EMEA | European Agency for the Evaluation of Medicinal Products |
| Generic product | Non-patented medicinal product of low molecular weight, and therapeutically equivalent |
| Low molecular weight drug | Classical medicinal product prepared by chemical synthesis |
| Second generation biopharmaceuticals | The second generation biopharmaceutical product is derived from an approved biopharmaceutical product which has been deliberately modified to change one or more of the product's characteristics. |

**Table 1** ■ Definitions.

batch-to-batch consistency in the manufacturing process. The entire process of drug identification, of establishing its safety and efficacy and guiding it through the drug approval procedures is lengthy, time consuming and costly.

A generic product is a copy of the brand name, innovator's product, except for the inactive ingredients. The required dossier for market authorization

| Patented product | Generic product |
|---|---|
| New drug application (NDA) | Abbreviated new drug application (ANDA) |
| Safety studies (pre-clinical, animal toxicity) Efficacy studies (in patients) | |
| Bioavailability/bioequivalence | Bioequivalence in healthy subjects |
| Chemistry, manufacturing controls | Chemistry, manufacturing controls |
| Dissolution (solid oral dosage forms) | Dissolution (solid oral dosage forms) |

**Table 2** ■ Drug approval process (for small, low molecular weight drugs).

**Pharmaceutically equivalent:**
- Same dosage form
- Same strength of active
- Same route of drug administration
- Same labeling

**Bioequivalent:**
- Pharmacokinetic profile the same[a]
- Pharmacodynamic profile the same
- Clinical comparison the same
- In vitro dissolution profile the same

**Therapeutically equivalent = Pharmaceutically equivalent + Bioequivalent = Interchangeable**

A generic product must be pharmaceutically equivalent and bioequivalent to be considered therapeutically equivalent and hence interchangeable with the brand name product.

[a] Within a narrow range of the reference (comparator) product (± 20%). *Source*: FDA Guidance for industry: Bioavailability and bioequivalence studies for orally administered drug products–general considerations, Rockville, MD, 2003 (http://www.fda.gov/cder/guidance/index.htm).

**Table 3** ■ Generic (small molecular weight) product and therapeutic equivalence.

focuses on only two aspects. The generic (small molecule) drug product should be pharmaceutically equivalent and bioequivalent to the brand name product, and therefore therapeutically equivalent and interchangeable with the brand name drug product (Table 3). A generic product is expected to have the same safety profile as the brand name product. The bioequivalence documentation of the generic product (generally through pharmacokinetic profiling) assures the efficacy of the generic product.

In the case of small molecules, the identity of the active substance is established through a validated chemical synthesis route, full analysis of the active agent and impurity profiling, and other techniques. In the case of biopharmaceuticals this is, generally speaking, not possible. A first challenge is the

| Small molecular weight drugs | Biopharmaceuticals |
|---|---|
| Low molecular weight | High molecular weight |
| Simple chemical structure | Complex three-dimensional structure |
| Chemically synthesized | Produced by living organism |
| Easy characterization | Difficult to impossible to fully characterize |
| Synthetically pure | Often heterogeneous |
| Rarely produce immune response | Prone to eliciting an immune response |

**Table 4** ■ Difference between small molecular weight drugs and biopharmaceuticals.

complex manufacturing process of biopharmaceuticals involving living organisms. The production process should be controlled in every minor detail. Moreover, in Chapter 2 a long list of analytical techniques is presented to characterize biopharmaceuticals, but in many instances full characterization is not possible with our current toolbox of analytical techniques (see Chapter 2 and Fig. 1).

A generic product (small molecule) contains the same active ingredient with inactive (most of the time) excipients as the reference product. As explained above, this is not always possible in biopharmaceutical protein products and therefore, these are not referred to as biogenerics. This biopharmaceutical product contains the active ingredient which is similar (but not necessarily equal) in characteristics to the reference product. For this reason, the generic biopharmaceutical products are referred to as follow-on proteins or follow-on biologics or biosimilar products. A biosimilar product has a pharmacological and therapeutic activity that is similar to the reference (comparator) product, but may differ in its pharmaceutical equivalence (characteristics). Biosimilar

products are not generic products since it could be expected that there may be subtle differences between the biosimilar and reference product from the innovator and are not interchangeable with brand name products.

## BIOSIMILAR AND FOLLOW-ON BIOLOGICS

Biosimilar products are expected to be comparable to an approved reference product in terms of quality, safety and efficacy profile. Approval of these products should be considered based on product comparisons and demonstration of comparability to the reference product.

Biopharmaceutical products may be currently manufactured by the same manufacturer at different sites. The "FDA Guidance on comparability" protocol is used for assuring product quality of the approved product after certain changes are made in the manufacturing process (comparability assessment, see below). The quality of these products is assured by chemical analysis and/or by using a comparability clinical study protocol.

A question often raised and debated by a generic manufacturer is whether the approach of using a comparability protocol can be extrapolated and adopted for approval of biosimilar products manufactured by a different manufacturer. The regulatory answer today is no, it cannot be used for the approval of a biosimilar product.

The requirements for approval of biosimilar products should be based on the structural complexity and clinical knowledge of and experience with the reference biopharmaceutical product. Products such as growth hormone and interferon, for example, have known and relatively simple chemical structures. In addition, extensive manufacturing and clinical experience is available for these products. On the other hand, monoclonal antibodies are large, glycosylated proteins and clinically less experience has been obtained with them so far. Because of the varying complexity of the biotech-derived products, the requirements for the approval process should be structured on a case-by-case basis. The following information is required for product approval.

- Structural information—Primary, secondary, tertiary, and if relevant, quaternary structure information, including information regarding the glycosylation pattern, if relevant.
- Manufacturing process
- Quality attributes and clinical activities
- Pharmacokinetic-Pharmacodynamic information, mechanism of drug action
- Clinical experience, efficacy and toxicity information

- UV absorption
- Circular dichroism spectroscopy
- Fourier transform IR
- Fluorescence spectroscopy
- NMR spectroscopy
- Calorimetric approaches
- Bio-assays
  - Immunochemical assays
    ELISA
    Immunoprecipitation
    Biosensor (SPR, QCM)
  - Potency testing
    In cell lines
    In animals
  - Chromatographic techniques
    RP-HPLC
    SEC-HPLC
    Hydrophobic interaction HPLC
    Ion-exchange HPLC
    Peptide mapping
  - Electrophoretic techniques
    SDS–PAGE
    IEF
    CZE
- Field flow fractionaction
- Ultracentifugation
- Static and dynamic light scattering
- Electron microscopy
- X-ray techniques
- Mass spectrometry

**Figure 1** Analytical techniques for monitoring protein structure. *Source*: From Crommelin et al., 2003.

## REGULATORY ROUTES

From a regulatory perspective, a copy of a biopharmaceutical product can be identified as a generic product. But in practice it is unlikely, due to additional complexity, particularly safety issues. The copy of a biopharmaceutical product is required to have a similar safety and efficacy profile as the brand name/innovator product, and therefore it is referred to as "biosimilar". Biosimilar products are non-interchangeable.

According to the U.S. Food, Drug and Cosmetic Act, the approval process can follow one of two routes: New Drug Application (NDA) with two subclasses, and Abbreviated New Drug Application (ANDA)

- *Section 505(b)(1)*: Full reports of investigations of safety and efficacy are needed. This results in a full NDA, with right of reference. This means that information about safety and efficacy can be used by others to document safety and efficacy of the product.
- *Section 505(b)(2)*: This requires clinical studies, without the right of reference, e.g., NDA for rDNA. Most of the biosimilar products fall into this category.
- *Section 505(3)*: This is the route for ANDA applications. This requires the dosage form to be pharmaceutically equivalent and requires only bioequivalent studies. It does not require clinical or pre-clinical studies. This is the route normally followed for small molecule generic products.

Biosimilar products are different from second generation biopharmaceuticals (Table 2). The second generation biopharmaceuticals have improved pharmacological properties/biological activity compared to an already approved biopharmaceutical product which has been deliberately modified. The second generation products are marketed with the claim of improved clinical superiority. The second generation biopharmaceuticals require a full New Drug Application and are not interchangeable with the brand name product.

## EQUIVALENCE

Biopharmaceutical products are injectables and include intravenous, intramuscular and subcutaneous products. For intravenous products, the question of bioavailability (and hence bioequivalence) does not arise. However, for intramuscular and subcutaneous products, the issue of bioavailability and hence bioequivalence is an important one. One should expect equivalence in availability and pharmacokinetic pattern.

Two "types" of equivalence can be envisioned.

- Within a manufacturer—changes in the manufacturing process, changes in the formulation or a change in manufacturing site by a given manufacturer. This requires assurance of pharmaceutical equivalence. At times, depending upon the nature of the change, a comparability study (see below) may be required. The FDA Guidance on Comparability is summarized in the insert box.
- Between manufacturers—This falls in the category of a biosimilar product and it requires confirmation of pharmaceutical equivalence as well as bioequivalence.

## KEY POINTS OF THE FDA GUIDANCE ON COMPARABILITY

The concept of comparability studies is described in the FDA Guidance on Comparability.

- The comparability study protocol is generally followed for changes related to existing products within a given manufacturer after the drug product is approved. The demonstration of comparability does not necessarily mean that the quality attributes of the pre-change and post-change products are identical; but that they are similar enough and that the existing knowledge is sufficiently predictive to ensure that any differences in quality attributes have no adverse impact upon safety or efficacy of the drug product.
- Process changes among biotech products frequently include changing master cell banks. The changes in manufacturing process are judged by characterization studies, possible preclinical, pharmacokinetic and pharmacodynamic and/or clinical studies. The principles of comparability are used to permit pioneer manufacturers to change the production process, cell line, formulations and manufacturing site.
- This concept takes into consideration the unique features of protein products including complexity of the structures to allow flexibility in comparability testing.
- The comparison relies heavily on analytical characterization. A determination of comparability can be based on a combination of analytical testing, biological assays, and in some cases non-clinical and clinical data.
- The comparability is based on the expectation that the safety and efficacy expected for the product from a modified process/formulation or site change is similar to that from the original process.
- The principal objective of the comparability protocol is to reduce or eliminate the need for human

clinical studies, especially after certain scale-up and post approval changes in composition, manufacturing process and change in manufacturing site. The comparability exercise is to demonstrate similarity.

## DRUG APPROVAL

The regulatory approval process for biosimilars is very different from that of typical generic pharmaceuticals (Table 5). With small molecule drugs, it is straightforward to prove that the two products are pharmaceutically equivalent, bioequivalent and therefore therapeutically equivalent. This is not the case with biosimilar products. The precise composition of a biosimilar product is dependent on the process used to make it, so a greater number of studies are needed to prove that a generic version is equivalent to the original. Omnitrope and Valtropin, for example, are biosimilars of somatropin, developed by using Pfizer's Genotropin and Eli Lilly's Humantrope, respectively. Sandoz' Omnitrope and Biopartners' Valtropin, both recombinant human growth hormones, were the first biosimilars to receive marketing authorization from European regulators, followed closely by Omnitrope receiving approval in the United States. Products which are in the pipeline or are presently dealt with by the regulatory authorities include insulin, erythropoietin, and granulocyte-colony stimulating factor (G-CSF).

For most of the approved biosimilars up until now clinical studies demonstrating similarity in terms of therapeutic outcome were performed. The safety and efficacy profile of biosimilar products is highly dependent on the robustness and the monitoring of the quality aspects. Moreover, one also has to keep in mind that the pharmacological and toxicological effects (e.g., immunogenicity) of quite a few biopharmaceuticals (e.g., interferons) are restricted to the human species. All three major regulatory authorities (from European Union, Japan and United States) have adopted a flexible, case-by-case, science-based approach to preclinical safety evaluation needed to support clinical development and marketing authorization. The primary goals of pre-clinical safety evaluation are: (*i*) to identify an initial safe dose and subsequent dose escalation scheme in humans, (*ii*) to identify potential target organs for toxicity and for the study of whether such toxicity is reversible, and (*iii*) to identify safety parameters for clinical monitoring.

## CHARACTERIZATION

Characterization of the active moiety and impurity/contaminant profiling plays a significant role in the development process of a biosimilar drug product. The technological advances in instrumentation have played a major role in improved identification and characterization of biotech products (Fig. 1). It is acknowledged that no single analytical method can fully characterize the biotech product. A collection of orthogonal analytical methods is needed to piece together a complete picture of a biotech product. Determining how a small homogeneous protein is folded in absolute terms can be accomplished using crystal X-ray diffraction. This can be difficult, expensive and non-realistic to perform in the formulated drug product and on a routine basis. Moreover, X-ray diffraction analysis doesn't pick up low levels of conformational contaminants. The most basic aspect of assessing its identity is to determine its covalent, primary structure using LC/MS/MS, or peptide mapping/amino acid sequencing (e.g., via the Edman-degradation protocol) and disulfide bond-locating methods. Using circular dichroism, Fourier transform infrared and fluorescence spectroscopy, immunological methods, chromatographic techniques, and others, differences in secondary and higher order structures can be monitored. Selective analytical methods are used to determine the purity as well as impurities of the biotech product. Methods here include again chromatographic techniques and gel electrophoresis, capillary electrophoresis, iso-electric focusing, static and dynamic light scattering, ultracentrifugation, and others. Inadequate characterization can result in failure to detect product changes that can impact the safety and efficacy of a product. The characterization factors that impact safety and efficacy of the product should be identified in the product development process.

Comparative analytical characterization of the reference and biosimilar product will provide a foundation for determining whether a clinical study is necessary. The sensitivity of the analytical techniques to detect subtle product differences is far superior to the ability of clinical trials to detect product differences. But, the impact of these (subtle)

| New drug approval | Biosimilar drug product (follow-on biologics, follow-on proteins) |
|---|---|
| Safety (pre-clinical) | Safety[a] |
| Efficacy (clinical) | Comparative clinical |
| Characterization | Complex and difficult |
| Regulations: 505(b)(1) | Regulations: 505(b)(2) |

[a]Established through appropriate characterization procedure and comparability protocol.

**Table 5** ■ Drug approval process (biopharmaceuticals).

changes on the performance of the protein in the clinical situation is not always clear. If a clinical study is warranted, the comparative data will help determine the study parameters. A well designed and focused clinical approach can typically confirm with relatively small patient numbers that the new, biosimilar product has the same pharmacological properties as the innovator's product.

## CLINICAL STUDIES

One of the key aspects in the approval process of biosimilar products will be the science-based rigorous determination of whether a (limited) clinical study will be required. The clinical studies should be required to assure safety and efficacy of the product.

The range of variation in the reference product used in clinical studies can be used for the definition of the boundaries within which the reference product has been shown to be safe and efficacious. These boundaries can be related to composition, or to processing/formulation parameters.

The clinical comparability exercise is a stepwise procedure that should begin with pharmacokinetic and pharmacodynamic studies followed by clinical efficacy and safety trials. The choice of the design of the pharmacokinetic study, i.e., single dose and/or multiple dose designs, should be justified. Normally comparative clinical trials are required for demonstration of clinical comparability. However, in certain cases, comparative pharmacokinetic/pharmacodynamic studies between the biosimilar product and the reference product using biomarkers may prove to be adequate.

## REGULATORY FRAMEWORK (EMEA OVERARCHING DOCUMENT)

There are three major parts of the application dossier—Safety, Efficacy and Quality (Table 6). In 2006, the EMEA has published a series of guidance documents on biosimilar medical products containing biotechnology-derived proteins as active substance, e.g., recombinant erythropoietin, somatropin, G-CSF and human insulin. These guidelines define key

concepts/principles of biotechnology derived proteins and discuss quality issues, as well as non-clinical and clinical issues. The overarching guideline for biosimilar drug products is CHMP/437/04. The EMEA has also adopted a "Guidelines on Comparability" protocol (2003). These guidelines provide information to the sponsor choosing to develop a new biological medicinal product claimed to be similar in terms of quality, safety and efficacy to an original approved reference medicinal product. The CMC part of the dossier should be worked out in detail along the lines mentioned above. It suffices here to pay attention to the paragraph on immunogenicity.

## IMMUNOGENICITY (RELATED TO OVERARCHING EMEA DOCUMENT)

Immunogenicity is a major concern for all biotech products (see Chapter 6). The immune response against therapeutic proteins differs between products since the immunogenic potential is influenced by many factors. These factors include, but are not limited to, the protein, the product and process related impurities, excipients, stability, dosing regimen and patient. Immunogenicity should be studied in patients. At present, neither animal studies nor physicochemical characterization can fully predict immunogenicity. All biotech products must be tested for their immunogenic response in humans. Our immune system can detect alterations in a product missed by analytical methods. Therefore, post marketing surveillance is essential to monitor immunological reactions.

## THE CHALLENGE AND THE FUTURE

A major problem today is the inadequate definition of the relationship between the complex structure and function of protein pharmaceuticals. Analytical tools are becoming increasingly sensitive and provide more detailed information regarding the molecular structure. This may allow for certain biotech products to be shown to be pharmaceutically equivalent, therapeutically equivalent and interchangeable on the basis of a validated analytical definition alone. Sufficient experience has been gained over the last two decades by the regulators and by the industry regarding risk assessment and determining if a clinical study is required when certain types of changes are made. And this expertise will keep on growing.

In the production of biopharmaceuticals, minor changes in production conditions may lead to subtle changes in the molecular structure of the protein. Folding might be different or glycosylation patterns might change. For relatively small molecules like insulin, a well characterized biopharmaceutical

| Quality: |
| --- |
| ◼ Characterization |
| **Safety:** |
| ◼ Non-clinical studies |
| **Efficacy:** |
| ◼ Clinical studies |
| ◼ Immunogenicity |

**Table 6** ◼ Regulatory framework.

product, equivalence can be established using available analytical tools. But for larger and complex proteins, it is not possible to fully characterize the molecule and establish equivalence. In such a scenario, clinical safety and efficacy studies are needed to establish equivalence.

Science based regulatory policies are being developed. They are dynamic and have evolved over many years and continue to evolve based on the development of superior analytical techniques to characterize the products, on introducing improved manufacturing practices and controls, and on growing clinical and regulatory experience. Rigorous standards of ensuring product safety and efficacy must be maintained. At the same time unnecessary and/or unethical duplication trials must be avoided. The approval of a biosimilar product should depend on the complexity of the molecule. A gradation scheme should be designed for the drug approval process rather than using a "one size fits all" model. Different regulatory regimens are required from simple chemically synthesized molecules to highly complex molecules, e.g., from a chemically synthesized simple molecule like acetaminophen to cyclosporine, to insulin, to human growth hormone, to interleukins, to erythropoietin-type growth factors, to albumin, to monoclonal antibodies, to factor VIII.

The regulatory processes for biopharmaceuticals are following an evolutionary route. We learn from the new information coming in every day, we evaluate the data, adjust the rules and develop new protocols to make sure that the patient keeps on receiving high quality, safe and effective biopharmaceuticals.

## ACKNOWLEDGMENTS

The authors would like to thank Dr. Tina Morris of USP and Dr. Hae-Young Ahn of the FDA for their constructive comments.

## REFERENCES

Crommelin DJA, Storm G, Verrijk R, de Leede L, Jiskoot W., Hennink WE. (2003). Shifting paradigms: biopharmaceuticals versus low molecular weight drugs. Int J Pharm 266:3—16.

EMEA Guidances. (Accessed at http://www.emea.eu.net).

FDA Guidance concerning demonstration of comparability human biological products, including therapeutic biotechnology-derived products. April 1996.

FDA Guidances. (Accessed at http://www.fda.gov/cder/guidance/index.htm).

ICH: Q5E Comparability biotechnological/biological products subject to changes in their manufacturing process. June 2005.

# Questions and Answers

## ■ Questions

1. A bacterial strain carrying a foreign structural gene with its own promoter on an appropriate plasmid does not yield a substantial amount of the encoded gene product. What factors could explain this failure?

2. What kind of bacterial plasmid is needed in order to function as an optimal vector for DNA cloning in a particular bacterial host?

3. Potential hosts for the biotechnological production by the recombinant DNA technology of a human protein, lacking functional post-translational modifications, and to be used as a biopharmaceutical are:
   a. *Escherichia coli* K-12
   b. *Bacillus subtilis*
   c. *Saccharomyces cerevisiae* (a yeast)
   d. *Aspergillus nidulans* (a fungus)
   e. Plant cells
   f. Animal cells
   Which one(s) would you prefer? Why?

4. Same question as above but now the protein is, for its biological activity, dependent on specific post-translational modifications.

5. To gain microbial products in biotechnology one may use batch cultures or alternatively continuous cultures. What are the differences between these culture methods and what are the practical consequences of these differences?

6. To use a batch culture for production, what kinds of measures must be taken in order to achieve an efficient production yield?

7. To isolate an animal gene for the purpose of isolating the gene product in a bacterial host, what would be the most appropriate isolation procedure?

8. A foreign product, encoded by a recombinant plasmid, will lead to fast killing of the bacterial host that should produce that product. What kind of measures should be taken, in order to gain substantial amounts of that product?

9. The PCR technology, using specific primers for *Salmonella typhimurium*, reveals a clear signal in a food product, or in a pharmaceutical product produced through biotechnology. What

conclusions can be drawn as to the safety of the food product, or of the pharmaceutical product?

10. DNA probes may reveal genetic diseases. Is this feasible with all genetic diseases?

## ■ Answers

1. There are various possible explanations. At each stage of the gene expression something may go wrong or occur with low efficiency. For example:
   a. The authentic promoter of the foreign gene does not (optimally) function in the specific host.
   b. The foreign gene contains introns. Since the bacterial host is not able to cope with introns, a functional gene product is not feasible.
   c. The construct may yield an mRNA without appropriate translational signals, e.g., a ribosome binding signal. Fusion of the gene toward a leading fragment of a functional bacterial gene might at least overcome the translational start problem. In that case a fused gene product may be produced in substantial amounts.
   d. The mRNA molecule may appear very unstable. In that case the gene expression is doomed to be low.
   e. The foreign gene product is produced in the bacterial host, but appears very unstable as it is degraded by one or more of the bacterial proteases. Therefore, bacterial strains are frequently used as production hosts with minimal proteolytic activity.

2. The crucial demands are that the plasmid is able to replicate (preferably as a multicopy plasmid) in the specific host and that it is maintained in a stable fashion in the host. Advantages for the optimal application are the presence on the plasmid of selective markers (mostly antibiotic resistance determinants) and a range of restriction sites. A relativly small size of the plasmid will allow rather simple experimental procedures.

3. The product should be produced in a safe and economic way. Since the product is not depending on post translational modifications, prokaryotic hosts like *E. coli* K-12 or *B. subtilis* are attractive (from the point of safety and economics) based on long lasting biotechnological

experience. The fact that *E. coli* is a Gram-negative host causes extra efforts when it comes to purification of the product. A safe biopharmaceutical should be completely free of LPS. Taking this into consideration *B. subtilis* is preferable. The eukaryotic micro-organisms *S. cereviseae* and *A. nidulans* could be options in companies with a lot of experience with these organisms (and most likely with specific patents around the application of such organisms). Plant and animal cells are, a priori, not specifically required and are not appropriate, since plant and animal cell cultures are production-wise very demanding.

4. In this case the prokaryotic organisms cannot be used, since they have only a very limited post-translational modification activity. Animal cells could fulfill the post-translational modifications as can the human cells responsible for the protein production. They are therefore, despite high costs, most desirable. However, it is known that *Aspergillus* species are remarkably active in post-translational modification, and it is certainly worthwhile to consider these organisms since they can be cultivated in an economic way.

5. In the batch culture device the medium is gradually depleted and various (unwanted) metabolites of the growing cells appear, while in the continuous culture device there is a continuous nutrient supply and removal of cells and growth inhibiting metabolites. The practical consequence for cultivation in a batch device is that the production inevitably comes to an end and regular restarts (time and money consuming) of the culture are required. Continuous cultures on the other hand do not need restarts and have a more economic outlook. However, the control and handling of a (large scale) continuous culture are complicated.

6. Prevent an extensive lag phase. This is achieved by using an inoculum for the culture that is optimally adapted to the conditions in the batch device. In addition, one may try to postpone an early onset of the stationary phase; for example, by adding extra nutrients after a while.

7. If the gene encodes a rather small protein with a known amino acid sequence, one may chemically synthesize the gene. If the gene product is a large protein, this is not feasible. Keeping in mind that the gene might be endowed with introns, it seems most appropriate to start by isolating mRNA from appropriate sources. mRNA should then be converted into cDNA.

8. In that case the foreign gene should be controlled by a bacterial promoter that can be switched "on" and "off" at will. Cultivation of the cells under conditions where the promoter is "off," allows

cells to grow. When cells are present in high amounts and still metabolically active, the promoter is switched "on"; for example, by addition of a specific inducing agent to the medium.

9. The signal achieved by PCR reveals specifically the presence of DNA. This DNA might be present as such or set free from *Salmonella* cells, either alive or dead. The safety of a food product depends on the presence of harmful bacterial cells that are alive or, in some instances, on the presence of a toxin produced by the bacterium. A PCR technology analysis is, therefore, not conclusive to answer the question whether the food is safe or not. As to the biopharmaceutical, the safety regulations are more stringent as drug safety may be jeopardized by the presence of bacterial constituents (e.g., endo- or exo-toxins). Therefore, PCR revealing *Salmonella typhimurium* DNA in a biopharmaceutical is very alarming.

10. No. A probe can be developed and used as a detection tool only for genetic diseases with a well-known and well-defined genetic basis. So far, most genetic diseases are not known at the level of the DNA. Some diseases are known to be the result of rather complex DNA changes and their detection will, therefore, not be amenable for straightforward DNA probing.

## CHAPTER 2: Biophysical and Biochemical Analysis of Recombinant Proteins (Pages 23–48)

### ■ Questions

1. What is the net charge of G-CSF at pH 2.0, assuming that all the carboxyl groups are protonated?
2. Based on the above calculation, do you expect the protein to unfold at pH 2.0?
3. Design an experiment using blotting techniques to ascertain the presence of a ligand to a particular receptor.
4. What is the transfer of proteins to a membrane such as nitrocellulose or PDVF called?
5. What is the assay in which the antibody is adsorbed to a plastic microtitration plate and then is used to quantify the amount of a protein using a secondary antibody conjugated with HRP named?
6. In two-dimensional electrophoresis, what is the first method of separation?
7. What is the method for separating proteins in solution based on molecular size called?

### ■ Answers

1. Based on the assumption that glutamyl and aspartyl residues are uncharged at this pH, all

the charges come from protonated histidyl, lysyl, arginyl residues, and the amino terminus, i.e., 5 His + 4 Lys + 5 Arg + N-terminal = 15.

2. Whether a protein unfolds or remains folded depends on the balance between the stabilizing and destabilizing forces. At pH 2.0, extensive positive charges destabilize the protein, but whether such destabilization is sufficient or insufficient to unfold the protein depends on how stable the protein is in the native state. The charged state alone cannot predict whether a protein will unfold.

3. A solution containing the putative ligand is subjected to SDS-PAGE. After blotting the proteins in the gel to a membrane, it is probed with a solution containing the receptor. The receptor, which binds the ligand, may be labeled with agents suitable for detection or, alternatively, the complex can subsequently be probed with an antibody to the receptor and developed as for an immunoblot. Note that the reciprocal of this can be done as well, in which the receptor is subjected to SDS-PAGE and the blot is probed with the ligand.

4. This method is called blotting. If an electric current is used then the method is called electroblotting.

5. This assay is called an ELISA (enzyme-linked immunosorbent assay).

6. Either IEF or native polyacrylamide electrophoresis. The second dimension is performed in the presence of the detergent SDS.

7. Size exclusion chromatography.

## CHAPTER 3: Production and Downstream Processing of Biotech Compounds (Pages 49–65)

### ■ Questions

1. Name four types of different bioreactors.
2. Chromatography is an essential step in the purification of biotech products. Name at least five different chromatographic purification methods.
3. What are the major safety concerns in the purification of cell-expressed proteins?
4. What are the critical issues in production and purification that must be addressed in process validation?
5. Mention at least five issues to consider in the cultivation and purification of proteins.
6. *True or false*: Glycosylation is an important post-translational change of pharmaceutical proteins. Glycosylation is only possible in mammalian cells.
7. Glycosylation may affect several properties of the protein. Mention three possible changes with glycosylation.

8. Pharmacologically active biotech protein products have complex three dimensional structures. Mention two or more important factors that affect these structures.

### ■ Answers

1. Stirred-tank; airlift; microcarrier; and membrane bioreactors.
2. Adsorption chromatography; ion-exchange chromatography; affinity chromatography; HIC; gel permeation; size-exclusion chromatography.
3. Removal of viruses, bacteria, protein contaminants, and cellular DNA.
4. *Production*: Scaling up and design. *Purification*: Procedures should be reliable in potency and quality of the product and in the removal of viral, bacterial and protein contaminants.
5. Grade of purity; pyrogenicity; N- and C-terminal heterogeneity; chemical modification/conformational changes; glycosylation and proteolytic processing.
6. *False*. Glycosylation is also possible, e.g. in yeast cells.
7. Solubility; pKa, charge; stability; and biological activity.
8. Amino-acid structure; hydrogen and sulfide bridging; post-translational changes; and chemical modification of the amino acid rest groups.

## CHAPTER 4: Formulation of Biotech Products, Including Biopharmaceutical Considerations (Pages 67–94)

### ■ Questions

1. How does one sterilize biotech products for parenteral administration?
2. A pharmaceutical protein, which is poorly water soluble around its pI, has to be formulated as an injection. What conditions would one select to produce a water soluble, injectable solution?
3. Why are most of the biotech proteins to be used in the clinic formulated in freeze-dried form? Why is, as a rule, the presence of lyoprotectants required? Why is it important to know the glass transition temperature or eutectic temperature of the system?
4. Why is it not necessarily wise to work at the lowest possible chamber pressures?
5. Why are (with the exception of oral vaccines) no oral delivery systems available for protein?
6. What alternative route of administration to the parenteral route would be the first to look into if a systemic therapeutic effect is pursued and if one does not wish to exploit absorption enhancing technologies?

7. If one considers using the iontophoretic transport route for protein delivery, what are the variables to be considered?

8. What are the differences among the endocrine, paracrine, and autocrine way of cell communication? Why is information about the way cells communicate important in the drug formulation process?

9. A company decides to explore the possibility of developing a feed back system for a therapeutic protein. What information should be available for estimating the chances for success?

10. Why is the selection of the dimensions of a colloidal particulate carrier system for targeted delivery of a protein of utmost importance?

11. Design a targeted, colloidal carrier system and a protocol for its use to circumvent the three hurdles to achieve successful treatment of solid tumors (mentioned in Table 14).

12. What are the options for inducing therapeutic actions upon attachment of immunoliposomes to (tumor) target cells?

## ■ Answers

1. Through aseptic manufacturing protocols. Final filtration through 0.2 or 0.22 μm pore filters into the vials/syringes further reduces the chances of contamination of the protein solutions.

2. One has to go through the items listed in Table 1. As the aqueous solubility is probably pH dependent, information on the preferred pH ranges should be collected. If necessary, solubility enhancers (e.g., lysine, arginine and/or surfactants) and stabilizers against adsorption/aggregation should be added. "As a last resort," one might consider carriers such as liposomes.

3. Chemical and physical instability of proteins in aqueous media is usually the reason to dry the protein solution. Freeze drying is then the preferred technology, as other drying techniques do not give rapidly reconstitutable dry forms for the formulation, and/or because elevated temperatures necessary for drying jeopardize the integrity of the protein. The glass transition/eutectic temperature should not be exceeded as otherwise collapse of the cake can be observed. Collapse slows down the drying process rate and collapsed material does not rapidly dissolve upon adding water for reconstitution.

4. Because gas conduction (one of the three heat transfer routes) depends on pressure and is reduced when the pressure is reduced.

5. Because of the hostile environment in the GI tract regarding protein stability and the poor

absorption characteristics of proteins (high molecular weight/often hydrophilic).

6. The pulmonary route.

7. Physical characteristics of the protein and medium, such a molecular weight, pI, ionic strength, and pH. And, in addition, electrical current options (pulsed, permanent, wave shape) and desired dose level/pattern (pulsed/constant/variable).

8. This information is important because, particularly with paracrine and autocrine acting proteins targeted delivery should be considered to minimize unwanted side effects.

9.   i. The desired pharmacokinetic profile (e.g., information on the PK/PD relationship/circadian rhythm).

  ii. Chemical and physical stability of the protein on long-term storage at body/ambient temperature.

  iii. Availability of a bio-sensor system (stability in vivo, precision/accuracy).

  iv. Availability of a reliable pump system (see Table 10).

10. The body is highly compartmentalized and access to target sites inside and outside the blood circulation is highly dependent on the size of the carrier system involved (and other factors such as the presence of diseased tissue, and surface characteristics such as charge, hydrophobicity/hydrophilicity, ligands).

11. The selection should be based on the induction of bystander effects, "cocktails" of homing devices (e.g., MAb), selection of non-modulating receptors and non-shedding receptors. Neutralization of free, shed tumor antigens with free, non-conjugated MAb by injection of these free antibodies before the administration of ligand-carrier-drug combinations would be an approach for avoiding neutralization of the carrier-homing device combination by shed antigen.

12. Figure 35 gives an overview of these options.

## CHAPTER 5: Pharmacokinetics and Pharmacodynamics of Peptide and Protein Drugs (Pages 95–123)

## ■ Questions

1. What are the major elimination pathways for protein drugs after administration?

2. Which pathway of absorption is rather unique for proteins after SC injection?

3. What is the role of plasma binding proteins for natural proteins?

4. How do the sugar groups on glycoproteins influence hepatic elimination of these glycoproteins?

5. In which direction might elimination clearance of a protein drug change when antibodies against the protein are produced after chronic dosing with the protein drug? Why?
6. What is the major driving force for the transport of proteins from the vascular to the extravascular space?
7. Why are protein therapeutics generally not active upon oral administration?
8. Many protein therapeutics exhibit Michaelis–Menten type, saturable elimination kinetics. What are the underlying mechanisms for this pharmacokinetic behavior?
9. Explain counterclockwise hysteresis in plasma concentration–effect plots.
10. Why is mechanism-based PK/PD modeling a preferred modeling approach for protein therapeutics?

■ **Answers**

1. Proteolysis, glomerular filtration followed by intraluminal metabolism or tubular reabsorption with intracellular lysosomal degradation, renal peritubular absorption followed by catabolism, and receptor-mediated endocytosis followed by metabolism in the liver and possibly other cells.
2. Biodistribution from the injection site into the lymphatic system.
3. Plasma proteins may act as circulating reservoirs for the proteins that are their ligands. Consequently, the protein ligands may be protected from elimination and distribution. In some cases, protein binding may protect the organism from undesirable, acute effects; in other cases, receptor binding may be facilitated by the binding protein.
4. In some cases, the sugar groups are recognized by hepatic receptors (galactose by the galactose receptor, for example), facilitating receptor-mediated uptake and metabolism. In other cases, sugar chains and terminal sugar groups (terminal sialic acid residues, for example) may shield the protein from binding to receptors and hepatic uptake.
5. Clearance may increase or decrease by forming antibody–protein complexes. A decrease of clearance occurs when the antibody–protein complex is eliminated slower than free protein. An increase of clearance occurs when the protein–antibody complex is eliminated more rapidly than the unbound protein, such as when reticuloendothelial uptake is stimulated by the complex.
6. Protein extravasation, i.e., transport from the blood or vascular space to the interstitial tissue

space, is predominantly mediated by fluid convection. Protein molecules follow the fluid flux from the vascular space through pores between adjacent cells into the interstitial space. Drainage of the interstitial space through the lymphatic system allows protein therapeutics to distribute back into the vascular space.
7. The gastrointestinal mucosa is a major absorption barrier for hydrophilic macromolecule such as proteins. In addition, peptide and protein therapeutics are degraded by the extensive peptidase and protease activity in the gastrointestinal tract. Both processes minimize the oral bioavailability of protein therapeutics.
8. Receptor-mediated endocytosis is the most frequent cause of nonlinear pharmacokinetics in protein therapeutics. Its occurrence becomes even more prominent if the protein therapeutic undergoes target-mediated drug disposition, i.e., if the receptor-mediated endocytosis is mediated via the pharmacologic target of the protein therapeutic. As the binding to the target is usually of high affinity, and the protein therapeutic is often dosed to saturate the majority of the available target receptors for maximum pharmacologic efficacy, saturation of the associated receptor-mediated endocytosis as elimination pathway is frequently encountered.
9. Counterclockwise hysteresis is an indication of the indirect nature of the effects seen for many protein drugs. It can be explained by delays between the appearance of drug in plasma and the appearance of the pharmacodynamic response. The underlying cause may either be a distributional delay between the drug concentrations in plasma and at the effect site (modeled with an indirect link PK/PD model), or by time consuming post-receptor events that cause a delay between the drug–receptor interaction and the observed drug effect, for example, the effect on a physiologic measure or endogenous substance.
10. Protein therapeutics are often classified as "targeted therapies" where the drug compound acts on one specific, well-defined response pathway. This well-documented knowledge on the mechanism of action can be translated relatively easily into a mechanism-based PK/PD modeling approach that incorporates the major physiological processes relevant for the pharmacologic effect. The advantage of mechanism based as compared to empirical PK/PD modeling is that mechanism-based models are usually more robust and allow more reliable simulations beyond the actually measured data.

## CHAPTER 6: Immunogenicity of Therapeutic Proteins (Pages 125–132)

### ■ Questions

1. Which factors contribute to unwanted immunogenicity of therapeutic proteins?
2. What are possible clinical consequences of antibody formation against biopharmaceuticals in patients?
3. Why do aggregates of recombinant human proteins induce antibodies that cross-react with the (non-aggregated) drug?
4. Explain the fundamental difference between (a) antibody formation in children with growth hormone deficiency treated against recombinant human growth hormone, and (b) antibody formation against rh erythropoietin in patients with chronic renal failure.
5. Give an example of a case that demonstrates that the formulation of a biopharmaceutical can affect the immune response.
6. Give at least three approaches that can be followed to reduce the immunogenicity of a biopharmaceutical.
7. Why is standardization of assays for detection of anti-drug antibodies important?
8. Why are antidrug–antibody titers against a monoclonal antibody more difficult to determine accurately than antibodies against interferon?

### ■ Answers

1. See Figure 2.
2. Reduction of therapeutic efficacy, enhancement of efficacy (seldom), anaphylactic reactions, cross-reactivity with endogenous protein.
3. Aggregates can break B-cell tolerance against native (-like) epitopes (repetitive epitopes); the more "native-like" the aggregate, the more likely cross-reactivity with the monomer will occur.
4. (a) is the classical immune response versus (b), the breaking of B-cell tolerance.
5. See examples given in the text for erythropoietin and interferon α.
6. Design another formulation, remove aggregates, pegylate or change the glycosylation pattern of the protein or use amino acid mutants, use human (ized) versions of the proteins or select another route of administration. *NB*: Some of these approaches will lead to a new bioactive drug molecule and that has implications for the way authorities will judge the procedure to be followed for obtaining marketing approval (see Chapter 24).
7. Different assay formats and blood sampling schedules give largely different answers and thus hamper direct comparison between studies. It is therefore difficult to compare the results obtained with different products that are tested for immunogenicity in different labs.
8. Monoclonal antibodies are often administered in high doses and have a long circulation time (days to weeks). This will likely cause interference with the assay by the circulating drug (resulting in false negatives or underestimation of antibody titers). Another possibility for interference is the occurrence of cross reactivity of the reagents in the test for the induced antibodies and the original drug-antibody. With interferon a different situation is encountered: Interferons are rapidly cleared and administered in low doses (microgram range); therefore, interferons will less likely interfere with the measurement of anti-interferon antibodies.

## CHAPTER 7: Genomics, Other "Omics" Technologies, Personalized Medicine, and Additional Biotechnology-Related Techniques (Pages 133–174)

### ■ Questions

1. What were the increasing levels of genetic resolution of the human genome planned for study as part of the HGP?
2. What is functional genomics?
3. What is proteomics?
4. What are SNPs?
5. What is the difference between pharmacogenetics and pharmacogenomics?
6. Define metabonomics.
7. What is a DNA microarray?
8. What phase(s) of drug action are affected by genetic variation?
9. Define personalized medicine.
10. What is a biomarker?
11. Define systems biology.
12. Why are engineered animal models valuable to pharmaceutical research?
13. What two techniques are commonly used to produce transgenic animals?
14. What is a knockout mouse?
15. What is site-directed mutagenesis?
16. What structural techniques can provide information about the 3-D structure of a protein?
17. Define the term peptidomimetic.
18. What is tissue engineering?
19. What are stem cells?
20. What are two approaches to high-throughput synthesis of drug leads and how do they differ?

# ■ Answers

1. HGP structural genomics was envisioned to proceed through increasing levels of genetic resolution: detailed human genetic linkage maps [approximately 2 megabase pairs (Mb = million base pairs) resolution], complete physical maps (0.1 Mb resolution), and ultimately complete DNA sequencing of the approximately 3.5 billion base pairs (23 pairs of chromosomes) in a human cell nucleus (1 base pair resolution).

2. Functional genomics is a new approach to genetic analysis that focuses on genome-wide patterns of gene expression, the mechanisms by which gene expression is coordinated, and the interrelationships of gene expression when a cellular environmental change occurs.

3. A new research area called proteomics seeks to define the function and correlate that with expression profiles of all proteins encoded within a genome.

4. While comparing the base sequences in the DNA of two individuals reveals them to be approximately 99.9 per cent identical, base differences, or polymorphisms, are scattered throughout the genome. The best-characterized human polymorphisms are SNPs occurring approximately once every 1000 bases in the 3.5 billion base pair human genome.

5. Pharmacogenetics is the study of how an individual's genetic differences influence drug action, usage, and dosing. A detailed knowledge of a patient's pharmacogenetics in relation to a particular drug therapy may lead to enhanced efficacy and greater safety. While sometimes used interchangeably (especially in pharmacy practice literature), pharmacogenetics and pharmacogenomics are subtly different. Pharmacogenomics introduces the additional element of our present technical ability to pinpoint patient-specific DNA variation using genomics techniques. While overlapping fields of study, pharmacogenomics is a much newer term that correlates an individual patient's DNA variation (SNP level of variation knowledge rather than gene level of variation knowledge) with his or her response to pharmacotherapy.

6. The field of metabonomics is the holistic study of the metabolic continuum at the equivalent level to the study of genomics and proteomics.

7. The biochips known as DNA microarrays and oligonucleotide microarrays are a surface collection of hundreds to thousands of immobilized DNA sequences or oligo-nucleotides in a grid created with specialized equipment that can be simultaneously examined to conduct expression analysis.

8. Genomic variation affects not only the pharmacokinetic profile of drugs (via drug metabolizing enzymes and drug transporter proteins), it also strongly influences the pharmacodynamic profile of drugs via the drug target.

9. Pharmacotherapy informed by a patient's individual genomics and proteomics information. Sometimes referred to as giving the right drug to the right patient in the right dose at the right time.

10. Biomarkers are clinically relevant substances used as indicators of a biologic state. Detection or concentration change of a biomarker may indicate a particular disease state physiology, or toxicity. A change in expression or state of a protein biomarker may correlate with the risk or progression of a disease, with the susceptibility of the disease to a given treatment, or the drug's safety profile.

11. Systems biology is the study of the interactions between the components of a biological system, and how these interactions give rise to the function and behavior of that system.

12. Engineered animal models are proving invaluable since small animal models of disease are often poor mimics of that disease in human patients. Genetic engineering can predispose an animal to a particular disease under scrutiny and the insertion of human genes into the animal can initiate the development of a more clinically-relevant disease condition.

13. (a) DNA microinjection and random gene addition; (b) homologous recombination in embryonic stem cells.

14. A knockout mouse, also called a gene knockout mouse or a gene-targeted knockout mouse, is an animal in which an endogenous gene (genomic wild-type allele) has been specifically inactivated by replacing it with a null allele.

15. Site-directed mutagenesis (also called site-specific mutagenesis) is a protein engineering technique allowing specifically (site-direct) alteration (mutation) of the primary amino acid sequence of proteins to create new chemical entities.

16. Protein X-ray crystallography and NMR spectroscopy.

17. Peptidomimetic (sometimes called peptide mimetics and nonpeptide mimetics) are defined as structures that serve as appropriate substitutes for peptides in interactions with receptors and enzymes. The mimetic must possess not only affinity, but also efficacy or substitute function.

18. Tissue engineering is the multidisciplinary field of varied strategies to regenerate natural or grow new human tissues and organs. Sometimes referred to as the more general term

"regenerative medicine," tissue engineering has integrated biotechnology, clinical medicine, cell biology, developmental biology, and biomaterials engineering into an effort to overcome the challenges associated with conventional surgical approaches to tissue and organ repair or replacement.

19. Stem cells are cells that possess the ability to divide into daughter cells and multiply for infinite periods in culture giving rise to daughter cells with identical developmental potential and/or a cell with less potential.

20. There are two overall approaches to high-throughput synthesis. True combinatorial chemistry applies methods to substantially reduce the number of synthetic operations or steps needed to synthesize large numbers of compounds. Combichem, as it is sometimes referred to, is conducted on solid supports (resins) to facilitate the needed manipulations that reduce labor. Differing from combinatorial chemistry, parallel procedures apply automation to the synthetic process, but the number of operations needed to carry out a synthesis is practically the same as the conventional approach. Thus, the potential productivity of parallel methods is not as high as combinatorial chemistries. Parallel chemistries can be conducted on solid-phase supports or in solution.

## CHAPTER 8: Gene Therapy (Pages 175–210)

### ■ Questions

1. What was the disease target for the first gene therapy clinical trial? What vector was selected for gene transfer?

2. Retroviral vectors are predominantly given by ex vivo methods in the clinic. What are the advantages associated with this method of delivery?

3. Several clinical trials involve gene transfer for the treatment of malignant glioma. One approach involves use of a recombinant retrovirus expressing the HSV-tk transgene. Another involves use of a recombinant adenovirus expressing the p53 transgene.
   a. Which of the four current strategies to treat cancer by gene therapy does each of these trials employ? Describe the principle behind each strategy.
   b. List two advantages and two disadvantages associated with the vector used in each of these trials.
   c. Outline potential drawbacks to the use of each of these strategies for cancer therapy.
   d. What other approaches could have been selected to prevent the growth and spread of

malignant tissue? Explain the principle behind each.

4. a. What is the purpose of the packaging cell line during the production of recombinant viral vectors for gene transfer?
   b. What is the risk associated with using packaging cell lines for vector production?

5. Provide at least two examples of how gene therapy is used to modulate the immune system to fight infection.

6. Briefly outline the primary approach to correct monogenetic diseases such as muscular dystrophy and cystic fibrosis. How might this be achieved in the future?

7. To date significant adverse effects have been reported in two gene therapy clinical trials.
   a. What was the focus of each of these trials?
   b. What adverse effects occurred?

8. It has been shown that non-viral vectors are, to some degree, also subject to recognition by the immune system.
   a. What is responsible for this effect?
   b. What has been done to avoid this in the context of vector design?

### ■ Answers

1. The first gene therapy clinical trial was initiated in 1990 for the treatment of adenosine deaminase (ADA) deficiency. In this trial, patients with ADA deficiency were given peripheral blood lymphocytes treated with a retroviral vector expressing the ADA transgene.

2. Advantages of ex vivo delivery are:
   a. Limited amounts of vector are needed for gene transfer.
   b. Selection methods allow for 100% transduction efficiency in the cell population given to the patient.
   c. Toxicity associated with gene transfer is significantly reduced due to removal of the vector prior to administration of cells.
   d. Recent use of regulated gene expression cassettes also allow for destruction and removal of cells in the event an adverse event does occur such as uncontrolled proliferation due to activation of oncogenic genes or graft-versus-host disease after adoptive transfer of T-cells.

3. a. *Retrovirus trial*: Gene directed enzyme prodrug therapy. Cells transduced by the virus express an enzyme capable of converting a drug (in this case ganciclovir) to a cytotoxic metabolite. This conversion cannot occur in cells that do not express the transgene, limiting the cytotoxic effect to transduced

cells and their neighbors through the by-stander effect.

*Adenovirus trial:* Correction of genetic mutations that contribute to a malignant phenotype. Cells transduced by the virus express a gene that is necessary for controlled cell division and development. This prevents the uncontrolled growth and division associated with malignant disease.

b. *Retrovirus:*

  i. Advantages:
- Retroviruses can infect dividing cells which are the therapeutic target in this trial. (Despite this fact, transduction efficiency of this vector in vivo has been low).
- Retroviruses are capable of inducing long-term gene expression which should be sufficient for effective removal of malignant tissue.

  ii. Disadvantages:
- Retroviruses have the potential for inducing insertional mutagenesis in normal, healthy cells.
- Transgene expression is sometimes limited by the host immune response to cellular components acquired by the virus during large scale production.

*Adenovirus:*

  i. Advantages:
- Adenoviruses can infect dividing cells which are the therapeutic target in this trial.
- Adenoviruses can induce high levels of transgene expression in short periods of time.
- Adenoviruses do not have the risk of insertional mutagenesis.
- It is relatively easy to produce large amounts of recombinant adenovirus sufficient for clinical use.

  ii. Disadvantages:
- Transgene expression is transient, making readministration necessary for continued effect.
- Adenoviral vectors are capable of inducing a potent immune response. This not only limits the success of gene transfer after a second dose of virus, but is also associated with severe toxicity at certain doses.
- Pre-existing immunity to adenovirus serotype 5 is common in the general population. This may also limit gene transfer.

c. *Drawbacks:*

  i. To gene directed enzyme pro-drug therapy:
- Efficacy relies on efficient transgene expression and drug bioavailablility.
- The therapeutic effect may spread to healthy cells through the bystander effect.

  ii. To gene replacement therapy:
- Gene replacement may stop tumor growth but not eliminate it.
- Expression is not limited to malignant tissue.

d. *Other approaches for cancer gene therapy:*

  i. *Immunotherapy:* A vector expressing pro-inflammatory cytokines, co-stimulatory molecules or tumor-specific antigens is injected directly into the tumor mass. This facilitates the formation of an anti-tumor immune response that targets and destroys malignant cells.

  ii. *Virotherapy:* A RCV that naturally targets cancers is directly injected in the tumor mass. The virus can induce cell death during replication in malignant tissue by producing cytotoxic proteins and subsequent cell lysis.

4. a. The primary purpose of the packaging cell line is to provide genetic elements that support virus replication and assembly. These have been eliminated from the vector to prevent it from causing disease in the patient.

  b. The recombinant virus can incorporate elements for replication into its genome through homologous recombination during the production process. The potential for generation of RCV in this manner does exist for each vector but can vary due to specific features of a given packaging cell line.

5. Examples of gene therapy for infectious disease:

  a. Ex vivo delivery of antigenic components of pathogens of interest (or vectors expressing these antigens) to stimulate and promote an immune reaction in peripheral blood mononuclear cells isolated from a patient.

  b. Overexpression of proteins that interfere with virus infection.

  c. Use of antisense and decoy molecules that block pathogen replication by binding to the pathogen genome.

  d. Overexpression of known antigenic epitopes of the pathogen to stimulate an immune response.

6. The primary approach to correct monogenetic disorders is to replace the missing gene with its functional counterpart to restore function and

reverse disease processes. This has not been accomplished to date due to the limited amount of genetic material that can be accommodated by the viral vectors available for gene transfer and inefficient gene expression in target tissues. In some cases, an immune response against the transgene, which is seen as foreign in a system where it never was present, also limits long-term correction.

The success of long-term gene expression lies in the continued:

a. Development of safe and efficient site-specific recombinase systems.
b. Inclusion of scaffold/matrix attachment regions from human gene clusters to promote episomal segregation of genetic sequences during cell division in constructs for gene transfer.
c. Use of artificial human chromosomes.

Many of these approaches are still in the early testing phase and are limited by inefficient delivery methods.

7.  a. One trial employed a recombinant adenovirus for the treatment of ornithine transcarbamylase (OTC) deficiency. The other trial employed a recombinant retrovirus for the treatment of SCID-X1.
    b. *OTC trial*: Severe immune response to the recombinant viral vector.
       *SCID-XI trial*: Uncontrolled lymphoproliferative syndrome due to retroviral integration near the LMO2 promoter at a time when the patients contracted chicken pox.

8.  a. Non-viral vectors can stimulate an immune response through:
       i. *Interaction/aggregation with serum components*: These large conglomerates localize in components of the RES that in turn activate the immune system.
       ii. *Immunostimulatory unmethylated CpG motifs in plasmid DNA*: Unmethylated DNA is a common feature of microbial genomic sequences and thus is recognized by the immune system as foreign.
       iii. *Route of administration*: The strongest immune reactions to non-viral vectors have been noted when they are given by the intravenous and intrapulmonary routes.
    b. *Efforts to minimize the immune response to non-viral vectors include*:
       i. Reducing interaction of vectors with serum components through covalent attachment of non-toxic polymers like poly(ethylene) glycol.
       ii. Elimination of CpG motifs through
          ▪ the use of special bacterial strains capable of methylated plasmid DNA

          ▪ site-directed mutagenesis
          ▪ design and use of CpG-free plasmids
          ▪ creation of "minimal" plasmids free of unnecessary prokaryotic sequences
    iii. Incorporation molecules that suppress the immune response in the vector.
    iv. Administration of vector components in a sequential manner instead of concurrently. For example, injecting cationic lipids alone prior to an injection of the plasmid DNA.

## CHAPTER 9: Oligonucleotides (Pages 211–224)

### ■ Questions

1. Which antisense-oligonucleotide modifications are able to recruit RNase H, and which are not?
2. Explain the principle of RNAi.
3. What are the major obstacles in therapeutic applications of oligonucleotides?
4. What is the difference between gene correction and gene silencing?
5. Are there any structural and functional differences between DNAzymes and aptamers? If so, name them.
6. What are the differences in requirements for antisense oligonucleotides that are made for exon skipping versus those that are made to inhibit translation of a mutated gene?

### ■ Answers

1. Only charged antisense oligodeoxyribonucleotide phosphodiesters and phosphorothioates elicit efficient RNase H activity. Non-charged oligonucleotides, including for example the peptide nucleic acids, morpholino-oligos, and 2′-O-alkyloligoribonucleotides do not recruit RNAse H activity and act by physical mRNA blockade.
2. RNAi is a mechanism for RNA-guided regulation of gene expression in which dsRNA inhibits the expression of genes with complementary nucleotide sequences. The RNAi pathway is initiated by the enzyme Dicer, which cleaves dsRNA to short double-stranded fragments of 20 to 25 base-pairs. One of the two strands of each fragment, known as the guide strand, is then incorporated into the RISC and base-pairs with complementary sequences. The most well-studied outcome of this recognition event is a form of post-transcriptional gene silencing, however the process also affects methylation of promoters, increases degradation of mRNA (not mediated by RISC), blocks protein translation, and enhances protein degradation.

3. Poor pharmacokinetics, instability, and inability to cross membranes.

4. Gene correction makes use of a homologous recombination process to permanently correct single or multiple point mutations within a region of the gene of interest and therefore acts at the level of DNA. Gene silencing aims at reducing the level of active transcripts of the gene of interest by targeted degradation of the mRNA.

5. Both oligonucleotides form complex three-dimensional structures that can bind their target molecule. However, DNAzymes possess a domain that catalyzes target molecule conversion, whereas aptamers act by physical blockade.

6. Exons can be skipped from the mRNA with antisense oligoribonucleotides. They attach inside the exon to be removed, or at its borders. The oligonucleotides interfere with the splicing machinery so that the targeted exons are no longer included in the mRNA. Classical antisense oligonucleotides are single-stranded DNA or RNA molecules that generally consist of 13 to 25 nucleotides. They are complementary to a sense mRNA sequence and can hybridize to it through Watson–Crick base-pairing. Translation inhibition can be achieved through physical mRNA blockade, or mRNA cleavage by recruitment of RNase H.

## CHAPTER 10: Hematopoietic Growth Factors (Pages 225–242)

### ■ Questions

1. What are the roles of hematopoietic factors?
2. What are the major lineages or types of mature blood cells?
3. Generally, chemically describe the HGFs.
4. How do HGFs function?
5. Define the difference between multilineage growth factors and lineage-specific growth factors.
6. What are the in vivo actions of rhG-CSF and rhGM-CSF in patients with advanced cancer?
7. What is the physiologic role of EPO?
8. What are the currently commercially available HGFs?
9. What are the indications for rhG-CSF?
10. What are the indications for rhGM-CSF?
11. What are the indications for rhEPO?
12. What are the indications for rhSCF?
13. What are the indications for rhIL-11?

### ■ Answers

1. Hematopoietic growth factors regulate both hematopoiesis and the functional activity of blood cells (including proliferation, differentiation, and maturation). Some HGFs mobilize progenitor cells to move from the bone marrow to the peripheral blood.

2. The myeloid pathway gives rise to red blood cells (erythrocytes), platelets, monocytes/macrophages, and granulocytes (neutrophils, eosinophils, and basophils). The lymphoid pathway gives rise to lymphocytes.

3. They are glycoproteins, which can be distinguished by their amino acid sequence and glycosylation (carbohydrate linkages). Hematopoietic growth factors have folding patterns that are dictated by physical interactions and covalent cysteine-cysteine disulfide bridges. Correct folding is necessary for biologic activity. Most HGFs are single-chain polypeptides weighing approximately 14 to 35 kDa. The carbohydrate content varies depending on the growth factor and production method, which in turn affects the molecular weight but not necessarily the biologic activity.

4. Hematopoietic growth factors act by binding to specific cell surface receptors. The resultant complex sends a signal to the cell to express genes, which in turn induce cellular proliferation, differentiation, or activation. An HGF may also act indirectly if the cell expresses a gene that causes the production of a different HGF or another cytokine, which in turn binds to and stimulates a different cell.

5. Multilineage growth factors (e.g., GM-CSF, IL-3, and SCF) affect multiple cell lineages and tend to act on early progenitor cells before they become committed to one lineage. Lineage-specific growth factors (e.g., G-CSF, M-CSF, EPO, and presumably thrombopoietin) predominantly affect one cell type and act later in the hematopoietic cascade.

6. Both growth factors cause a transient leucopenia that is followed by a dose-dependent increase in the number of circulating mature and immature neutrophils. Both growth factors enhance the in vitro function of neutrophils obtained from treated patients. rhGM-CSF, but not rhG-CSF, also increases the number of circulating monocytes/macrophages and eosinophils, as well as in vitro monocyte cytotoxicity and cytokine production.

7. EPO maintains a normal red blood cell count by causing committed erythroid progenitor cells to proliferate and differentiate into normoblasts. EPO also shifts marrow reticulocytes into circulation.

8. Five HGFs are commercially available: rhG-CSF (filgrastim, lenograstim, pegfilgrastim), rhGM-CSF (molgramostim, sargramostim), rhEPO

(epoetin alfa, epoetin beta, darbepoetin alfa), rhSCF (ancestim), and rhIL-11 (oprelvekin).

9. Approval for marketing varies by country and not all countries have all labeled uses. rhG-CSF is indicated for neutropenia associated with myelosuppressive cancer chemotherapy, bone marrow transplantation, and severe chronic neutropenia; rhG-CSF is also indicated to mobilize PBPC for PBPC transplantation; rhG-CSF is indicated for the reversal of clinically significant neutropenia and subsequent maintenance or adequate neutrophil counts in patients with HIV infection during treatment with antiviral and/or other myelosuppressive medications.

10. rhGM-CSF is indicated for neutropenia associated with bone marrow transplantation and antiviral therapy for AIDS-related cytomegalovirus. rhGM-CSF is also indicated for failed bone marrow transplantation or delayed engraftment, and for use in mobilization and after transplantation of autologous PBPCs.

11. rhEPO is indicated to treat anemia associated with chronic renal failure, zidovudine-induced anemia in HIV-infected patients, and chemotherapy-induced anemia. rhEPO is also indicated to reduce allogeneic blood transfusions and hasten erythroid recovery in surgery patients.

12. rhSCF is used in combination with filgrastim to increase PBPC yield in hard-to-mobilize patients.

13. rhIL-11 is indicated to prevent thrombocytopenia and to reduce the need for platelet transfusions in patients with cancer receiving chemotherapy.

## CHAPTER 11: Interferons and Interleukins (Pages 243–264)

### ■ Questions

Decide whether each of the statements below is *true* or *false*. If you believe a statement is false explain why.

1. Interferons (IFNs) are defined:
   a. by the cell type which produces them
   b. by their anti-inflammatory properties
   c. by their antiviral activity
   d. by their protein structure
   e. by their genetic structure

2. Human IFN alpha:
   a. is produced selectively by leukocytes
   b. is a virucidal substance
   c. triggers antiviral effects in cells expressing appropriate receptors
   d. acts on the immune system to booster specific antiviral response
   e. comprises twelve subtypes

3. Interleukins (ILs) are characterized by:
   a. their action on target cells
   b. their protein structure
   c. their genetic structure
   d. pro- or anti-inflammatory effect
   e. their cell of origin

4. The following ILs are generally considered to be "proinflammatory," i.e. induce and/or be part of a Th1 response:
   a. the IL-1 family, IL-2, -8, -12
   b. IL-3
   c. IL-4, -5, -9
   d. IL-10, -19, -20, -22, -24, -26, -28A, -28B and -29
   e. IL-15, -16, -17, -18, -22, -23, and -32

5. ILs are:
   a. secreted specifically by leukocytes to act on other leukocytes
   b. bound to a specific receptor complex to exert their effect
   c. a family of proteins which regulate the immune response
   d. nontoxic products of the body in response to pathogens and other potentially harmful agents
   e. long-acting immune modulators

6. IFNs and ILs can be toxic. Several (patho-) physiological containment mechanisms exist to counteract excessive production:
   a. soluble receptors (sR)
   b. binding to cell surface receptors
   c. neutralizing antibodies
   d. negative feedback mechanisms
   e. naturally occurring IL receptor antagonists

7. The following IFNs are used as approved therapy:
   a. IFNα2
   b. IFNβ
   c. IFNγ
   d. IFNω
   e. IFNα8
   Where appropriate, specify some of the indications for use.

8. The following ILs are approved for therapeutic use:
   a. IL-1
   b. IL-2
   c. IL-10
   d. IL-11
   e. IL-12
   Where appropriate, specify some of the indications for use.

9. a. Protein PEGylation:
   b. prolongs circulation half-life of the PEGylated protein
   c. decreases antigenicity of the PEGylated protein
   d. protects the protein from proteolysis

e. is difficult due to the toxicity of polyethylene glycol (PEG)
   improves the therapeutic efficacy of the PEGylated protein

10. The following PEGylated IFNs and ILs have been approved for therapeutic use:
    a. IFN α2
    b. IFN β
    c. IL-1
    d. IL-2
    e. IL-12

## ■ Answers

1. Interferons definitions:
   a. *False.* Although IFNα used to be called "leukocyte IFN" and IFNβ "fibroblast IFN" because they were initially produced from buffy coats (leukocytes) infected with Sendai virus and human diploid fibroblasts stimulated with poly(I)-poly(C) or Newcastle disease virus (NDV), respectively, IFNs and their units (IU) are *defined* by their antiviral activity.
   b. *False.* While they can act as immune-modulators and on occasion have anti-inflammatory properties (e.g. IFNβ for the treatment of multiple sclerosis), they will more often induce a Th1 or proinflammatory response. IFNγ is one of the classical proinflammatory markers.
   c. *True.*
   d, e. *False.* The full protein and genetic sequences of the different IFNs and their subtypes were only defined long after the initial crude IFN mixtures had been tested in the clinic initially against viral diseases and subsequently against cancers.
      Today, however, the protein and genetic sequences are necessary to specify an IFN and its purity during production by biotechnologies. Also, new IFNs or ILs will be accepted as such by the Human Genome Nomenclature Committee (HGNC) based on their function and a previously unknown genetic sequence.

2. Human IFN alpha:
   a. *False.* IFN alpha is produced by many cell types, including T-cells and B-cells, macrophages, fibroblasts, endothelial cells, and osteoblasts among others.
   b. *False.* By interacting with their specific heterodimeric receptors on the surface of cells, the IFNs initiate a broad and varied array of signals that induce antiviral state.
   c. *True.*
   d. *True.*
   e. *True.* See Table 1. Each IFNα subtype has a distinct antiviral, antiproliferative, and stimulation of cytotoxic activities of NK and T-cells. To date only one recombinant subtype, IFNα2, has been predominantly used therapeutically.

3. ILs characterization:
   a. and e) *False.* ILs are characterized by their protein and gene structures registered in the HCGN database (and similar centralized databases). Their names and symbols must be approved by the HGNC.
   b. *True.*
   c. *True.*
   d. *False.* While some ILs can be classified as pro- or anti-inflammatory, this is not what basically defines them.

4. "Anti-inflammatory" ILs:
   a. *True.*
   b. *False.* IL-3 is a multicolony stimulating, hematopoietic growth factor (GF) which stimulates the generation of hematopoietic progenitors of every lineage.
   c. *False.* These three ILs all play a role in the differentiation and activation of basophils and eosinophils leading to a Th2 response.
   d. *False.* These ILs are all part of the IL-10 family. However IL-10,-19, and -20 are "anti-inflammatory", IL-22, -24, -26, -28A, -28B and -29 are considered "proinflammatory."
   e. *True.*

5. ILs are:
   a. *False.* ILs are mainly secreted by leukocytes and primarily affecting growth and differentiation of hematopoietic and immune cells. They are also produced by other normal and malignant cells and are of central importance in the regulation of hematopoiesis, immunity, inflammation, tissue remodeling, and embryonic development.
   b. *True.*
   c. *True.*
   d. *False.* Many ILs, primarily those with proinflammatory function, are intrinsically toxic either directly or indirectly, i.e., through induction of toxic gene products.
   e. *False.* ILs usually have a short circulation time, and their production is regulated by positive and negative feedback loops.

6. IFNs and ILs containment mechanisms to counteract excessive production:
   a. *True.*
   b. *False.* Binding to cell surface receptor is a physiological process and has negligible effect on "circulating" IFNs or ILs.
   c–e. *True.*

7. The following IFNs are used as approved therapy.
   a. *True*. IFNα (Roferon® A, IntronA®, Infergen®) is indicated for the treatment of chronic hepatitis B and C, Kaposi's sarcoma, renal cell carcinoma, malignant melanoma, carcinoid tumor, multiple myeloma, non-Hodgkin lymphoma (NHL), hairy cell leukemia, chronic myelogenous leukemia, thrombocytosis associated with chronic myelogenous leukemia, and other myeloproliferative disorders.
   b. *True*. IFNβ (Betaseron®, Betaferon®, Avonex®, Rebif®) is indicated for the treatment of multiple sclerosis.
   c. *True*. IFNγ (Actimmune®) is indicated for the treatment of chronic granulomatous disease, severe, malignant osteopetrosis.
   d. *False*. IFNω has only been studied in vitro and in the nude mouse model where it has shown anticancer activity against several tumor cell lines and transplants.
   e. *False*. IFNα8 has only been studied in various cell lines where it has however consistently shown the most powerful antiviral effect of the subtypes tested.
8. The following ILs are approved for therapeutic use:
   a. *True*. An IL-1 analog/antagonist (Kineret®) is indicated for the treatment of rheumatoid arthritis.
   b. *True*. IL-2 (Proleukin®) is indicated for the treatment of adults with metastatic renal cell carcinoma or metastatic melanoma.
   c. *False*. Clinical development of IL-10 (Tenovil™) as an anti-inflammatory drug for several indications such as psoriasis, Crohn's disease (CD), and rheumatoid arthritis was discontinued in phase III due to insufficient efficacy to warrant further development.
   d. *True*. IL-11 (Neumega®) is indicated for the prevention of severe thrombocytopenia following myelosuppressive chemotherapy.
   e. *False*. Early clinical trials have been performed in patients with chronic hepatitis C. The program was, however, discontinued in early phase II due to toxicity.
9. Protein PEGylation:
   a. *True*.
   b. *True*.
   c. *True*.
   d. *False*. PEG is inert, nontoxic, nonimmunogenic and in its most common form either linear or branched terminated with hydroxyl groups that can be activated to couple to the desired target protein.
   e. *True*.

10. The following PEGylated IFNs and ILs have been approved for therapeutic use:
    a. *True*: For chronic hepatitis C and B. Limited clinical trials have also been conducted in renal cell carcinoma, malignant melanoma, and NHL.
    b. c, d, and e) *False*. Although early clinical trials have been conducted with PEGylated IL-2 in RCC and malignant melanoma and pharmacokinetic studies with PEGylated IFNβ in animal models.

## CHAPTER 12: Insulin (Pages 265–280)

### ■ Questions

1. Which insulin analog formulations cannot be mixed and stored? Why?
2. What are the primary chemical and physical stability issues with human insulin formulations?

### ■ Answers

1. Lantus®, a long-acting insulin formulation which is formulated at pH 4.0, should not be mixed with rapid- or fast-acting insulin, which are formulated under neutral pH. If Lantus is mixed with other insulin formulations, the solution may become cloudy due to pI precipitation of both the insulin glargine and the fast- or rapid-acting insulin resulting from pH changes. Consequently, the pharmacokinetic/pharmacodynamic profile (e.g., onset of action, time to peak effect) of Lantus and/or the mixed insulin may be altered in an unpredictable manner.
2. The two primary modes of chemical degradation are $Asn^{B3}$ deamidation and HMWP formation. These routes of chemical degradation occur in all formulations; however, they are generally slower in suspension formulations. Physical instability is most often observed in insulin suspension formulations and pump formulations. In suspension formulations, particle agglomeration can occur resulting in the visible clumping of the crystalline and/or amorphous insulin. The soluble insulin in pump formulations can also precipitate.

## CHAPTER 13: Growth Hormones (Pages 281–291)

### ■ Questions

1. One molecule of hGH is required to sequentially bind to two receptor molecules for receptor activation. What consequences might the requirement for sequential dimerization have on observed dose-response relationships?

2. Growth hormone is known or presumed to act directly upon which tissues?

3. You are investigating the use of hGH as an adjunct therapy for malnutrition/wasting in a clinical population which also has severe liver disease. What effects would you expect the liver disease to have on the observed plasma levels of hGH after dosing and on possible efficacy (improvement in nitrogen retention, prevention of hypoglycemia, etc.)?

### ■ Answers

1. Sequential dimerization will potentially result in a "bell-shaped" dose response curve, i.e., response is stimulated at low concentrations and inhibited at high concentrations. The inhibition of responses at high concentrations is due to blocking of dimerization caused by the excess hGH saturating all the available receptors. Inhibition of in vitro hGH binding is observed at high hGH (mM) concentrations. Reductions in biological responses (total IGF-1 increase and weight gain) have also been seen with increasing hGH doses in animal studies. However, inhibitory effects of high concentrations of hGH are not seen in treatment of human patients since hGH dose levels are maintained within normal physiological ranges and never approach inhibitory levels.

2. Growth hormone is known to act directly on both bone and cartilage and possibly also on muscle and adipose tissue. Growth hormone effects on other tissues appear to be mediated through the IGF-1 axis or other effectors.

3. Severe liver disease may reduce the clearance of the exogenously administered hGH and observed plasma levels may be higher and persist longer compared to patients without liver disease. However, the increased drug exposure may not result in increased anabolic effects. The desired anabolic effects require the production/release of IGF-1 from the liver. Both IGF-1 production and the number of hGH receptors may be reduced due to the liver disease. To understand the results (or lack of results) from the treatment, it is important to monitor effect parameters (i.e., IGF-1 and possibly IGF-1 binding protein levels, liver function enzymes, etc.) in addition to hGH levels.

### CHAPTER 14: Recombinant Coagulation Factors and Thrombolytic Agents (Pages 293–307)

### ■ Questions

1. A number of second-generation thrombolytic agents have either been approved or are in late stages of development. Discuss some of the limitations that the second-generation thrombolytic agents are designed to address.

2. Design an rFVIII therapeutic regimen for a 35 kg patient with a laceration. Assume that the desired plasma concentration of Factor VIII is 30 IU/dL.

3. What criteria should Factor VIII dosage be based on?

### ■ Answers

1. Although alteplase demonstrated an increased patency rate in the infarct-related artery and a decrease in mortality, several areas were identified where further improvements could be made in the treatment of AMI. Second-generation thrombolytic agents are designed to address some of these shortcomings.

   Due to the rapid clearance of rt-PA from the circulation by the liver, the current administration is via intravenous infusion over 90-minutes or 3 hours. Second-generation thrombolytic agents have a slower plasma clearance allowing administration as a single or double bolus regimen (see Tables 1 to 3).

   Although alteplase is more fibrin-selective compared to streptokinase and urokinase, there is still a 30% to 50% fall in systemic fibrinogen levels. Second-generation thrombolytic agents are more fibrin specific and could result in further reduction in systemic fibrinogenolysis.

2. Dose = 30 IU/dL × 50 mL/kg (volume of distribution) × 35 kg = 525 IU.

3. Dosage should be individualized based on the needs of the patient, severity of deficiency, presence of inhibitors, and the desired increase in factor VIII.

### CHAPTER 15: Monoclonal Antibodies: From Structure to Therapeutic Application (Pages 309–337)

### ■ Questions

1. What are the structural differences among the five immunoglobulin classes?

2. a. What are key differences in PK/PD between mAbs and small molecule drugs?

   b. Why do IgGs typically show non-linear PK in the lower plasma (serum) concentration range?

3. What is a surrogate mAb and how can it potentially be used in the drug development process of mAbs?

4. Which other modes of action apart from antibody-dependent cellular cytotoxicity (ADCC) are known for mAbs? What are the key steps of ADCC?

5. Why do IgGs have a longer in vivo half-life compared with other Igs?

6. What are the development phases for antibody therapeutics? What major activities are involved in the each phase?

## ■ Answers

1. The following structural properties distinguish mAbs:

   a. The molecular form can be different for the five immunoglobulin classes: IgG, IgD and IgE are monomers; IgM appears as pentamer or hexamer; and IgA as either a monomer or a dimer.

   b. Consequently, the molecular weight of the different Ig is different (IgG 150-169 kD, IgA 160-300 kD, IgD 175 kD, IgE 190, IgM 950 kD).

2. a. Metabolism of mAbs appears to be simpler than for small molecules. In contrast to small molecule drugs, the typical metabolic enzymes and transporter proteins such as cytochrome P450, multi-drug resistance efflux pumps are not involved in the disposition of mAbs. Therefore, drug-drug interaction studies for those disposition processes are only part of the standard safety assessment for small molecules and not for mAbs. Monoclonal antibodies, which have a protein structure, are metabolized by proteases. These enzymes are ubiquitously available in mammalian organisms. In contrast, small molecule drugs are primarily metabolized in the liver.

   Because of the large molecular weight, intact mAbs are typically not cleared by the renal elimination route in the kidneys; however, renal clearance processes can play a major role in the elimination of small molecule drugs.

   Pharmacokinetics of mAbs usually are dependent on the binding to the pharmacological target protein and show non-linear behavior as consequence of its saturation kinetics.

   In general, mAbs have longer half-life (in the order of days and weeks) than small molecule drugs (typically in the order of hours).

   The distribution of mAbs is very restricted (volume of distribution in the range of 0.1 L/kg). As a consequence, mAbs do have limited access to tissue compartments as potential target sites via passive, energy-independent distribution processes only (e.g., brain).

   b. At lower concentrations, mAbs generally show non-linear pharmacokinetics due to receptor-mediated clearance processes, which are characterized by small capacity of the clearance pathway and high affinity to the target protein. Consequently at these low concentrations, mAbs exhibit typically shorter half-life. With increasing doses, these receptors become saturated and the clearance as well as elimination half-life decreases until it becomes constant. The clearance in the higher concentration range, which is dominated by linear, non-target related clearance processes, is therefore also called non-specific clearance in contrast to the target-related, specific clearance.

3. A surrogate mAb has similar antigen specificity and affinity in experimental animals (e.g., mice and rats) compared to those of correspondent human antibody in humans. It is quite common that the antigen specificity limits ADME studies of humanized monoclonal antibodies in rodents. Studies using surrogate antibodies might lead to important information regarding safety, mechanism of action, disposition of the drug, tissue distribution, and receptor pharmacology in the respective animal species, which might be too cumbersome and expensive to be conducted in non-human primates. Surrogate mAbs (from mouse or rat) provide a means to gain knowledge of ADME and PD in preclinical rodent models and might facilitate the dose selection for clinical studies.

4. Apart from ADCC, monoclonal antibodies can exert pharmacological effects by multiple mechanisms that include direct modulation of the target antigen, complement–dependent cytotoxicity (CDC), and apoptosis.

   The key steps of ADCC are: 1) opsonization of the targeted cells; 2) recognition of antibody-coated targeted cells by Fc receptors on the surface of monocytes, macrophages, natural killer cells and other cells; 3) destruction of the opsonized targets by phagocytosis of the opsonized targets and/or by toxic substances released after activation of monocytes, macrophages, natural killer cells, and other cells.

5. IgG can bind to neonatal Fc receptor (FcRn) in the endosome, which protects IgG from catabolism via proteolytic degradation. This protection results into a slower clearance and thus longer plasma half-life of IgGs. Consequently, changing the FcRn affinity allows to adjust the clearance of mAbs (higher affinity–lower clearance), which can be employed to tailor the pharmacokinetics of these molecules.

6. Pre-IND, Phase I, II III and IV are the major development phases for antibody therapies. Safety pharmacology, toxicokinetics, toxicology, tissue cross reactivity, local tolerance, PK support for molecules selection, assay support for PK/PD, and PK/PD support for dose/route/regimen are major activities in the Pre-IND phase. General toxicity, reproductive toxicity, carcinogenicity, immunogenicity, characterization of dose-concentration-effect relationship, material comparability studies, mechanistic modeling approach, and population pharmacokinetics/predictions are major activities from Phase I to Phase III. Further studies might be performed as needed after the mAb got market authorization. These studies are called Phase IV studies.

## CHAPTER 16: Monoclonal Antibodies in Cancer (Pages 339–363)

### ■ Questions

1. From the name TOSITUMOMAB AND 131I TOSITUMOMAB, what can one infer about the type of drug and its origin?
2. The epidermal growth factor receptors inhibitors (both monoclonal antibodies and tyrosine kinase inhibitors, such as gefinitib), have a very unique side effect profile which may also demonstrate a pharmacodynamic effect. Describe the profile and what development of this side effect may mean in terms of treatment effectiveness.
3. Describe the theory of angiogenesis and how vascular endothelial growth factor(VEGF) inhibitors may counteract this important mechanism of cancer development.
4. Evaluate the following order for alemtuzumab. Is there anything wrong with this order? *Note*: The answer may include dosage, route, regimen, or ancillary medications.
   1. Alemtuzumab, 30 mg IV over 2 hr Monday through Friday
   2. Premedication: Benadryl, 50 mg IV × 1
   3. Famciclovir, 250 mg PO BID
5. Which of the following four cell types will not be affected by gemtuzumab ozogamycin and why: T-lymphocytes, platelets, monocytes, or neutrophils?
6. Bevacizumab is an angiogenesis inhibitor. List what is known about bevacizumab in terms of thrombotic and bleeding concerns. Are there any guidelines on duration of time between bevacizumab use after major surgery? What are they?
7. Describe the clinical literature that supported the FDA approval of panitumumab? What indication does it currently have?

8. Keeping rituximab's mechanism of action in mind, which of the following disease states would rituximab likely not show any benefit and why?
   a. Autoimmune hemolytic anemia
   b. Cutaneous T-cell lymphoma
   c. Immune thrombocytopenic purpura
   d. Rheumatoid arthritis
9. Which of the epidermal growth factor inhibitors require that patients test positive for the EGFR receptor?
10. List the three black box warnings associated with rituximab use.

### ■ Answers

1. From the name TOSITUMOMAB AND 131I TOSITUMOMAB, one can infer that it is a monoclonal antibody (MAb) of murine origin, as designated by its suffix of "omab," and that it is conjugated or radio-labeled, since the drug name contains a second word containing one of the periodic elements.
2. The epidermal growth factor receptors (EGFR) inhibitors all share a common side effect profile that is dermatologic in origin. Generally patients will present with an acneiform rash that can not be successfully treated with over-the-counter acne agents. This rash is due to the fact that EGFR is overexpressed in many cancers as well as normal skin and hair follicles. Therefore, in some cases, the development of a rash may be associated with clinical efficacy of the drug.
3. For tumors to grow larger than 2 mm$^3$, they must begin to grow their own blood supply, both to provide oxygen and carry away wastes, a process known as angiogenesis. Several growth factors are necessary to stimulate angiogenesis; one of the most potent is VEGF. Bevacizumab is a VEGF inhibitor that prevents VEGF from binding to receptors, which subsequently prevents angiogenesis and tumor growth. Many think that VEGF inhibitors will be very successful in early stage disease where they can prevent large tumor growth, although bevacizumab is currently used more in a metastatic and late stage setting.
4. There are two main points incorrect about this order. First, the alemtuzumab weekly dose should not exceed 90 mg. Second, *Pneumocystis carinii* prophylaxis is missing. Since alemtuzumab causes a profound t-cell depletion, patients are at an unacceptable risk of developing opportunistic infections, such as *P. carinii* and CMV reactivation. Patients require prophylaxis with both antibacterials and antivirals to prevent

these complications. An additional order for acetaminophen would be acceptable to prevent administration- associated side effects.

5. T-lymphocytes will not be affected by gemtuzumab because they do not express the 67-kDa glycosylated transmembrane protein CD33, like the rest of the cell lines do.

6. Evidence suggests that at least 28 days must elapse between a major surgery and subsequent bevacizumab administration. This is because antiangiogenesis inhibitors are associated with vascular dysfunction by their mechanism of action. There have been wound healing concerns, excessive bleeding and even clotting concerns with the use of bevacizumab in clinical trials. Concomitant use of warfarin was shown to be safe in one recent clinical trial.

7. Panitumumab is currently indicated for "the treatment of patients with EGFR-expressing, metastatic colorectal carcinoma with disease progression on or following fluoropyrimidine-, oxaliplatin-, and irinotecan-containing chemotherapy regimens" (i.e., third- or fourth-line use). This approval was based on a phase III trial ($n = 463$) that was randomized for panitumumab monotherapy or best supportive care (BSC). The mean progression-free survival was 96 days for the panitumumab group and 60 days for the BSC alone group. Eight percent of patients in the treatment arm exhibited a partial response (PR) and no observable response was observed in the control arm.

8. Cutaneous T-cell lymphoma. This is because rituximab is a chimeric MAb that binds to the antigen CD20 (cluster of differentiation 20), which is found on B-lymphocytes (B-cells).

9. Use of trastuzumab require a positive test for the HER-2/neu protein (i.e., either a positive result on fluorescence in situ hybridization (FISH) or immunohistochemistry (IHC) 2+) as clinical efficacy in the pivotal approval trials were related to overexpression of this protein.

10. Fatal infusion reactions, tumor lysis syndrome (TLS), and severe mucocutaneous reactions.

## CHAPTER 17: Monoclonal Antibodies in Solid Organ Transplantation (Pages 365–375)

### ■ Questions

1. Monoclonal antibodies are used for several reasons in solid organ transplantation. What benefit do they provide over polyclonal antibodies?

2. The rationale behind the development and use of monoclonal antibodies in solid organ transplantation is focused on the prevention of host recognition of donor tissue (rejection). What are the two ways in which the host immune system recognizes donor tissue and may cause tissue damage?

3. What are the molecular targets for monoclonal antibodies currently used in solid organ transplantation?

4. Monoclonal antibodies are used in solid organ transplantation. Describe the reasons why a monoclonal antibody would be administered before transplant, at the time of transplant, or following transplant.

5. There are several important pharmacokinetic parameters that must be considered when administering monoclonal antibodies to solid organ transplant recipients. What are they and their pharmacokinetic parameters?

6. Muromonab has a characteristic infusion-related reaction. Why does this reaction occur and how can it be attenuated?

7. Daclizumab and basiliximab are two monoclonal antibodies directed against the alpha subunit of the interleukin-2 receptor. What is the difference between these two antibodies?

8. There are several benefits as well as several risks associated with the use of monoclonal antibodies in solid organ transplantation. What are these benefits and risks?

### ■ Answers

1. Monoclonal antibodies provided targeted immunosuppression. The advantage monoclonal antibodies offer over polyclonal antibodies is that the receptor target is known. Polyclonal antibody development involves the introduction of human lymphocytes into an animal host immune system. The animal will then develop polyclonal antibodies directed against human lymphocyte cell surface targets. As a consequence, each inter-batch variability and potency may vary. Although significant outcome data exist with the use of polyclonal antibodies, monoclonal antibodies have a known target allowing for in vivo and in vitro pharmacokinetic and pharmacodynamic data to aid incorporation into novel immunosuppression regimens.

2. The two ways in which the host immune system recognizes donor tissue are:
   a. Complement dependent antibody mediated rejection occurs when the host (recipient) develops or has preformed antibodies against the donor tissue. Pre-formed antibodies will aggregate to the implanted tissue and initiated the complement cascade, which facilitates cell lysis. The majority of these antibodies are usually directed against the MHC located on

the surface of the donor tissue. An absolute contraindication to transplantation is the presence of pre-formed antibodies against MHC complex I, which is located on the surface of all nucleated cells.

b. The second way in which the host immune system attacks donor tissue is through T-cell mediated rejection. This occurs when the donor tissue is recognized as foreign by host antigen presenting cells. Antigen presenting cells present donor tissue antigens to the T-cells which stimulates T-cell proliferation and graft infiltration leading to inflammation and arteritis.

3. Alemtuzumab (Campath-1H®) targets the CD52 receptor, located on peripheral blood lympho-cytes, natural killer cells, monocytes, macro-phages, and thymocytes.

   Daclizumab (Zenapax®) targets the CD25 alpha subunit of the IL-2 receptor, located on activated T-lymphocytes.

   Basiliximab (Simulect®) targets the CD25 alpha subunit of the IL-2 receptor, located on activated T-lymphocytes.

   Muromonab-OKT3 (Orthoclone-OKT3®) targets the CD3 receptor located on CD2, CD4, and CD8 positive lymphocytes.

   Rituximab (Rituxan®) targets the CD20 recep-tor located on B-lymphocytes.

4. The administration of monoclonal antibodies prior to transplant is called desensitization. This strategy is reserved for "highly sensitized" patients, meaning they have high titers of circulating antibodies against donor specific antigens. Monoclonal antibodies that target cells which produce these antibodies are employed in conjunction with plasmapheresis and pooled human immune globulins. Removal of these antibodies may facilitate successful transplantation across this immunologic barrier.

   Monoclonal antibodies administered at the time of transplant are called induction. Induction is pro-vided at the time of transplant to decrease the ability of the host immune system to respond to implanta-tion of foreign tissue. In addition, monoclonal antibodies which provide profound T-cell depletion given at the time of transplant may facilitate the need for certain maintenance immunosuppressants.

   Following transplantation, monoclonal antibodies may be used to treat cell-mediated or antibody-mediated rejection. Cell and antibody infiltrates found in biopsy specimens, in correlation with the clinical status of the patient, will dictate the type, dose and duration of the monoclonal antibody chosen.

5. The volume of distribution, biological half-life and total body clearance can differ significantly between solid organ transplant recipients. Careful consideration of these pharmacokinetic para-meters must be employed to maximize the efficacy and minimize the toxicity associated with administration of these agents. For example, weight-based dosing in obese patients must be carefully considered and biological markers of efficacy should be evaluated to determine the appropriate dose and dosing schedule. In addi-tion, monoclonal antibodies are also removed by plasma exchange procedures, such as plasma-pheresis, which may be performed during the perioperative period. Therefore, it would be prudent to administer the monoclonal antibody following the plasma exchange prescription to avoid removal of the drug and avoid a possible decrease in efficacy.

6. Muromonab's infusion-related reaction occurs because, when the molecule binds to the CD3 receptor, it actually activates the cell prior to inducing apoptosis. T-cell activation leads to increased production of inflammatory cytokines and when the cell undergoes apoptosis these cytokines are released causing a "cytokine release syndrome." This cytokine release syndrome is characterized by fever, chills, rigors, diarrhea, and, potentially, capillary leak leading to pulmon-ary edema. Often times this reaction is the worst when the largest number of cells are present, namely the first dose. However, this reaction can occur after several days of dosing. This reaction can be attenuated by administration of corticos-teroids, histamine blockers, and cyclooxegenase antagonists. Pharmacotherapy aimed at reducing the production or the interaction of cytokines with their receptors may decrease the severity of the cytokine release syndrome.

7. *Structure activity relationship*: Daclizumab has a binding capacity of $3 \times 10^9 \, M^{-1}$ versus basiliximab which has a binding capacity of $1 \times 10^{10} \, M^{-1}$. Therefore, basiliximab is three times more potent than daclizumab.

   *Dosing*: Daclizumab is dosed based on weight, while basiliximab is given as a 20 mg dose. The dosing schedule varies based on the type of solid organ to be transplanted as well as concomitant immunosuppression given. These agents, how-ever, are only approved for prevention of acute rejection in kidney transplant recipients.

8. Benefits include targeted immunosuppression, no batch variability, and low antigenicity in humanized products. The risks associated with any type of immunosuppression include an increased risk for infection, as well as malignancy. Patients who receive monoclonal antibodies which specifically target a cell line, such as muromonab, are associated with a significantly increased risk of post-transplant

lymphoproliferative disease. Appropriate antimicrobial prophylaxis and vigilant screening for post-transplant malignancy may allow for safe and effective use of these monoclonal antibodies in solid organ transplantation.

## CHAPTER 18: Monoclonal Antibodies in Anti-inflammatory Therapy (Pages 377–385)

### ■ Questions

1. Are targeted biologic therapies for autoimmune diseases to be used only after drugs like steroids and methotrexate have had an adequate trial of use and have failed to control the patient's symptoms?
2. What is the primary clinical concern with the immunogenicity of biologic therapies?
3. What is the most likely explanation for why a patient who receives a dose of omalizumab might have an increase in their total serum IgE level for many weeks after the first dose?
4. Why do some cell subsets in the peripheral blood increase after dosing with efalizumab or natalizumab?
5. If a trial reports an ACR70 of 20% on active drug, what does that mean?
6. Progressive multifocal leucoencephalopathy (PML) is an opportunistic brain infection typically seen in the context of severe immunosuppression. The point of the treatment with natalizumab was to block the trafficking of inflammatory cells into the brain in MS patients. Why was the 1:1000 occurrence of PML in patients treated with natalizumab unexpected?
7. Given that there are currently three anti-TNF agents on the market, how do you determine which one to use? How would you compare and contrast them?
8. What are the key differences in the indication for use of rituximab versus abatacept in rheumatoid arthritis?

### ■ Answers

1. Although the standard of care in diseases like rheumatoid arthritis is still to start with older DMARDs like methotrexate, the decision of when to start or switch therapies is complex and impacted by individual issues linked to clinical response like tolerance/adherence to a particular therapeutic regimen, severity and course of disease and its progression, and concomitant medications and medical issues. It is likely that the standard of care will continue to change and incorporate earlier use of biologic therapies that can modify the disease course with fewer generalized side effects.

2. If a biologic therapy is highly immunogenic there is a concern about the increasing number of patients exposed to the drug, particularly upon repeat exposure after a hiatus, because their anti-drug antibodies could neutralize the majority of the drug and they would not likely get the full dose or effect. Though less likely, there are also rare examples of anti-drug antibodies resulting in an autoimmune or allergic-type reaction.

3. Therapeutic monoclonal antibodies that target soluble molecules like IgE form complexes. Though immune complexes are typically cleared from the blood more quickly than monomeric IgG, soluble target molecules typically have a shorter serum half-life than IgG. So an assay detecting the soluble target (in this case IgE) that can detect the target even when it is bound to the drug (which is typically an longer-lived IgG) will show more target present in the serum post-dosing as compared to baseline. This is called a carrier effect. Assuming the drug neutralized the bound target, then the test detecting the target can be misleading, because the target, though present, is effectively inactive.

4. Efalizumab and natalizumab are both monoclonal antibodies that block lymphocyte movement between the blood and tissues ("trafficking"). When this movement is effectively blocked in one direction (from the blood into the tissues), an apparent increase in the peripheral lymphocyte population will be evident on assessment by flow cytometry (or perhaps even on a CBC with differential) post dosing.

5. An ACR70 of 20% means that 20% of the patients had a 70% improvement in their rheumatoid arthritis disease.

6. Though natalizumab was recognized as a very potent and efficacious anti-inflammatory drug in multiple sclerosis (MS), until the PML cases with natalizumab treatment were reported, PML was typically seen in patients thought to be much more severely immunosuppressed (typically with AIDS or post-bone marrow transplant, for example). These cases suggested that there was a much greater degree of immunosuppression with natalizumab (at least to the CNS, and possibly to the GI tract as well) than previously appreciated. This new information provided some additional evidence for the importance of T-cell immune surveillance in controlling PML. Much active debate occurred about weighing of the relative risks of this rare but potentially fatal outcome *versus* the effect of not effectively treating the underlying MS disease. Given the high unmet medical need in MS, regulatory authorities

eventually approved a conservative plan to allow limited access to the drug.

7. Although the three anti-TNF biologics have broadly similar efficacy and safety profiles in rheumatoid arthritis (RA) there are significant differences in the three anti-TNF agents particularly with respect to dosing characteristics and also in the details of the approved indications for use.

Infliximab is the only anti-TNF agent given intravenously, has the longest potential dosing interval, and as the first FDA approved anti-TNF agent, has approvals in the most indications (RA, PsA, AS, UC, adult and pediatric CD, and PP). For RA it is approved in combination with methotrexate "for reducing signs and symptoms, inhibiting the progression of structural damage and improving physical function in patients with moderately to severely active" disease.

Etanercept is a dimeric soluble fusion protein, is FDA approved for use in patients with moderately to severely active RA (either used alone or in combination with methotrexate), as well as in polyarticular JRA, PsA, AS, and PP. For adult patients with RA, PsA, or AS the recommended dose of etanercept is 50 mg SC weekly, given either as one 50 mg injection or as two 25 mg injections on the same day or up to 4 days apart.

Adalimumab is a monoclonal antibody that neutralizes TNF-$\alpha$ and lyses cells expressing TNF-$\alpha$ on their surface in the presence of complement proteins. It is currently FDA approved for use in patients with RA, PsA, and AS as a 40 mg dose SC every other week. It may be used in combination with glucocorticoids, salicylates, non-steroidal anti-inflammatory drugs (NSAIDs), analgesics, methotrexate or other DMARDs. In addition, an increased dosing frequency of 40 mg SC every week is on label for RA patients not receiving methotrexate in combination with adalimumab

8. Rituximab in combination with methotrexate is indicated for the treatment of adult patients with moderate to severe rheumatoid arthritis who have had an inadequate response to one or more TNF antagonist therapies. Abatacept is indicated for use as monotherapy or in combination with DMARDS in patients with moderate to severe active rheumatoid arthritis who have had an inadequate response to DMARDs or TNF antagonists.

## CHAPTER 20: Follicle-Stimulating Hormone (Pages 399–403)

### ■ Questions

1. What makes the formulation process of recombinant FSH difficult?

2. What makes the profile of glycoprotein hormone preparations so complex?

### ■ Answers

1. Recombinant proteins are highly purified preparations, not stabilized by the presence of other (contaminating) proteins. Urinary FSH preparations contain, for instance, more than 95% of proteins of largely undetermined origin. Recombinant protein formulations can be protected against the destabilizing effect of the freeze-drying process and against the effect of adsorption losses by the addition of albumin or gelatin in their formulations. However, this addition is not desirable, since it unnecessarily contaminates the highly purified protein, and may lead to immunological and/or local tolerance problems. Formulations based on low molecular weight compounds allow for more simple and reliable quality control. This formulation however requires optimization of the formulation and the freeze-drying process.

2. FSH is a glycoprotein existing of a large array of isohormones, differing in the composition of their four carbohydrate side chains. The fate of such an isohormone in an organism is a function of its intrinsic activity and its pharmacokinetics. It has been demonstrated that for recombinant FSH isohormone fractions, a clear correlation exists between their pI value and their receptor binding activity on the one hand and their pharmacokinetic behavior on the other. The relatively basic isoforms display high receptor binding and high intrinsic bioactivity with a short plasma residence time. Relatively acidic isohormones, that are more heavily sialyiated, combine low receptor binding and low intrinsic bioactivity with a long plasma residence time. Increasing acidity of the isohormone leads to an increase in absorption rate and elimination half-life, and to a decrease in clearance rate. The longer blood residence times of the acidic isohormones counterbalance their relatively lower intrinsic activities.

## CHAPTER 21: Vaccines (Pages 405–427)

### ■ Questions

1. What are the characteristics of the ideal vaccine? Which aspects should be addressed in the design of a vaccine in order to approach these characteristics?

2. How do antibodies neutralize antigens?

3. How do T-cells discriminate between exogenous (extracellular) and endogenous (intracellular)

antigens? What is the eventual result of these differences in responsiveness?

4. Which categories of conventional vaccines exist and what are their characteristics?

5. Which technological approaches for modern vaccine development can be discerned? Mention at least one example of each category.

6. Mention two main problems related with the immunogenicity of peptide-based vaccines. How are these problems dealt with?

7. Mention at least three advantages and three disadvantages of nucleic acid vaccines. Give one advantage and one disadvantage of RNA vaccines over DNA vaccines.

8. Which stages are discerned in the manufacture of cell-derived vaccines?

9. Mention two or more examples of currently available combination vaccines. Which pharmaceutical and immunological conditions have to be fulfilled when formulating combination vaccines?

## ■ Answers

1. The characteristics of the ideal vaccine are given in Figure 1. The first step in vaccine development is the identification of protective antigens. These antigens form the basis of the vaccine. Structures that cause deleterious effects should be eliminated. The antigens should be expressed by a safe expression system with high expression levels. The desired immunological effect as well as the route of administration are pivotal factors in the choice of a formulation form. The antigens may either be formulated as part of a live vaccine (either attenuated bacteria or viruses or live vectors), or isolated and formulated as a subunit vaccine, by using one of the modern strategies (including anti-idiotype, synthetic peptide, and nucleic acid vaccines) discussed in this chapter. An adjuvant is usually added to enhance the immune response. The immunogenicity of subunit vaccines can be improved by proper presentation forms, e.g., by incorporation of protein antigens into carrier systems such as liposomes or ISCOMs, or by chemical conjugation of peptide or polysaccharide antigens to carrier proteins. The physico-chemical stability of the vaccine components should also be addressed. The overall production process should be easy, consistent and cheap.

2. Antibodies are able to neutralize antigens by at least four mechanisms:
   a. Fc mediated phagocytosis
   b. Complement activation resulting in cytolytic activity

   c. Complement mediated phagocytosis and
   d. Competitive binding on sites that are crucial for the biological activity of the antigen.

3. T-cells are able to distinguish exogenous from endogenous antigens by the type of self-antigen (MHC antigen) that is associated with processed antigen on the surface of the antigen-presenting cell. Processed antigen binds to MHC molecules, resulting in a cell surface located antigen/MHC complex. The complex is recognized by the TCR/CD4 or CD8 complex. A cell infected with a virus presents partially degraded viral antigen (i.e., endogenous antigen) complexed with class I MHC. The complex is recognized by CD8 positive T-cells, resulting in the induction of cytotoxic T-cells. Professional antigen-presenting cells like macrophages phagocytose exogenous antigen and present it in conjunction with class II MHC. CD4 positive T-cells bind to the MHC-antigen complex. Subsequent B-cell or macrophage activation leads to antibody or inflammatory responses, respectively.

4. Conventional vaccines consist of either live attenuated vaccines or non-living vaccines. For non-living vaccines we discern three generations. The first generation comprises suspensions of inactivated, pathogenic organisms. Second generation vaccines contain purified components, varying from whole organisms or extracts of organisms to purified single components. Third generation vaccines are either well-defined mixtures of purified components or protective components formulated in an immunogenic presentation form. Examples of these categories are given in Table 2.

5. Improved live vaccines are obtained by genetic engineering. The two main strategies are:
   a. Genetic attenuation of organisms (e.g., oral cholera vaccine)
   b. Use of live vectors expressing proteins from pathogenic species (e.g., live recombinant vaccinia vaccines carrying viral or tumor antigens).

   Subunit vaccines can be improved by rDNA technology as follows:
   a. genetic detoxification of proteins (e.g., genetically detoxified pertussis toxin)
   b. expression of proteins in host cells (e.g., recombinant hepatitis B vaccine)
   c. genetic fusion of peptide epitopes with carrier proteins (e.g., experimental malaria vaccines based on epitopes genetically fused with hepatitis B surface antigen). Strategy (b) can be combined with (a) or (c).

   Subunit vaccines also can be based on molecular mimicry according to two strategies:

a. Anti-idiotype antibodies (e.g., experimental *Pseudomonas* and *Streptococcus* vaccines)

b. Synthetic peptides (e.g., experimental influenza vaccine).

Most recently, nucleic acids coding for pathogen-derived antigens have emerged as potential vaccine candidates. In particular, plasmid DNAs coding for viral antigens (e.g., hepatitis B, influenza, HIV) are being explored.

6. The first problem concerns the low immunogenicity of plain peptide vaccines. The immunogenicity can be improved by constructing multiple antigen peptides or by chemical coupling of peptides to carrier proteins. Alternatively, peptide epitopes can be incorporated into carrier proteins through genetic fusion of the peptide DNA with that of the carrier protein. The second problem of peptide antigens is that their conformation does not necessarily correspond to that of the epitope in the native protein, which may lead to poor immune responses or responses to irrelevant peptide conformations. Solutions to this problem are sought in constraining the conformation of the synthetic peptide by chemical cyclization methods.

7. The advantages and disadvantages of nucleic acid vaccines are given in Table 5. An advantage of RNA is that there is no risk of incorporation into host DNA. On the other hand, RNA is less stable than DNA.

8. The three production stages are:
   a. Cultivation of cells and/or virus
   b. Purification of the desired components
   c. Formulation of the vaccine.

9. Examples of combination vaccines include diphtheria-tetanus-pertussis(-polio) vaccines and measles-mumps-rubella(-varicella) vaccines. Prerequisites for combining vaccine components are:
   a. Pharmaceutical compatibility of vaccine components and additives
   b. Compatibility of immunization schedules; and
   c. No interference between immune responses to individual components.

## CHAPTER 22: Dispensing Biotechnology Products: Handling, Professional Education, and Product Information (Pages 429–438)

### ■ Questions

1. What are some of the causes of pharmacist reluctance to handling biotech products?
2. In what areas of study do pharmacists and pharmacy students need to engage to be best prepared to provide pharmaceutical care services to patients receiving biotechnology therapeutic agents?
3. What resources are available to pharmacy practitioners to learn more about biotechnology and the drug products of biotechnology?
4. How do the storage requirements of biotech products differ from the majority of products pharmacists normally dispense?
5. What is the most common temperature for the storage of biotech pharmaceuticals?
6. Why is human serum albumin added to the solution of many biotech drugs?
7. Why should biotech products not be shaken when adding any diluent?
8. During travel, what precautions should also be observed with biotech products?
9. Should biotech products be filtered prior to administration?
10. What assessments must be done by the pharmacist before a patient can be considered a candidate for home therapy with a biotech product?
11. What types of professional services information are provided by manufacturers of biotech drugs?

### ■ Answers

1. Lack of understanding of the basics of biotechnology, lack of understanding of the therapeutics of recombinant protein products; unfamiliarity with the side effects and patient counseling information; lack of familiarity with the storage, handling and reconstitution of proteins; and the difficulty of handling reimbursement issues.
2. Basic biotechnology/immunological methods; protein chemistry; therapeutics of biotechnology agents; storage, handling, reconstitution and administration of biotechnology products.
3. Biotechnology/immunology texts, continuing education programs, manufacturers' information and toll-free assistance, biotechnology-oriented journals, the Internet.
4. The shelf life of these products is often considerably shorter than has been the case with more traditional compounds. These products need to be kept at refrigerated temperatures. There are, of course, exceptions to this rule.
5. In general, most biotech products are shipped by the manufacturer in gel ice containers and need to be stored at 2°C to 8°C. Once reconstituted, they should be kept under refrigeration until just prior to use.
6. Most biotech products may adhere to either plastic or glass containers such as syringes and polyvinyl chloride intravenous bags reducing effectiveness of the product. Human serum albumin is usually added to the solutions to prevent adherence.

7. Shaking may cause the product to break down (aggregation). Usually when this happens one can observe physical separation or frothing within the vial of liquid products.

8. They should be stored in insulated, cool containers. This can be accomplished by using ice packs to keep the biotech drug at the proper temperature in warmer climates, whereas the insulated container in colder climates may be all that is required. In fact, when traveling in sub-freezing weather, the products should be protected from freezing.

9. Filtering biotech products is not generally recommended since most of the proteins will adhere to the filter.

10. Before a patient can be a candidate for home therapy, an assessment of the patient's capabilities must occur. The patient, family member, or care giver will need to be able to inject the medication and comply with all of the storage, handling, and preparation requirements.

11. Medical information services provided by manufacturers of biotech drugs are similar to the product, medical and patient management services provided by drug companies for traditional drug products. Information provided via this service generally includes appropriate indications, side effects, contraindications to use, results of clinical trials and investigational uses. Upon request, manufacturers can supply a product monograph and selected research articles that provide valuable information about each product.

## CHAPTER 24: Regulatory Issues and Drug Product Approval for Biopharmaceuticals (Pages 447–453)

### ■ Questions

1. Human growth hormone has a molecular weight of around 22 kDa (see Chapter 13), and erythropoietin of 34 kDa (see Chapter 10). Why does the EMEA request different clinical protocols for approval of a biosimilar product for these protein drugs?

2. A company wishes to market an erythropoietin product in the United States. Are both the 505(b)(1) and 505(b)(2) routes open to be followed?

3. a. When an U.S. company builds a second manufacturing plant to increase the supply of its biopharmaceutical product, does it have to follow the biosimilar-approval route to obtain market authorization for the product produced in its new plant?

   b. Does it have to perform clinical studies to show equivalence?

### ■ Answers

1. Human growth hormone is a non-glycosylated protein with a well established primary sequence; erythropoietin is heavily glycosylated with a number of isoforms with more analytical challenges. The EMEA Guidance documents giving more details can be found on the EMEA website.

2. In principle, both routes are open. The main difference will be in the clinical study part of the dossier. The NDA route using 505(b)(2) route may involve less extensive clinical testing, but that has to be discussed with the authorities prior to starting the full development program.

3. a. No, the FDA Guidance on Comparability will apply.

   b. That depends on the complexity of the molecule. For relatively simple, non-glycosylated biopharmaceuticals the clinical study requirements will be different than for large, highly glycosylated biopharmaceuticals.

# Index